Family Violence and Nursing Practice

Janice Humphreys, RN, PhD, CS, NP
Associate Professor
Department of Family Health Care Nursing
University of California, San Francisco
San Francisco, California

Jacquelyn C. Campbell, PhD, RN, FAAN
Anna D. Wolf Endowed Professor
Associate Dean for Faculty Affairs
Johns Hopkins University School of Nursing
Baltimore, Maryland

D0506977

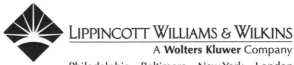

LIPPINCOTT WILLIAMS & WILKINS
A **Wolters Kluwer** Company
Philadelphia • Baltimore • New York • London
Buenos Aires • Hong Kong • Sydney • Tokyo

Senior Acquisitions Editor: Patricia Casey
Editorial Assistant: Megan Klim
Senior Production Editor: Rosanne Hallowell
Senior Production Manager: Helen Ewan
Managing Editor / Production: Erika Kors
Art Director: Carolyn O'Brien
Manufacturing Manager: William Alberti
Indexer: Victoria Boyle
Compositor: Lippincott Williams & Wilkins
Printer: Maple/Binghamton

ISBN: 0-7817-4220-X

Library of Congress Cataloging-in-Publication Data is available upon request.

LWW.com

To Rick and Jack, with love.

—Janice

For women of courage everywhere—and
especially those I love the most: Constance Morrow,
Dorothy Bowman, Christy Endrud, Deborah
Bowman, Shelley Kirk, Nadia Boulos, and
Grace Endrud—and the men who love them.

—Jackie

Contributors

Sara A. Barrett, RN, MA
School Nurse
East Detroit Public School System
East Pointe, Michigan

Helene Berman, RN, PhD
Associate Professor
School of Nursing
University of Western Ontario
London, Ontario, Canada

Diane Bohn, RN, CNM, DNS
Assistant Professor
School of Nursing
University of Minnesota
Minneapolis, Minnesota

Linda Bullock, PhD, RN
Assistant Professor
Sinclair School of Nursing
Columbia, Missouri

Doris Campbell, PhD, RN, FAAN
Professor
University of South Florida
Tampa, Florida

Mary Ann Curry, RN, PhD, FAAN
Professor
School of Nursing
Oregon Health & Science University
Portland, Oregon

Nancy J. Fishwick, PhD, RN
Associate Professor
University of Maine School of Nursing
Orono, Maine

Terry Fulmer, PhD, RN, FAAN
Professor of Nursing
Head, Division of Nursing
The Steinhardt School of Education
New York University
Co-Director
Hartford Institute for Geriatric
   Nursing
New York, New York

Faye A. Gary, EdD, RN, FAAN
Professor
University of Florida College of
   Nursing
Gainesville, Florida

Nancy Glass, PhD, MPH, RN
Assistant Professor
School of Nursing
Oregon Health & Science University
Portland, Oregon

Jennifer Hardesty, PhD
Post-Doctoral Fellow
Johns Hopkins University
Baltimore, Maryland

Dena Hassouneh-Phillips, RN, PhD
Assistant Professor
School of Nursing
Oregon Health & Science University
Portland, Oregon

Angela Henderson, RN, PhD
Associate Professor
University of British Columbia
   School of Nursing
Vancouver, British Columbia, Canada

M. Christine King, EdD, RN
Associate Professor
University of Massachusetts,
    Amherst, School of Nursing
Amherst, Massachusetts

Kären Landenburger, PhD, RN
Associate Professor
University of Washington, Tacoma
Tacoma, Washington

Kathryn Laughon, RN
Doctoral Candidate
Johns Hopkins University School of
    Nursing
Baltimore, Maryland

Laura Smith McKenna, DNSc, RN
Assistant Professor
School of Nursing
Samuel Merritt College
Oakland, California

Barbara Parker, PhD, RN, FAAN
Professor and Director
Center for Nursing Research and
    Doctoral Program
University of Virginia School of
    Nursing
Charlottesville, Virginia

Rachel Rodriguez, PhD, RN
Assistant Professor
University of Wisconsin–Madison
    School of Nursing
Madison, Wisconsin

Josephine M. Ryan, DNSc, RN
Associate Professor
University of Massachusetts,
    Amherst, School of Nursing
Amherst, Massachusetts

Mary Cay Sengstock, PhD
Professor
Wayne State University
Detroit, Michgan

Daniel J. Sheridan, PhD, RN, CNS
Assistant Professor
Johns Hopkins University School
    of Nursing
Baltimore, Maryland

Janette Y. Taylor, PhD, RN
Assistant Professor
University of Iowa School of Nursing
Iowa City, Iowa

Sara Torres, PhD, RN, FAAN
Dean and Professor
School of Nursing
The University of Medicine and
    Dentistry of New Jersey
Newark, New Jersey

Yvonne Campbell Ulrich, PhD, RN
Department of Psychosocial &
    Community Health
University of Washington School of
    Nursing
Seattle, Washington

Joan C. Urbancic, PhD, RN, APRN
Professor
McAuley School of Nursing
University of Detroit Mercy
Detroit, Michigan

Reviewers

Jane E. Corrarino, MS, RN
Assistant Director of Nursing
Suffolk County Department of
    Health Services
Hauppauge, New York

Angela C. Frederick, RN, CS
Doctoral Student, Teaching Assistant
University of Pennsylvania
Philadelphia, Pennsylvania

**Arlene Kent-Wilkinson, RN,
    BSN, MN**
Forensic Nurse Educator
Calgary, Alberta, Canada

**Ann Malecha, PhD, MSN,
    BSN**
Assistant Professor
Texas Woman's University, Houston
    Center
Houston, Texas

**Cindy A. Peternelj-Taylor, RN,
    BScN, MSc**
Professor
University of Saskatchewan
Saskatoon, Saskatchewan, Canada

Bonnie Price, RN, BSN
Program Coordinator
Forensic Nurse Examiners of Saint
    Mary's Hospital
Glen Allen, Virginia

Mable H. Smith, RN, JD, PhD
Associate Professor
Old Dominion University
Norfolk, Virginia

Kim Wieczorek, RN, BSN
Assistant Program Coordinator
Forensic Nurse Examiners of Saint
    Mary's Hospital
Glen Allen, Virginia

Preface

A woman enters the emergency department with facial bruises and severe abdominal pain. She is asked how her injuries occurred, and she mumbles that she fell down a flight of stairs. Her male companion glowers in the doorway of the cubicle. The nurse firmly asks him to wait outside and gently proceeds with obtaining a detailed history from the woman, including assessment for family violence.

In another part of the hospital, a newly postpartum battered mother in the obstetrical unit fears going home and does not know where to go. Her nurse-midwife helps arrange her discharge directly to an abused woman shelter.

A 14-year-old daughter of a woman who has five other children is being seen in the outpatient clinic with her mother. The mother voices the concern, "I don't want to have to 'do time' for what I might do to her." Mother and daughter are counseled by the nurse.

These are three illustrations of the multitude of possible interfaces of nursing and family violence. Family violence is widespread in American society. Americans are more likely to be hurt or killed in the home by another family member than at any other place by any other person (Straus & Gelles, 1990). Long-term physical and psychological health consequences are documented from all forms of family violence (Felitti et al., 1998; Campbell & Lewandowski, 1997). Nursing has an important role to play in the prevention, identification, treatment, and scholarly investigation of this health concern.

A violent act is physical force that results in injury or abuse to the recipient. Within the family, violence can be directed toward any member by another, and can include sexual acts as well as other forms of physical aggression. Regardless of whether the violent action is perpetrated by the father against the mother, the mother against the child, or the adolescent against the grandfather, violence in the family is a profound event that affects the whole family. To consider the abuse of a woman, a child, or an elderly family member as an isolated event is to see only an aspect of the effects of violence in American families. The problem of violence must be addressed in its totality to see the full picture with all its ramifications.

There is growing recognition of the potential and actual contributions of nursing to the needs of survivors of family violence (Humphreys, Parker, & Campbell, 2001; Campbell, 1998). Nurses can play a unique role in assisting battered children, women, men, and elders as they respond to the trauma of physical and psychological assaults. Nursing as a predominantly female profession, and as a discipline based on holistic (addressing physiological, psychological, societal, cultural and spiritual needs) and client-based theories and models, is ideally suited to understanding the needs of family violence survivors.

Much of the literature on health care system response to family violence fails to separate various discipline approaches. *Family Violence and Nursing Practice* specifically addresses the role of nursing in response to family violence (Campbell, 1998). Since the first version of this text was published in 1982, thousands of nurses have become involved in a variety of ways in the care of survivors of family violence. Nurses provide direct care to survivors in shelters, homes, hospitals, and community settings. Nurses are frequently members of boards of directors at shelters and other agencies assisting survivors. Nursing research on family violence has evolved rapidly and is reported in the literature with ever greater frequency (Humphreys, Parker, & Campbell, 2001; Campbell & Parker, 1999).

One of the most visible outcomes of nursing's greater awareness and contribution to the area is the development of the Nursing Network on Violence Against Women International (NNVAWI). This grassroots organization was a direct outgrowth of the 1985 Surgeon General's Workshop on Violence and Public Health. Immediately following that meeting and every 2 years since, the NNVAWI has held a conference where participants exchange practice ideas, research findings, theory, and policy initiatives related to all forms of violence against women. Over time the group has become truly international; the 2003 meeting is in Adelaide, Australia (see www.NNVAWI.org).

Forensic nursing and the Forensic Nursing Association have grown in importance in recent years, with the forensic nursing role in family violence increasingly recognized (see Chapter 13). The American Nurses' Association has also adopted a resolution addressing the nursing role in violence against women, as has the Emergency Nurses' Association, the Black Nurses' Association, the Hispanic Nurses' Association, the Association on Women's Health and Obstetrical Nursing, and the College of Nurse Midwives. The American Academy of Nursing has formed a

policy task force on violence. These are exciting developments—yet much more can be done. (See Chapter 14, Future Directions for Nursing, for further discussion of nursing education, research, and social policy issues.)

This new version of *Family Violence and Nursing Practice* has been almost completely rewritten, with new chapters, new research from all disciplines (with an emphasis on nursing research), and new appendices containing helpful assessment instruments and approaches. The book maintains an emphasis on all levels of prevention of family violence as well as immediate nursing care.

All of the clients in examples at the beginning of this Preface are "victims" of family violence in that they are "subjected to oppression, deprivation, or suffering" within violent families, whether or not they are the actual recipients of the aggressive acts. At the same time, the philosophy of this text is that these people and their family units have significant strengths on which appropriate nursing care will build. This is why the term *survivor* replaced *victim* in the previous edition of the book, and remains the philosophy as well as terminology in this edition. We wish to reiterate the need to move from a nursing care perspective of feeling sorry for victims to nursing care that forms partnerships with survivors and potential survivors. The other basic assumptions of the book are that nursing care of survivors of family violence considers the whole family, is based on a firm theoretical and research foundation, and can be a significant force at all levels of prevention. The main objective of this book is to integrate nursing practice in relation to family violence with existing theory and research. The need for increased nursing scholarship and research toward evidence-based practice in this area is also a consistent theme.

Culture and Family Violence

Because of the increased availability of information on racial, ethnic, and cultural aspects of family violence, we have made a concerted effort to discuss these variables in each chapter. While there are obvious similarities in both influencing factors and responses of all survivors of family violence, there are, nevertheless, aspects that are unique to certain racial and cultural groups. In order to give culturally competent nursing care, it is imperative that nurse researchers continue to explore these variations and to incorporate findings into their work with violent and potentially violent families (Torres, Campbell, et al., 2000). At the same time, nurses can form alliances with organizations from various ethnic groups to learn from them how best to provide culturally competent care in these sensitive areas (Rodriguez, 1999). We are also beginning to better understand that violence also occurs in same-sex relationships (Relf, 2001). Working with survivors of this form of family violence also necessitates cultural competence.

Community Collaboration

Professional nurses develop a plan of care only after thorough consideration of the client's community. In turn, nursing as a profession must adapt to the ever-changing needs of the community and society. For example, if violence in the family is common and possibly increasing, then the professional nurse must alter the process by which she develops, initiates, and evaluates her care to include the likelihood of violence in families. The actual and potential alterations in individual and family health that are associated with violence are immense, complex, and in need of nursing consideration if maximum levels of wellness are to be achieved. Stress on the family is a major contributing factor to the occurrence of violence in families. The professional nurse, aware of this influence and practicing in an area of increasing unemployment, would be remiss if she failed to consider and adapt to the increased potential for family violence when conducting her assessment.

The mere awareness of the problem of family violence is not enough. Nurses must act as client advocates. In the case of family violence, the nurse may begin by educating other professionals about the dynamics of the problem. For instance, she may help others who become involved in a case of child abuse to understand that physical harm inflicted on a dependent child by a parent is really just an isolated act in the interactions of a complex family unit. Nursing is furthermore in an excellent position to prevent, identify, and intervene against family violence. In hospitals, nurses may administer nursing care to patients with a wide range of needs related to potential or actual family violence (such as the adolescent with a gunshot wound, the infant who has been abandoned, and the chronically ill elderly woman who is preparing to move in with her daughter's family). Mental health and obstetrical inpatient units are also areas where patient needs arising out of violence can be found if nurses know how to look for them. Client advocacy in the clinic, community, and hospital involves active searching for victims and attention to prevention as well as education and direct intervention. The professional nurse has always focused primarily on the client rather than "the problem."

Relevance to Nursing

The definition of nursing given by the American Nurses Association in its Social Policy Statement is, "the diagnosis and treatment of human responses to actual or potential health problems." Nursing care of survivors of family violence fits well within the scope of this definition and thereby includes the prevention of family violence, as well as detection and treatment. Nursing from the time of Nightingale has been concerned with the individual, the family, and the community. Such a focus allows the nurse to be perceived as more helping and better prepared than many other professionals to assist clients who experience family violence.

Because of their sheer numbers, variety of practice locations, and client needs, and in particular the nature of their practice, nurses are in an ideal position to take action to decrease the likelihood of family violence and to mitigate its effects. Nurses provide care to families in more settings than probably any other health care provider. Nurses see family members in the hospital, clinic, school, community, and private practice. They have traditionally provided care to whole families, even though the initial request for care may have come from an individual. The nurse routinely includes information about the individual's family, culture, and health attitudes and practices when doing an assessment. She is frequently seen as helpful and trustworthy by families when they feel they cannot trust other health or criminal justice or social service professionals. Nurses, because they are often less threatening than other professionals, are in a much better position to elicit information from a battered woman or abusing parent, and to ensure that

the individual client or family has the paramount role in decision making beyond what the law requires.

When the setting, agency, family, or situation indicates that another professional would be better suited as coordinator, the nurse, when well informed and aware, is still an integral member of the team. This book is designed to give the nurse the necessary background to understand, identify, assess, coordinate care of, and provide interventions for potential and actual victims of family violence.

The Nurse as Coordinator of Care

The problem of family violence is multidimensional. The professional nurse cannot be expected to meet the needs of every member of a violent family in every respect without help. Rather, violent families require a broad range of interventions and teamwork. Many other professionals are likely to have contact with the members of the violent family. Social workers, physicians, lawyers, police officers, dentists, and community advocates all may be involved in their own form of intervention with the violent family. It is often necessary that one professional coordinate these varied interventions. The professional nurse is in an excellent position in many instances to initiate and coordinate interventions, and to be the ongoing case manager.

Unit of Focus: The Family

The purpose of this book is to address the nursing care of survivors of family violence, including victims of child abuse, wife abuse, and abuse of the elderly. Violence, therefore, is examined as an indicator of family needs and issues. Often, abuse of a family member has been viewed as an isolated interaction or incident involving at the most the survivor and the perpetrator. However, as shown in *Family Violence in Nursing Practice*, every violent act within a family affects each of its members, and violence in the family is an ongoing pattern of behavior. The family and its functioning are the major unit of focus.

If the violent family is to be the major focus of the present work, it is necessary to examine the consequences of violence on each family member. The type of abuse perpetrated against a family members is not limited to physical violence. Sexual abuse, emotional abuse, threats and intimidation, other controlling behavior, incest, and neglect are all included.

Summary

Violence in the American family is a common health problem of possibly tremendous magnitude. Violence occurs against all family members and is an indicator of complex family needs and issues. Nursing is in an excellent position to be actively involved with other professionals by initiating, coordinating, and evaluating the multidisciplinary approach to violent families, but traditionally has had a limited knowledge base about family violence. *Family Violence in Nursing Practice* conveys knowledge to nurses in a format that covers nursing interventions based on existing theories and research about families and violence; extends nursing care to all members of violent families and all forms of family violence; and emphasizes the strengths and health potential of victims and families—an approach that empowers nursing to contribute to the prevention of this major health concern.

Acknowledgments

This book evolved out of our professional interest in and commitment to survivors of family violence. For the existence of this text we owe a great many thanks:

- To our many friends and colleagues who provided support and indulgence.

- To our expert contributing authors who share our concern for survivors of family violence.

- To our invaluable funding sources, including the National Institute of Nursing Research, the National Institute of Justice, the Centers for Disease Control, the National Institute of Mental Health, and the National Institute of Drug Abuse.

- To Liz Schaeffer, Freelance Editor, for her advice, counsel, and patience.

- To our students who have challenged us to grow.

- To the battered women and children who freely shared their problems and concerns.

- To the profession of nursing for providing an opportunity to care about the needs of other human beings.

- To each other for continuing friendship and sharing of ideas.

Janice Humphreys, RN, PhD, CS, NP
Jacquelyn C. Campbell, PhD, RN, FAAN

References

Campbell, J. C. (1998). *Empowering survivors of abuse: Health care for battered women and their children.* Thousand Oaks, CA: Sage.

Campbell, J. C. & Lewandowski, L. A. (1997). Mental and physical health effects in intimate partner violence on women and children. *The Psychiatric Clinics of North America, 20,* 353–375.

Campbell, J. C. & Parker, B. (1999). Clinical nursing research on battered women and their children. In A.S.Hinshaw, S. L. Feetham, & J. L. F. Shaver (Eds.), *Handbook of clinical nursing research* (pp. 535–559). Thousand Oaks: Sage.

Felitti, V. J., Anda, R. F., Nordenberg, D., Williamson, D. F., Spitz, A. M., Edwards, V., Koss, M. P., & Marks, J. S. (1998). Relationship of childhood abuse and household dysfunction to many of the leading causes of death in adults. The Adverse Childhood Experiences (ACE) Study [see comments]. *American Journal of Preventive Medicine, 14,* 245–258.

Humphreys, J. C., Parker, B., & Campbell, J. C. (2001). Intimate partner violence against women. In D.Taylor & N. Fugate-Woods (Eds.), *Annual Review of Nursing Research* (pp. 275–306). New York: Springer Publishing Company.

Relf, M. V. (2001). Battering and HIV in men who have sex with men: A critique and synthesis of the literature. *Journal of the Association of Nurses in AIDS Care, 12,* 41–48.

Rodriguez, R. (1999). The Power of the Collective: Battered migrant farmworker women creating safe spaces. *Health Care for Women International, 20,* 417–426.

Straus, M. A. & Gelles, R. J. (1990). *Physical violence in American families: Risk factors and adaptations to family violence in 8,145 families.* New Brunswick, NJ: Transaction Publishers.

Torres, S., Campbell, J. C., Campbell, D. W., Ryan, J., King, C., Price, P., Stallings, R., Fuchs, S., & Laude, M. (2000). Abuse during and before pregnancy: Prevalence and cultural correlates. *Violence and Victims, 15,* 303–322.

Contents

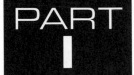

PART I

Theoretical Background

harm others, regardless of gender. A representative definition of this school of thought is Moyer's (1987) description of aggression as "overt behavior involving intent to inflict noxious stimulation or to behave destructively toward another organism." Scholars now include psychological injury as one of the possible results of aggression.

Nursing literature also has addressed aggression, distinguishing assertiveness from aggression. Herman (1978) describes aggression as getting what is wanted at the expense of others. Aggressive behavior is seen as dominating, deprecating, humiliating, and embarrassing to others, whereas "assertion is the direct, honest, and appropriate expression of one's thoughts, feelings, opinions, and beliefs . . . without infringing on the right of others" (Herman, 1978). This distinction seems useful and is accepted as a basic premise of this book. Aggression therefore is seen as destructive in intent, either physically or psychologically, and as infringing on the rights of others.

Violence

Aggression can be seen on a continuum with violence at the extreme end, encompassing destructive results as well as aggressive intent. Webster defines violence as the "exertion of any physical force so as to injure or abuse." The word originates from the Latin *violare*, to violate, rape, or injure. Consistent with the official definition and its Latin root, common associations with violence are much more negative than those associated with aggression. Yet much violence is socially tolerated, for instance, police violence, war, and self-defense. Whether violence is deemed appropriate depends on the agent, circumstances, status of the victim, and degree of harm inflicted. Some authors have even insisted that violence is necessary as a reflection of conflicting groups and interests in any society. Yet entire cultures are totally nonviolent, wherein violence in any form is absolutely disallowed (Levinson, 1989).

American culture officially condemns violence, but it is covertly sanctioned in many ways. Violent characters are glorified on television, in books, and in music; threats to hurt and kill each other are made in jest as a constant part of common language. One of the most well-known and honored homicide researchers, Marvin Wolfgang (1978), said, "When war is glorified in a nation's history and included as part of the child's educational materials, a moral judgment about the legitimacy of violence is firmly made." American society is undecided whether hitting a child is legitimate punishment or a form of violence. Societal ambivalence about attitudes and values toward violence are undoubtedly reflected in the high rate of violent crime and in problems with violence in the family.

HISTORICAL BACKGROUND

Anthropologists are uncertain about the prevalence of violence in early civilizations. Some scholars have used the historical record to argue in favor of the inevitability of violence. For instance, Kolb (1971) observes that "at best, only 10 generations in the era of recorded history have avoided war." These arguments stress that peoples of peace are relatively rare in the ethnographic record and assert that they were usually backward and submissive to a powerful and overtly aggressive neighbor. In refutation, Malinowski (1973) showed that wars cannot be traced back to the earliest beginnings of human culture, only to the start of written history. Others add that only a small percentage of the population took part in any but the "world" wars of the 20th century and that people have to be indoctrinated in war. As for the contention that peaceful peoples were always in the minority, there is evidence that the majority of the peoples living in the "cradle of civilization" (Asia Minor) from approximately 9000 to 5000 B.C. were hunter-gatherers and apparently lived in a predominantly peaceful manner. None of the hundreds of skeletons unearthed shows evidence of violent death. Far from being backward, this culture was one of the most advanced of its time (Eisler, 1988).

It has often been noted that the United States has a long history of violence used as a means to achieve socially acceptable ends. The favorite period of many Americans is the era of the Old West, which is characterized as violent as much as anything else. Harris polls have consistently found that Americans tend to romanticize their early wars and to admire the violent heroes of the past. Some scholars have correlated the fascination with our violent past with the fact that there are only a few countries (usually where there is war or civil unrest) that have a higher homicide rate than the United States (Archer 1977). Thus, historical examination of violence shows a predilection for violence among human beings from at least very early in civilization but a propensity that is by no means equally distributed among individuals, cultures, or all periods of time. Historical background gives an overview to the problem of violence but does not illuminate causation. Theories of aggression and violence are summarized in Box 1-1, and important points about aggression and violence are listed in Box 1-2.

THEORETICAL FRAMEWORKS EXPLAINING VIOLENCE

The theoretical frameworks that attempt to illuminate the causative factors of violence can be divided in a variety of ways. The broad categories chosen to organize material for this text are biological, psychological, sociological, and anthropological. This review of theoretical frameworks cannot be considered exhaustive but indicates the problems with determining causality of problems of violence and points out some of the inconsistencies, gaps, and difficulties in the traditional theoretical field. It also underpins the theoretical information concerned with specific aspects of violence in the family. Note that the various theories are not mutually exclusive. There are likely multiple explanations for violent behavior (see Figure 1-1).

Biological Perspective: Instinctivist Theories

Lorenz's (1966) theory on aggression is the best known in the field. He views aggression as a fighting instinct common to men and animals; it serves important species-preservation functions by favoring genes for strength and preventing too much population density. Ardrey (1966), who also sees aggression as innate and within species, uses observations of animals to postulate that dominance and subordination are inevitable and that aggression and competition ensure the genetic transmission of useful traits. He believes that humans and animals are fundamentally motivated by aggression and the acquisition and defense of territory. Much time and space, from all perspectives, has been used to refute the simplistic theories of Ardrey and Lorenz. They have been criticized severely for poor

BOX 1-1 **SUMMARY OF THEORIES OF AGGRESSION AND VIOLENCE**

Biological Theories: Aggression is an innate characteristic that is either an instinctual drive (the instinctivist school of thought) or neurologically based (neurophysiological theories). The latter examines how brain functioning, hormones, or both influence degrees of aggressive tendencies and violent behaviors. Research evidence links increased testosterone levels to increases in aggression, but the studies do not indicate a causal relationship. Factors such as mood, sampling difficulties, and environment must be considered as intervening characteristics.

Role of Alcohol: Research indicates that alcohol facilitates aggression because of the negative affect it has on conscious cognitive processing, yet violence occurs as frequently without the presence of alcohol. For example, neither are most criminals alcoholics nor the majority of alcoholics violent criminals. Research has not substantiated the theory that alcohol directly causes aggression, but it is suggested that alcohol detrimentally affects certain psychological and physiological processes that then lead to aggressive behavior.

Psychological Theories: These theories include the following: *Frustration–aggression theory* is no longer in favor; it is, however, of historical importance as the first use of learning theory to explain aggression. *Cognitive neoassociation theory* expands frustration–aggression theory to include a wide variety of stressors as precipitants for aggressive behavior. *Social cognitive theory* holds that aggressive behavior is learned through either modeling or personal experience and that an individual's use of aggression depends upon cognitive interpretation of the triggering event as well as the reactions of others. *Social information processing theory* is a cognitive theory that incorporates scripts (highly associated concepts that both explain and guide behavior) to explain aggression. The *general aggression model* incorporates elements of all of the aforementioned theories to explain how personal and situational factors influence an individual's internal state and predict the use of aggression.

Cultural Attitudes Fostering Violence: Tacit acceptance of violence as a means to resolve conflict is common. War and weapons are justified as protection. Excessive and aggressive behavior is so pervasive that previously stigmatized behavior is now considered normal.

Structural Violence of Society: Violence has been institutionalized. State-sanctioned killing through executions is positively related to an increase in homicide. Poverty and unemployment appear to be associated with increased rates of violence. The notion of a subculture of violence in various groups has been explored by researchers. Evidence is conflicting, and it appears that other factors better explain increased rates of aggression in particular subgroups.

scholarship; anthropomorphizing; equating hunting with aggression; ignoring evidence of cultures where violence is unknown; failing to recognize that the fighting of animals of the same species (highly ritualized, defensive, stereotyped, and seldom fatal) cannot be compared to the cruel, destructive, and attacking violence of humans; and disregarding the evidence that the early hunting-and-gathering populations were predominantly peaceful (Montagu, 1978). It has also been found that in nonhuman primates, male aggression, territoriality, and dominance battles are only a small fraction of the total interaction, and the group cohesively strives to keep these disruptive incidents to a minimum (Tracy & Crawford, 1992). Wallace (1973) points out that many animals are almost entirely passive and yet are thriving as species. Aggression leading to violence has been shown by other anthropologists to be maladaptive in early human civilizations and thereby hardly genetically favored (Leavitt, 1975).

BOX 1-2 **SUMMARY OF IMPORTANT POINTS ABOUT THEORIES OF AGGRESSION AND VIOLENCE**

- Aggression is not an instinctual drive but must be viewed as destructive behavior with intent to harm physically or emotionally. Our notions of aggression are grounded in our perceptions of men and women. We often see aggressive behavior as different depending on the gender of the person.
- Violence is a complex and multifaceted phenomenon that is tolerated and socially sanctioned throughout American society. We justify war and physical punishment of children.
- Biological, psychological, social, and cultural explanations of violence add to a growing body of knowledge about violence, yet none of the explanations alone answer satisfactorily the question of why violence occurs. Each approach has strengths and weaknesses, all of which should be considered.
- Social and cultural explanations about aggression and violence are the most comprehensive, because they consider factors that are beyond the individual and address issues of how our social world influences behaviors.
- Race and poverty are correlated variables; thus, in studies of poverty and violence one must avoid the faulty assumption that violence occurs more frequently in certain racial groups. Poverty is a condition that often sustains violence.

There is evidence that evolutionary psychology can help explain some of the patterns of homicide. Daly and Wilson (1998) interpret much of the homicide between young men and between spouses in terms of men's need to control women and their reproduction to ensure their genetic continuation. However, these researchers also emphasize that their analysis is not designed to provide an answer to homicide questions in terms of motive, nor do they claim that biological theory should replace social or circumstantial explanations for violence.

Neurobiological Perspective

Violence as defined earlier in this chapter is aggression that has harm as the outcome (e.g., death). The environmental and psychological roots of aggressive behavior have been studied for centuries, but it is only in the past 30 years that scientists have systematically explored biological links to aggressive behavior. Recent studies using both animal and human models suggest a role of endocrine and neurotransmitter systems as inhibitors and facilitators of aggressive behavior (Kavoussi, Armstead, & Coccaro, 1997). Evidence also points to testosterone as

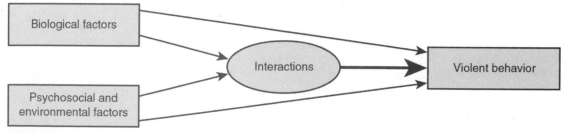

FIGURE 1–1 • Model of multiple antecedents of violent behaviors.

having a role in aggressive behavior (Rubinow & Schmidt, 1996; Scerbo & Kolko, 1994). There has also been extensive research on the role of substances such as alcohol and drugs on the neural mechanisms for aggression (Giancola, 2002). Although biological factors play a significant role in the development of aggressive behaviors, all experts stress the importance of environmental and learning factors in combination with biology (Kavoussi et al., 1997). All human beings experience anger and may behave aggressively under enough provocation, so sorting out the interactions of psychological and environmental factors with basic genetics and physiology is complex . Furthermore, much of the neurobiology research on aggression has used animal models; applying those findings to human aggression is always problematic (Kavoussi et al., 1997).

Neurochemical Factors

During the last 30 years, a vast number of studies have suggested that several neurotransmitters have a role in modulation of animal and human aggressive behavior. The neurotransmitters include serotonin, dopamine, and norepinephrine.

Serotonin. The connection between serotonin (5-HT) and aggression has been established by the repeated observation that abnormalities in central serotonin function correlated with impulsive aggression (Kavoussi et al., 1997). Several studies have demonstrated the major metabolite of serotonin, 5-hydroxyindolacetic acid (5-HIAA), is reduced in the cerebrospinal fluid (CSF) of subjects with a history of aggression (e.g., violence toward others and violent suicide attempts; see, for example, Dolan, Anderson, & Deakin, 2001). Further evidence of the important role that serotonin plays in regulating aggression comes from studies suggesting that serotonergic-enhancing drugs can be effective in reducing impulsive aggression (Kavoussi et al., 1997; Salzman et al., 1995). There is also preliminary evidence for a genetic disturbance in serotonergic function that might predispose individuals to aggressive behaviors (Nielson et al., 1994).

Dopamine and Norepinephrine. The brain's dopaminergic and noradrenergic systems also appear to play a role in aggressive behavior. Animal studies suggest that an increase in brain dopamine activity creates a state in which animals are more prepared to respond impulsively and aggressively to stimuli in the environment (Blackburn, Pfaus, & Phillips, 1992).

An increase in noradrenergic functioning also has been found to correlate with aggressive behavior in human beings as well as animals. Involvement of the noradrenergic system in aggression is supported by the finding that blockage of noradrenergic receptors is a clinically useful treatment for aggressive behaviors. Beta-adrenergic blockers have been effective in reducing aggressive behavior in chronic psychiatric inpatients (Sorgi, Ratey, & Polakoff, 1986), patients with brain injuries (Yudofsky, Williams, & Gorman, 1981), and adults with attention-deficit disorder (Mattes, 1986).

Sex Steroids

In human beings, androgens (male hormones naturally produced in the body) appear to play a role in the regulation of aggressive behavior, although the nature of the role remains unclear (Rubinow & Schmidt, 1996; Kavoussi et al., 1997). Testosterone has been studied extensively in relation to human assertiveness, dominance, and aggression.

Archer (1991) conducted a comprehensive literature review of studies comparing the testosterone levels of violent and nonviolent offenders. The studies examined employed various research designs and statistical techniques; however, the study results identified that those prisoners convicted of violent crimes had higher testosterone levels than those who committed nonviolent crimes. Most of the studies reviewed by Archer used samples of male offenders, but the few studies completed with female offenders reported similar findings. More recent studies have provided further support for the role of testosterone in aggressive behavior. Dabbs, Carr, Frady, and Riad (1995) reported that violent offenders have higher testosterone levels than offenders who commit nonviolent crimes (e.g., burglary, theft, and drug dealing) and that those with a higher level of testosterone are more aggressive in prison settings. In violent alcoholic offenders, high testosterone concentration in CSF is associated with increased aggressiveness and sensation seeking (Virkkunen et al., 1994). Furthermore, a relationship between higher salivary testosterone and observed aggression was documented in a sample of aggressive children (Scerbo & Kolko, 1994).

In spite of the evidence that testosterone levels may be elevated in aggressive offenders, the use of testosterone-lowering agents has been of limited benefit in reducing aggressive behaviors (Kavoussi et al., 1997). The exception to this is men convicted of sex offenses, where antiandrogens appear to lower both deviant and nondeviant sexual drive and activity and the behavior improvement was associated with testosterone level (Kravitz, Haywood, Kelly et al., 1995). In spite of the large body of evidence about testosterone, it is important to realize that these findings have seldom been replicated in samples of persons who are not criminals. In addition, recent studies have shown that elevated testosterone alone does not account for aggressive behavior (Bernhardt, 1997).

Brain Lesions

The study of patients who suffer brain injuries can provide important evidence to the neurobiology of aggressive behavior. In one study, 70% of patients with brain injuries secondary to blunt trauma exhibited irritability and aggression (McKinlay, Brooks, & Bond et al., 1981). A history of head trauma is significantly more common in male batterers than in nonviolent men (Rosenbaum, Hoge, & Adelman et al., 1994). Although there is a relationship between aggressive behavior and brain injury, the injury may not be responsible for the increased aggression (Kavoussi et al., 1997). The increased incidence of brain injuries in violent populations may be due to the increased likelihood that violent individuals are in more situations where they can be injured (e.g., fights in the community). Studies are inconsistent regarding the location of aggression-enhancing lesions from brain injuries (Kavoussi et al., 1997). In studies where CT scans were employed, different regions, including the temporal, prefrontal, and frontal lobes, have been identified as areas with lesions that resulted in increased physical and verbal aggression (Kavoussi et al., 1997). Another limitation in brain-imaging research is the inability to determine the underlying cause of the structural and functional brain abnormalities identified. Few studies with children have been conducted, so it is unclear when difficulties first occur. Even so, targeting pharmacologic interventions to treat brain lesions resulting from head trauma in violent offenders may result in decreased aggression and violence in this population.

Interaction Between Systems

There have been few studies on the interaction between the different brain systems that contribute to the regulation of aggressive behavior. As stated by

Kavoussi and colleagues (1997), "Hypothesizing that only one neurobiologic system influences aggressive behavior would be naïve." For instance, animal model studies have shown an interaction between testosterone and serotonin in the regulation of aggressive behavior (Bonson, Johnson, Fiorella, Rabin, and Winter, 1994). As the empirical evidence suggests, there is considerable credence to the position that neurobiologic systems do influence aggressive behavior. However, a direct causal link is difficult to establish with the existing evidence. Studying the interactions among biological, social, environmental, and psychological factors related to aggression is the most promising approach (Fishbein, 2001; Susman, 1997). Raine's (Raine & Liu, 1998; Raine, Reynolds, Venables, & Mednick, 1997) useful biosocial model of violence proposes direct predisposition to aggression from both biological and psychosocial sources, but the most important pathways are from interactions between factors (see Box 1-1).

Role of Alcohol and Drugs in Aggressive Behavior

The general population and researchers have long associated substance abuse with violence, but the relationships are extremely complex. Preventive interventions should be based on empirical research that clarifies the relationship between alcohol, drugs, and aggression.

Alcohol-Related Aggression. Violent crime and alcohol are associated in research, but, as first pointed out by Moyer (1987), most criminals are not alcoholics, and the majority of alcoholics are not violent criminals. Laboratory experiments have shown increased aggression with alcohol ingestion, but there is variability in the studies, and not all subjects react the same. Research has not substantiated the "direct-cause paradigm," the theory that alcohol directly causes aggression. Rather, alcohol detrimentally affects certain psychological and physiological processes that then lead to aggressive behavior (Giancola, 2002).

The cognitive effects of alcohol ingestion have been examined in several studies. For several decades, theorists (e.g., Pernanen, 1976) have hypothesized that alcohol consumption increases the probability of an aggressive reaction by reducing the number of available psychological coping mechanisms that rely on conceptual/abstract reasoning. Cognitive models of violence postulate that aggressive behavior is determined by the relative balance of instigative (e.g., threats, insults) and inhibitory cues (e.g., anxiety, norms of reciprocity) present in hostile interpersonal situations. Instigative cues increase the probability of an aggressive act, whereas inhibitory cues decrease the probability of an aggressive act (Giancola, 2002). Steele and Josephs (1990) proposed that alcohol interferes with information processing so that the ability to allocate attention to multiple aspects of a situation is inhibited. The person's ability to evaluate social and environmental information that provides feedback concerning appropriate forms of behavior is disrupted. All these cognitive abilities are components of a more general construct termed "executive functioning" (Giancola, 2002). Executive functioning is defined as higher-order cognitive processes involved in planning, initiation, and regulation of behavior. Giancola (2002) argues that executive functioning mediates the alcohol–aggression relationship and that acute alcohol consumption disrupts executive functioning, which then heightens the probability of aggression. However, only one study (of college-age males) has assessed the relationship between executive functioning, acute alcohol consumption, and aggression (Lau, Pihl, & Peterson, 1995). Alcohol and low executive functioning had independent effects on aggression; however, an interaction between executive functioning and alcohol consumption was not observed in the sample (Lau et al., 1995).

Currently, little is known about the acute effects of alcohol on testosterone and serotonin in the human brain (Giancola, 2002). Animal models suggest that low doses of alcohol tend to enhance blood testosterone levels, whereas high doses tend to have a suppressing effect (Giancola, 2002). Although limited research exists that examines the relationship between alcohol and testosterone in humans, acute alcohol consumption has been suggested in the depletion in brain serotonin (Giancola, 2002).

There is a limited number of published studies on alcohol-related aggression in women. Recent studies have examined the manner in which acute alcohol consumption and provocation effect aggressive behavior in men and women (Giancola, Helton, Osborne, Fuss, Terry, & Westerfield, 2002). In a sample of 102 healthy social drinkers between 21 and 35 years of age (54% male), provocation was a stronger elicitor of aggression than either gender or alcohol (Giancola et al., 2002). Under low provocation, men were more aggressive than were women; however, under high provocation men and women were equally aggressive, except in cases of extreme aggression, in which men again exhibited higher levels than women (Giancola et al., 2002). Furthermore, alcohol increased aggression for men but not for women. These results are consistent with other recent studies that indicate provocation and alcohol are effective in eliciting aggression for men; however, only provocation seems to be an effective aggression elicitor for women.

Findings are mixed about the relationship of preassault drinking to outcomes experienced by both offenders and victims. In two path analyses conducted with self-reported data from college women (Ullman, Karabatsos, & Koss, 1999a) and college men (Ullman, Karabatsos, & Koss, 1999b), victim drinking was related to greater sexual victimization. Victim drinking was associated with less offender aggression in the female college sample (Ullman et al., 1999a), but it was related to more offender aggression in the male college sample (Ullman et al., 1999b). Furthermore, in a national sample of college women, offender preassault drinking was weakly associated with sexual victimization severity but strongly associated with offender aggression, whereas offender aggression was the strongest predictor of sexual victimization severity (Ullman et al., 1999a). Based on these results, it appears that victim drinking may not play as substantial a role as offender drinking in sexual assault outcomes (Brecklin & Ullman, 2002). Brecklin and Ullman (2002) recently analyzed the data from 859 female sexual assault victims identified through the National Violence against Women Survey. The analysis showed that offender behavior (e.g., drinking and aggression), not victim behavior, is an important determinant of sexual assault outcomes of women (Brecklin & Ullman, 2002). Offender drinking predicted rape completion, and offender aggression predicted both victim injury and medical care outcomes in multivariate analysis, controlling for demographic, drinking, and assault characteristics (Brecklin & Ullman, 2002). Similar findings were recently reported in a study of intimate partner femicide (Sharps et al., 2000), where male drinking was associated with domestic violence as well as attempted and actual murders of female partners, but the alcohol use of the females was not. These findings imply that attention should be paid to offender interventions to reduce negative health outcomes for women.

Drug Use and Aggression. The literature on illicit drug use and crime often find strong associations between illicit drug use and both violent and property offenses (Martin & Bryant, 2001). Goldstein's (1985) conceptual framework for the relationship between drugs and violence identified three factors through which they may be linked: the drugs' psychopharmacological effects, the user's economic needs, and the violence associated with the distribution and control of illicit drugs.

In their literature review, Gelles and Strauss (1988) concluded that although drugs such as cocaine and marijuana have been associated with violence, opiates such as heroin have not. As with alcohol, effects of drugs on violent behavior appear to be associated with social, individual, and situational factors rather than neurophysiological causes. The majority of studies have found little evidence of a psychopharmacologic basis for an illicit drug–violence association (Martin & Bryant, 2001). A potential exception is amphetamines. In studies completed with primates, stump-tail macaques (monkeys) were given amphetamines. It was noted that the monkeys' aggressive behaviors increased significantly after they received the drug. According to Gelles and Strauss (1988), some investigators are pursuing the link between human amphetamine use and violence, but currently there is no conclusive evidence suggesting a causal link between this drug and violence. Recent data from a nationally representative sample indicated that although about 25% of the victims of violent crime perceived their offenders to have been drinking, less than 10% stated that the offender was under the influence of an illicit drug (Greenfield, 1998). Investigators are challenged to disentangle the relationships among alcohol, illicit drug use, and violence. Often the studies fail to distinguish between the many different substances used by the individuals and the combined effects of multiple drugs on aggression (Martin & Bryant, 2001).

Limitations of the Neurobiological Approach

As earlier noted, the majority of research examining the relationship between neurobiology and aggression has been conducted with men. Except for the evidence on the influence of hormones on aggression (which, as noted, is fragmentary and not totally conclusive), the neurophysiologists have not adequately explained the differences between male and female behavior. Females of all species are generally more difficult to stimulate to aggression and, once stimulated, express hostility somewhat differently than males (Rosoff & Tobach, 1991). It has been found that previous social experience and acquired learning of hierarchical rules are more important than sex hormones in aggressiveness and dominance pattern formation in monkeys (Laborit, 1978).

The most important determining factor in aggressive behavior in humans is gender, and although gender is obviously a physical factor the explanation of that difference is primarily found in the fields of sociology and psychology. Sociologists and psychologists generally acknowledge the neuronal and blood chemistry basis for aggression but differ in their perspectives on the major determinants of violence.

As demonstrated several decades ago, patients with implanted electrodes display hostility when stimulated, "but it is always expressed according to the subject's previous experience and evaluation of his present environment" (Delgado, 1971). Brain researchers have been criticized for diverting attention from social dilemmas, which some have said "contributes to unwillingness to undertake the political solutions to violence, which promise to achieve much more" (Coleman, 1974). However, neurophysiological bases for aggression are important for holistic understanding and can be viewed as background for psychological, sociological, and cultural influences that may lead to violent expression of the aggression.

Psychological Perspective

Psychological explanations of violence vary greatly. Many psychologists echo Freud's theories that aggression is a basic instinct or drive (Freud, 1932). Others de-emphasize or refute that view and identify other psychological traits that characterize the violent person. The theories addressed in this section include the frustration-aggression theory, the cognitive neoassociation theory, the social cognitive theory, the social information processing theory, and the general aggression model. Psychoanalytic frameworks, whose basic premise is that some basic need has been thwarted in the violent individual, usually by some form of faulty child rearing (Warren & Hindelang, 1979), is not addressed here.

Frustration-Aggression Theory

The frustration-aggression theory was first proposed by Dollard, Doob, Miller, and colleagues in 1939. They postulated that frustration, or an obstacle to achieving a desired goal, was the cause of all aggression. Although this theory has largely fallen out of favor, it is historically important because it is the first time researchers used current learning theories to attempt to understand aggression (Geen, 1998).

Cognitive Neoassociation Theory

Frustration as the sole antecedent to aggression has been discredited; however, stress related to noxious stimuli triggers memories, emotions, and behaviors that lead to fight (anger) or flight (fear) responses. The cognitive-neoassociation theorist holds that thoughts, affect, and behavior are linked in memory and triggered by an unpleasant and stressful condition or feeling (Anderson & Bushman, 2002; Berkowitz, 1989, 1993, 1998.) In an example offered by Anderson & Bushman (2002), the concept of "gun" is related to "anger," the desire to "harm" and the behavior of "shoot," which can lead to gun use. The cues that lead to gun use in a particular situation become associated with that event and further reinforce the cognitive associations among the emotions and behaviors.

Whether the ultimate response to a given trigger is fight or flight depends, according to Berkowitz (1993), on prior conditioning, genetic predisposition, and an appraisal of the best course of action for the situation. Berkowitz (1998) suggests that a wide range of stressors such as physical pain, excessive heat, economic uncertainty, and political unrest can all lead to an increase in aggressive behaviors in humans.

There is some evidence that activating violent thoughts and feelings can, at least in the short term, result in increased aggressive behavior. Smith and Donnerstein's review of the literature (1998) concludes that a variety of studies demonstrate that "priming" aggressive thoughts through viewing violent movies and television immediately results in greater propensity toward aggression in a wide variety of settings.

Social Cognitive Theory

Bandura is the originator and best-known proponent of the social cognitive theory as an explanation for aggression. He calls the theory psychological because it grows out of the school of behavioral psychology, yet it obviously contains aspects of sociological framework. Bandura (1973) originally named the theory "social learning theory." He reformulated the theory, however, to include more cognitive processes to account for observational learning and renamed the theory accordingly (Bandura, 1986). Okun (1986) notes that the majority of the general violence literature and, more specifically, the research on abuse of women use learning theory either explicitly or implicitly to explain why violence occurs.

Bandura defines aggression as "behavior that results in personal injury and in destruction of property," allowing that the injury "may be psychological." He also notes that the behavior must be labeled as aggressive by society, as determined by the action's intensity, the intentions attributed to the performer by others, and the characteristics of the labeler. Bandura believes that aggressive behavior may be considered adaptive or destructive, depending on the situation in which it is used. He acknowledges the role of biological subcortical structures in producing destructive behavior but believes that the social situation is most important in determining the frequency, form, circumstances, and target of the action.

Bandura postulates that rather than arising from instinct or frustration, aversive experiences result in emotional arousal, which is perceived in the individual as fear, anger, sorrow, or even euphoria, depending on prior learning, cognitive interpretation, and other people's reaction to the same experience. Moreover, "frustration or anger arousal is a facilitative but not a necessary condition for aggression" (Bandura, 1973). Bandura concludes that the majority of events that stimulate aggression (such as insults, status threats, or unjust treatment) "gain activating capacity through learning experiences." To illustrate this, he notes the many people who have experienced divorce, parental rejection, poverty, mental illness, or brain damage and have never become violent. He perceives the motivation for aggression as reinforcement based, not biologically determined. "The social learning theory of aggression distinguishes between acquisition of behaviors that have destructive and injurious potential and factors that determine whether a person will perform what he has learned . . . because not all that people learn is exhibited in their actions."

The acquisition of aggressive behavior can be learned through modeling or observational learning or by direct experience or practice. Performance is determined by both internal (biological and cognitive) and external instigators (Bandura, 1973, 1979). Bandura showed this through experiments with children. He notes also that observation of other's behavior also provides clues as to whether an action will be rewarded or punished when it occurs. If a child sees a parent or peer gain status, dominance, resources, or power by using violence, he or she will be more likely to use it (Bandura, 1973). It has often been noticed that violent men are more likely to have been abused as children, and these ideas also help to explain why some peer groups (such as gangs) and subcultures are known for violence (Bandura, 1973). Bandura found that the parents of aggressive boys from middle-class homes "repeatedly modeled and reinforced combative attitudes and behavior," even though they neither abused their children nor displayed antisocial violence (Bandura, 1973). Huesmann and colleagues' (Huesmann, Eron, Lefkowitz, & Walder, 1984) 22-year longitudinal analysis showed that aggressive behavior in men at age 30 was associated with early viewing of television violence as boys, even when controlling for intelligence, socioeconomic status, and parenting variables. Pettit (1997), in his review of the literature on the developmental course of aggression, concluded that there is substantial support in the literature for a relationship between parental use of aggressive disciplinary techniques and greater aggressive behavior in children.

Bandura (1979) explains that behavior learned from models is reinforced if the imitative actions are perceived as useful to the person. Laborit (1978) explains that if aggression is successful and dominance achieved by it, then the aggression is reinforced. A study of highly aggressive, incarcerated male adolescents showed that witnessing severe violence was related to perceived positive outcomes for the use of aggression. A year-long study of schoolchildren showed that children who demonstrated aggression-encouraging cognitions in the fall and perceived more support in the environment for these cognitions were more likely to demonstrate aggressive behavior through the school year (Egan, Monson, & Perry, 1998).

Various applications of the full social cognitive model have been tested as explanations of aggression and have generally been supported. A test of an application of a social cognitive model to men who physically abused their intimate partners found support for the model (Copenhaver, 2000). These men did not have fewer coping skills than nonviolent men, but the abusive men tended to interpret ambiguous situations negatively and thus respond with violence. Researchers found support for proposed cognitive mediators (self-efficacy and response-outcome expectancies) between exposure to aggression and aggressive behavior in children in one study (Perry, Perry, & Rasmussen, 1986).

Social cognitive theory incorporates biological, psychological, and sociological factors of causation of violence. Other theorists (Goldstein, 1974; Holtzworth-Munroe, 1992; Straub, 1971) have modified or amplified Bandura's basic propositions, but the thrust of the arguments remains the same. It has been used to explain various types of aggression, from schoolyard bullying to serial murder (Castle & Hensley, 2002). Empirical evidence supports the theoretical proposition that aggressive behavior is learned, at least in many cases, and growing research explains the mediating and moderating variables through which this may occur.

Social Information Processing Theory

Another cognitive theory, social processing theory, holds that all human behavior, including aggression, is mediated by cognitive processes (Dodge & Coie, 1987). Huesmann purports that behavior is modeled within a hierarchical system. Biological and neurochemical processes are at the lowest level, whereas higher-order information retrieval and cognitive processing are required for more complex behaviors. Within biological constraints, social information processing theory postulates that human behaviors include the following four steps: behavioral cues are recognized and interpreted, scripts (described subsequently) are retrieved (and enacted), the script is evaluated, and the environmental response is evaluated.

Huesmann (1986) incorporates script theory in the social information processing model. Scripts, highly associated concepts that both explain and guide behavior in a particular situation, were first proposed by Schank & Abelson (1977). Scripts are both learned by observation and reinforced by conditioning. Thus, society's response to an individual's use of a particular script will influence if and how that script is used in the future. Huesmann (1998) stated that "more aggressive people are presumed to have encoded a larger number of aggressive scripts" (p. 87). The longer scripts persist as a response, the more refined and resistant to modification they become. Although this is a primarily cognitive model, Huesmann postulates that negative emotional arousal (such as feeling angry) will "prime" individuals to retrieve more aggressive scripts and result in the individual retrieving the most well-learned scripts and evaluating the scripts less carefully.

In several studies, social information processing has been found to explain the link between the early experience or witnessing of violence and later aggressive behavior. An examination of children found that both violent victimization and witnessing violence were associated with aggressive behavior and mediated through social information processing rather than emotional factors (Schwartz & Proctor, 2000). Dodge and colleagues (Dodge, Price, Bachorowski, & Newman, 1990) found that the social information processing model explained higher rates of aggressive behavior in maltreated versus nonmaltreated children. Replication of this research by the same team (Dodge, Pettit, & Bates, 1995) again found that, even when controlling for potentially confounding factors, social information processing patterns explained the link between early maltreatment and later aggression in children.

Social information processing has been particularly studied as a potential causal mechanism between viewing of violent content in the media, particularly television, and subsequent violent behavior. A longitudinal study following 570 children from preschool to adolescence found support for cognitive models such as social information processing to explain the relationship between preschool television viewing and adolescent behavior, including aggression (Anderson, Huston, Schmitt, Linebarger, & Wright, 2001).

General Aggression Model

Synthesizing elements from the previous models, as well as several others, Anderson and Bushman (2002) proposed the general aggression model (GAM). In this model, inputs from the person (traits, sex, beliefs, attitudes, values, and scripts) and the situation (aggressive cues, provocation, frustration, discomfort, drugs, and incentives) both influence the person's internal state (affect, cognition, and arousal) and thereby determine the outcomes (appraisal and decision processes that lead to either thoughtful or impulsive action). The authors of this chapter hope that this model will be the basis for creating multisystem violence interventions. However, the newness of the theory precludes the existence of research testing its components.

Sociological Forces Affecting Violence

The sociological theories of violence generally consider some biological and psychological aspects of causation, but their basic proposition is that social structure and conditions are more important (West, 1979). They vehemently reject the notion that aggression is an instinct or drive and postulate that most violent offenders do not generally act destructively (Chatterton, 1976). Except for these areas of agreement, sociologists vary widely in their approach. There are theorists who emphasize any one of the following aspects: cultural attitudes fostering violence, the structural violence inherent in our society, the role of power, and the influence of poverty.

Cultural Attitudes Fostering Violence

The United States has a long history of violence used as a means to achieve socially approved ends. American culture reflects at least a covert acceptance of violence in the media, in attitudinal surveys, and in choice of heroes. Farrell (2000) notes that there is a tendency toward excess in American culture, including excessive violence (what he terms "berserk" behavior) that is encouraged through the spectrum of entertainment and news media. Senator Moynihan (1993) suggests that aggression and other deviant behavior have become so pervasive in American society that, rather than address the behaviors, the boundaries of deviancy have been refined so that previously stigmatized behavior is now considered normal. A cross-cultural analysis of wife beating found that sanctions at the community level against wife battering were extremely important in keeping occasional acts of violence against wives from escalating to severe abuse (Counts, Brown, & Campbell, 1999). Further discussion of the role of culture in violence can be found later in the section entitled "Insights from Anthropology."

Structural Violence of Society

A closely related theme is that violence in America reflects the violence inherent in our way of life. Gil (1978) notes that the structure of our capitalist society prevents individuals from attaining their full potential. Others believe that the existence of state-sanctioned killing through capital punishment has a brutalizing effect that results in an increase in violent crime. Studies by a variety of scientists using different methods have in fact found that homicide and other violent crime rates increase when criminals are executed (Bailey, 1998; Harries & Cheatwood, 1997; Lester, 2000; Thompson, 1999).

Poverty

To explain the greater amounts of urban violence, particularly among poor, young black men, sociologists have proposed extensive theories. Berkowitz (1998), in his review, noted that poverty, or a more complex variable of economic deprivation, was a good predictor of aggressive behavior in adolescents. Anderson and Anderson's (1998) model testing found that socioeconomic status was positively related to violent crime, independent of other factors. Jewkes' (2002) review of the relationship between intimate partner violence and poverty found that there is a strong positive correlation between poverty and rates of violence and that this relationship may be mediated through stress or a crisis in male role identity. Campbell and colleagues' (in press) analysis of risk factors for intimate partner femicide found that the male partner's unemployment significantly increased the risk of lethal violence among battered women.

Subculture of Violence

Researchers have postulated the concept of a subculture of violence—wherein violence becomes part of the social norms and may, under some conditions, be a socially desirable behavior—to explain regional differences in aggression (Wolfgang and Ferracuti, 1982). More specifically, some researchers have theorized that within the United States there exists a "southern culture of violence" that arises from a culture of honor (Nesbit, 1993).

Anderson and Anderson's (1998) review of the literature, however, does not find strong support for either a culture of violence or a southern culture of honor. They noted that empirical support for the theories was weak and that variables for a culture-of-honor model had not been clearly operationalized, and suggested that there are other historical and environmental factors that explain the increased rates of violence in the South, findings echoed by Pridemore's (2002) review. Some studies have found support for the theory of a subculture of violence (Harer & Steffensmeier, 1992; Rice & Goldman, 1994; Kposowa & Breault, 1993), particularly for an increase in violence in the southern U.S. and among African Americans. However, studies that more rigorously controlled for confounding variables and that directly tested the theorized mediating relationships have failed to support the theory (Cao, Adams, & Jensen, 1997; Hensley, Tung, Xu, Gray-Ray, & Ray, 1999; Kposowa & Breault, 1995; Tedeschi & Felson, 1994). Nevertheless, some studies still find that certain types of honor-related violence may remain high in certain geographic regions (the western and southern U.S.) despite other factors (Cohen, 1998; Cohen & Nisbett, 1997). Although the subculture-of-violence theory does not appear to explain most types of violence, it may explain specific honor-related violence in some regions.

INSIGHTS FROM ANTHROPOLOGY

The Meaning of Violence Cross-Culturally

The meaning of the term "violence" within a culture varies through time as well as from culture to culture. Historically in the United States, the *Journal of Marriage and the Family* first mentioned family violence after 1970, and not until after 1973 were there references to wife abuse in *The New York Times*. The first official declaration of violence as a health problem was by former Surgeon General Dr. C. Everett Koop in 1985 (U.S. Department of Health and Human Services, 1986).

Behaviors generally understood as abuse in one culture may be considered legitimate in another. Torres' (1991) comparison of Mexican Americans and Anglo-Americans demonstrated differences in behaviors that were considered abusive. Although there was no difference in the severity and frequency of violence between the two groups, Mexican Americans less frequently labeled their experience of being hit as abuse. Whether the differences were related to ethnicity or to sociocultural factors such as religion, education, and economic factors characteristic of each group, it is apparent that abuse occurs within a context that influences interpretation (Counts, Brown, & Campbell, 1999; Torres, 1991). The absence of reports of abuse in a culture does not mean it does not exist. An unstated assumption in much of the anthropological literature is that if the persons interviewed or observed did not know, acknowledge, or admit there was abuse, it was not classified as abuse (Korbin, 1991). If abuse is a function of a person's perception of being victimized, the culture's beliefs and norms become important in understanding the influence of culture on recognition of violence as well as the culture's definition of violence. In fact, because of different cultures' perceptions of what constitutes abuse and the complexity of different cultural systems, it may not be possible to attain a universal definition of family violence that is culturally specific (Korbin, 1991).

Sensitivity of the observer may also reflect societal differences about the meaning of violence. Female anthropologists may be more sensitive to the occurrence of violence against women or may have had women more readily disclose violence to them (Campbell, 1985). An ethnographer may report only the positive about a culture either because she or he has "fallen in love" with the people or because he or she wants to maintain the trust with the society, which has been established over time (Erchak, 1999). However, some societies are totally nonviolent both interpersonally and in terms of warfare, according to many different anthropologists and other reporters. The existence of such cultures provides powerful evidence that cultural forces and learning are at least as important as biology in explaining the occurrence of violence. The characteristics of such societies are important in identifying possible primary prevention approaches. Nonviolent societies tend to be more egalitarian (either in terms of power or economics) than hierarchical in sex role and ethnic group arrangements, treat children with kindness and without corporal punishment, value cooperation over competition, and have definitions not tied to violence and control of women (Counts, Brown, & Campbell, 1999; Eisler, 1988; Levinson, 1989; Paddock, 1975; Whiting, 1965).

In this discussion, "culture" refers to homogeneous nations, political subdivisions within nations, ethnic groups, or small-scale societies (Levinson, 1989). The culture of an individual is one's "social heredity." The role of culture in relationship to violence must be understood (Campbell, 1985; Torres, 1991; Torres et al., 2000). The problem of whether to view culture as a causative influence is complex because there are probably multiple mingled antecedents associated with violence. Three major theoretical frameworks purport to explain the cultural influences on violence: social organization, with its premises related to sexual inequality; cultural patterning; and cultural consistency, with a cultural spillover hypothesis. Each theoretical framework is described briefly with support for its claims. Although cultural determinants of violence have not been totally established, there is beginning support for each of these theories.

Social Organization and Sexual Inequality

"Social organization" is defined in sociology as the pattern of relationships between and among individuals and social groups and how the individuals are related to each other and the whole group (Straus, 1974). Social-organization theories of family violence claim causes of violence can be found in the structure of the society and its effect on how the family members relate to each other. Levinson (1989) found more severe physical punishment of children in more complex societies and in societies with more single-parent families. He also noted more wife beating and child beating in societies where men have multiple wives (polygenous households). One of the aspects of social organization is gender relationships.

Traditionally patriarchal societies have viewed violence toward wives as a male prerogative, stemming from the idea that women are the property of men (Dobash & Dobash, 1979; Dobash & Dobash, 1998; Heise, Ellsberg, & Gottemoeller, 1999). There is inconsistent evidence about any direct correlation between the status of women and violence against women cross-culturally (Counts, Brown, & Campbell, 1999; Heise, Ellsburg, & Goettemoeller, 1999; Lester, 1980). The following issues complicate research in this realm:

- There are many spheres and indicators of women's status (Whiting, 1965).
- There has been a failure to measure women's status at the cultural or ethnic group level rather than at the couple level.

- The relationship may be curvilinear (Campbell, 2001). In other words, in cultures where women are totally subjugated, women may not be beaten often because other societal mechanisms are in place that keep women's status low. In societies where there is equality between men and women, wife beating is limited. Domestic violence is highly prevalent in societies where women's status is disputed or changing rapidly.

In the United States, Yllo (1983) found that violence against women was greater in the states where women's status, measured by economic, educational, political, and legal rights, was especially low or especially high (Yllo, 1983; 1984). In two cross-cultural analyses of less complex societies, control of the wealth, authority in the home, and women's economic autonomy were related to frequency of wife beating (Counts, Brown, & Campbell, 1999; Levinson, 1989).

The concept of women's status is complex. Status may differ in the public and private spheres of a culture, as well as among dimensions of power, prestige, and rewards, which are indicators of status in the United States. Cross-cultural indicators related to women's status that have been associated with wife beating are female autonomy, matrilocality, virtue as honor, the male perception of females as male property, male sexual jealousy, strong association of women with nature, cultural sanctions allowing wife beating, other violence against women, female entrapment in marriage (divorce restrictions), male control of production, and male domestic decision-making (Campbell, 1985; Counts, Brown & Campbell, 1999; Levinson, 1989).

The effect of gender inequality can also be seen culturally in the maltreatment of female children. Female infants and young girls are more likely to be malnourished and receive inadequate medical care than are their brothers in societies where there is male gender preference (Heise, Ellsberg, & Gottemoeller, 1999; Korbin, 1991). In India and the People's Republic of China, amniocentesis has been used for sex determination and then followed by abortion of female fetuses. There is also some indication that sexual inequality is related to societies known for warfare (Eisler, 1988; Montagu, 1978). Understanding these complex questions is important to the prevention of violence.

Cultural Patterning

Cultural patterning starts with the assumption that people have an innate drive for aggression but postulates that they are patterned culturally to discharge their aggression in particular ways. Cultural patterning uses social learning theories to understand how cultures and subcultures transmit the preference for violence to be expressed in particular ways. The subculture-of-violence theory is a branch of cultural patterning theory and was discussed earlier.

Cultural Consistency Theory of Violence

Elements of a culture tend to be interdependent. Knowledge of the interdependent factors within a culture and their relationship to violence can ultimately provide a framework of cultural norms. This knowledge not only provides a greater understanding of what leads to abuse, but it can also help influence the development of cultures that are free of violence (Levinson, 1989). The cultural consistency theory explains that even cultural norms not directly related to violence can have an effect on violence that occurs within the culture. An example of this concept is that Mexican American boys may be so afraid of their fathers' punishment that there is little communication between father and son. Because of the poor communication, the boys unwittingly act in such a way that they offend their fathers and are punished severely. Family structure that contains stress and physical abuse models violence, which is then acted out by the next generation. In the cultural consistency theory, the norms of this family behavior reflect the values of the society as a whole. The norms are tied to the structure of the systemic properties of the culture (Whyte, 1978). In this way, violence tends to be consistent with the norms and values of the society (Carroll, 1980). This explanation thus helps in understanding the causation of violence within a culture. Paddock's (1975) description of nonviolent communities in Mexico is consistent with the cultural consistency theory. Paddock reported differences in child-raising practices between violent and nonviolent communities, including differences in punishment. Attitudes of men in the less violent community reflected less machismo. The violent community was authoritarian, but in the nonviolent cultural system the authority was shared. The consensus of the group reflected a shared attitude against interpersonal violence. Cultural consistency theory explains why societies known for warfare are also associated with high rates of individual violence.

Cultural Spillover Hypothesis

According to the cultural spillover hypothesis of the cultural consistency framework, the more a society tends to use physical force toward socially approved ends, the greater the likelihood that this legitimization of force will be generalized to other areas of life (Baron, Straus, & Jaffee, 1988). Examples of the use of force in a society are in maintaining order in schools, controlling crime, or dominating international events for the country's self-interest. There is evidence that in states where there is a strong emphasis on physical punishment of children, strict or corporal punishment in schools, and high levels of incarceration, there is more interpersonal violence (Baron, Straus, & Jaffee, 1988).

Ethnic Groups in the United States

There are many different cultures in the United States. All the theories presented may at least partially explain the effect of culture on violence, yet studies of differences among ethnic groups within the United States indicate the complexity of the influences. To be useful, variables implicated in abuse must have explanatory power both within and between cultures. It is also important to refrain from assuming that members of ethnic groups can be characterized similarly in terms of characteristics related to abuse. One of the variables that has been shown important to consider is level of acculturation of the family or couple into the United States in conjunction with socioeconomic status. Several investigations have shown that increased acculturation is associated with an increase in intimate partner violence and child abuse, at least for Hispanic families (Sorenson & Telles, 1991; Torres et al., 2000). An interactional approach is needed to understand the effect of cultural differences on ethnic groups (Gelfand & Fandetti, 1986; Sorenson, 1996). That is, ethnic groups need to be assessed according to language, generation of the immigrant, cultural homogene-

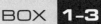

BOX 1-3 STRENGTHS AND WEAKNESSES OF THEORETICAL APPROACHES

BIOLOGICAL THEORIES

STRENGTHS

- Aggression and violence are due to brain or hormonal imbalances and thus are treatable or manageable with treatment.
- Neurobiological bases for aggression are important to provide a holistic understanding and can be viewed as background for psychological, sociological, and cultural influences that may lead to violence.

WEAKNESSES

- Social or environmental conditions that may influence or mediate violence or aggression are not considered.
- There is the risk of diverting attention from social issues and undertaking political solutions to violence.
- Animal models are used in many research studies examining the neurobiological bases of aggression.
- Human research has been done primarily on men and prisoners.

PSYCHOLOGICAL/ COGNITIVE THEORIES

STRENGTHS

- These theories incorporate how environmental influences such as television, exposure to violence, and peer reactions affect behavior. By monitoring such societal influences, violence can be mediated.
- This theoretical approach has a growing body of literature confirming key parts of some theories and suggests plausible and often empirically supported mediating factors.

WEAKNESSES

- This approach minimizes the role that power has in violent interactions.

- This perspective sometimes implies that once the violence is modeled and observed, violent actions will automatically follow.

SOCIOLOGICAL EXPLANATIONS

STRENGTHS

- Conditions such as unequal power relations and poverty create situations where violence is an outcome.
- Structural changes, such as creating equal status between men and women and minimizing the financial gap between the rich and the poor, will eradicate the need for violent actions to occur.

WEAKNESSES

- The solutions are long term and do not address the immediate health concerns resulting from violent behaviors.
- The explanations tend to focus on the general "macrosociological" level and do not hold individuals accountable for their violent behaviors.

CULTURAL EXPLANATIONS

STRENGTHS

- Violent behaviors in certain cultures tend to be associated with factors such as child-rearing techniques and beliefs, attitudes about women, warfare, and crime. By examining cultural practices, we can gain understanding of how violence fits and what purposes it serves.

WEAKNESSES

- Analysis of culture does not offer any solutions about how to change specific behaviors of individuals or groups.

ity of the neighborhood, degrees of activity in traditional religions, socioeconomic status, and the interaction of these factors with the institutions of work, school, social services, medical services, and community. Ethnic identity and levels of oppression have also been found to be important variables in relation to violence, but there has yet to be sufficient study to specify their exact roles and the interactions of these variables with other factors. Several studies have shown that socioeconomic status accounts for differences in prevalence of husband-to-wife abuse among U.S. ethnic groups (Dearwater et al., 1998; DeMaris, 1990; Lockhart, 1987; Torres, 1991). Many investigations find that apparent differences in levels of violence between ethnic groups diminish considerably or disappear in the United States when socioeconomic class is the same or statistically controlled (Hawkins, 1990).

Box 1-3 summarizes strengths and weaknesses of various theories of violence.

SUMMARY

Violence and abuse cannot be understood out of context. The complexity of factors related to violence is magnified by varied cultural systems. Further complicating the issue in the United States is the difference in the level of acculturation and oppression of the various cultures and ethnic groups. Membership in a culture or ethnic group cannot forecast the person's perception of or reaction to violence. Important differences between one's beliefs and those of persons from other cultures or ethnic groups will probably exist. It is important to examine assumptions (Torres, 1991). The influence of spiritual, moral, somatic, psychological, metaphysical, economic, kinship, and territoriality issues needs to be taken into account to discern the individual and family's views of violence and abuse. Only then can nurses and other health practitioners structure their approaches to ethnic groups for perception and management of the problem (Flaskerud, 1984).

References

Anderson, C. A., & Anderson, K. B. (1998). Temperature and aggression: Paradox, controversy, and a fairly clear picture. In R.G. Geen & E. Donnerstein (Eds.), *Human aggression: Theories, research, and implications for social policy.* San Diego: Academic Press.

Anderson, C. A., & Bushman, B. J. (2002). Human aggression. *Annual Review of Psychology, 53,* 27–51.

Anderson, D. R., Huston, A. C., Schmitt, K. L., Linebarger, D. L., & Wright, J. C. (2001). Early television viewing and adolescent behavior: The recontact study. *Society for Research on Child Development Monograph, 66*(19), I–VIII.

Anderson, R. N. (2001). Deaths: Leading causes for 1999. *National Vital Statistics Report, 49*(11).

Archer, J. (1991). The influence of testosterone on human aggression. *British Journal of Psychology, 82,* 1–28.

Archer, J. (1977). The psychology of violence. *New Society, 42,* 63–66.

Arnold, S. E. (1993). Estrogen for refractory aggression after traumatic brain injury. *American Journal of Psychiatry, 150,* 1564–1656.

Ardrey, R. (1966). *The territorial imperative.* New York: Atheneum.

Bailey, W. (1998). Deterrence, brutalization, and the death penalty: Another examination of Oklahoma's return to capital punishment. *Criminology, 36,* 711–733.

Bandura, A. (1973) *Aggression: A social learning analysis.* New York: General Learning Press.

Bandura, A. (1979). The social learning perspective. In H. Toch (Ed.), *Psychology of crime and criminal justice.* New York: Holt, Rinehart, and Winston.

Bandura, A. (1986). Social foundations of thought and action: A social-cognitive theory. Englewood Cliffs, NJ: Prentice-Hall.

Baron, L., Straus, M., & Jaffee, D. (1988). A test of the cultural spillover theory. *Annals of the New York Academy of Sciences, 528,* 79–110.

Berkowitz, L. (1989). Frustration-aggression hypothesis: Examination and reformulation. *Psychological Bulletin, 106*(1), 59–73.

Berkowitz, L. (1993). Pain and aggression: Some findings and implications. *Motivation and Emotion, 17,* 277–293.

Berkowitz, L. (1998). Affective aggression: The role of stress, pain, and negative affect. In R. G. Geen & E. Donnerstein (Eds.), *Human aggression: Theories, research and implications for practice.* San Diego: Academic Press.

Bernhardt, P. (1997). Influences of serotonin and testosterone in aggression and dominance: Convergence with social psychology. *Current Directions in Psychological Science, 6,* 44–48.

Blackburn, J. R., Pfaus, J. G., & Phillips, A. G. (1992). Dopamine functions in appetites and defensive behaviors. *Progress in Neurobiology, 39,* 247–279.

Bonson, K. R., Johnson, R. G., Fiorella, D., Rabin, R. A., & Winter, J. C. (1994). Serotonergic control of androgen-induced dominance. *Pharmacology, Biochemistry and Behavior, 49,* 313–322.

Brecklin, L. R., & Ullman, S. E. (2002). The roles of victim and offender alcohol use in sexual assaults: Results from the National Violence Against Women Survey. *Journal of Studies on Alcohol, 63,* 57–64.

Brennan, W. (1998). Aggression and violence: Examining the theories. *Nursing Standard, 12,* 36–37.

Campbell, J. (1985). The battering of wives: A cross-cultural perspective. *Victimology, 10,* 174–185.

Campbell, J. C. (2001). Global perspectives on wife beating and health care. In M. Martinez (Ed.), *Prevention and control of aggression and its impact on victims* (pp. 215–228). New York: Kluwer Publishers.

Campbell, J. C., Webster, D., Koziol-McLain, J., Block, C., Campbell, D., et al. (in press). Risk factors for femicide in abusive relationships: Results from a multi-site case control study. *American Journal of Public Health.*

Cao, L., Adams, A., & Jensen, V. J. (1997). A test of the black subculture of violence thesis: A research note. *Criminology, 35*(2), 367–379.

Castle, T., & Hensley, C. (2002). Serial killers with military experience: Applying social learning theory to serial murder. *International Journal of Offender Therapy and Comparative Criminology, 46*(4), 453–465.

Chatterton, M. R. (1976). The social contexts of violence. In M. Borland (Ed.), *Violence in the family* (pp. 15–36). Atlantic Highlands, NJ: Humanities Press.

Cohen, D. (1998). Culture, social organization, and patterns of violence. *Journal of Personality and Social Psychology, 75* (2), 408–419.

Cohen, D., & Nisbett, R. E. (1997). Field experiments examining the culture of honor: The role of institutions in perpetuating norms about violence. *Personality and Social Psychology Bulletin, 23*(11), 1188–1199.

Coleman, L. S. (1974). Perspectives on the medical research of violence. *American Journal of Orthopsychiatry, 44,* 685–692.

Copenhaver, M. M. (2000). Testing a social-cognitive model of intimate abusiveness among substance-dependent males. *American Journal of Drug and Alcohol Abuse, 26,* (4), 603–628.

Counts, D., Brown, J., & Campbell, J. C. (1999). *To have and to hit: Cultural perspectives on wife beating.* Chicago: University of Illinois Press.

Dabbs, J. M., Carr, T. S., Frady, R. L., & Riad, J. K. (1995). Testosterone, crime, and misbehavior among 692 male prison inmates. *Personality and Individual Differences, 18,* 627–633.

Daly, M., & Wilson, M. (1998). An evolutionary psychological perspective on homicide. In M. D. Smith & M. Zahn (Eds.), *Homicide: A sourcebook of social research* (pp. 58–71). Thousand Oaks, CA: Sage Publications.

Dearwater, S. R., Coben, J. H, Campbell, J. C., Nah, G., Glass, N. E., McLoughlin, E., & Bekemeier, B. (1998). Prevalence of intimate partner abuse in women treated at community hospital emergency departments. *Journal of the American Medical Association, 280*(5), 433–438.

Delgado, J. (1971). The neurological basis of violence. *International Social Science Journal, 33,* 33–48.

DeMaris, A. (1990). The dynamics of generational transfer in courtship violence: A biracial exploration. *Journal of Marriage and the Family, 52,* 219–231.

Dobash, R. E., & Dobash, R. P. (1979). *Violence against wives.* New York: The Free Press.

Dobash, R. E., & Dobash, R. P. (1998). *Rethinking violence against women.* Thousand Oaks, CA: Sage Publications.

Dodge, K. A., & Coie, J. D. (1987). Social information-processing factors in reactive and proactive aggression in children's peer groups. *Journal of Personal and Social Psychology, 53,* 1146–1158.

Dodge, K. A., Pettit, G. S., & Bates, J. E. (1995). Social information processing patterns partially mediate the effect of early physical abuse on later conduct problems. *Journal of Abnormal Psychology, 104,* 632–643.

Dodge, K. A., Pettit, G. S., Bates, J. E., & McClaskey, C. L. (1986). Social competence in children. *Society for Research into Child Development Monograph, 51.*

Dodge, K. A., Price, J. M., Bachorowski, J. A., & Newman, J. P. (1990). Hostile attributional biases in severely aggressive adolescents. *Journal of Abnormal Psychology, 104,* 632–643.

Dolan, M.C. (1994). Psychopathy: a neurobiological perspective. *British Journal of Psychiatry, 165,* 151–159.

Dolan, M. C., Anderson, I. M., & Deakin, J. F. W. (2001). The relationship between 5-HT function and aggression in highly aggressive personality. *British Journal of Psychiatry, 178,* 352–359.

Dolan, M., Deakin, J. F., Roberts, N., & Anderson, I. (2002). Serotonergic and cognitive impairment in impulsive aggressive personality disordered offenders: Are there implications for treatment? *Psychological Medicine, 32,* 105–117.

Dollard, J., Doob, L., Miller, N., Mowrer, O., & Sears, R. (1939). *Frustration and aggression.* New Haven, CT: Yale University Press.

Egan, S. K., Monson, T. C., & Perry, D. G. (1998). Social-cognitive influences on change in aggression over time. *Developmental Psychology, 34*(6), 1155.

Eisler, R. (1988). *The chalice and the blade: Our history, our future*. San Francisco: Harper & Row.

Elliott, F. A. (1982). Neurobiological finding in adult minimal brain dysfunction and the dyscontrol syndrome. *Journal of Nervous and Mental Disease, 170*, 680–687.

Erchak, G. M. (1999). In D. Counts, J. Brown,, & J. C. Campbell, (Eds.), *To have and to hit: Cultural perspectives on wife beating*. Chicago: University of Illinois Press.

Farrell, K. (2000). The berserk style in American culture. *Cultural Critique, 46*, 179–209.

Fishbein, D. (2001). *Biobehavioral perspectives in criminology*. Belmont, CA: Wadsworth/Thomson Learning.

Flaskerud, J. H. (1984). A comparison of perceptions of problematic behavior by six minority groups and mental health professionals. *Nursing Research, 33*(4), 190–197.

Fox, J. A., & Zawitz, M. W. (2002). *Homicide trends in the U.S.* Washington, D.C.: Bureau of Justice Statistics, U.S. Department of Justice.

Freud, S. (1932). Why war? In R. Maple & D. R. Matheson (Eds.), *Aggression, hostility and violence* (pp. 118–132). New York: Holt, Rinehart and Winston.

Garza-Trevino, E. S. (1994). Neurobiological factors in aggressive behavior. *Hospital & Community Psychiatry, 45*, 690–699.

Geen, R. G. (1998). Processes and personal variables in affective aggression. In R. G. Geen & E. Donnerstein (Eds.), *Human aggression: Theories, research and implications for social policy*. San Diego: Academic Press.

Gelfand, D. E., & Fandetti, D. V. (1986). The emergent nature of ethnicity: Dilemmas in assessment. *Social Casework: The Journal of Contemporary Social Work*, 542–550.

Gelles, R. & Straus, M. (1988). *Intimate violence*. New York: Simon & Schuster.

Giancola, P. R. (2000). Neuropsychological functioning and antisocial behavior: Implications for etiology and prevention. In D. Fishbien (Ed.), *The science, treatment and prevention of antisocial behavior: Application to the criminal justice system* (pp. 1–16). Kingston, NJ: Civic Research Institute.

Giancola, P. R. (2002). Alcohol-related aggression during the college years: Theories, risk factors, and policy implications. *Journal of Studies on Alcohol, 63*, 129–139.

Giancola, P. R., Helton, E. L., Osborne, A. B., Terry, M. K., Fuss, A. M., & Westerfield, J. A. (2002). The effect of alcohol and provocation on aggressive behavior in men and women. *Journal of Studies on Alcohol, 63*, 64–74.

Gil, D. G. (1978). Societal violence and violence in families. In J. M. Eckelaar & S. N. Katz (Eds.), *Family Violence* (pp. 16–27). Toronto: Butterworth.

Goldstein, M. (1974). Brain research and violent behavior. *Archives of Neurology, 30*, 2–81.

Goldstein, P. J. (1985). The drugs/violence nexus: A tripartite conceptual framework. *Journal of Drug Issues, 15*, 493–506.

Greenfield, L. A. (1998). *Alcohol and crime: An analysis of national data on the prevalence of alcohol involvement in crime*. Washington, DC: U.S. Department of Justice (NCJ 168632).

Harer, M. D., & Steffensmeier, D. (1992). The differing effects of income inequality on black and white rates of violence. *Social Forces, 70*, 1035–1054.

Harries, K., & Cheatwood, D. (1997). *The geography of execution: The capital punishment quagmire in America*. Lanham, MD: Rowan and Littlefield.

Hawkins, D. F. (1990). Explaining the black homicide rate. *Journal of Interpersonal Violence, 5*(2), 151–163.

Heise, L., Ellsberg, M., & Gottemoeller, M. (1999). *Ending violence against women*. Baltimore, MD: Johns Hopkins University Population Reports.

Hensley, C., Tung, Y. Y., Xu, X., Gray-Ray, P., & Ray, M. (1999). A racial comparison of Mississippi's juvenile violent and property crime rates: A test of self-control and subculture of violence theories. *Journal of African American Men, 4*(3), 21–44.

Herman, S. J. (1978). *Becoming assertive: A guide for nurses*. New York: Van Nostrand Reinhold.

Holtzworth-Munroe, A. (1992). Social skills deficits in maritally violent men: Interpreting the data using a social information processing model. *Clinical Psychological Review, 12*, 605–617.

Hoyert, D. L., Arias, E., Smith, B. L., Murphy, S. L., & Kochanek, K. D. (2001). Deaths: Final data for 1999. *National Vital Statistics Report, 49*(8), 1–114.

Huesmann, L. R. (1986). Psychological processes promoting the relation between exposure to media violence and aggressive behavior by the viewer. *Journal of Social Issues, 42*, (3), 125–140.

Huesmann, L. R. (1998). The role of information processing and cognitive schema in the acquisition and maintenance of habitual aggressive behavior. In R. G. Geen & E. Donnerstein (Eds.), *Human aggression: Theories, research, and implications for social policy*. New York: Academic Press.

Huesmann, L. R., Eron, L. D., Lefkowitz, M. M., & Walder, L. O. (1984). The stability of aggression over time and generations. *Developmental Psychology, 20*(6), 1120–1134.

Hull, J. G. (1981). A self-awareness model of the causes and effect of alcohol and consumption. *Journal of Abnormal Psychology, 90*, 586–600.

Hull, J. G., & Bond, C. F. (1986). Social and behavioral consequence of alcohol consumption and expectancy: a recta-analysis. *Psychological Bulletin, 99*, 347–360.

Jewkes, R. (2002). Intimate partner violence: Causes and prevention. *The Lancet, 359*(9315), 1423–1429.

Kavoussi, R., Armstead, P., & Coccaro, E. (1997). The neurobiology of impulsive aggression. *Anger, Aggression, and Violence, 20*, 395–403.

Kolb, L. (1971). Violence and aggression: An overview. In J. Fawcett (Ed.), *Dynamics of violence* (pp. 40–50). Chicago: American Medical Association.

Korbin, J. E. (1991). Cross-cultural perspectives and research directions for the 21st century. *Child Abuse and Neglect, 15*, 67–77.

Kposowa, A. J., & Breault, K. D. (1995). Reassessing the structural covariates of violent and property crimes in the USA: A county level analysis. *British Journal of Sociology, 46*(1), 79–105.

Kravitz, H. M., Haywood, T. W., Kelly, J., et al. (1995). Medroxyprogesterone treatment for paraphiliacs. *Bulletin of the American Academy of Psychiatry and the Law, 23,* 19–33.

Laborit, H. (1978). Biological and sociological mechanisms of aggression. *International Social Science Journal, 30,* 738–745.

Lau, M. A., Pihl, R. O., & Peterson, J. B. (1995). Provocation, acute alcohol intoxication, cognitive performance, and aggression. *Journal of Abnormal Psychology, 104,* 150–155.

Leavitt, R. (1975). *Peaceable primates and gentle people: Anthropological approaches to women's studies.* New York: Harper & Row.

Lester, D. (1980). A cross-culture study of wife abuse. *Aggressive Behavior, 6,* 361–364.

Lester, D. (2000). Executions as a deterrent to homicide. *Perceptual and Motor Skills, 91*(2), 696.

Levinson, D. (1989). *Family violence in cross-cultural perspective.* Newbury Park, CA: Sage Publications.

Linnoila, M., Virkkunen, M., Scheinin, M., Nuutila, A., Rimon, R., & Goodwin, F. K. (1983). Low cerebrospinal fluid 5-hydroxyindoleacetic acid concentration differentiates impulsive from non-impulsive violent behavior. *Life Science, 33,* 2609–2614.

Lockhart, L. L. (1987). A reexamination of the effects of race and social class on the incidence of marital violence: A search for reliable differences. *Journal of Marriage and the Family, 49,* 603–610.

Lorenz, K., (1966). *On aggression.* New York: Bantam Books.

Malinowski, B. (1973). An anthropological analysis of war. In E. Maple & O. Matheson (Eds.), *Aggression, hostility and violence* (pp. 76–100). New York: Holt, Rinehart, and Winston.

Markowitz, P. I., & Coccaro, E. F. (1995). Biological studies of impulsivity, aggression and suicidal behaviour. In E. Hollander & D. Stein (Eds.), *Impulsivity and aggression* (pp. 71–91). Chichester, England: John Wiley & Sons.

Martin, S. E., & Bryant, K. (2001). Gender differences in the association of alcohol intoxication and illicit drug abuse among persons arrested for violent and property offenses. *Journal of Substance Abuse, 13,* 563–581.

Mattes, J. A. (1986). Propranolol for adults with temper outbursts and residual attention deficit disorder. *Journal of Clinical Psychopharmacology, 6,* 299–302.

McKinlay, M. W., Brooks, D. N., Bond, M. R., et al. (1981). The short-term outcome of severe blunt head injury as reported by the relatives of the injured person. *Journal of Neurology, Neurosurgery and Psychiatry, 44,* 527–533.

Merriam-Webster (1993). *Merriam-Webster's collegiate dictionary* (10th ed.). Springfield, MA: Author.

Montagu, A. (1978). *Learning non-aggression.* New York: Oxford Press.

Moyer, K. E. (1987). *Violence and aggression.* New York: Paragon House.

Moynihan, D.P. (1993). Defining deviancy down. *American Scholar, 62,* 17–30.

Nesbitt, R. E. (1993). Violence and U.S. regional culture. *American Psychologist, 48,* 441–449.

Nielson, D. A., Goldman, D., Virkkunen, M., Tokola, R., Rawlings, R., & Linnoila, M. (1994). Suicidality and 5-hydroxyindoleacetic acid concentration associated with a tryptophan hydroxylase polymorphism. *Archives of General Psychiatry, 51,* 34–38.

Okun, L. E. (1986). *Woman abuse: Facts replacing myths.* Albany, NY: SUNY Press.

Paddock, J. (1975). Studies on antiviolent and "normal" communities. *Aggressive Behavior, 1,* 217–233.

Pernanen, K. (1976). Alcohol and crimes of violence. In B. Kissin & H. Begleiter (Eds.), *The biology of alcoholism: Social aspects of alcoholism* (pp. 351–444). New York: Plenum Press.

Perry, D. G., Perry, L. C., & Rasmussen, P. (1986). Cognitive social learning mediators of aggression. *Child Development, 57*(3), 700–711.

Pettit, G. S. (1997). The development course of violence and aggression. *Psychiatric Clinics of North America, 20*(2), 283–299.

Pridemore, W. A. (2002). What we know about social structure and homicide: a review of the theoretical and empirical literature. *Violence and Victims, 17*(2), 127–156.

Raine, A., & Liu, J. H. (1998). Biological predispositions to violence and their implications for biosocial treatment and prevention. *Psychology, Crime and Law, 4,* 107–125.

Raine, A., Brennan, P. A., Farrington, D. P., Mednick, S. A. (1997). NATO ASI Series A: *Life sciences* (Vol. 292). Plenum Publishing Corporation.

Raine, A., Reynolds, P., Venables, P. H., & Mednick, S. A. (1997). Biosocial bases of aggressive behavior in childhood: Resting heart rate, skin conductance orienting and physique. *Biosocial Bases of Violence, 107*–126.

Rennison, C. M. (2001). *Criminal victimization 2000: Changes 1999-2000 with trends 1993-2000.* Washington, DC: Bureau of Justice Statistics, National Crime Victimization Survey, (Publication No. NCJ 187007).

Renzetti, C. M., Edleson, J. L., & Bergen, R. K. (Eds.) (2001). *Sourcebook on violence against women.* Thousand Oaks, CA: Sage Publications.

Reza, A. Mercy, J. A., & Krug, E. (2001). Epidemiology of violent deaths in the world. *Injury Prevention, 7,* 104–111.

Rice, T. W., & Goldman, C. R. (1994). Another look at the subculture of violence thesis: Who murders whom and under what circumstances. *Sociological Spectrum, 14*(4), 371–384.

Rosenbaum, A., Hoge, S. K., Adelman, S. A., et al. (1994). Head injury in partner-abusive men. *Journal of Consulting and Clinical Psychology, 62,* 1187–1193.

Rosoff, B., & Tobach, E. (1991). *On peace, war and gender: A challenge to genetic explanations.* New York: The Feminist Press.

Rubinow, D. R., & Schmidt, P. J. (1996). Androgens, brain, and behavior. *American Journal of Psychiatry, 153,* 974–984.

Salzman, C., Wolfson, A. N., Schatzberg, A., et al. (1995). Effect of fluoxetine on anger in symptomatic volunteers with borderline personality disorder. *Journal of Clinical Psychopharmacology, 15,* 23–29.

Scerbo, A. S., & Kolko, D. J. (1994). Salivary testosterone and cortisol in disruptive children: Relationship to aggressive, hyperactive, and internalizing behaviors. *Jour-*

nal of the American Academy of Child and Adolescent Psychiatry, 33, 1174–1184.

Schwartz, D., & Proctor, L. J. (2000). Community violence exposure and children's social adjustment in the school peer group: The mediating roles of emotion regulation and social cognition. *Journal of Consulting Clinical Psychology, 68*(4), 670–683.

Shahinfar, A., Kuppersmidt, J. B., & Matza, L. S. (2001). The relation between exposure to violence and social information processing among incarcerated adolescents. *Journal of Abnormal Psychology, 110*(1), 136–141.

Shanck, R. C., & Abelson, R. P. (1977). *Scripts, plans, goals and understanding: An inquiry into human knowledge structures.* Hillsdale, NJ: Erlbaum.

Sharps, P. W., Campbell, J. C., Campbell, D. W., Gary, F. A., & Webster, D. (2001). The role of alcohol use in intimate partner femicide. *American Journal on Addictions 10,* 122–135.

Siann, G. (1985). *Accounting for aggression: Perspectives on aggression and violence.* London: Allen Unwin.

Smith, S. L., & Donnerstein, E. (1998). Harmful effects of exposure to media violence: Learning of aggression, emotional desensitization, and fear. In R. G. Geen & E. Donnerstein (Eds.), *Human aggression: Theories, research, and implications for social policy.* San Diego: Academic Press.

Sorenson, S. (1996). Violence against women: Examining ethnic differences and commonalities. *Evaluation Review 20*(2), 123–145.

Sorenson, S., & Telles, C. A. (1991). Self-reports of spousal violence in a Mexican-American and non-Hispanic white population. *Violence & Victims 6*(1), 3–15.

Sorgi, P. J., Ratey, J. J., & Polakoff, S. (1986). Beta adrenergic blockers for the control of aggressive behaviors in patient with chronic schizophrenia. *American Journal of Psychiatry, 143,* 775–776.

Steele, C. M., & Josephs, R. A. (1990). Alcohol myopia: Its prized and dangerous effects. *American Psychology, 45,* 921–933.

Straub, E. (1971). The learning and unlearning of aggression. In J. Singer (Ed.), *The control of aggression and violence.* New York: Academic Press.

Straus, M. (1974). Leveling, civility, and violence in the family. *Journal of Marriage and the Family, 36,* 18–25.

Susman, E. J. (1997). Modeling developmental complexity in adolescence: Hormones and behavior in context. *Journal of Research on Adolescence, 7,* 283–306.

Tedeschi, J. T., & Felson, R. B. (1994). *Violence, aggression, and coercive actions.* Washington, DC: American Psychological Association.

Thompson, E. (1999). Effects of an execution on homicides in California. *Homicide Studies, 3,* 129–150.

Torres, S. (1991). A comparison of wife abuse between two cultures: Perceptions, attitudes, nature and extent. *Issues in Mental Health Nursing, 12*(1), 20–21.

Torres, S., Campbell, J. C., Campbell, D. W., Ryan, J., King, C., Price, P., Stallings, R., Fuchs, S., & Laude, M. (2000). Abuse during and before pregnancy: Prevalence and cultural correlates. *Violence and Victims, 15*(3), 303–322.

Tracy, K. K., & Crawford, C. B. (1992). Wife abuse: Does it have an evolutionary origin? In D. A. Counts, J. K. Brown & J. C. Campbell (Eds.), *Sanctions and sanctuary: Cultural perspectives on the beating of wives* (pp. 19–42). Boulder, CO: Westview Press.

Ullman S. E., Karabatsos, G., & Koss M. P. (1999a). Alcohol and sexual assault in a national sample of college women. *Journal of Interpersonal Violence, 14,* 603–625.

Ullman S. E., Karabatsos, G., & Koss M. P. (1999b). Alcohol and sexual aggression in a national sample of college men. *Psychology of Women Quarterly, 23,* 673–689.

U.S. Department of Health and Human Services. (1986). *Surgeon general's workshop on violence and public health.* Washington, DC: Health Resources and Services Administration (HRSA).

Valzelli, L. (1981). *Psychobiological aggression and violence.* New York, NY: Raven Press.

Virkkunen, M., Kallio, E., Rawlings, R., Tokola, R., Poland, R. E., Guidotti, A., Nemeroff, C., Bissette, G., Kalogeras, K., Karonen, S., & Linnoila, M. (1994). Personality profiles and state aggressiveness in Finnish alcoholic, violent offenders, fire setters, and healthy volunteers. *Archives of General Psychiatry, 51,* 28–33.

Walker, L. O., & Avant, K. C. (1995). *Strategies for theory construction in nursing* (3rd ed.). Norwalk, CT: Appleton & Lange.

Wallace, C. (1973). Why do animals fight? In T. Maples & D. R. Matheson (Eds.), *Hostility and violence* (pp. 126–135). New York: Holt, Rinehart & Winston.

Wallman, J. (1999). Serotonin and impulsive aggression: Not so fast. *The Henry Frank Guggenheim Review 3*(1), 25–29.

Warren, M. Q., & Hindelang, M. J. (1979). Current explanation of offender behavior. In H. Toch (Ed.), *Psychology of crime and criminal justice* (pp. 62–80). New York: Holt, Rinehart& Winston.

West, D. J. (1979). The response to violence. *Journal of Medical Ethics, 5,* 128–136.

Whiting, B. B. (1965). Sex identity conflict and physical violence: A comparative study, part 2. *American Anthropology, 67,* 128–135.

Whyte, M. K. (1978). Cross-cultural code dealing with the relative status of women. *Ethnology, 17,* 214–225.

Wolfgang, M. (1978). Violence in the family. In I.L. Kutash et al. (Eds.), *Violence: Perspectives on murder and aggression.* San Francisco: Jossey-Bass.

Wolfgang, M. E., & Ferracuti, F. (1982). The subculture of violence: Towards an integrated theory in criminology. Beverly Hills, CA: Sage Publications.

Yllo, K. (1983). Sexual equality and violence against wives in American states. *Journal of Comparative Family Studies, 14*(1), 67–86.

Yllo, K. (1984). The status of women, marital equality, and violence against wives. *Journal of Family Issues, 5*(3), 307–320.

Yudofsky, S., Williams, D., & Gorman, J. (1981). Propranolol in the treatment of rage and violent behavior in patients with chronic brain syndromes. *Journal of American Psychiatry, 138,* 218–220.

Theories of Intimate Partner Violence

• Nancy J. Fishwick, Jacquelyn C. Campbell, and Janette Y. Taylor

DEFINITIONS AND SCOPE

The issue of abuse and violence within intimate adult relationships began to receive public attention in the 1970s, largely through the efforts of grass-roots women's groups (Schecter, 1982). Scholarly attention to this significant social and health problem has increased dramatically over the past 3 decades. This chapter provides an overview of theoretical frameworks that attempt to explain the causes of abuse within intimate adult relationships and women's responses to abuse and violence over time. The historical roots and traditional and contemporary theoretical approaches to the phenomenon are analyzed, and the concept of machismo is described as a theoretical construct providing gender-related insight into the abuse of women. The chapter concludes with suggestions for a theoretical base for nursing research on and practice with women in abusive relationships.

Definition of Terms

We have adopted the term "intimate partner violence" to encompass the diverse realities of abuse within the intimate relationships of adults. The Centers for Disease Control and Prevention (CDC) definition for intimate partner violence (IPV) can be summarized as follows: physical or sexual violence (use of physical force) or threat of such violence; or psychological/emotional abuse and/or coercive tactics when there has been prior physical and/or sexual violence between persons who are spouses or nonmarital partners (dating, boyfriend-girlfriend) or former spouses or nonmarital partners (Saltzman, Fanslow, McMahon, & Shelley, 1999). Thus, IPV can occur in all kinds of intimate relationships, including marriage, committed same-sex or opposite-sex relationships, and dating relationships of adults and adolescents. Intimate partner violence has been conceptualized as comprising two separate phenomena that Johnson (1995) called "common couple violence" and "patriarchal terrorism." The low-level violence between intimate partners (i.e., common couple violence) is often more bilateral and less often includes forced sex and controlling behaviors. Even with this type of violence, the injuries inflicted by women are less severe than those they receive (Tjaden & Thoennes, 2000).

However, the type of domestic violence that is seen in wife abuse shelters, in the criminal justice system, among women with mental health problems from IPV, and in emergency departments is primarily directed toward women and characterized by coercive control. In these relationships, women may, indeed, use physical violence, but it is almost always in self-defense (Dobash, Dobash, Wilson, & Daly, 1992). We use the term "battering of female partners" to characterize these relationships to make clear the severity of the abuse and its gender specificity. "Battering" has been defined as deliberate and repeated physical aggression or sexual assault inflicted on a woman by a man with whom she has or has had an intimate relationship, within a context of coercive control (Campbell, 1989; Campbell & Humphreys, 1993). Battering is thus a pattern, not a single incident, and the underlying dynamic is power and control of the female victim. Although it is true that, in some small proportion of cases, a woman may be the primary perpetrator of battering against a male partner, the preponderance of evidence suggests that the incidence is very low. The consensus of most experts on intimate partner violence is that the repetitive, prolonged, serious assault involving severe injury, done intentionally with minimal provocation and in the interest of coercive control, is almost exclusively perpetrated against women (Dobash & Dobash, 1998).

"Coercive control" refers to the variety of strategies in which the abusive partner keeps the woman fearful of future harm to herself and her children and, in fact, even keeps the woman doubtful of her own reality. Examples of controlling strategies include emotional and verbal abuse, restriction of her contact with others (social isolation), control of her personal and household finances (economic abuse), and intimidating and threatening behavior. These controlling behaviors are depicted in the "Power and Control Wheel" developed by Duluth, Minnesota's Domestic Abuse Intervention Project; the wheel is widely used in public and professional education literature (see, for example, Warshaw & Ganley, 1995).

Intimate partner violence and battering are not restricted to heterosexual relationships. Battering in lesbian and gay-male relationships has been described in the literature, but relatively little data-based research on the subject has been conducted (Lobel, 1986; Renzetti, 1992; Turell, 2000; West, 1998a). The one random-sample survey of IPV that included same-sex couples indicated that the prevalence of IPV among same-sex male couples was significantly higher than among same-sex female couples (Tjaden & Thoennes, 1999). There is also one nursing investigation in a population-based survey of same-sex male couples that included IPV; this survey revealed a significant occurrence of prior sexual assault, substance abuse, and forced sex in those relationships (Greenwood et al., 2002). Furthermore, in smaller, more qualitative studies, evidence suggests that among violent same-sex couples (female and male) the fundamental dynamic of intimate partner violence, or threats thereof, is similar to that experienced in a battering heterosexual relationship (NiCarthy, 1986; Renzetti, 1992). However, the theoretical and empirical literature conducted with heterosexual couples cannot be assumed to translate directly to the experiences of same-sex couples; much more research is needed in this area (Relf, 2001).

Scope of the Problem

To describe the extent of IPV, most experts give percentages of lifetime and past-year prevalence; acute trauma from abuse is a third way to describe prevalence of the problem (e.g., Dearwater, Coben, Nah, Campbell, McLoughlin, & Glass, 1998). Although IPV has decreased in the past decade, the numbers of women reporting such violence are still high. In 1998, approximately 900,000

U.S. women reported physical or sexual assault by intimates in a criminal justice survey, compared to 1.1 million in 1993 (Rennison, 2001). Between 1993 and 1998, IPV accounted for 22% of violent crimes against women (versus 3% for men) (Rennison, 2001). Rates of past-year IPV range from 1.8% to 14% in population-based studies and up to 44% in health care settings (Jones et al., 1999; Tjaden & Thoennes, 2000), although the more usual prevalence in health care settings is between 10% and 23%. Lifetime estimates vary from 5% to 51% (Tjaden & Thoennes, 2000), with the most usual range between 25% and 35%. Women are significantly more likely to be physically or sexually assaulted by a current or former intimate partner than by an acquaintance, family member, friend, or stranger (Tjaden & Thoennes, 2000). As high as these figures are, it is commonly accepted that they (particularly crime data) are underestimates. For nurses, it is important to remember that at least 1 in every 10 women encountered in a health care setting is currently in a violent relationship (Sampselle, 1991). Poor women and young women are particularly at risk (Tjaden & Thoennes, 2000). Divorced or separated women are also at increased risk, but because these are cross-sectional surveys, it is not clear whether the marital dissolution occurred before or after the violence.

Abuse and Homicide of Female Partners and Homicide of Abusers

One of the most frightening aspects of abuse of female partners is its connection with homicide of women. The danger for women in abusive relationships is verified by U.S. Crime Report data, which indicate that one third of all female homicide victims were murdered by a husband, an ex-husband, or a boyfriend (Greenfield et al., 1998). The percentage is even higher (40% to 50%) if ex-boyfriends are included among perpetrators. Between two thirds and four fifths of these femicides were preceded by IPV of the female partner before she was killed (Campbell, 1992; Campbell, Sharps, & Glass, 2000; Morocco, 1998). In a recently completed nursing study of risk factors for intimate partner femicide, 70% of the total sample and 79% of the women killed between the ages of 18 and 50 were physically abused by their murderes before they were killed (Campbell et al., in press).

Battered women are acutely aware that they are in danger of being killed. One of the strongest risks for femicide in battering relationships occurs when women take deliberate action to sever a dangerously abusive relationship (Campbell et al., in press; Wilson & Daly, 1993). Women frequently remain in the relationship because of the realistic fear of life-threatening consequences should they attempt to leave, but their fear has not always been treated as valid by the public (Langford, 1996). Battering men feel that the departure of an intimate partner is the ultimate loss of control, and many chillingly have been heard to say something like, "If I can't have you, no one can." Approximately one third of femicides by intimate partners are followed by suicide of the male partner. This phenomenon almost never occurs when a woman kills a man.

Nationwide, approximately 2,000 women are incarcerated for murdering their batterers (Grossfeld, 1991). Women do not usually kill people; they perpetrate about 15% of the homicides in the United States. When women do kill, it often involves a male partner and is done in self-defense. Traditionally, women who killed their batterers were charged with first- or second-degree murder or a reduced charge of manslaughter, or they had to plead temporary insanity

(Gillespie, 1989). Because a battered woman's lethal act typically does not happen immediately after the assaults directed at her, she usually cannot claim self-defense as the motive for her action. From a legal standpoint, self-defense requires the reasonable belief of imminent danger of death or serious injury; furthermore, the action taken must have been a reasonable response to perceived danger rather than an overreaction. Fortunately, many courts have broadened the definition of self-defense to take into account the circumstances of battered women. In the 1980s and early 1990s, governors in several states granted clemency to battered women serving prison sentences, because their actions were subsequently considered justifiable (Grossfeld, 1991).

There have been few studies of women who killed their batterers. In a classic early study, Angela Browne (1987) interviewed 42 women facing murder or attempted-murder charges in the death or serious injury of their mates. Compared with wife batterers who had not been killed, the men who had been killed had a significantly greater history of frequent drug and alcohol abuse, extensive police records for a variety of criminal offenses, reports of threatening to kill someone, and abuse of their own children. Furthermore, the women who were charged with murder had sustained a significantly higher degree of and frequency of injury, including forced sex from their partners, than women whose abusive partners were still living. The women had made many attempts to obtain outside intervention for the violence directed at them, but the responses received from the criminal justice system were ineffective. Browne (1987) concluded that women who murder their abusers have become trapped in a seemingly inescapable spiral of escalating violence against them and desperately fear for their lives and the lives of their children, and therefore take lethal action for survival. A smaller nursing study of 12 women incarcerated for killing their batterers supported most of Browne's conclusions, with the exception that these women did not note an escalation in the frequency or severity of the physical or sexual abuse directed at them before murdering the batterer (Foster, Veale, & Fogel, 1989).

During the 1990s, the rate of women killing their intimate partners decreased substantially. In 1975 in the United States, approximately the same number of men were killed by an intimate partner as had killed their spouse or ex-wife. In 2000, the ratio was 1:4 (i.e., one male killed by an intimate partner for every four women killed by an intimate partner). The change has been shown to be associated with the introduction in some states of strong laws that protect battered women, as well as more substantial resources, including shelters (Browne, Williams, & Dutton, 1998). Apparently, in states where such protective resources and laws exist, battered women are less likely to feel that their only recourse is to kill their abuser.

HISTORICAL PERSPECTIVE

Intimate partner violence (and violence against women in general) has deep historical roots, and continues to be condoned and even legally sanctioned in many societies. In their classic early study of wife-beating, Dobash and Dobash (1979, p. 31) placed such abuse in its historical context as a form of behavior that has "existed for centuries as an acceptable and, indeed, a desirable part of a patriarchal family system within a patriarchal society, and much of the ideology and many of the institutional arrangements which supported the patriarchy through the subordination, domination, and control of women are still reflected in our culture and our social institutions."

Current cultural support of abuse of women stems in large measure from the historical and contemporary use of violence to maintain patriarchal social structure. Patriarchy can be defined as "any type of group organization in which males hold dominant power and determine what part females shall and shall not play" (Rich, 1979, p. 78). Referring to the United States, hooks (1984, p. 118) extended the definition of patriarchy and located it within the dynamics of violence when she observed that

[domestic violence] is inextricably linked to all acts of violence in this society that occur between the powerful and the powerless, the dominant and the dominated. While male supremacy encourages the use of abusive force to maintain male domination of women, it is the Western philosophical notion of hierarchical rule aPnd coercive authority that is the root cause of violence against women, of adult violence against children, of all violence between those who dominate and those who are dominated.

This analysis of power dynamics allows us to better see the foundations on which oppression and colonization are grounded. Isolated acts of wife abuse do not keep our society sexist, but when the acts are multiplied and coupled with the frightening incidences of rape, homicide of women, and genital mutilation, and considered along with the historical precedents of suttee, witch-burning, foot-binding, mutilating surgery, and female infanticide, patriarchy's power can be seen as based ultimately on violence.

Early Violence Against Women

The Bible provides the early written prescription for the physical punishment of wives. Deuteronomy 22:13–21 lists a law condemning brides to death by stoning if unable to prove virginity (Davidson, 1977). In early Rome, husbands and fathers could legally beat women or put them to death for many reasons, but especially for adultery or suspected infidelity, reflecting "not so much thwarted love but loss of control and damage to a possession" (Dobash & Dobash, 1979, p. 37). Jesus was more egalitarian in his thinking, but the sexist statements of Saint Paul set the tone for the Christian Church. Constantine, the emperor and religious leader of the Byzantium branch of Christianity, set the example for treatment of wives by putting his own young wife to death by scalding (Davidson, 1977). By medieval times, the widespread and varied nature of wife-beating had been documented. In Spanish law, a woman who committed adultery could be killed with impunity. In France, female sexual infidelity was punishable by beating, as was disobedience. Italian men punished unfaithful women with severe flogging and exile for 3 years (Dobash & Dobash, 1979). A medieval theological manual refers to the necessity, according to Church doctrine, of wife-beating "for correction." A Catholic abbé in the Middle Ages decried the common cruelty to and murder of wives of prominent Christian men (Davidson, 1977).

The medieval "age of chivalry" promoted the ideal of female chastity before marriage and fidelity after marriage, which was an important aspect of male property rights and outward signs of the master maintaining control (Dobash & Dobash, 1979). This glorification and objectification of women as weak, asexual adornments actually contributed to their subjugation and was associated with the use of male force in rescues and tournaments. The close of the Middle Ages saw the rise of the nuclear family, the development of modern states, and the beginning of capitalism, all of which eroded the position of women and strengthened the authority of men. In 16th-century England, allegiance to fathers and husbands was equated with loyalty to the king and to God (Dobash & Dobash, 1979).

One of the best-documented forms of systematic violence against women is the "witch-hunts" in western Europe from the 1500s to the 1700s. Though the actual number can never be known, authoritative estimates range from 200,000 to 9 million women murdered, often by hanging or burning, as punishment for their perceived healing abilities, assumed to have been acquired through "consorting with Satan" (Achterberg, 1991). Feminist analysis of this practice has revealed that the main crime of the women involved was a lack of submission to the stereotyped role of the subservient medieval woman.

The Effects of Capitalism and Protestantism

Capitalism and Protestantism developed simultaneously. The basic unit of production moved outside of the family, and for the first time wages were paid for work on a regular basis. Because domestic work received no wages, it became devalued. The Protestant religion idealized marriage and equated wifely obedience with moral duty. The head of the household gained much of the power that formerly belonged to priests (Dobash & Dobash, 1979).

Martin Luther is considered less misogynistic than most of the men of his time, but even he equated female subservience with the woman's role and admitted to boxing his wife's ear when she got "saucy" (Davidson, 1977). John Knox insisted that the "natural" subordination of women was ordained by God. Wife-beating was discouraged by the Protestant theologians, but the husbands' right to beat his wife was acknowledged, and the practice was widespread (Dobash & Dobash, 1979). As May explained, "children, property, earning, and even the wife's conscience belonged to the husband" (May, 1978, p. 38). During the 17th, 18th, and 19th centuries in the Western world, there was little objection to the husband using force as long as it did not exceed certain limits. The wife could be beaten if she "caused jealousy, was lazy, unwilling to work in the fields, became drunk, spent too much money, or neglected the house" (May, 1978, p. 138). While the Reformation set the tone in the rest of Europe, Napoleon influenced France, Holland, Italy, and sections of Switzerland and Germany. He thought of wives as "fickle, defenseless, mindless beings, tending toward Eve-like evil" and deserving of punishment for misdeeds as "causing" bankruptcy or criminality in her husband (Davidson, 1977, pp. 14–16). He is quoted as saying to the Council of State, "The husband must possess the absolute power and right to say to his wife, 'Madam, you shall not go out, you shall not go to the theater, you shall not receive such and such a person; for the children you bear shall be mine'" (Davidson, 1977, p. 15).

The common saying of the time was "Women, like walnut trees, should be beaten every day" (Davidson, 1977, p. 14). In the few short years between the French Revolution and the reign of Napoleon, many women petitioned the courts for divorce because of wife-beating, but with Napoleon's regime, this recourse was again ended for central European women.

Many forms of violence against women have been carried out throughout the world. During the same time period as the witch-burnings in Europe, the practice of suttee, or inclusion of the widow and concubines in a man's funeral pyre, was being carried out in India. The women were often drugged or coerced to the pyre. Even when she was not forced, the widow knew that her alternatives to death on the pyre consisted of prostitution or a life of servitude and starvation with her husband's relatives. Cultural beliefs held the widow to blame for the man's death because of her actions during her present life or in a past life. The Chinese custom of foot binding was forced by male insistence that women were not attractive unless their feet were tiny stumps caused by years of excruciatingly painful binding and breaking of the bones. As a result, women were forced to be absolutely dependent on men, because they could take only a few tottering steps without assistance. The practice of female genital cutting (mutilation) began prior to colonization in several countries of Africa and the Middle East (Boddy, 1998). The practice continues in many countries, although change is occurring in some villages, as grassroots women's groups have successfully substituted nonviolent, meaningful ways to celebrate girls' transition to womanhood.

In eerily similar practices, Western medicine in the late 19th century used the surgical procedures of clitoridectomy, oophorectomy, and hysterectomy to "cure" masturbation, insanity, deviation from the "proper" female role, heightened sexual appetites, and rebellion against husband or father (Daly, 1978). Radical feminists argued that the medical practices of superfluous hysterectomies, unnecessarily mutilating surgery for breast cancer, the use of IUDs (intrauterine devices), and coercive sterilization of impoverished or mentally retarded women in the 1960s and 1970s were evidence of continued violence against women by male-dominated medicine. More recently, the latest forms of contraception control (e.g., Norplant and anitfertility "vaccines") have come into question as part of an ongoing discrimination against women, especially poor women and women of color (Roberts, 1997; Silliman, 1992).

Legalization of Violence Against Women

Lest we think that the practices of violence against women are confined to other countries and other times, we need to remember that the United States was founded on the equal rights of white *men*, not of women (and not of persons of color). John Adams rejected his wife's plea for better treatment of women in the new government. Sir William Blackstone's interpretation of English law, which upheld the husband's right to employ moderate chastisement in response to improper wifely behavior, was used as a model for American law. In 1824, Mississippi legalized wife-beating, and in 1886 a proposed law for punishment of husbands who beat their wives was defeated in Pennsylvania. North Carolina passed the first law against wife-beating in 1874, but the court pronounced that it did not intend to hear cases unless there was permanent damage or danger to life (Davidson, 1977). British common law in the 18th century also established the legal right of a man to use force with his wife to ensure that she fulfilled her wifely obligations: "the consummation of marriage, cohabitation, conjugal rights, sexual fidelity, and general obedience and respect for his wishes" (Dobash & Dobash, 1979, pp. 14, 74). John Stuart Mill petitioned Parliament to end the brutal treatment of British wives in 1869. The legal changes that followed were directed not toward eliminating the practice of wife-beating but toward limiting the amount of damage that was being done. The 19th century in England was also marked by a greater tolerance of conjugal violence in the lower classes, whereas chivalry was expected of the upper classes (May, 1978).

As late as 1915, a London police magistrate reaffirmed that wives could be beaten at home legally as long as the stick used was no bigger than the man's thumb ("the rule of thumb" from a 1782 judge's proclamation) (Dobash & Dobash, 1979; May, 1978). It was legal for a husband to rape his wife in every state in the United States until the early 1970s, and laws preserving the legality of marital rape were common in the United States until the late 1980s and early 1990s (Russell, 1990). It continues to be difficult for women to prosecute their husbands for rape (Kirkwood & Cecil, 2001). Clearly, the law has been condoning violence toward wives for centuries. Dobash and Dobash (1979, p. 31) summarized this relationship: "The ideologies and institutions that made such treatment both possible and justifiable have survived, albeit somewhat altered from century to century, and have been woven into the fabric of our culture and are thriving today."

Widespread cultural tolerance of violence against women, and intimate partner violence in particular, continued through the 1980s (Carmody & Williams, 1987; Dibble & Straus, 1980). There was clearly a cultural shift in the late 1980s and early 1990s, with far fewer Americans believing that domestic violence is a private matter and far more believing that the police should intervene, at least if there is injury to the victim (Klein, Campbell, Soler, & Ghez, 1997). However, men are still less convinced than women that domestic violence is a serious problem that needs societal attention.

Contemporary Forms of Violence Against Women

Female infanticide, homicide of women, and genital mutilation are rooted in history and continue today. They are found in their most blatant forms in societies that rigidly adhere to a tradition of male dominance. Because of the higher life expectancy of females, the number of females in the population should be higher than the number of males; however, world statistics show fewer females than males (Janssen-Jurreit, 1982). The number of females in proportion to males is lowest in Arab and Islamic countries and in India. The statistics seem to indicate negligent care of female newborns at the very least. India and the Arabic and Islamic nations also practice the killing of adult women with frightening regularity. Men can kill wives and daughters in India for "public embarrassment," especially "habitual disobedience"; for having illegitimate children; and for having insufficient dowries (Driver, 1971; Heise, Ellsberg, & Gottemoeller, 1999). In some Arabic and Muslim communities, a woman who has had sex before marriage can be killed as a matter of family honor, a practice that was also common in non-Muslim Mediterranean countries until recently (Janssen-Jurreit, 1982; Malik & Salvi, 1976).

Genital mutilation is a widespread form of female abuse practiced in much of East, West, and Central Africa and in parts of the Middle East. The mutilation can take the form of removal of the tip of the clitoris, complete clitoridectomy, or excision of all the external genitalia except the labia majora and may be accompanied by infibulation—the closure of the wound by sewing with catgut or by using thorns, leaving a small opening for urination and menstrual flow. After infibulation, the aperture can be opened further for intercourse and childbirth and resewn at the husband's command. The practices are often carried out without anesthesia, with crude instruments, and with no regard for prevention of infection; complications are rampant (Hosken, 1977–78). In Egypt, the majority of girls between ages 8 and 10 have a clitoridectomy performed. In these cultures, such practices are considered necessary for a woman to be marriageable; without marriage, a woman is considered worthless (Janssen-Jurreit, 1982).

Rape is a form of violence against women more in the realm of public awareness. In her classic work entitled *Our Blood: Prophecies and Discourse on Sexual Politics*, Andrea Dworkin (1976, p. 46) stated, "Rape is no excess, no aberration, no accident, no mistake—it embodies sexuality as the culture defines it." Rape takes many forms: sexual abuse of children, gang rape, forced intercourse with wives, sexual torture of female prisoners, intercourse with therapists, forced sexual initiation, bride capture and group rape as a puberty rite, as well as the more commonly identified form of sexual assault on a female by an unknown male (Brownmiller, 1975; Heise, Ellsberg, & Gottemoeller, 1999). Across all patriarchal societies, rape is "an exercise of domination and the infliction of degradation upon the victim," restricts the independence of women, and reminds them of their vulnerability, thereby keeping them subjugated (Schram, 1978, p. 78). Rape is a crime of violence, not sex, and continues to be used as an instrument of war (WHO, 2002). Rape and forced sex across a continuum of relationships and contexts continues to be common in the United States as well as in developing countries (Tjaden & Thoennes, 2000). See also Chapter 7.

THEORETICAL FRAMEWORKS

At various times, social reform groups have recognized intimate partner violence as a serious threat to the safety, health, and well-being of women, children, and families. For example, concern for the plight of abused women and children was intertwined with the primary goals of the suffragists in Great Britain and the United States, of those who promoted temperance in the late 1800s, and of those who promoted family planning and women's reproductive rights in the early and mid-1900s (Pleck, 1987). Abuse was blamed on poverty, drunkenness, and "brutish" men. The second wave of the women's movement in the 1960s raised awareness that violence against women was more prevalent than had been realized, and that attributions to poverty and alcohol could not account for the abuse experienced by women from all walks of life.

Scholarly attention to the issue has increased exponentially in the past 3 decades, as public and private funds have been allocated for research, education, treatment services, and prevention programs. Many theories have been offered to explain the social structures, cultural traditions, and personal behaviors that create and perpetuate abuse and violence. Feminist critiques remind us that focusing exclusively on individual and couple dynamics fails to explain why so many women are abused by their intimate partners. Additional important critiques of existing theoretical frameworks have come from those who point out the questionable relevance of current theories to members of racial and ethnic minority groups (Barnes, 1999; Phillips, 1998; West, 1998b). Only recently have researchers and policy makers begun to explore with persons of color and varied ethnicity the adequacy of current theories. Race and ethnicity shapes the experience and interpretation of intimate partner violence in myriad ways, including the influence of culturally based family structures and subordinate roles of women. The poverty experienced by racial and ethnic minorities in the United States clearly complicates women's experience, particularly in terms of unequal access to social resources and financial independence (West, 1998b). Recent efforts that integrate research findings and theoretical explanations from many disciplines hold promise in the search for theories that help explain, predict, ameliorate, and ultimately prevent intimate partner violence.

Theories of Causation

Contemporary theories of causation attempt to explain and predict the motivations, circumstances, and other factors that characterize individuals who perpetrate abuse and violence within intimate partner relationships. In general, current frameworks for understanding the causes of intimate partner violence fall into one of several categories (Cunningham et al., 1998):

- Biological theories of criminal behavior
- Theories of psychopathology of individual perpetrators
- Family systems theories
- Social learning theories
- Feminist theories of gender-related power imbalances

Ecological frameworks and theories of masculinities integrate research findings from many disciplines and perspectives.

Psychobiological Perspectives

Until the 1970s, studies of intimate partner violence, generally from the field of psychiatry, tended to focus on the individual psychopathology of both the abuser and his victim. The notion of masochism dominated early explanations of intimate partner violence, with abuse conceptualized as deliberately provoked by women who required this behavior to meet their need for suffering. For example, in response to 12 case studies, a group of psychiatrists concluded, "We see the husband's aggressive behavior as freeing masochistic needs of the wife and to be necessary for the wife's (and the couple's) equilibrium" (Snell, Rosenwald, & Robey, 1964, p. 110). This type of study generally used small samples, often drawn from already diagnosed mentally ill patients, and was biased by adherence to the Freudian conceptualization that all women have masochistic tendencies. Research published after 1970, based on population-based data, refutes the myth of female masochism. Vestiges of beliefs in female masochism do linger, however, in many popular victim-blaming explanations of why a woman remains in an abusive relationship. Explanations such as "she must like it" or "she must have provoked it" are rooted in the concept of female masochism.

Psychobiological explanations of the perpetrator's abusive and violent behavior have focused on mood disorders, personality disorders, the psychoneurological effects of head injury, and the neurochemical effects of posttraumatic stress disorder (PTSD). The complex neurophysiological brain functions influenced by neurochemical balances and connections and how they relate to aggression are just beginning to be determined through animal and human investigations. Clearly, neurological damage from injury and neurochemical alterations from PTSD are implicated in increased aggression, including increased aggression toward intimate partners (Jordan et al., 1992; Cohen, Rosenbaum, Kane, Warnken, & Benjamin, 1999; see also Chapter 1). However, research suggests that although all these conditions may be correlated with intimate partner violence, they are not necessarily causative of that particular form of violence. That is, not all men with psychoneurological conditions or personality disorders are abusive or violent toward anyone. Furthermore, men who suffer from psychological or neurological conditions in which aggression or violence may be a component do not necessarily target only their intimate partners; they may, in fact, be aggressive or violent in a variety of situations.

In a related line of inquiry, the field of evolutionary psychology contends that contemporary male aggression against intimate female partners is at least partially determined by genetic factors or "heritable predispositions"; the aggressive behavior of modern-day humans reflects the normative adaptive and survival behaviors in our ancestral past. In this perspective, the extreme sexual jealousy of the intimate female partner and subsequent violence of abusive men dates back to evolutionary forces to reproduce and pass along genes for survival of the species (Cunningham et al., 1998; Wilson & Daly, 1993). Again, there is evidence supporting hypotheses generated by evolutionary psychology (Daly, Singh, & Wilson, 1999), but not definitive proof that these biological processes are more important than sociological and anthropological factors. Most theorists see interactive processes between psychoneurological and sociocultural factors.

Alcohol and Drugs as Causes of Intimate Partner Violence

The use or abuse of alcohol by perpetrators of abuse has consistently been noted in connection with IPV, but investigators point out that alcohol is only one factor among many. Alcohol is commonly believed to have a biochemically "disinhibiting effect," whereby a person's usual voluntary behavioral constraints are temporarily removed, resulting in aggressive behavior. Other theorists speculate that intoxicated behavior is, to some extent, learned. Individuals are excused and forgiven for violent behavior that occurs while drinking; drinking thus provides a period of time during which one may behave in ways that would be unacceptable if sober (Kantor & Straus, 1987; Testa & Leonard, 2001). More-recent evidence has found that cognitive processes are altered by alcohol, resulting in less-effective problem-solving and a greater tendency to interpret interpersonal cues as threatening. Therefore, abusive partners who already find it difficult to resolve conflicts without aggression and who perceive their partners as threatening may be even more likely to be violent when drunk (Kantor, 1993).

New evidence suggests that alcohol and drug abuse are risk factors for IPV occurrence, for move severe IPV, for men to reassault even after intervention, and for intimate partner femicide (Gondolf, 1997a; Sharps et al., 2001; Testa & Leonard, 2001). Abused women report, however, that batterers are not always drunk when abusive and not always abusive when drunk (Kub, Campbell, Rose, & Soeken, 1999). Again, it appears as though alcohol and drugs generally potentiate abusive tendencies in batterers but do not cause them.

Social Learning Perspectives

Much theoretical and empirical attention has focused on the idea that abusive behavior is behavior learned in childhood—a notion derived from social learning theory. The hypothesis states that children observe and imitate the behavior that adults model for them. Behaviors learned in the home, or modeled by significant adults, can become entrenched in adulthood, especially if those behaviors are consistently reinforced by the broader society. In terms of explaining the perpetrator's behavior in intimate partner violence, social learning theory suggests that boys who are reared in violent homes learn to use aggression to cope with a variety of negative feelings. This leads to long-term consequences of becoming an abusive parent or spouse or developing other criminally abusive behaviors in adulthood. Substantive bodies of research support these premises (e.g., Maxfield & Widom, 2001; Straus & Gelles, 1990).

Family Systems Theory and Family Stress Theory

In the family systems approach, the family is viewed as a dynamic organization made up of individual family members and subsystems, in constant interaction with the broader community and social systems. Role expectations, communication patterns, and power status of family members are examples of some aspects of family functioning affected by the responses and feedback of family members. Explanations of IPV rooted in family systems theory tend to analyze the behavior of both the perpetrator and the victim, often apportioning responsibility equally to each partner. Interventions such as couples counseling arise from a family systems perspective. Criticism has been leveled at this approach for its tendency to minimize the degree of responsibility of the male perpetrator and to exaggerate the responsibility of the victim (Cunningham et al., 1998). In general, couples counseling, which is based on the assumption of dual responsibility for relationship difficulties, has been found ineffective in resolving intimate partner violence and may, in fact, place the woman at risk for further harm from her batterer.

Feminist or Power Imbalance Theories

Articulated most eloquently by Rebecca and Russell Dobash (1979, 1993, 1998) and by Ellen Pence and colleagues (Pence, Paymer, Ritmeester, & Shepard, 1993), the feminist theories of IPV emphasize the underlying premises of the need for power and control on the part of batterers, and of the societal arrangements of patriarchy and tolerance of (not support for) violence against women. This model also uses aspects of social learning theory, with the premise that perpetrating abusive behavior is a choice to use a set of learned behaviors. Although it is difficult to prove individual abuser's assimilation of these abstract premises, the continuing gender differences in perceptions about IPV (Klein, Campbell, Soler, & Ghez, 1998), as well as the historical and international record of violence against women associated with cultural norms of male ownership of women and lack of equal power relationships within homes, are evidence in support of this theoretical framework (Counts, Brown, & Campbell, 1999; Levinson, 1989). Furthermore, several international studies from South Africa, India, and China associate male justification for hitting women and male domination of household affairs with reported wife-beating (Abrahams, 2002; Martin, Tsui, Maitra, & Marinshaw, 1999; Wood & Jewkes, 2001; Xu, Campbell, & Zhu, 2001).

Integrated Frameworks to Explain Intimate Partner Violence

Sociocultural Model

A multifactorial model of intimate partner violence, which combines elements of family systems theory, social learning theory, social structures, and cultural factors, was first developed by Murray Straus and his colleagues (Straus & Gelles, 1990). This model recognizes the societal background of the high level of violence in our culture, the sexist organization of the society and its family system, and cultural norms legitimizing violence against family members. With this background of societal influences, the family is believed to be inherently at high risk for violent interaction by virtue of the great amount of time family members spend interacting; the broad range of activities over which conflict can occur; the intensity of emotional involvement of the members; the involuntary nature of family membership; the impingement of family members on each other's personal space, time, and lifestyles; and the assumption of family members that they have the right to try to change each other's behavior (Straus, 1980). Within these societal and family contexts, Straus and others believed that people can be socialized to use violence for conflict resolution. Children learn this by observing parental violence, by experiencing physical punishment, by seeing their parents tolerate sibling fighting, and, if boys, by being taught to value violence. This socialization teaches the association of love with violence and justifies the use of physical force as a morally correct means of solving disputes.

Ecological Framework

More recently, an ecological framework has been proposed that integrates research findings from several disciplines, including feminist theory, into an explanatory framework of the origins of gender-based intimate partner violence (Heise, 1998). The ecological approach views intimate partner violence as a multifaceted phenomenon that is the result of a dynamic interplay among personal, situational, and sociocultural factors; these factors may be imagined as concentric circles nested within a larger circle (World Health Organization, 2002). At the individual level, the person who perpetrates abuse and violence possesses a set of developmental experiences and personality factors that shape interactions with other individuals (e.g., with the intimate partner and with other family members) and with the broader community and society. Individual-level factors that have been demonstrated as partially predictive of becoming abusive include witnessing domestic violence as a child, experiencing physical or sexual abuse as a child, and, to a lesser extent, having an absent or an emotionally abusive father.

Factors identified at the level of the microsystem, or situational-level factors, refer to the interactions between the abuser and other individuals and systems and to the abuser's subjective interpretation of those interactions. Several aspects of the microsystem, especially in terms of family structure and functioning, have been identified as risk factors for the development of intimate partner violence. They include male economic and decision-making authority in the family; male control of wealth and resources in the family; marital conflict, especially in relationships with an asymmetrical power structures; and excessive use or abuse of alcohol by the perpetrator.

The third level of factors, the exosystem, refers to characteristics of influential social structures, including the rules, norms, and social expectations that govern personal behavior. For example, research has consistently demonstrated that, although violence against women occurs in all socioeconomic groups, abuse is more common in low-income families and in households in which the man is unemployed. The reason for the increased risk for abuse in these situations is unclear, but it is possible that poverty may underlie much stress and conflict between an intimate couple. A second factor at the exosystem level is social isolation of the woman and the family; sources of support and assistance may not be readily available to women who have been socially or geographically cut off from a social network.

The fourth and final ecosystem level, the macrosystem, refers to the values, beliefs, and rules of the broader culture in which the individual, family, and community operate. Here, the patriarchal roots of intimate partner violence are illuminated; the need for treatment and prevention strategies that move beyond the individual and couple level becomes clear when these deep roots are appreciated. At this level, risk factors for future violent behavior include cultural definitions of manhood that are linked to dominance, toughness, aggression, male honor, and machismo; male adherence to rigid and traditional gender roles for both sexes; the sense of ownership or entitlement men have over women; cultural approval of physical chastisement of women; and cultural approval of the use of violence to settle interpersonal disputes. Similar risk factors were revealed in an analysis of preliterate and peasant societies. The incidence and frequency of wife-beating was found to be greatest in societies in which men control the family wealth, adults engage in violent conflict resolution, men hold domestic authority, and divorce is restricted for women (Campbell, 1985; Levinson, 1989). In another cross-national investigation, factors associated with lower and less serious levels of IPV across small-scale and more complex societies included female work groups, community-level sanctions against serious wife-beating with indigenous strategies to address low-level incidents, and sanctuary for abused women.

In summary, the ecological approach integrates research findings from various disciplines into a comprehensive framework that improves our understanding of the origins of intimate partner violence.

Machismo or Masculinity as a Synthesizing Framework

Another synthesizing framework is machismo or macho behavior. The concept of machismo, or compulsive masculinity, can be found in psychological, sociological, and anthropological literature and is also mentioned in much of the domestic violence research. Contemporary scholarship addresses it within the study of masculinity (e.g., Archer, 1994; Connell, 1995; Gilmore, 1990; Miedzian, 1991). Machismo cannot be said to be a direct cause of wife abuse, but study of it can help in understanding the phenomenon. This section examines explanations for machismo, delineates characteristics associated with it, briefly describes some of the related general violence literature, and explains the association of macho attitudes with violence against women.

Origins. Psychoanalytic literature attributed compulsive masculinity to dominating mothers, but in reality, as anthropologist Beatrice Whiting (1965) stated, "an individual identifies with that person who is perceived as controlling those resources that he wants" (p. 126). Relegation of most early childcare to females results in first identification with mothers, but when boys realize that the world is obviously still dominated by males, they try to change allegiance. In small-scale societies when fathers are completely separated from women and children, a more violent society results (Whiting, 1965). In our country, the pattern of men excluding themselves from childcare predominated over all groups until the 1970s; even now, it is primarily well-educated, middle class men who participate to any great degree. Even boys from female-headed households find models of tough masculine behavior on television, from other adult males, and "on the street" (Anderson, 1999). When boys come under social pressure to establish their own masculine identity, they reject their own feminine natures and overemphasize the traditional male values of toughness and hardness and may commit deviant acts "as a public pronouncement" that they are "real men" (Gibbons, 1970).

All-male groups across societies become a factor in the breaking of ties with mothers and in maintaining dominance over and social distance from females

(Gilmore, 1990). All-male groups in any culture, such as gangs in our inner cities today, tend to facilitate the expression of aggression and provide group standards for maleness, such as bravery and toughness (Miedzian, 1991). Yet male bonding can only be regarded as a manifestation of machismo, not as a cause.

Socialization for Masculinity. The training for the male role starts early when more stringent demands are made of and enforced more harshly on boys than on girls. Around the world, even preschool boys are more aggressive than girls, yet the amount of aggression demonstrated is culturally dependent. Male school and peer group activities are explicitly organized around struggle. Boys are encouraged to restrict their activities to masculine pursuits even in kindergarten, and boys are encouraged to hunt, fight, play sports, and play violent video games in all-male company (Miedzian, 1991). Violence can be viewed "as a clandestine masculine ideal in Western culture" (Toby, 1966, p. 19). The ideal male wields authority, especially over women, has unlimited sexual prowess, is invulnerable, has competition as his guiding principle, never discloses emotion, is tough and brave, has great power, is adept at one-upsmanship, can always fight victoriously if he needs to, and doesn't really need anyone. These standards are almost universal around the world and almost impossible to reach (Gilmore, 1990).

Characteristics. Many characteristics have been cited as representative of macho behavior. Whiting (1965) identified "a preoccupation with physical strength and athletic prowess, or attempts to demonstrate daring and valor or behavior that is violent and aggressive" (p. 127). Thrill-seeking behavior, inability to express emotions, independence, egotism, and support of the military have been noted by other authors. Attitudes that value sexual virility, the treatment of women as commodities and conquest objects, the insistence on female subjugation, the inability to cooperate with women, and the adherence to the "unwritten law" that female sexual infidelity must be avenged are all characteristic of macho attitudes. Macho characteristics, therefore, can be defined as the male attitudes and behavior arising from and supported by the patriarchal social structure, which express sexism and male ownership of women, glorify violence, emphasize virility, and despise gentleness and the expression of any emotions except anger.

Machismo, Violence, and Culture. There is considerable evidence of linkages between macho attitudes and violent behavior. Laboratory experiments among college males show connections between aggressiveness and macho characteristics (Archer, 1994). Another characteristic of macho behavior that has been investigated is owning or carrying a gun. The most significant correlation with gun ownership is the approval of and willingness to use violence, rather than having been a victim of violent crime (Williams & McGrath, 1978). Two of the countries with the highest homicide rates in the world, Columbia and Mexico, also have strong machismo ethics (World Health Organization, 2002). The highest rates of homicide in the United States are found in the deep South (Mississippi, Alabama, and Louisiana) and in the West (Texas, New Mexico, and Nevada), both areas characterized by an ethic of macho behavior. These six states have an average homicide rate of almost four times greater than the rate in all of New England. Arizona, Texas, and Mississippi also have the highest number of guns per capita while New England and the eastern United States have the lowest. Reviews of the evidence indicate that violence in the United States is better explained by a "subculture of masculinity" than the "subculture of violence" (Erlanger, 1974). Several studies of murderers have also noted macho characteristics (e.g., Gillies, 1976).

Cross-nationally, macho attitudes are often strongest where other forms of violence against women are the most severe and patriarchy the strongest. The machismo ethic is very similar to the "honor code" of many Arab and other Mediterranean cultures, wherein the woman is defined as property and the man must defend that property with violence, if necessary, toward other men and toward the woman (Counts, Brown, & Campbell, 1999; Gilmore, 1990).

One of the forms that the violence associated with machismo may take is wife abuse; the male who holds strong macho values will usually consider it his right to beat his wife. The other factors theorized to contribute to intimate partner violence, which have been previously reviewed, can be understood within this context. Alcohol can be seen as a disinhibiting agent that weakens the social prescription against doing physical harm to women except in certain situations. Intoxication can then be used as a convenient excuse for battering a woman because our society teaches that such behavior is less reprehensible when under its influence. Alcohol, therefore, can give a man the courage, the excuse, and the convenient loss of social veneer necessary to behaviorally express his need for power and macho attitudes.

Macho attitudes also fit into social learning theory and the idea that stressors or frustration may result in wife abuse. The patriarchal family arrangement makes it clear that the man may appropriately express his frustration toward his wife. Dobash and Dobash explained this connection as follows: "Thus, all men see themselves as controllers of women, and because they are socialized into the use of violence they are [all] potential aggressors against their wives" (Dobash & Dobash, 1979, p. 22). Television is also replete with male heroes using violence, without sanctions, to achieve goals.

Machismo and Powerlessness. In a classic framework, Goode (1971) explained family violence within a framework of social systems and social stratification. According to Goode, the family is a power system like all other social units, which "all rest to some degree on force and its threat" to operate. There are four ways by which people can be made to serve the ends of those in authority: force and its threat (power), economic variables, prestige or respect, and likability, attractiveness, friendship, or love. Within a male–female relationship, a combination of these factors is used to preserve male dominance. The threat of force is used more frequently than actual violence. Physical abuse enters into the picture more often when the other three persuasive mechanisms fail or when the male feels his authority is threatened. Thus, battering behavior is more likely to appear when the man's control, and therefore his macho pride, is challenged by the woman's job, education, pregnancy, or possible infidelity, if the man feels insecure about his own power.

The man who feels inadequate or is powerless in the male world is most likely to use force and violence where he can, in the home and in his neighborhood. Only a few men actually achieve dominance in work and economically, and their traditional male role in the home is being threatened. The less educated and poorer male is the farthest from the ideal in society and is therefore likely to be more overt in his machismo and violent behavior (e.g., Anderson, 1999; Tolson, 1977). The disenfranchised male is more likely to insist on his "conjugal right" to authority in the home, and violence is used when his power seems to be slipping. The data on the association of unemployment, poverty, lack of skills, and lower levels of education with intimate partner violence illustrates this mechanism. It has also been suggested that the high incidence of child abuse or excessive physical punishment in the background of many batterers has contributed to a sense of inadequacy and problems in identification with the father, which is later expressed as compulsive masculinity (Lystaad, 1975).

When a woman gets married in a patriarchal culture or neighborhood, her primary responsibility becomes child-rearing, housework, and "taking care of" her mate. The household responsibilities are seen as a service to the person in authority, the husband, and how well they are done is a symbol of "commitment and subservience" (Dobash & Dobash, 1979). This helps explain the often trivial nature of the incident preceding battering frequently described by abused women, typically about performance of a small household chore. If performed poorly or reluctantly (in the abuser's perception), it becomes a symbol of rebellion against his control. Such revolt must be quelled swiftly, with force if necessary, and such force has great symbolic meaning for the future.

From Goode's (1971) basic premises, we note that to use prestige or love to influence, a husband needs to be verbally persuasive. Several researchers have listed poor communication skills as a factor that predisposes males to abuse. Males with lower education may have fewer verbal skills, less prestige, and fewer economic resources, and therefore may perceive a need to rely more frequently on brute power to maintain their position. In contrast, the middle class male is characterized as follows: "The greater the other resources an individual can command, the more force he can muster, but the less he will actually deploy or use force in an overt manner" (Goode, 1971, p. 628). The only difference according to class may be in terms of degree and frequency of violence; the issue is still control and dominance. The middle class male may be more likely to hit his wife only once at a time because of the consequences to his position if he were known as a batterer. Yet even one blow is a powerful symbol of force and authority. As described by Stark and Flitcraft, "complex social factors may determine whether and in what combination physical, ideological, political, and economic force will be used to control women" (Stark, Flitcraft, & Frazier, 1979, p. 481).

Jealousy and Machismo. Jealousy is frequently associated with wife-beating and femicide and is most logically viewed within the context of the husband's macho attitudes and his effort to maintain control over his wife. One of the dictionary definitions of "jealous" is "zealous in guarding" (Gove, 1961). Ownership is implied. Because women are considered the possession of a husband, real or imagined sexual infidelity is the gravest threat to male dominance. Jealousy over women's jobs, children (even unborn), friends, other family, and anything that takes her attention away from him has often been described in interview data from battered women (Campbell, Rose, & Kub, 1998; Dobash & Dobash, 1979; Landenburger, 1998; Walker, 1979). From a macho viewpoint, jealousy is part of male dominance and control.

Sexual Relationships as Part of Macho Attitudes. The macho attitudes of wife beaters are also reflected in their sexual relationships with their wives. Conquest is an integral part of sex. Forced sex and sexual abuse is usually part of the pattern of victimization (Campbell & Soeken, 1999; Finkelhor & Yllo, 1983; Russell, 1990). Stark, Flitcraft, and Frazier (1979) felt that the deliberate, sexual nature of wife abuse is shown in the predominance of injuries to the face, chest, breast, and abdomen. Batterers see control of all aspects of sex, including contraception and "safe sex," as a part of their masculine definition (Davilla & Brackley, 1999). Refusal of sex becomes a provocation for abuse.

TYPOLOGIES OF BATTERERS AND OF DOMESTIC VIOLENCE

An important conclusion reached by many who work with men who batter their female partners is that there is no single personality profile, social characteristic, or "type" of man who batters, and there may be at least two distinct types of IPV. As advanced by Michael Johnson (1995; 2000) and briefly noted earlier, IPV can be separated into "terroristic battering" (formerly "patriarchal terrorism") and "common couple violence." Macho and feminist theories explain terroristic battering better than they do common couple violence. With terroristic battering, the violence is almost entirely perpetrated toward females, increases in severity and frequency over time, is motivated by desire for power and control, and is characterized by perpetrators who are unrepentant and whose behavior is difficult to modify. Terroristic batterers are more familiar to advocates in domestic-violence shelters and, until recently, to the criminal justice system. Johnson hypothesized that common couple violence is more common, with perpetrators more amenable to interventions, and is more likely to have females as well as males as perpetrators.

Aside from type of IPV, variability in abuse has also been described in relation to other aspects of abuse, such as motives for the abuse or violence; the nature, severity, and frequency of the violence; whether the perpetrator commits violence outside the family; and whether the perpetrator is affected by a psychological or personality disorder (Holtzworth-Munroe, 2000; Johnson & Ferraro, 2000). This insight is particularly important for programs that reduce men's abuse in their intimate relationships. Program developers and clinicians want to know what works for whom and under what circumstances (Gondolf, 1997b).

Although the conceptual labels differ, the core characteristics of subtypes of men who batter are remarkably similar and are extremely useful in advancing our understanding of the causes of intimate partner violence.

Holtzworth-Munroe and Stuart (1994) identified three subtypes of batterers. The least violent is the "family-only" batterer. These men use the lowest levels of physical, psychological, and sexual abuse against their partners, are the least likely to be violent outside the home, and do not show evidence of psychopathology. The second subtype of batterer, the "dysphoric-borderline batterer," perpetrates a moderate or severe degree of physical abuse against their intimate partner. They may also be violent outside the family, and they are likely to show characteristics of depression, anxiety, or borderline personality disorder. The third subtype, the "generally violent antisocial batterer," is the most violent type of batterer, both to his intimate partner and to those outside the family. This type of batterer is also most likely to show evidence of antisocial personality disorder—for example, by criminal behavior and arrests (Holtzworth-Munroe, 2000; Holtzworth-Munroe and Stuart, 1994).

In another study, couples who had experienced severe violence were not only interviewed and observed but also physiologically monitored during arguments induced in a laboratory setting. The results provided evidence of two types of batterers (Jacobson & Gottman, 1998). One group of men displayed an overall internal calmness during verbally aggressive arguments, a "cold physiology," with low heart rates and other measures; men in this group were called "cobras." The other group of men displayed the expected higher heart rates and other measures of emotional distress and were called "pit bulls." The investigators further described "pit bulls" as those men who deprive their partners of any independence and closely monitor their daily activities; they suspect sexual betrayal in the most innocuous contexts and eventually lose control of their emotions, erupting in violence. In contrast, the cobras are described as sociopaths with a high degree of criminal behavior and violence. They resemble the "generally violent, antisocial batterers" of Holtzworth-Munroe, whereas the pit bulls resemble "dysphoric, borderline batterers" (Johnson & Ferraro, 2000).

Our understanding of the causes of men's violence against women in intimate relationships has significantly improved over the past 3 decades of research and theory development. Theoretical explanations started with simplistic, single-factor attributions (for example, men's witnessing abuse in childhood or men's alcohol abuse). From there, explanations became more nuanced, taking into account how factors interact, and then developed into more complicated typologies of batterers as a heterogeneous group. Researchers then integrated research findings and theoretical models from disparate fields of study into synthesizing explanatory frameworks, which led finally to ongoing research that, to enhance efficacy of treatment approaches, is making important distinctions among men who batter. Frameworks that better address the intersections of intimate partner violence, gender, race, and ethnicity are still clearly needed, as are frameworks that address violence between same-sex partners. It is important to remember that these 3 decades of scientific work were inspired by women telling stories of abuse and violence inflicted on them by the person who claimed to love them most. It is equally important to keep future empirical and theoretical work grounded in women's realities, in which safety from further harm and empowerment for difficult decisions are integral to all work with women in abusive relationships.

THEORIES OF WOMEN'S RESPONSES TO INTIMATE PARTNER VIOLENCE

One of the most difficult dynamics of intimate partner violence for professionals and the general public to understand is why a woman would stay with an abusive partner, sometimes for many years. The question has been addressed from many perspectives, some of which have promoted victim-blaming attributions. Overall, however, the past 3 decades of research have resulted in growing appreciation for the complexity and resourcefulness of women's strategic actions as they attempt to resolve the abuse or, if needed, to break free of the abusive relationship, even in the face of ongoing danger and hardship. A majority of abused women do, in fact, leave the abusive relationship or manage to make the violence end, but it may take many years (Campbell et al., 1994). The important question is not, "Why does she stay?" Instead people should ask, "Why do so many men beat their wives?" and "What is preventing her from staying safe?"

This section of the chapter examines theoretical formulations of response under three major headings: sociocultural responses to women who experience intimate partner violence, psychological responses of women to the abuse and violence, and contemporary descriptions of patterns of women's responses to intimate partner violence.

An important caveat is that many women undoubtedly *do* extricate themselves from relationships at the onset of abuse, or soon after. Because most research has not addressed this issue, our knowledge of women who quickly break free is very limited. Therefore, the theoretical and empirical work accomplished thus far is more useful in understanding the responses of women who endure abuse over a longer period of time.

Sociocultural Perspectives

Sociocultural explanations of the perpetuation of violence against female partners focus on society's explicit and implicit rules that legitimize violence under certain circumstances. Privacy of the family and sanctity of all that transpires within a family's home have traditionally been protected in American culture (Straus & Gelles, 1990). As described earlier, male dominance within the family often is culturally unquestioned and may be embedded in a cultural context of machismo, overt or covert male power and entitlement over women, and male authority within the community (Heise, 1998). With these sociocultural factors in mind, women are believed to remain in abusive relationships because of the social barriers that keep them there. Family, friends, and neighbors are reluctant to become involved in a family's "private business." Although this is changing, official helping agencies such as the police, the court system, clergy, psychology, and health care professionals all may be unresponsive to the battered woman's needs in the name of keeping the sanctity of the family.

Psychological Perspectives

Research and theory from psychological perspectives have extensively explored personality and psychological factors related to women's responses to abusive relationships. Low self-esteem is often suggested in popular literature as a reason for women's continued involvement in abusive relationships. Women with low self-esteem are thought to be vulnerable to abuse, more tolerant in permitting the abuse to continue, and less likely to seek outside intervention. Research, however, has failed to support this persistent notion. The conclusion of most research in this area is twofold. First, as with most psychological attributes characteristic of battered women, the low self-esteem that many abused women experience is likely the consequence of the abuse and of the stigma associated with it rather than a preexisting condition. Second, women with low self-esteem are no more likely to become involved in an abusive relationship than are women with higher levels of self-esteem.

Similarly, symptoms of depression, posttraumatic stress disorder (PTSD), and alcohol and drug abuse are consistently found to be more prevalent among abused women than women not battered (Campbell et al., 1997; Dieneman, Boyle, Baker, Resnick, Wiederhorn, & Campbell, 2000; Golding, 1999). Again, most evidence sees these symptoms as sequelae of trauma rather than precursors. The more trauma women have experienced in their lifetimes, such as abuse in childhood or sexual assault in addition to intimate partner violence, the more symptoms they exhibit. Even though these symptoms are a consequence of the violence, they may interfere with a woman's problem-solving and coping abilities. Therefore, interventions need to take these potential problems into account. (See Chapter 11.)

Learned Helplessness

In the late 1980s, Martin Seligman's theory of learned helplessness was promoted as a reasonable explanation of women's psychological and behavioral responses to abuse (Walker, 1979, 1984). The original model, based on controlled laboratory experiments with animals, stated that passivity results when uncontrollable bad events occur and when future responses are expected to be futile. Learning that outcomes are uncontrollable results in motivational deficit (passivity), cognitive deficit (poor problem-solving), and emotional deficit (depression). An attributional component was later added to the model, with persons blaming themselves for the adversity and being more likely to become more helpless.

Learned helplessness theory suggests that repeated abuse leads to the development of a cognitive perception that the victim is unable to resolve her current abusive situation, accompanied by depression and apathy, which then results in an inability to leave the relationship. Walker (1984) found some support for learned helplessness in a sample of battered women, especially in terms of depression. However, many did not perceive a loss of control of events in their lives, nor did they show low self-esteem. Rather than becoming passive and immobilized over time, as predicted by the learned helplessness model, women's help-seeking activities increased as the frequency and severity of violence increased.

Grief Model

A grief model has also been advanced to explain the depression as a normative resolution process of personal loss and grief that accompanies the dissolution of any valued intimate relationship. In this model, depression of battered women is in response to the anticipated termination of the relationship, and the temporary separations and reunions with the abusive partner are comparable to the ambivalent behavior in any troubled marriage or significant relationship. In a comparison of learned helplessness and grief models, Campbell (1989) compared 97 battered women with 96 women who were in troubled but nonviolent relationships. Both theoretical models were nearly equal in explanatory power, and more of the battered women were severely depressed than the nonabused women and also experienced more frequent and severe physical symptoms of stress. Even so, few of the battered women blamed themselves, and they had considered or tried significantly more solutions to their relationship problems than had women in troubled but nonviolent relationships, showing the strength and creativity of trying to end abuse.

Survivor Models

Contemporary research most strongly supports models in which battered women are viewed as active survivors rather than helpless victims (Campbell, Rose, & Kub, 1998; Gondolf & Fisher, 1988; Hoff, 1990). Data from 6,612 records from 50 battered-women's shelters in Texas showed battered women persistently seeking help to end the abuse directed at them (Gondolf & Fisher, 1988). Help-seeking efforts increased rather than decreased when the batterer's level of violence increased, particularly when he engaged in more antisocial or criminal behavior in general. The inadequate response of social agencies to the needs of battered women was the most notable impediment to safety, rather than internal characteristics of the women. This suggests that helping agencies must strengthen their advocacy role for women and remove the barriers that keep women trapped in abusive relationships, rather than concentrating on treating victims.

Patterns of Women's Responses

The notion of women as survivors rather than victims has been further developed in contemporary research that has examined the process of women leaving an abusive relationship. These studies, often based on qualitative data from in-depth interviews, have illuminated the complexity of women's experiences with and responses to intimate partner violence. An important unifying theme in this growing body of research is that women's responses to abuse reflect a dynamic process that evolves according to the nature of the abuse, their interpretations of the abuse, and the relationship as a whole, as well as to their expectations of the pragmatic consequences of remaining in or severing the relationship. Nurse researchers have made particularly important contributions to this body of knowledge.

Cycle Theory of Violence

Lenore Walker was one of the first researchers to describe a dynamic process in abusive relationships that she called the "cycle theory of violence" (Walker, 1979, 1984). From extensive interviews with battered women in which they described battering incidents, Walker described a three-phase cycle of violence. The first or "tension-building phase" is characterized by an escalation of tension, with verbal abuse and minor battering incidents. The woman engages in placating behavior, trying desperately to avoid serious incidents. This phase may last for weeks or years, until the tension has mounted to the breaking point. Phase two, "the acute battering incident," is the outbreak of serious violence that may last from two to twenty-four hours. The woman is powerless to affect the outcome of the second phase and can only try to protect herself and her children. In the third phase, the man becomes contrite, loving, and promises to reform, reinforcing the woman's hope that the beatings will end. Unfortunately, the cycle almost always repeats itself. Over time, the third phase occurs less often, leaving the woman trapped between the preoutburst tension and the battering episodes.

Empirical tests of Walker's cycle of violence theory lend inconsistent support for the three phases. Sixty-five percent of Walker's sample gave evidence of a tension-building phase prior to the battering, and 58% described loving contrition after the battering (Walker, 1984). Dobash and Dobash (1984) used similar research methods but did not find support for Walker's third phase of the cycle of violence; only 14% of the batterers in their sample apologized after the worst incident of assault. Painter and Dutton (1985) found unpredictable postbattering behavior on the part of the men. Nevertheless, advocates and the women themselves have accepted Walker's cycle of violence theory as a plausible explanation for the behavior of abused women. The three-phase cycle often appears in clinical protocols for professional education and in community education efforts by women's groups.

The Process of Becoming Involved In and Recovering From an Abusive Relationship

Several researchers have documented the experience of becoming embroiled in, coping with, and extricating oneself from an abusive relationship, from the perspective of women who have lived through intimate partner violence. The research demonstrates the strengths and creative resistance strategies that women draw upon in the face of intimate partner violence.

In a nursing investigation of women's experiences with intimate partner violence, Landenburger (1989, 1998) described factors that influence women's choices about the relationship over time, including factors that assisted or hindered women's departure from the relationship. The four phases of binding, enduring, disengaging, and recovering emerged from a qualitative analysis of in-depth interviews. Women went through the four phases, but not necessarily in a linear fashion, as they experienced changes in the meaning ascribed to the abuse, in interactions with the abusive partner, and in perceptions of themselves.

In the first phase, the binding phase, when the relationship is new and promising, a woman responds to abuse with redoubled efforts to make the relationship work and to prevent future abuse. Logical, creative strategies are employed to appease the abusive partner.

In the second phase, or time of enduring, a woman tolerates the abuse because of the positive aspects of the relationship and because she feels at least partially responsible for the abuse. Landenburger described a "shrinking of self" in which women's personal needs, desires, and goals are put aside to fully attend to the abusive partner's needs, desires, and goals, in an effort to prevent or reduce further abuse. Though a woman may tentatively seek outside help at this time, she does not openly disclose her circumstances to others for fear of the consequences to her safety and to her partner's social status.

The phase of disengaging involves the woman labeling her situation as being abusive and herself as undeserving of abusive treatment. A breaking point may be reached at which the woman is cognizant of the danger she is in and of the possibility that she might attempt to kill the abuser. As the woman struggles with independent-living and safety concerns, she may leave and return to the abusive relationship several times.

After a time of readjustment and successfully dealing with the many barriers that could trap her in the abusive relationship, a woman may enter a phase of recovery in which she remains separated from the abuser. An important point for nurses and other helpers to realize is that, from the woman's perspective, the abuse was just one aspect of a whole relationship that may still have some positive elements. The woman wants the abuse to stop but wants to maintain the good aspects of the relationship.

Many elements of the process explicated by Landenburger of becoming involved in, coping with, and, for some, eventually becoming disentangled from an abusive intimate relationship are supported by the findings of other researchers. For example, in a qualitative study of women's accounts of coping with abusive partners, Mills (1985) found that as women separated from the abusive relationship their outlook for future success was affected by whether they took on the negative self-identity of "victim" or the positive self-identity of "survivor." This can be seen as analogous to Landenburger's "shrinking of self" and the later reemergence of self during the recovery phase. Another nursing researcher, Yvonne Ulrich (1991), found that for some women the realization that achieving their self-potential would never be possible within the abusive relationship was an important catalyst for leaving. Using Gilligan's theory of women's moral development as framework for interpreting women's narratives about intimate partner violence, Belknap found that women's sense of self played a role in their silence. Women maintained secrecy about many abuses in their lives in the belief that they were somehow responsible for the abuse. Self-blame, combined with the fear that no one would believe their stories, kept women silent (Belknap, 1999, 2000).

"Reclaiming self" is the explanatory core of women's responses to intimate partner violence in the nursing research program of Wuest and Merritt-Gray (Merritt-Gray & Wuest, 1995; Wuest & Merritt-Gray, 1999). Using methods grounded in feminist theory, with narrative data from 13 rural women who had left abusive relationships, Wuest and Merritt-Gray told of women who described the process of living in and eventually leaving an abusive relationship. A variety of strategies were employed in three stages of reclaiming the self: "counteracting abuse," "breaking free," and "not going back" to the relationship. The strategic actions that women employed in resisting the abuse contradict the view of battered women as passive victims. Women described "relinquishing parts of self" early in the process when their partner became abusive; they minimized the abuse in a variety of ways, but they also began "fortifying defenses." Fortifying defenses refers to a variety of personal activities that promoted self-reflection, enhanced their capabilities for independence, and improved their knowledge of ways to achieve freedom from abuse.

Sustaining the separation from the abusive partner, or not going back, is an important stage best explicated in this framework (Wuest & Merritt-Gray, 1999). The process of leaving an abusive relationship can be so long and arduous that, after leaving, women experience ambivalence, uncertainty, and depleted reserves of emotional and physical energy. Sustaining freedom from abuse requires establishing and maintaining a safe place to live and learning to navigate through the maze of searching for employment, applying for financial assistance, and enlisting the assistance of law enforcement and the court system in custody issues or on-going stalking or harassment from the abusive partner.

Using a longitudinal design in which women were interviewed at three different time points over 3 years, Campbell and colleagues (1998) described the resourcefulness of women's approaches to resolving the violence in their relationships. A majority of the sample were still in the abusive relationship at the beginning of the study, so the results do not rely on women's reflections on a past abusive relationship. In contrast to other explications of women's responses to abuse, the overall goal of women in this study was to resolve the abuse (achieve nonviolence) rather than necessarily leaving the intimate relationship. Women's stories revealed that the notion of "staying" or "leaving" an abusive relationship is a gross oversimplification of women's status in the relationship. For example, an "in/out" category was developed to describe women who were ambivalent about maintaining or leaving the relationship. These women may have left, or had the abuser thrown out, more than once; however, they continued to have positive feelings for the partner and, though certain that they wanted the abuse to end, were not convinced that the entire relationship had to be sacrificed.

Another important insight gained from the study is that leaving the intimate relationship and ending the violence were often independent outcomes. For some women, violence continues, and may even escalate, after they leave the abusive partner. Women are easily stalked by their ex-partner and can be harassed for years by virtue of legal proceedings, child-custody and visitation rules, and other reasons for continued contact. It is essential for nurses and the public to understand that ending the abusive relationship does not necessarily end the violence for women and their children. Efforts to assist and support women must be made with full cognizance of this dangerous reality. Statements such as "Why don't you just leave?" need to be eliminated from our set of responses to women's disclosure of abuse.

Although the complexity of women's stories over three years did not support description of a process with distinct phases, women did describe various circumstances and events that played pivotal roles in their quest for nonviolence. For example, achieving financial independence provided an important psychological and pragmatic boost that helped some women leave the relationship. For others, the realization that their children's well-being was in jeopardy or that they were becoming violent in response was a catalyst for leaving the abusive partner.

In summary, theoretical frameworks of women's responses to intimate partner violence have evolved in complexity and explanatory power over the past thirty years. Contemporary research refutes the image of women as passive victims in abusive relationships. Rather, women actively respond to the abusive behaviors with creative and intelligent strategies, the goal being to be free of violence, perhaps while maintaining the relationship, but, more often, requiring dissolution of the relationship. Though this is a complicated process, a pattern of normative stages or phases have been described in qualitative research; detailed knowledge of the process can be used to develop phase-specific nursing assessments and interventions with women who are experiencing intimate partner violence. The reality of ongoing danger and harassment from the perpetrator has been illustrated in women's narrative accounts and in review of homicide data. Those who are in positions to help women must remain aware that leaving an abusive relationship does not necessarily ensure the safety of women and their children. Rather, the level of danger may increase for some time after leaving; evaluation of danger and review of safety plans must be an integral component of work with women, even after they have left an abusive partner. Clearly, further research on the typologies of batterers, described earlier in this chapter, will improve the accuracy of danger assessments and appropriate safety plans for women and their children.

SUMMARY

Intimate partner violence is clearly a public health problem of considerable magnitude in North America and around the world. Nurses have many roles to play in primary prevention efforts as well as in the application of appropriate interventions with those who have experienced abuse in intimate relationships. Although attention to the issue is fairly recent in the nursing and health care community, the problem is not a new phenomenon. Historical records reveal that wife-beating has been socially sanctioned in patriarchal societies throughout history, and, indeed, there continues to be cultural support, to varying degrees, for men to dominate and control their wives and partners through aggressive means (Dobash & Dobash, 1979, 1993; Heise, 1998; WHO, 2002).

This chapter has reviewed the evolution of theoretical frameworks that explain the causes of intimate partner violence, including psychobiological explanations, socialization theories, family system stressors, and an ecological framework. The concept of machismo was seen to be important in explaining the behavior of abusive men. Recent progress was described in understanding the types of men who batter, which is extremely important knowledge for those who work with such men and who wish to improve the safety of women and children. Theoretical frameworks that describe and explain women's responses to intimate partner violence were presented chronologically, beginning with victim-blaming perspectives, followed by theories in which the victim is viewed as passive and helpless, and concluding with more recent frameworks that highlight the strength and creativity of women's resistance to and resolution of intimate partner violence.

Though our knowledge remains imperfect, contemporary understanding of the causes of men's violence against women and women's responses provides an important base for the development of nursing assessment tools and interventions for primary prevention and early detection of intimate partner violence, and for therapeutic approaches for those who experience it.

References

Abrahams, N. (2002). *Men's use of violence against intimate partners: A study of working men in Cape Town.* Cape Town, South Africa: University of Cape Town.

Achterberg, J. (1991). *Woman as healer.* Boston: Shambhala.

Anderson, E. (1999). *Code of the Streets.* New York: W. W. Norton.

Archer, J. (Ed.) (1994). *Male violence.* London: Routledge.

Barnes, S. Y. (1999). Theories of spouse abuse: Relevance to African Americans. *Issues in Mental Health Nursing, 20,* 357–371.

Belknap, R. A. (1999). Why did she do that? Issues of moral conflict in battered women's decision making. *Issues in Mental Health Nursing, 20,* 387–404.

Belknap, R. A. (2000). Eva's story: One woman's life viewed through the interpretive lens of Gilligan's theory. *Violence Against Women, 6,* 586–605.

Boddy, J. (1998). Violence embodied? Circumcision, gender politics, and cultural aesthetics. In R. E. Dobash & R .E. Dobash (Eds.), *Rethinking violence against women* (pp. 77–110). Thousand Oaks, CA: Sage.

Browne, A. (1987). *Battered women who kill.* New York: Free Press.

Browne, A., Williams, K. R., & Dutton, D. R. (1998). Homicide between intimate partners. In M. D. Smith & M. Zahn (Eds.), *Homicide: A sourcebook of social research,* pp. 149–164. Thousand Oaks, CA: Sage.

Brownmiller, S. (1975). *Against our will: Men, women, and rape.* New York: Bantam Books.

Cohen, R. A., Rosenbaum, A., Kane, R. L., Warnken, W. J., & Benjamin, S. (1999). Neuropsychological correlates of domestic violence. *Violence & Victims, 14,* 397–411.

Campbell, J. C. (1985). Beating of wives: A cross-cultural perspective. *Victimology, 10,* 174–185.

Campbell, J. C. (1989). A test of two explanatory models of women's responses to battering. *Nursing Research, 38*(1), 18–24.

Campbell, J. C. (1992). "If I can't have you, no one can": Power and control in homicide of female partners. In J. Radford & D. E. H. Russell (Eds.), *Femicide: The politics of woman killing* (pp. 99–113). New York: Twayne.

Campbell, J. C., & Humphreys, J. (1993). *Nursing care of survivors of family violence.* St. Louis: Mosby.

Campbell, J. C., Kub, J., Belknap, R. A., & Templin, T. (1997). Predictors of depression in battered women. *Violence Against Women, 3*(3), 276–293.

Campbell, J. C., Miller, P., Cardwell, M. M., & Belknap, R. A. (1994). Relationship status of battered women over time. *Journal of Family Violence, 9,* 99–111.

Campbell, J., Rose, L., & Kub, J. (1998). Voices of strength and resistance: A contextual and longitudinal analysis of women's responses to battering. *Journal of Interpersonal Violence, 13,* 743–761.

Campbell, J. C., Sharps, P. W., & Glass, N. E. (2000). Risk assessment for intimate partner homicide. In G. F. Pinard & L. Pagani (Eds.), *Clinical assessment of dangerousness: Empirical contributions* (pp. 136–157). New York: Cambridge University Press.

Campbell, J., & Soeken, K. (1999). Forced sex and intimate partner violence: Effects on women's health. *Violence Against Women, 5,* 1017–1035.

Campbell, J., Webster, D., Koziol-McLain, J., Block, C. R., Campbell, D. W., Curry, M. A., Gary, F., McFarlane, J., Sachs, C., Sharps, P., Ulrich, Y., Wilt, S. A., Manganello, J., Xu, X., Schollenberger, J., Frye, V. A., & Laughon, K. (in press). Risk factors for intimate partner femicide. *American Journal of Public Health.*

Connell, R. (1995). *Masculinities.* Cambridge: Polity Press.

Carmody, D. C., & Williams, K. R. (1987). Wife assault and perceptions of sanctions. *Violence and Victims, 2*(1), 25–38.

Counts, D. A., Brown, J. K., & Campbell, J. C. (1999). *To Have and To Hit: Cultural Perspectives on Wife Beating.* Chicago: University of Illinois Press.

Cunningham, A., Jaffe, P., Baker, L., Dick, T., Malla, S., Mazaheri, N., & Poisson, S. (1998). Theory-driven explanations of male violence against female partners: Literature update and related implications for treatment and evaluation. [On-line]. Available: www.lfcc.on.ca/maleviolence.pdf.

Daly, M. (1978). *Gyn/Ecology: The metaethics of radical feminism.* Boston: Beacon Press.

Daly, M., Singh, L. S., & Wilson, M. (1999). Children fathered by previous partners: A risk factor for violence against women. *Canadian Journal of Public Health, 84*(3), 209–210.

Davidson, T. (1978). *Conjugal crime: Understanding and changing the wifebeating problem.* New York: Hawthorne Books.

Davila, Y. R., & Brackley, M. H. (1999). Mexican and Mexican-American women in a battered women's shelter: Barriers to condom negotiation for HIV/AIDS prevention. *Issues Mental Health Nursing, 20*(4), 333–355.

Dearwater, S., Coben, J., Nah, G., Campbell, J., McLoughlin, E., & Glass, N. (1998). Prevalence of domestic violence in women treated at community hospital emergency departments. *Journal of the American Medical Association, 280*(5), 433–438.

Dibble, U., & Straus, M. (1980). Some social structural determinants of inconsistency between attitudes and behavior. *Journal of Marriage and the Family, 42,* 72, 79.

Dienemann, J., Boyle, E., Baker, D., Resnick, W., Wiederhorn, N., & Campbell, J. (2000). Intimate partner abuse among women diagnosed with depression. *Issues in Mental Health Nursing, 21,* 499–513.

Dobash, R. E., & Dobash, R. P. (1979). *Violence against wives.* New York: Free Press.

Dobash, R . E., & Dobash, R. P. (1984). The nature and antecedents of violent events. *British Journal of Criminology, 23,* 269–288.

Dobash, R. E., & Dobash, R. P. (1993). *Women, violence, and social change.* London: Routledge.

Dobash, R. E., & Dobash, R. P. (1998). *Rethinking violence against women.* Thousand Oaks, CA: Sage.

Dobash, R. P., Dobash, R. E., Wilson, M., & Daly, M. (1992). The myth of sexual symmetry in marital violence. *Social Problems, 39*(1), 71–91.

Driver, E. D. (1971). Interaction and criminal homicide in India. *Social Forces, 60,* 155–156.

Dworkin, A. (1976). *Our blood: Prophecies and discourses on sexual politics.* New York: Harper & Row.

Erlanger, H.S. (1974). The empirical status of the subculture of violence thesis. *Social Problems, 22,* 289.

Finkelhor, D., & Yllo, K. (1983). Rape in marriage: A sociological view. In D. Finkelhor, R. J. Gelles, G. T. Hotaling, & M. A. Straus (Eds.), *The dark side of families: Current family violence research* (pp. 119–130). Beverly Hills: Sage.

Foster, L. A., Veale, C. M., & Fogel, C. I. (1989). Factors present when battered women kill. *Issues in Mental Health Nursing, 10,* 273–284.

Ganley, A. L. (1995). Understanding domestic violence. In C. Warshaw & A. L. Ganley (Eds.), *Improving the health care response to domestic violence: A resource manual for health care providers* (pp. 15–45). San Francisco: Family Violence Prevention Fund.

Gibbons, D. C. (1970). *Delinquent behavior.* Englewood Cliffs, NJ: Prentice-Hall.

Gillespie, C. K. (1989). *Justifiable homicide.* Columbus, OH: Ohio State University Press.

Gillies, H. (1976). Homicide in the west of Scotland. *British Journal of Psychology, 28,* 116.

Gilmore, D. D. (1990). *Manhood in the making: Cultural concepts of masculinity.* New Haven, CT: Yale University Press.

Golding, J. M. (1999). Intimate partner violence as a risk for mental disorders: A meta-analysis. *Journal of Family Violence, 14,* 99–132.

Gondolf, E. W. (1997a). Patterns of reassault in batterer programs. *Violence and Victims 12*(4), 373–387.

Gondolf, E. W. (1997b). Batterer programs: What we know and need to know. *Journal of Interpersonal Violence, 12*(1), 83–98.

Gondolf, E. W., & Fisher, E. R. (1988). *Battered women as survivors: An alternative to learned helplessness.* Lexington, MA: Lexington Books.

Goode, W. (1971). Force and violence in the family. *Journal of Marriage and the Family, 33,* 624–636.

Gove, P. B. (Ed.). (2002). *Webster's Third New International Dictionary, Unabridged.* Springfield, MA: Merriam-Webster.

Greenfield, L. A., Rand, M. R., Craven, D., Klaus, P. A., Perkins, C. A., Ringel, C., Warchol, G., & Matson, C. (1998). *Violence by intimates: Analysis of data on crimes by current or former spouses, boyfriends and, girlfriends.* Washington, DC: US Department of Justice.

Greenwood, G. L., Relf, M. V., Huang, B., Pollack, L. M., Canchola, J. A., & Catania, J. A. (2002). Battering victimization among a probability-based sample of men who have sex with men (MSM). *American Journal of Public Health 92*(12), 1964–1969.

Grossfeld, S. (1991, September 2). "Safer" and in jail: Women who kill their batterers. *Boston Globe,* pp. 1, 12, 13.

Heise, L. (1998). Violence against women: An integrated, ecological framework. *Violence Against Women, 4,* 262–290.

Heise, L. L., Ellsberg, M. C., & Gottemoeller, M. (1999). Ending violence against women. *Population Reports, 27*(4), 1– 43.

Hoff, L. A. (1990). *Battered women as survivors.* London: Routledge.

Holtzworth-Munroe, A. (2000). A typology of men who are violent toward their female partners: Making sense of the heterogeneity of husband violence. *Current Directions in Psychological Science* [On-line], *9* (4). Available at: http://www.psychologicalscience.org.

Holtzworth-Munroe, A., & Stuart, G. L. (1994). Typologies of male batterers: Three subtypes and the differences among them. *Psychological Bulletin, 116,* 476–497.

hooks, b. (1984). *Feminist theory: From margin to center.* Boston: South End Press.

Hosken, F. P. (1977-78). Female circumcision in Africa. *Victimology, 2,* 487–498.

Jacobson, N., & Gottman, J. (1998). *When men batter women: New insights into ending abusive relationships.* New York: Simon & Schuster.

Janssen-Jurreit, M. (1982). *Sexism: The male monopoly on history and thought (V. Moberg, Trans.).* New York: Farrar, Straus, & Giroux.

Johnson, M. P. (1995). Patriarchal terrorism and common couple violence: Two forms of violence against women. *Journal of Marriage and the Family, 57,* 283–294.

Johnson, M. P. (2000). Conflict and control: Images of symmetry and asymmetry in domestic violence. In A. Booth, A. C. Crouter, & M. Clements (Eds.), *Couples in conflict.* Hillsdale, NJ: Erlbaum.

Johnson, M. P., & Ferraro, K. J. (2000). Research on domestic violence in the 1990s: Making distinctions. *Journal of Marriage and the Family, 62,* 948–963.

Jones A., Campbell, J., Gielen, A., O'Campo, P., Dienemann, J., Kub, J., & Schollenburger, J. (1999). Annual and lifetime prevalence of partner abuse in a sample of female HMO enrollees. *Women's Health Issues, 9,* 295–305.

Jordan, B. K. Marmar, C. R., Fairbank, J. A., Schlenger, W. E., Kulka, R. A., Hough, R. L., & Weiss, D. S. (1992). Problems in families of male Vietnam veterans with posttraumatic stress disorders. *Journal of Clinical and Consulting Psychology, 60*(6), 916–926.

Kantor, G. K. (1993). Refining the brushstrokes in portraits on alcohol and wife assaults. In *APA, alcohol and interpersonal violence: Fostering multidisciplinary perspectives* (pp. 281–290). Washington, DC: National Institute on Alcohol Abuse and Alcoholism, NIH.

Kantor, G. K., & Straus, M. A. (1987). The "drunken bum" theory of wife beating. *Social Problems, 34,* 213–230.

Kirkwood, M. K., & Cecil, D. K. (2001). Marital rape: A student assessment of rape laws and the marital exemption. *Violence Against Women, 7*(11), 1234–1253.

Klein, E., Campbell, J., Soler, E., & Ghez, M. (1997). *Ending domestic violence: Changing public perceptions.* Newbury Park, CA: Sage.

Kub, J., Campbell, J. C., Rose, L., & Soeken, K. (1999). Role of substance use in the battering relationship. *Journal of Addictions Nursing, 11*(4), 171–179.

Landenburger, K. (1989). A process of entrapment in and recovery from an abusive relationship. *Issues in Mental Health Nursing, 3,* 209–227.

Landenburger, K. M. (1998). Exploration of women's identity: Clinical approaches with abused women. In J. C. Campbell (Ed.), *Empowering survivors of abuse: Health care for battered women and their children* (pp. 61–69). Thousand Oaks, CA: Sage.

Langford, D. R. (1996). Predicting unpredictability: A model of women's processes of predicting battering men's violence. *Scholarly Inquiry for Nursing Practice, 10* (4), 371–385.

Levinson, D. (1989). *Family violence in cross-cultural perspective.* Newbury Park, CA: Sage.

Lobel, K. (Ed.). (1986). *Naming the violence: Speaking out about lesbian battering.* Seattle, WA: The Seal Press.

Lystaad, M. H. (1975). Violence at home. *American Journal of Orthopsychiatry, 45,* 339.

Malamuth, N., Sockloskie, R., Koss, M., & Tanaka, J. (1991). Characteristics of aggressors against women: Testing a model using a national sample of college students. *Journal of Consulting and Clinical Psychology, 59,* 670–681.

Maletzky, B. M. (1973). The episodic dyscontrol syndrome. *Diseases of the Nervous System, 34,* 179–180.

Malik, M .O. A., & Salvi, O. (1976). A profile of homicide in the Sudan. *Forensic Science, 7,* 141–150.

Martin, S. L., Tsui, A. O., Maitra, K., & Marinshaw, R. (1999). Domestic violence in northern India. *American Journal of Epidemiology, 150,* 417–426.

Maxfield, M. G., & Widom, C. S. (2001). An update on the "cycle of violence." In *National Institute of Justice research in brief* (pp. 1–7). Washington, DC: U.S. Department of Justice.

May, M. (1978). Violence in the family: An historical perspective. In J. P. Martin (Ed.), *Violence and the family* (pp. 135–163). Chicester: John Wiley & Sons.

McFarlane, J., & Parker, B. (1994). *Abuse during pregnancy: A protocol for prevention and intervention.* White Plains, NY: March of Dimes Birth Defects Foundation.

Merritt-Gray, M., & Wuest, J. (1995). Counteracting abuse and breaking free: The process of leaving revealed through women's voices. *Health Care for Women International, 16,* 399–412.

Miedzian, M. (1991). *Boys will be boys: Breaking the links between masculinity and violence.* New York: Anchor Doubleday.

Mills, T. (1985). The assault on the self: Stages in coping with abusive husbands. *Qualitative Sociology, 8,* 103–123.

Moracco, K. E., Runyan, C. W., & Butts, J. (1998). Femicide in North Carolina. *Homicide Studies, 2,* 422–446, 1998.

NiCarthy, G. (1986). *Getting free.* Seattle: The Seal Press.

Painter, S. L., & Dutton, D. (1985). Patterns of emotional bonding in women: Traumatic bonding. *International Journal of Women's Studies, 8,* 363–375.

Pence, E., Paymar, M., Ritmeester, T., & Shepard, M. (Eds.) (1993). *Education groups for men who batter: The Duluth model.* New York: Springer.

Phillips, D. S. H. (1998). Culture and systems of oppression in abused women's lives. *JOGNN, 27,* 678–683.

Pleck, E. (1987). *Domestic tyranny: The making of American social policy against family violence from colonial times to the present.* New York: Oxford University Press.

Relf, M. V. (2001). Battering and HIV in men who have sex with men: A critique and synthesis of the literature. *Journal of the Association of Nurses in AIDS Care, 12*(3), 41–48.

Rennison, C. (2001). *Violent victimization and race, 1993–98.* Washington, DC: Bureau of Justice Statistics, US Department of Justice.

Renzetti, C. M. (1992). *Violent betrayal: Partner abuse in lesbian relationships.* Thousand Oaks, CA: Sage.

Rich, A. (1979). *On lies, secrets, and silence.* New York: W.W. Norton.

Roberts, D. (1997). *Killing the Black body.* New York: Pantheon.

Russell, D. (1990). *Rape in marriage.* Bloomington, IN: Indiana University Press.

Saltzman, L. E., Fanslow, J. L., McMahon, P. M., & Shelley, G. A. (1999). *Intimate partner violence surveillance: Uniform definitions and recommended data elements, version 1.0.* Atlanta, GA: National Center for Injury Prevention and Control, Centers for Disease Prevention.

Sampselle, C. M. (1991). The role of nursing in preventing violence against women. *Journal of Obstetric and Gynecological Nursing, 20,* 481–487.

Schecter, S. (1982). *Women and male violence: The visions and struggles of the battered women's movement.* Boston: South End Press.

Schram, D. (1978). Rape. In J. R. Chapman & M. Gates (Eds.), *The victimization of women* (pp. 53–79). Beverly Hills: Sage.

Sharps, P. W., Campbell, J. C., Campbell, D. W., Gary, F. A., & Webster, D. (2001). The role of alcohol use in intimate partner femicide. *The American Journal on Addictions, 10,* 122–135

Silliman, J. M., & King, Y. (Eds.). (1999). *Dangerous intersections: Feminist perspectives on population, environment, and development.* Boston: South End Press.

Smith, M. D. (1987). The incidence and prevalence of woman abuse in Toronto. *Violence & Victims, 2*(3), 173–188.

Snell, J. E., Rosenwald, R. J., & Robey, A. (1964). The wife-beater's wife. *Archives of General Psychiatry, 11,* 107–112.

Stark, E., & Flitcraft, A. (1996). *Women at risk: Domestic violence and women's health.* Thousand Oaks, CA: Sage.

Stark, E., Flitcraft, A., & Frazier, W. (1979). Medicine and patriarchal violence: The social construction of a "private" event. *International Journal of Health Services, 9,* 461–493.

Straus, M. (1980). Wife-beating: How common and why? In M. A. Straus & G. T. Hotaling (Eds.), *The social causes of husband-wife violence* (pp. 23–38). Minneapolis, MN: University of Minnesota Press.

Straus, M., & Gelles, R. J. (1990). *Physical violence in American families.* New Brunswick, NJ: Transaction.

Testa, M., & Leonard, K. E. (2001). The impact of husband physical aggression and alcohol use on marital functioning: Does alcohol "excuse" the violence? *Violence and Victims, 16*(5), 507–516.

Tiger, L. (1969). *Men in groups.* New York: Random House.

Tjaden, P., & Thoennes, N. (2000). *Full report of the prevalence, incidence, and consequences of violence against women* (Publication No. NCJ-183781). Washington, DC: National Institute of Justice.

Tjaden, P., Thoennes, N., & Allison, C. J. (1999). Comparing violence over the life span in samples of same-sex and opposite-sex cohabitants. *Violence & Victims, 14*(4), 413–426.

Toby, J. (1966). Violence and the masculine ideal. *American Academy of Political and Social Science, 364,* 19.

Tolson, A. (1977). *The limits of masculinity.* New York: Harper & Row.

Turrell, S. C. (2000). A descriptive analysis of same-sex relationship violence for a diverse sample. *Journal of Family Violence, 15*(3), 281–293.

Ulrich, Y.C. (1991). Women's reasons for leaving abusive spouses. *Health Care for Women International, 12,* 465–473.

Walker, L. E. (1979). *The battered woman.* New York: Harper and Row.

Walker, L. E. (1984). *The battered woman syndrome.* New York: Springer.

Warshaw, C., & Ganley, A. (1995). *Improving the health care response to domestic violence: A resource manual for health care providers.* San Francisco: Family Violence Prevention Fund.

West, C. M. (1998a). Leaving a second closet: Outing partner violence in same-sex couples. In J. L. Jasinski & L. M. Williams (Eds.), *Partner violence: A comprehensive review of 20 years of research* (pp. 163–183). Thousand Oaks, CA: Sage.

West, C. M. (1998b). Lifting the "political gag order": Breaking the silence around partner violence in ethnic minority families. In J. L. Jasinski & L. M. Williams (Eds.), *Partner violence: A comprehensive review of 20 years of research* (pp. 184–209). Thousand Oaks, CA: Sage.

Whiting, B. (1965). Sex identity conflict and physical violence: A comparative study. *American Anthropologist, 67,* 126.

Williams, J. S., & McGrath, J. (1978). A social profile of urban gun owners. In J. A. Lonciardi & A. E. Pottieger (Eds.), *Violent Crime.* Beverly Hills: Sage.

Wilson, M., & Daly, M. (1993). An evolutionary psychological perspective on male sexual proprietariness and violence against wives. *Violence and Victims, 8,* 271–294.

Wood, K., & Jewkes, R. (2001). Dangerous love: Reflections on violence among Xhosa township youth. In R. Morrell (Ed.). *Changing men in southern Africa* (pp. 317–336). Pietermaritzburg, South Africa: University of Natal Press.

World Health Organization (2001). *Violence against women* [On-line]. Available: www5.who.int/violence_injury_prevention/main.cfm?p=0000000072.

World Health Organization (2002). *World report on violence and health.* Geneva, Switzerland: World Health Organization.

Wuest, J., & Merritt-Gray, M. (1999). Not going back: Sustaining the separation in the process of leaving abusive relationships. *Violence Against Women, 5,* 110–133.

Xu, X., Campbell, J. C., & Zhu, F. (2001). *Domestic violence against women in China: Prevalance, risk factors and health outcomes.* Paper presented at the Annual American Public Health Association, Atlanta, GA.

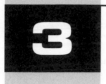

3

Theories of Child Abuse

• Faye A. Gary, Doris W. Campbell, and Janice Humphreys

EPIDEMIOLOGY AND CONSEQUENCES

Child maltreatment is found in all societies throughout the world and is typically shrouded in secrecy. Making inferences about child maltreatment prevalence and incidence worldwide is difficult because of the differences in definitions, methods of reporting the incidence, and various approaches to interpreting the occurrence of abuse. It is suggested, however, that child maltreatment is at epidemic proportions in developed and less-developed countries (Sedlak & Broadhurst, 1996). International data related to child maltreatment suggests that global prevalence is similar to data in North America, with about 20% of females and between 3% and 11% of males having been involved in sexual abuse before age 18. Little data are available from Africa, the Middle East, and the Far East nations (Finkelhor, 1994). The concern for about 1 million children who are yearly forced into prostitution, pornography, and other devastating acts throughout the world continues (Wolfe & Yuan, 2001).

In the United States, according to the National Center on Child Abuse and Neglect (NCCAN), about 3 million cases of child abuse were reported (NCCAN, 1997). Neglect is the most common complaint of maltreatment; it affects about 30 of every 1,000 children and represents 70% of all reported cases of abuse. Physical abuse occurs in 22% of reported cases, sexual abuse in 11%, and emotional maltreatment in 18% of all child abuse incidents. Critical data about the circumstances and outcomes of child maltreatment are not yet available from worldwide or national sources but will be important for surveillance and public policy promulgation. Future inquiry should include more details about antecedents of maltreatment, the role of the child in the maltreatment dynamics of abuse, the severity of physical and psychiatric disorders present in the victim and the perpetrator, parent and caregiver inadequacy, the nature of the abuse (frequency, duration, severity), and circumstances surrounding the maltreatment, including methods used to avoid disclosure and retain secrecy (Wolfe & Yuan, 2001).

This chapter presents content on the prevalence and associated costs of child maltreatment. It highlights theories used to conceptualize and understand child maltreatment and provides information about assessment, including specific clinical and research measures that can be administered to the child and parents or caregivers at various points during the management of child maltreatment. It concludes with implications for clinical and policy matters.

Long-Term Costs of Child Abuse and Neglect

Child abuse and neglect have documented physical, psychological, and behavioral consequences on children (Sedlak & Broadhurst, 1996). Examples of the consequences of abuse include physical injuries (including brain injury), low self-esteem, interrupted bonding with limited capacities to develop and maintain relationships, developmental delays, learning disabilities, and a variety of antisocial behaviors (Kerr, Black, & Krishnakumar, 2000). Child abuse and neglect have correlations with other severe psychiatric disorders, such as depression, posttraumatic stress disorder, and conduct disorders. Other deleterious childhood conditions, such as low academic achievement, early substance use and abuse, early sexual activity and adolescent pregnancy, and juvenile delinquency and subsequent involvement in the juvenile justice system have been linked to child abuse and neglect. Children who have experienced abuse or neglect may also go on to become adult criminals (Pomeroy, Green, & Kiam, 2001).

An average of three children die each day because of child abuse and neglect in this country. This is a tragic loss. Other direct costs of child abuse are difficult to calculate because they include numerous agents and agencies, among which are the child welfare, juvenile justice, law enforcement, judicial, health care, and mental health systems. Within the health care and mental health systems are costs linked to health assessments, hospitalization, and subsequent services to treat the plethora of outcomes: abuse, posttraumatic stress syndromes, foster care, homebound care, rehabilitation of individuals and families, and intensive treatment programs. Child Protective Services (CPS) and related investigative supportive services are typically associated with all aspects of child abuse and neglect (Fromm, 2001; Sedlak & Broadhurst, 1996).

Indirect costs can be conceptualized in terms of long-term consequences associated with child abuse and neglect. Special learning needs; health care, mental health, and substance abuse services; teen pregnancy; juvenile delinquency; and domestic violence are factors that need to be considered when calculating the long-term consequences of child abuse and neglect. Many, although not all, children who have experienced abuse and neglect enter the adult criminal justice system later in life (Wiese & Daro, 1995). The total direct and indirect cost associated with child maltreatment is estimated to be about $92 billion each year. But this staggering figure does not begin to state the catastrophic consequences that the abused children of this nation suffer (Fromm, 2001; Sedlak & Broadhurst, 1996).

Demographics of Child Maltreatment

Research has documented that age and gender are associated with maltreatment risk. Younger children are at higher risk for neglect. For example, infants and toddlers are dependent on their caretakers; with increasing age and independence, the risk for neglect decreases. Developmental phases during which the child asserts independence bring risks for abuse. Specifically, toddler, preschool, and early adolescent transitional periods require new behaviors from the child and adult. As a rule, these developmental transitional periods can place the child in jeopardy for maltreatment. The highest rates of physical abuse occur during adolescence with children aged 12 to 17 years, perhaps because of the conflicts that exist between parent and adolescent child.

Sexual abuse occurs somewhat differently; it becomes a threat to the child at age three and continues (Kaplan, Sadock, & Grebb, 1994; Sedlak & Broadhurst, 1996). Girls are more often abused than boys, with one in every four female children having been abused by age 18, as compared to one in every six boys (Kaplan et al., 1994). In many instances, vulnerable children know and have some type of relationship with the adults who abuse them. Male children are more likely to be abused by people outside the family, whereas females are more vulnerable to male family members. This finding has specific implications for nurses and other health professionals who have clinical assessment responsibilities and who assist with informing public policy (Kaplan et al., 1994; Sedlak & Broadhurst, 1996).

Race or ethnicity is not a significant variable in child maltreatment incidence. However, a few trends are noteworthy. Among children who were sexually abused, Caucasians tended to be more abused by their birth parents than are children of other ethnic and racial groups. In the category of physical abuse, Caucasian children were more often abused by parent substitutes than by birth parents (Sedlak & Broadhurst, 1996).

Clinical and research evidence has suggested that child mistreatment is an antecedent to many social problems in this country. Children who run away from home indicate maltreatment as the major reason for their decision to leave their homes (Gary, Moorhead, and Warren, 1996; Gary & Lopez, 1996). Furthermore, the prison population consists of a large portion of adults who were abused as children (Pomeroy et al., 2001).

Family characteristics are important factors as well in understanding the demographics of child maltreatment. If a child lives in a single-parent household, there is a 77% increased risk for being physically harmed, an 87% greater chance of being physically neglected, and an 89% greater risk of suffering injury or harm related to abuse or neglect, when compared with children who live with two parents. Families with annual incomes of less than $15,000 are about 22 times more likely to have a child who experiences maltreatment within the family, compared with families with annual incomes of $30,000 or more (Sedlak & Broadhurst, 1996). Hence, poverty is an important factor that is associated with child maltreatment.

DEFINITIONS OF CHILD MALTREATMENT

Child maltreatment is not an isolated event but instead takes place within the context of other familial and societal events, such as domestic violence, financial stress, emotional and psychiatric problems, and substance abuse (Hester, Pearson, & Harwin, 2000; Kaplan et al., 1994). Four types of child maltreatment have been clearly documented in the literature: emotional maltreatment, neglect, physical abuse, and sexual abuse (McGleughlin, Meyer, & Baker, 1999; Sedlak & Broadhurst, 1996; Administration of Children and Families, 2002; Weise & Daro, 1995; Wolfe & Yuan, 2001).

Emotional Maltreatment

This type of abuse, though devastating, is difficult to document. It involves attacking the child's self-esteem and sense of self. Verbal threats are typical in this category, as are belittling statements, name-calling, and scapegoating. Parents and caregivers who make unreasonable demands on the child, prescribe an adult role for the child within the household, or terrorize and exploit the child are practicing child emotional maltreatment. Extreme or bizarre forms of punishment, such as washing the child's mouth with soap or a bleach solution, or locking the child in a dark closet for a long period, are other examples. Withholding treatment, refusing to assist a child with a medical regimen, or any other acts of omission that cause or could cause harmful behavioral, cognitive, emotional, or mental disorders fall into this category as well.

Neglect

Food, shelter, clothing, health care, education, guidance, and protection constitute the child's basic needs; the failure of a parent or caregiver to provide for these needs is neglect. Refusal or delay in seeking health care, abandonment, expulsion from home, refusal to allow a runaway child to return home, and inadequate oversight are examples of physical neglect. Emotional neglect can be present too; it exists when the child lives in an environment that does not provide safety, love, self-worth, and a sense of being wanted. Though physically present, the parents or caregivers can be emotionally absent by not responding to these basic emotional needs. Spousal abuse in the child's presence is also a form of child emotional abuse. Educational abuse is likely to occur when the parent or caretaker tolerates truancy, fails to enroll the child in school, or neglects special-education needs required because of the child's physical or psychological challenges.

Physical Abuse

Physical abuse can be confused with physical punishment and behavior modification, although, corporal punishment, if overdone, can be physical abuse. Signs of physical abuse sometimes indicate differences in cultural child-rearing practices, as well as variations in definitions of aberrant behaviors, and responses to those behaviors. (For a more detailed discussion, see Mezzich, Kleinman, Fabrega, & Parron, 1996.) Physical abuse involves the purposeful use of force to the child's body that results or could result in an injury. Hitting, shaking, choking, burning, biting, kicking, poisoning, forcefully restraining a child against his will, and holding the child under water are typical examples of physical abuse.

Sexual Abuse

Sexual abuse involves incest, rape, sodomy, exhibitionism, pornography, prostitution, and the attempted or actual fondling of a child's genitals. It also includes sexual intercourse between a child and an adolescent or adult. These acts can also be considered emotional and physical acts of abuse. They are devastating betrayals of the child's trust and compromise personal safety. Sexual abuse has long-term consequences (Azar, 1989; Faller, 1996; Steward & Steward, 1996; Wachter & Aaron, 1983; Wolfe & Yuan, 2001).

THE ROLE OF THE CHILD IN ABUSE

The child's role in the abuse is usually not explored or discussed, though it is an important aspect to consider in abuse situations (Friedrich & Boriskin, 1976). Certain types of children may be more vulnerable and thus at heightened risk for sexual abuse—for example, children with intellectual disabilities or physical limitations, and children with particular physical characteristics (Balogh et al., 2001). These children may play a passive role in the abuse dynamic. Three conditions need to be in place for the child to be categorized as more vulnerable to abuse, according to Helfer (as reported in Friedrich & Boriskin). First, the child must have certain physical, emotional, or psychological needs (e.g., mental retardation, a health condition that requires additional attention, or clinging or anxious behavior) or must otherwise be perceived to be special or unusual, by the parents. Second, a crisis or a series of crises must have occurred, with the parent or caregiver experiencing more than the usual amount of stress. For example, consider the child with special physical needs who places additional burdens on the family's limited financial resources and requires more time for basic care. Third, an abiding potential in the parent to abuse or display pathological aggression toward the child must be present. Single parents without support networks or additional resources in times of need are more likely to express their aggression toward a vulnerable child. A child who is perceived to interfere with the goals of a parent or caregiver may become a source of frustration; certain events can trigger within the parent or caregiver the urge to harm that source.

The parent's or caregiver's tolerance for and belief about corporal punishment should also be considered. Child maltreatment must be separated from cultural beliefs and practices. Nurses and other health care professionals can explore with parents and caregivers their feelings, thoughts, and actions toward a child. If the health care professional determines that a child is at risk, he or she can administer additional assessment instruments or further inquire about the child's well-being. The child's safety should always be of paramount importance to the nurse and other health care providers.

SPECIFIC THEORIES

Over the past 3 decades, scientists have begun to explore child maltreatment from an empirical perspective, applying more rigid methodological approaches. However, the lack of universally acceptable definitions of child maltreatment has slowed the advancement of scientific knowledge until more recently. Research has aided health and social welfare professionals in better understanding that the theories of child maltreatment that utilize a single-cause model (individual or family tension) is not sufficient to explain such a complex phenomenon. A more integrated point of view is currently endorsed for the exploration of all types of abuse. However, our understanding of emotional maltreatment and neglect, to date, remains underdeveloped and does not allow for in-depth study, due to limited elucidation (Azar, Povilaitis, Lauretti, & Pouquette 1998).

One researcher, Azar (1991), developed a useful framework for identifying the different dimensions related to child abuse. She posited that one should consider the abuse's origins (group, individual, and culture), complexity (single or multiple causes), antecedent and consequence paradigm, and other factors. Azar assumed that theorists and clinicians make decisions based on all the preceding factors, though those decisions may be implicit.

Definitions of abuse guide the theorist's thinking and the subsequent assumptions. For instance, if child maltreatment is viewed by the theorist as being based on aggression, then theories about aggression are used to explain these behaviors. On the other hand, if the theorist thinks the context or environment is

BOX 3-1 **STAGES OF CHILD MALTREATMENT**

Stage 1: Parent or caregiver holds unrealistic standards regarding what are appropriate behaviors for the child.
Stage 2: Parent perceives the child's behavior as falling below expectations and standards.
Stage 3: Caregiver misinterprets the child's behavior but does not question her or his assigned meanings to the child's behavior. The adult does not query self when interventions fail to change the child's behavior.
Stage 4: The caregiver overreacts to the child's behavior after he or she has made some ineffective attempt to bring about the desired behavior in the child. The caregiver proceeds to severely punish the child.

important in explaining abuse, then family and environment are explored. Yet other theorists explain child maltreatment as the outer edge of normal parenting, with the other end of the continuum being optimal or effective parenting (Azar, 1989).

A useful method for conceptualizing the stages of child maltreatment is presented in Box 3-1 (Azar, 1989).

Efforts to prevent abuse and enhance adequate assessment and management of the victim and perpetrator are determined by clearly articulated and tested etiological theories. Theories guide the creation of interventions that target the cause and maintenance of the abuse. Five theories are briefly presented here: social learning theory, ecological theory, attachment theory, family systems theory, and resiliency theory.

Social Learning Theory

The social learning theory posits that behavior is learned (Bandura, 1977). Two basic methods of learning are proposed. First, the individual learns by rewards for a particular behavior, which reinforce that behavior. Second, the individual observes and then imitates the behavior prevalent in the environment. It has been suggested that abused children learn about aggression through modeling; that is, they imitate the behaviors they observe and are sometimes forced to participate in. Children who observe and participate in aggressive acts may continue to participate in them in their adult lives. The term "cycle of violence" suggests that there is an intergenerational transmission of violence through this system of learning (Flay, Allred, & Ordway, 2001; Widom, 1989; National Institute of Justice, 2002).

Social learning theory does not account for the majority of adults who, though abused as children, do not abuse others. Approximately 20% to 30% of abused children become abusers during adulthood. Social learning theory may not account for the multiple factors that could also help to explain child abuse, among which are levels of family functioning. For this complex problem, social learning theory appears simplistic (Flay et al., 2001; National Institute of Justice, 2002).

Intervention programs that embrace this model tend to have two basic approaches: discussion and interaction. The discussion aspect is less likely to work well with families from lower socioeconomic groups (National Institute of Justice, 2002). The action-oriented focus can occur during numerous therapeutic interactions between nurses and parents or caregivers. When the parents or caregivers are interacting with the nurse, the nurse can use this time to model nurturing, communicating, caring, and other age-appropriate responses (Knap & Deluty, 1989). Social learning theory is sometimes compared to ecological theory, but there are differences (Bandura, 1977).

Ecological Theory

Ecological theory suggests that multiple factors are associated with child maltreatment. Four systems are employed to describe the ecological theory approach: individual, family, community, and culture. Individual components are internal to the person, and behaviors manifest themselves based on the person's realities. The family system encompasses child-rearing history, socioeconomic factors, and child and parental characteristics. Components of the community include its level of safety and the values of its members. The sociopolitical milieu within which one lives and works, the characteristics of the neighborhood, and the influence of schools and churches interact to create a culture that ultimately influences the family (Belsky, 1980; National Institute of Justice, 2002; Young, 1964).

Ecological theorists postulate that child maltreatment is due to multiple factors that influence the family. Community violence is often cited as a causative agent in situations where the general milieu is hostile to children and their parents. Violence in a community can cause a family to isolate itself for reasons of safety. Isolation might bring some protection, but it can also create devastating outcomes; when families that are stressed or that have some maladaptive beliefs and behaviors become isolated, the children could be at greater risk. Isolation is the breeding ground for "family secrets." Weak ties with others in the community can cut off the family and allow child maltreatment, when it exists, to continue and even escalate (Granovetter, 1973). If a family develops a code of silence regarding child abuse, its isolation and weak ties with other family resources are likely to prevent intervention (Azar, 1989; Faller, 1996; Administration of Children and Families, 2002; Finkelhor, 1994; Wachter & Aaron, 1983).

Like social learning theory, ecological theory presents a rather rigid or linear approach to child maltreatment. It does not focus enough on individual adult or child variations. Just as significantly, it does not account for the intensity or density with which one or several of these levels might influence the behaviors of the adults and the child. Children can continue to be abused regardless of familial involvement at any level. That is to say, a child who is heavily involved with peers, participates in school activities, and continues to achieve academically might be sworn to silence or secrecy within the family about being abused. On the other hand, another child and family that is socially isolated from peers or adults at school and has a history of poor school performance could also be hiding abuse. Family secrecy would probably be a driving force in this familial dynamic. The developmental stage of the child can also have an impact on the ecological system at any given time.

One feature of the ecological model is that it requires the nurse and other health professionals to examine the child's plight beyond the immediate family and consider other circumstances that could influence the family. Programs that employ this model are likely to focus on parents' groups, home and school visitation, coordination of services with other agents and agencies within the community, and economic support as available (Belsky, 1980). One popular intervention program, the National Head Start and Public School Early Childhood Demonstration Project is an example.

Attachment Theory

The attachment theory suggests that children and their caregivers develop behavioral interactions that are mutually beneficial to each other. At the core of positive interpersonal relationships is the degree to which children and caregivers experience positive interactions that lay the foundation for future trusting human associations (Healey & Garrett, 1997). Attachment theory further categorizes attachment relationships as secure, anxious and ambivalent, anxious and avoidant, and disorientated and disorganized. If, for example, a child is secure and resolute about the attachment with caregivers, he or she feels unrestrained when exploring the environment and is eager to learn and continue to interact with others. This type of relationship is most desirable and is considered healthy. In the anxious and ambivalent relationship, the child does not easily differentiate between the capacity of the primary caregiver and of a stranger to provide comfort and solace. A child with an anxious and avoidant attachment relationship is likely to experience more psychological discomfort that is associated with distrust of the caregiver, as well as a stranger. That child is less likely to explore his or her environment and sometimes presents with clinging behaviors. It is difficult to bring comfort to this child. This type of child could occasionally present with physical problems, such as stomachache or colic, or could be a frequent crier. A child who has disoriented and disorganized patterns of attachment is experiencing high levels of stress and discomfort, in part, because of the confusion about how he or she should behave to gain approval and strengthen the attachment with the caregiver. This child is at high risk for other physical and psychological problems during his or her formative and adult years (Bowlby, 1969, 1973; Healey & Garrett, 1997; McGleughlin et al., 1999).

Children who are in the latter two categories are more likely to have experienced maltreatment and are less sure about whether it is safe to trust others. Such children should be monitored for low self-esteem. As adults they may unconsciously seek out pathological or deleterious relationships, and their lives could be entwined with violence and abuse. Maltreatment during childhood may create internal patterns that manifest in adulthood in interactions with one's own children and other adults. Hence, the nurse should suspect abuse in children who present with attachment problems, and should work to rule out violence in intimate relationships.

This theory is based on one factor: child–caregiver interactions. The importance of this factor should be considered in assessments, but it should not be a single predictor of child abuse. Furthermore, not all children who have experienced inadequate attachment patterns will grow up to become abusers. The perpetrator model (Azar, 1991; Hester et al., 2000) does not explain the plethora of other factors that could be in the abuse model.

Programs based on this theory suggest that the focus should be on strengthening attachment bonds between child and caregiver, even if it means placing the child in another home environment. A second perspective is to allow the child to remain in the existing home and teach the caregiver how to relate more appropriately and effectively with the child. The goal here is to overhaul the behavioral patterns in the relationship (Azar, 1991; Hester et al., 2000; Vulliamy & Sullivan, 2000; Wolfe & Yuan, 2001).

Family Systems Theory

Family systems theory considers the structure of the family and roles of all family members. The intent of interventions based on this theory is to transform the interactions among family members, strengthen specific roles and functions, and diminish or eliminate other roles and functions, with an eye toward creating a more functional or healthier family (Minuchin & Fishman, 1981).

Each family member's perceptions about the presenting problem is of interest to the nurse and other health care providers. A stepfather, for example, who abuses a child is viewed as only one part of the system within which the abuse occurs. The roles and functions of the mother, siblings, and other close relatives would also be explored. If the others did not intervene, that would be explored with the understanding that it was unspoken approval of the abuse. Family systems theory has grown in popularity over the past 3 decades and has received much attention for its usefulness when treating children and adolescents with mental health problems such as depression, suicidal tendencies, and schizophrenia.

The nurse will need to consider some key points when determining the utility of this model for the management of child maltreatment (Healey & Garrett, 1997; Minuchin & Fishman, 1981; Sedlak & Broadhurst, 1996; Wolfe, 2001). For example, the perpetrator is usually an adult who has power and authority over the child. The size of the adult relative to the child must be considered, as it has a profound influence on the child's capacity to take control (or not take control) of an abusive situation. Others in the family system may be unable or unwilling to take action. Therefore, the influence of power and authority and its potential consequences ought to be a component of the assessment.

Family systems models do not, traditionally, account for the use and abuse of power and authority that the perpetrator exercises over the victim and others in the immediate environment. In the scenario described, the child, mother, and other siblings are all victims of the father's predatory behaviors. Family systems theories would suggest exploring these issues with the family.

Programs that employ the family systems model highlight interfamilial relationships and communications. The therapist would convene the family members and, during the assessment, ask for clarifications about communications, decision-making, supports, subsystems, roles, functions, alliances, and points of tension. In most instances, conversations about sexual expressions would probably begin in an adult–adult discussion with children out of the session. However, depending on the topic and the nature of the abuse, children may be asked to join the session (Healey & Garrett, 1997; Minuchin & Fishman, 1981; Sedlak & Broadhurst, 1996; Wolfe, 2001).

This model also allows for the integration of other theories, such as attachment or social learning approaches. The attachment theory within the family systems context, for example, would highlight methods of strengthening the bonding between child and parent within the family context. If systems theory were used, the focus would be on learned behaviors.

Resiliency Theory

Resiliency theory seeks to explain how children survive abuse and are not damaged because of it. This theoretical approach does not explain why and under what circumstances the maltreatment occurred. The "cycle of violence" can be explored from this theoretical perspective because it explores the key elements that prohibit or forestall the abuse. Resiliency theory does not focus on the perpetrator of the abuse.

Resiliency can best be understood as focusing on those factors that help protect the child and provide the stimulus for continuous healthy growth and development. Research studies detail specific key elements that can be included in clinical trials where interventions and treatment are tested in controlled settings and definitive statements are made about the utility of the interventions over the short and long term.

Child maltreatment interventions are based on the premise that the child is harmed by the trauma. Mediating factors were not originally discussed as a method of defense against the trauma. Recent thinking suggests that variables such as severity and frequency of abuse, age of the victim at the time of the abuse, and the relationship of the perpetrator to the child can influence overall adjustment in later years. A specific mediating element that provides protective mechanism against abuse is support from a caring adult (Testa, Miller, Downs, & Panek, 1992). Healthy support systems can aid the child in framing the experience and enhancing self-esteem and can encourage future positive relationships with adults.

Resiliency theory and its accompanying interventions are not sufficient in themselves to deal with the complexities of child maltreatment. Although the approach centers on reducing the deleterious effects of child maltreatment, it does not address prevention of specific abuse and methods to counter the prevalence of abuse in general.

Intervention programs that utilize this theoretical orientation center on methods designed to enhance the protective features in an abused child's life. These intervention programs emphasize the use of community resources and reliance on inner strength, as well as the therapeutic effects of healthy adults working with children and teaching/demonstrating healthy coping strategies useful in problem solving and stress management. A key factor in this approach is the development of close relationships with trusting adults (Pomeroy et al., 2001; Runtz & Schallow, 1997; Testa et al., 1992; Wolfe & Yuan, 2001). Programs grounded in resiliency theory utilize mentors to help children in school and other community-based activities. A mentor helps the child with competencies necessary to navigate the activities of daily living at a particular age. Mentors can help with schoolwork, decision-making, enhanced self-esteem, crisis management, and coping skills. One program that utilizes resiliency underpinnings is the PACT (Parents and Children Together) program. This intervention was originally funded by the Department of Juvenile Justice, State of Florida (S. Hankinson, personal communication, 1998).

SCREENING FOR CHILD MALTREATMENT

In 2000, approximately 1,200 children in the United States died because of abuse and neglect—1.71 per 100,000 children. Of the 1,200 deaths, 44% were children younger than 1 year of age; 85% were younger than 6 years old (National Child Abuse and Neglect Data System, 2000). These facts are compelling evidence that early identification of child maltreatment is one of the major components of prevention. It is important for all clinicians, and others who

BOX 3-2	SCREENING AND TREATMENT OF MALTREATED CHILDREN

GENERAL SIGNS AND SYMPTOMS OF CHILD MALTREATMENT

- Displays symptoms of anxiety or depression
- Demonstrates social withdrawal and clinging behaviors
- Displays aggressive behaviors
- Exhibits low self-esteem
- Has attention deficit; poor school achievement
- Is fearful, anxious, and highly critical of self
- Has insatiable need for attention from others
- Shows a mismatch between behaviors and age
- Exhibits role-reversal behaviors
- Demonstrates a sudden change in behavior
- Develops psychiatric disorders in adolescence: eating disorders, runaway behaviors, posttraumatic stress syndrome, major depression and suicidal tendencies, anxiety disorders, psychosis

RECOMMENDED ACTIONS

- Interview the parent or caregiver
- Interview the child: trauma history and mental-status examination

SYMPTOM-SPECIFIC MEASURES: CHILD

- Brief Assessment of Traumatic Events (BATE)
- UCLA Loneliness Scale
- Children's Depression Inventory (CDI)
- Revised Children's Manifest Anxiety Scale (RCMAS)
- Conners' Rating Scale
- Child and Adolescent Psychiatric Assessment (CAPA)
- Denver Developmental Screening Test II
- Trauma Symptom Checklist–Children
- Piers-Harris Self Concept Scale

SYMPTOM-SPECIFIC MEASURES: PARENT/CAREGIVERS

- Symptom Checklist-90-R
- Family History and Relationships
- Parenting Stress Index
- Family Assessment Measure
- Recent Life Changes Questionnaire
- General Health Questionnaire
- Mental Status Examination

Data from Ambuel, B. (1995). *Family peace project.* Family and Community Medicine, Medical College of Wisconsin [Online]; Swenson, C., & Hanson, R. (Eds.). (1998). *Handbook of child abuse research and treatment.* New York: Plenum Press; and Zarin, D., & Ryan, N. (2000). *Handbook of psychiatric measures.* Washington, DC: American Psychiatric Association.

work with children, to be aware of the basic signs and symptoms of child maltreatment.

Useful areas to examine during assessment are trauma history, child health and mental health symptoms, and family history, conflicts, and relationships.

The measures listed in Box 3-2 are selected because of their particular value in aiding in the screening and treatment of child maltreatment. For a more detailed review of these instruments, consult the references as listed. A brief discussion of the three areas follows.

Trauma History

A clinical interview with the child is an important component of the overall assessment. The interviewer should remember not to rush the child but instead allow time for rapport to develop and be aware of the child's readiness to discuss the trauma. Play therapy is an excellent method to use when working with children who have experienced, or are suspected of having experienced, trauma. Puppets, drawings, anatomically correct dolls, family dolls, and pictures are essential tools for the interview (Goodman & Aman, 1990; Swenson & Hanson, 1998). The Brief Assessment of Traumatic Events (BATE) provides a structured process that helps to determine the child's exposure to physical abuse, sexual abuse, and domestic violence. It is important for the interviewer to ask the child about other types of violent acts, such as fires, car accidents, life-threatening illnesses, and natural disasters (Azar et al., 1998; Swenson & Hanson, 1998).

A clinical interview with the parents or caregivers is of equal importance. The parent or caregiver should be asked to provide detailed information about the maltreatment incident as well as historical information about the child that is considered relevant. Information about the child's educational, medical, mental health, developmental, and family history before and after the abuse incident should be elicited from the parent or caregiver. The interviewer should then shift to the parents or caregivers, and determine whether trauma has been a component in their lives. If prior maltreatment of parents or caregivers has not been resolved, the child may be compromised (MacFarlane & Waterman, 1986; Mierendorf & Sarandon, 2000; Steward and Steward, 1996; Wolfe & Yuan, 2001).

Child Mental Health and Behaviors

Self-report assessment instruments should be used to obtain information from the child. Numerous instruments exist to elicit information about the child. It is important to document general mental health symptoms as well as trauma-specific symptoms. The Children's Depression Inventory (CDI) is a widely used 27-item instrument used to assess the affective, cognitive, and behavioral dimensions of depression in the child (Kovacs, 1992; Swenson & Hanson, 1998). The Revised Children's Manifest Anxiety Scale (RCMAS) contains 37 items that query the child about anxiety-related symptoms (Zarin & Ryan, 2000). Self-concept can be assessed with the Piers-Harris Self-Concept Scale, which measures behavior, intelligence and school performance, physical appearance and other attributes, anxiety, popularity, happiness, and satisfaction (Piers, 1984; Zarin & Ryan, 2000).

The Trauma Symptom Checklist—Children (TSC—C) can be administered to children for the determination of trauma-specific symptoms such as posttraumatic stress syndrome. This instrument consists of six domains (Anxiety, Depression, Posttraumatic Stress, Sexual Concerns, Dissociation, and Anger) and can be administered to children between the ages of 8 and 15 (Bierie, 1995; Swenson & Hanson, 1998).

Mental health symptoms and behaviors manifested by the parent or caregiver are of paramount importance as well. Once the parent or caregiver knows that the child has been maltreated and that agents and agencies are involved with the assessment and overall management, a different level of concern is likely to surface. Parental or caregiver response to the reporting of the child's maltreatment can range from little concern to the manifestation of pathological mental health behaviors and a plethora of physical health problems. The Symptom Checklist (SCL-90-R) is a frequently used measure that documents the parent's or caregiver's overall symptomatology. This instrument contains 90 items of self-report that pertain to symptoms experienced over the previous week. The nine subscales in this measure are Somatization, Obsessive-Compulsive, Interpersonal Sensitivity, Depression, Anxiety, Hostility, Phobic Anxiety, Paranoid Ideation, and Psychoticism. It also contains three global scales: Global Severity, Positive Symptom Distress, and Positive Total (Derogatis, 1977; Swenson & Hanson, 1998; Zarin & Ryan, 2000).

Family History of Relationships

Other assessment tests administered to adults and the child can give a more complete understanding of the child–adult relationship. This information is of value because positive familial relationships assist with disclosure, the coping skills of the child and adults, the establishment of a more trusting relationship with the nurse and other professionals, and the overall treatment approach (MacFarlane & Waterman, 1986; Mierendorf & Sarandon, 2000; Minuchin & Fishman, 1981; Striefel, Robinson, & Truhn, 1998; Swenson & Hanson, 1998).

The 25-item Child's Attitude Towards Mother/Father Scale (CAM/CAF) is designed to measure the degree, severity, and magnitude of problems that the child perceives to be present in the relationship with parents and caregivers (Giuli & Hudson, 1977; Hester et al., 2000; Zarin & Ryan, 2000). This instrument can also be administered to siblings in the household. Clinicians should take special interest in determining whether the parental/caregiver relationship to a nonabused child is different than to the abused child. Observing for differences and similarities can sometimes lead to important information that can be used in constructing comprehensive and culturally relevant treatment plans.

A similar instrument, designed for parents and caregivers, is the Index of Parental Attitudes (IPA), which evaluates the parent–child relationship from the adult's point of view. It contains 25 items that query the adults about family relationships (Giuli & Hudson, 1977; Hudson, Wung, & Borges, 1980).

A thorough and accurate assessment of the child's and adults' perceptions and experiences are the key elements for the development of a relevant and comprehensive treatment plan. Formal measures provide excellent data at any phase of the treatment and can be used as baseline and termination points in the treatment. Comparing the difference in data generated at the beginning and ending of the process will generate important clinical data about evidence-based outcomes (Azar, 1991; Barnett, Miller-Perrin, & Perrin, 1997; Swenson & Hanson, 1998; Tzeng, Jackson, & Karlson, 1991).

PUBLIC POLICY AND FUTURE IMPLICATIONS

Substance abuse, mental health problems, physical health problems, disabilities, spouse abuse, unemployment, and alienation and isolation are but some of the experiences that constantly confront children who have been abused (Chalk, Gibbons, & Scarupa, 2002; Fagan & Wexler, 1987; Administration of Children and Families, 2002; Finkelhor, 1994; Gary-Hopps, Penderhughes, & Shunkar, 1995). Local, state, and national efforts should be intensified to reduce the devastating experiences that children and families confront on a daily basis.

Intensified research efforts are needed to improve the quality of data collection and dissemination to clinicians and other researchers. One focus for improved research should be in the area of prevention or unraveling the antecedent factors that are associated with child maltreatment. Currently, many of the resources available for the child abuse problem are applicable only after the child has been maltreated, with less emphasis on prevention and prior intervention. Schools, nurseries, social service agencies, and faith-based communities are examples of places where teaching about prevention of child maltreatment can occur. Communities could establish indicators of well-being to estimate risk or potential risk, develop strategic plans, articulate positive milestones for at-risk populations, and monitor the overall development of children (Chalk et al., 2002; Coohey & Braun, 1997; Finkelhor, 1994; Fromm, 2001; Gary, Moorhead, & Warren, 1996; Neglect, 1997; Wolfe & Yuan, 2001).

Strengthening the prevention, assessment, and treatment aspects of care could advance the clinical and research aspects of child maltreatment. Utilizing specific formal measures in the overall screening and treatment process could help clinicians, social service agencies, and researchers with program development that is specific for the child and family and available for evidence-based evaluations and outcomes.

Health care providers, law enforcement personnel, social service professionals, teachers, and other individuals who are in frequent contact with children should have more exposure to a universal curriculum that outlines the major indicators of child abuse and to a delineation of the best practices for the prevention and treatment of child maltreatment. This important information should be made available at all health and social service institutions, as well as at public and private schools.

SUMMARY

Child maltreatment is a major public health problem in the United States and the world. Theories that address this phenomenon should be strengthened and used to guide and direct clinical care and research programs. Theory-based best-practice guidelines could aid communities in the implementation of child maltreatment indicators, databases generated from formal research measures administered over time to children and parents/caregivers. Nurses and other health care providers are natural advocates for the promulgation of theories, public policy, and improved clinical practice for abused children and their families.

References

Administration of Children and Families. (2002). *What is child maltreatment?* U.S. Department of Health and Human Services. [Online]. Available: www.healthfinder.gov/orgs/HR0078.htm.

Ambuel, B. (1995). *Family peace project.* Family and Community Medicine, Medical College of Wisconsin [Online]. Available: www.family.mcw.edu/FamilyPeaceProject.

Azar, S. (1991). Models of child abuse: A metatheoretical analysis. *Criminal Justice and Behavior, 18,* 37.

Azar, S. T. (1989). Training parents of abused children. In J. M. Briesmeister (Ed.), *Handbook of parent training* (pp. 414–441). New York: Wiley.

Azar, S., Povilaitis, T., Lauretti, A., Pouquette, C. (1998). The current status of etiological theories in intrafamilial child maltreatment. In J. R. Lutzker (Ed.), *Handbook of child abuse research and treatment* (pp. 3–30). New York: Plenum Press.

Balogh, R., Bretherton, K., Whibley, S., Berney, T., Graham S., Richold, P., Worsley, C., & Firth, H. (2001). Sexual abuse in children and adolescents with intellectual disability. *Journal of Intellectual Disability Research, 45,* 194–201.

Bandura, A. (1977). *Social learning theory.* Upper Saddle River, NJ: Prentice-Hall.

Barnett, O. W., Miller-Perrin, C. L., & Perrin, R. D. (1997). *Family violence across the lifespan: An introduction.* Thousand Oaks, CA: Sage.

Belsky, J. (1980). Child maltreatment: An ecological integration. *American Psychologist, 35,* 320–335.

Bierie, J. (1995). *Trauma symptom inventory professional manual.* Odessa, FL.: Psychological Assessment Resources.

Bowlby, J. (1969). *Attachment and loss I.* New York: Basic Books.

Bowlby, J. (1973). *Attachment and loss II.* New York: Basic Books.

Chalk, R., Gibbons, A., & Scarupa, H. (2002). *Trends: Child research brief.* Washington, DC: Child Trends.

Coohey, C., & Braun, N. (1997). Toward an integrated framework for understanding child physical abuse. *Child Abuse & Neglect, 21*(11), 1081–1094.

Derogatis, L. (1977). *The SCL-90R: Administration, scoring and procedure manual for the r (revised) version.* Baltimore: Johns Hopkins University School of Medicine.

Fagan, J., & Wexler, S. (1987). Crime at home and in the streets: The relationship between family and stranger violence. *Violence and Victims, 2*(1), 5–23.

Faller, K. C. (1996). *Evaluating children suspected of having been sexually abused.* Thousand Oaks, CA: Sage.

Finkelhor, D. (1994). The international epidemiology of child sexual abuse. *Child Abuse and Neglect, 18,* 409–417.

Flay, B. R., Allred, C. G., & Ordway, N. (2001). Effects of positive action program on achievement and discipline: Two matched-control comparisons. *Preventive Science, 2*(2), 71–89.

Friedrich, W., & Boriskin, B. (1976). The role of the child in abuse: A review of the literature. *American Journal of Orthopsychiatry, 46*(4), 580–590.

Fromm, S. (2001). *Total estimated cost of child abuse and neglect in the United States statistical evidence* [Online]. Available: www.preventchildabuse.org.

Gary, F., & Lopez, L. (1996). The smart life: A community-based approach to assisting troubled youth. *Journal of Primary Prevention, 17*(1), 175–200.

Gary, F., Moorhead, J., & Warren, J. (1996). Characteristics of troubled youths in a shelter. *Archives of Psychiatric Nursing, 10*(1), 41–48.

Gary-Hopps, J., Penderhughes, E., & Shunkar, R. (1995). *The power to care: Clinical effectiveness with overwhelmed clients.* New York: Free Press.

Giuli, C., & Hudson, W. (1977). Assessing parent–child relationship disorders in clinical practice: The child's point of view. *Journal of Social Science Research, 1,* 77–92.

Goodman, G. S., & Aman, C. (1990). Children's use of anatomically detailed dolls to recount an event. *Child Development, 61*(6), 1859–1871.

Granovetter, M. (1973). Strength of weak ties. *American Journal of Sociology, 78,* 1360–1380.

Healey, K., & Garrett, A. (1997). Child abuse interventions strategic planning meeting. Washington, DC: National Institute of Justice [Online]. Available: http://www.ojp.usdoj.gov/nij/childabuse/about.html.

Hester, M., Pearson, C., & Harwin, N. (2000). *Making an impact: Children and domestic violence.* Philadelphia: Jessica Kingsley Publishers.

Hudson, W., Wung, B., & Borges, M. (1980). Parent–child relationship disorders: The parent's point of view. *Journal of Social Service Research, 3,* 283–294.

Kaplan, H. I., Sadock, B. J., & Grebb, J. A. (1994). *Kaplan and Sadock's synopsis of psychiatry: Behavioral sciences, clinical psychiatry* (7th ed.). Baltimore: Williams & Wilkins.

Kerr, M., Black, M., & Krishnakumar, A. (2000). Failure-to-thrive, maltreatment and the behavior and development of 6-year-old children from low-income, urban families: A cumulative risk model. *Child Abuse & Neglect, 24*(5), 587–598.

Knap, P., & Deluty, R. (1989). Relative effectiveness of two behavioral parent training programs. *Journal of Child Psychology, 18,* 314–322.

Kovacs, M. (1992). *The children's depression inventory.* North Tonawanda, NY: Multihealth Systems.

Lutzker, J. (Ed.). (1998). *Handbook of child abuse research and treatment.* New York: Plenum Press.

MacFarlane, K., & Waterman, J. (1986). *Sexual abuse of young children: Evaluation and treatment.* New York: Guildford Press.

McGleughlin, J., Meyer, S., & Baker, J. (Eds.). (1999). *Assessing sexual abuse allegations in divorce, custody, and visitation disputes.* New York: John Wiley & Sons.

Mezzich, J., Kleinman, A., Fabrega, H., & Parron, D. (1996). *Culture and psychiatric diagnosis: A DSM-IV perspective.* Washington, DC: American Psychiatric Press.

Mierendorf, M. (Producer, Director, Writer), & Sarandon, S. (Narrator). (2000). *Broken child* [Film]. (Available from Films for the Humanities & Sciences, P.O. Box 2053, Princeton, NJ 08543-2053.)

Minuchin, S., & Fishman, H. (1981). *Family therapy techniques.* Cambridge, MA: Harvard University Press.

National Center on Child Abuse and Neglect. (1997). *Child maltreatment 1996: Reports from the states to the National Center on Child Abuse and Neglect* [Online]. Available: www.eccac.org/other/fcan.htm.

National Child Abuse and Neglect Data System. (2000). Summary of key findings from calendar year 2000. U.S. Department of Health and Human Services. [Online]. Available: www.governmentguide.com/govsite. adp?bread=*Main&url=http%3A//www.governmentguide. com/ams/clickThruRedirect. adp%3F55076483%2C16920155%2Chttp%3A//www.calib.com/nccanch/prevmnth/index.cfm.

National Institute of Justice (2002). Child abuse intervention strategic planning meeting. U.S. Department of Justice, [Online]. Available: www.ojp.usdoj.gov/nij/childabuse/bg2_01.html.

Piers, E. (1984). *Piers-Harris Children's Self-Concept Scale. Revised manual.* Los Angeles: Western Psychological Services.

Pomeroy, E., Green, D., & Kiam, R. (2001). Female juvenile offenders incarcerated as adults. *Journal of Social Work, 1*(1), 101–115.

Runtz, M., & Schallow, J. (1997). Social support and coping strategies as mediators of adult adjustment following childhood maltreatment. *Child Abuse & Neglect, 21,* 211–226.

Sedlak, A., & Broadhurst, B. (1996) *Executive summary of the third national incidence study of child abuse and neglect* [Online]. Available:www.calib.com/nccanch/pubs/statinfo/nis3.cfm.

Steward, M. S., & Steward, D. S. (1996). *Interviewing young children about body touch and handling.* Chicago: Society for Research in Child Development.

Striefel, S., Robinson, M., & Truhn, P. (1998). Dealing with child abuse and neglect within a comprehensive family-support program. In J. Lutzker (Ed.), *Handbook of child abuse research and treatment* (pp. 267–289). New York: Plenum Press.

Swenson, C., & Hanson, R. (1998). Sexual abuse of children: Assessment, research, and treatment. In J. Lutzker (Ed.), *Handbook of child abuse research and treatment* (pp. 475–500). New York: Plenum Press.

Testa, M., Miller, B., Downs, W., & Panek, D. (1992). The moderating impact of social support following childhood sexual abuse. *Violence and Victims, 7,* 173–186.

Tzeng, O. C. S., Jackson, J. W., & Karlson, H. C. (1991). *Theories of child abuse and neglect: Differential perspectives, summaries, and evaluations.* New York: Praeger.

U.S. Department of Health and Human Services. Fact sheets-Administration for children and families programs. [Online]. Available: www.acf.dhhs.gov/programs/opa/facts/.

Vulliamy, A., & Sullivan, R. (2000). Reporting child abuse: Pediatricians' experiences with the child protection system. *Child Abuse & Neglect, 24*(11), 1416–1470.

Wachter, O., & Aaron, J. (1983). *No more Secrets for me.* Boston: Little Brown.

Widom, C. (1989). The cycle of violence. *Science 244,* 160–165.

Widom, C. S. (1992) The cycle of violence. *Research in Brief,* Washington, DC: U.S. Department of Justice, National Institute of Justice.

Wiese, D., & Daro, D. (1995). *Current trends in child abuse reporting and fatalities: The results of the 1994 annual fifty-state survey* [Online]. Available: www.vix.com/men/abuse/studies/child-ma.html.

Wolfe, D., & Yuan, L. (2001). *A conceptual and epidemiological framework for child maltreatment surveillance.* Ottawa: Minister of Public Work and Government Services Canada. Published by authority of the Minister of Health.

Young, L. R. (1964). *Wednesday's children: A study of child neglect and abuse.* New York: McGraw-Hill.

Zarin, D., & Ryan, N. (2000). *Handbook of psychiatric measures.* Washington, DC: American Psychiatric Association.

PART II

Nursing Practice

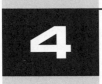

Abuse During Pregnancy

• Barbara Parker, Linda Bullock, Diane Bohn, and Mary Ann Curry

Pregnancy is a time when friends, family, and health professionals expect a woman's partner to be particularly concerned about and attentive to her health and well-being. It is difficult to imagine that anyone, especially the father of the baby, would intentionally injure a pregnant woman, thereby jeopardizing her health and the health of the fetus. However, many pregnant women experience abuse from their male partners. The purpose of this chapter is to summarize current research on abuse during pregnancy and to provide guidance to nurses who work with affected clients.

Nurses, nurse-midwives, and nurse practitioners can play a crucial role in breaking the cycle of violence in the lives of the pregnant women they serve. Pregnancy may be the only time an abused woman has frequent, ongoing contact with someone capable of assisting her. Nursing, as applied to survivors of domestic violence, includes identification, assessment, planning, intervention, and follow-up. The primary role of the nurse is that of advocate. Advocacy with the abused woman includes providing accurate information regarding abusive relationships, domestic-abuse laws, resources, and options, and providing ongoing emotional support regardless of the choices she makes.

Because of the unique aspects of pregnancy, abuse during pregnancy has been a topic of a significant amount of nursing research and clinical interventions. Early research on this topic focused on establishing the rate of abuse in pregnancy, including rates in specific ethnic groups. Early inquiry also included comparing disclosure rates attained through different instruments and different modalities (e.g., interview versus written questionnaire). Subsequent research established the effects of abuse during pregnancy on maternal and infant health and established predictors of abuse in pregnancy. Later research validated previous findings, included new variables, and tested beginning nursing interventions. This growing body of research provides a strong basis for nursing practice with abused pregnant women.

STUDIES OF INCIDENCE RATES

Early prospective surveys of pregnant women in public prenatal facilities (n = 1,203) in Maryland and Texas found 19% of African-American and Caucasian women and 14% first-generation Mexican-American women were abused while they were pregnant (McFarlane, Parker, Soeken, & Bullock, 1992; McFarlane, Parker, & Soeken, 1995). Abuse in the year prior to the pregnancy was a major predictor of abuse during pregnancy, with 55% of women who were abused while pregnant reporting abuse before pregnancy. Additionally, in this sample of women, the frequency and severity of abuse during pregnancy was greatest for the Caucasian women. When the same data set was analyzed by age, the investigators found that 22% of the pregnant adolescents reported abuse in pregnancy, compared to 16% of the adults (Parker, McFarlane, & Soeken, 1994). Rates in the year prior to pregnancy were 32% for teens and 24% for adults. Curry, Perrin, and Wall (1998) found similar rates: 38% of teens and 23% of adults. Both Curry (Curry, Perrin, & Wall, 1998) and Parker et al. (1994, 1996; McFarlane, Parker, & Soeken, 1996b) found a relationship between abuse and subsequent low birth weight (LBW) of the infant, validating the original work documenting this relationship, first described by Bullock and McFarlane (1989). In a large review of studies in the United States, Gazmarian and colleagues (2000) found an incidence range of 0.9% to 20.1%, with most estimates between 4% and 8%. The range of prevalence rates of abuse in pregnancy may reflect differences in specific clinical populations, geographic locations, definitions of abuse, methods of questioning, and time period of inquiry.

Several other nursing studies have examined rates of abuse in specific populations. Kershner, Long, and Anderson (1998) conducted a descriptive survey of 1,693 women at medical clinics and Women, Infants, and Children (WIC) sites in west-central (rural) Minnesota. The survey instrument was given to a sample of women (94% Caucasian and 4% Native American). Through the Abuse Assessment Screen (AAS), 21% of respondents reported abuse in the past 12 months, of which 89% was perpetrated by a current or former intimate partner. Bohn (2002) studied 30 urban pregnant Native-American women in the Midwest and found that 60% of women were in a relationship in which they had been abused and that 33% reported abuse during the index pregnancy.

Mattson and Rodriguez (1999) surveyed 450 pregnant Latina women to determine prevalence and type of abuse, level of acculturation to the American community, and self-esteem. Based on the AAS, 6.2% indicated abuse during the past year. Self-esteem for abused women was significantly lower than for nonabused women ($p < .05$), and acculturation scores for abused women were significantly higher.

A different approach to the study of abuse in pregnancy was undertaken by Sampselle, Petersen, Murtland, and Oakley (1992); they used survey data to compare the amounts of reported abuse between women who chose to obtain prenatal care from a certified nurse-midwife or a physician. They found a much lower rate of reported abuse than other studies, but they attributed this to the method of data collection (two questions on a written questionnaire that was given to the woman on the first visit). Additionally, the questions asked about experiences of abuse rather than specific violent incidents. Sampselle, however, was able to determine that women who selected a nurse-midwife for care had a higher reported rate of past abuse than women receiving prenatal care from a physician. Additionally, as this was a relatively affluent population, the study provides further evidence that abuse is not restricted to women in lower socioeconomic classes.

Campbell and others (1999) used a multisite case-control design with a sample of 1,004 women to determine the relative risk of LBW associated with intimate partner abuse. Women were purposely recruited to represent six different ethnic groups (African-American, Anglo-American, Cuban, Central-American, Mexican-American, and Puerto Rican groups). They were interviewed during the 72 hours after delivery, with abuse determined by the written Index of Spouse Abuse (ISA) and a modification of the AAS. Puerto Rican women reported abuse during pregnancy in response to the AAS questions in a significantly greater proportion than the other three Latina groups who had the lowest prevalence of all groups (Torres et al., 2000). More acculturation was associated with more physical abuse during pregnancy, as were several of the indicators of cultural norms, such as belief in wife/mother role supremacy for women and cultural-group belief in the acceptability of men hitting women. Physical and nonphysical abuse were both significant risk factors for LBW for the term but not the preterm infants, but the risk estimates became nonsignificant in the adjusted statistical models. This suggested a confounding or mediating effect of other abuse-related maternal health problems (notably low weight gain and poor obstetrical history) and further described the path by which abuse affects birth weight.

SUBSTANCE USE OR ABUSE

For many women, substance use may be a way of self-medicating the pain of involvement in an abusive relationship. Increased rates of substance use during pregnancy have been noted among abuse survivors (Campbell et al., 1999; McFarlane, Parker, & Soeken, 1996b). Significantly increased rates of tobacco use during pregnancy have been found among battered women, compared with non-battered women (Bullock & McFarlane, 1989; McFarlane, Parker, & Soeken, 1996b). An increased rate of drug use during pregnancy among abuse survivors also has been reported (McFarlane et al., 1996b).

Of recent concern during pregnancy is polysubstance use; that is, the use of tobacco, alcohol, and other drugs (Chasnoff, Neuman, Thornton, Callaghan, & Angela, 2001). Although there is some debate about the relative effects of drug, alcohol, and tobacco exposure during pregnancy (Frank, Augustyn, Knight, Pell, & Zuckerman, 2001), negative fetal/infant effects from maternal drug use may include LBW, preterm birth (PTB), congenital malformation, intrauterine growth retardation, intrauterine fetal demise (IUFD), asphyxia, sudden infant death syndrome (SIDS), seizures, hyaline membrane disorders, abnormal behavior and state control, mental retardation, cerebral infarcts, and withdrawal symptoms (Delaney-Black et al., 2001; Wilbourne, Dorato, Yeo, and Curet, 2000). Maternal problems related to drug use during pregnancy may include miscarriage, abruptio placentae, delayed prenatal care, and parenting problems (Brady, Posner, Lang, & Rosati, 1994; McCaul, 1998).

Smoking during pregnancy is associated with a number of adverse effects on the fetus and developing child. These outcomes include LBW, miscarriage, stillbirth, fetal death, SIDS, intrauterine growth retardation, ear and lower-respiratory-tract infections, negative behaviors, and behavioral problems (Freid, Watkinson, & Gray, 1998; Griesler, Kandel, & Davies, 1998; Lipscomb et al., 2000; Thomas, 2001; Varisco, 2001).

Studies that examined alcohol use during pregnancy among abused women have yielded conflicting results. Two studies found increased usage (Amaro, Fried, Cabral, & Zuckerman, 1990; Hillard, 1985), whereas two others report decreased usage (Bullock & McFarlane, 1989; Campbell, Poland, Walker, & Ager, 1992). Alcohol consumption during pregnancy, especially if chronic or heavy, is associated with numerous fetal/infant problems. These problems may include growth and neurodevelopment disorders and deficits; LBW; microcephaly; behavioral, facial, limb, cardiac, genital, and neurological abnormalities; and other anomalies and problems frequently associated with fetal alcohol syndrome or fetal alcohol effect (Jacobs et al., 2000; Lipscomb et al., 2000; Shu, Hatch, Mills, Clemens, & Susser, 1995).

Curry (1998) conducted a prospective study of the interrelationship between abuse during pregnancy, substance use, and psychosocial stress. A total of 1,937 women receiving care were recruited, with abuse being measured by the AAS. Psychosocial stress was measured by the 11-item Prenatal Psychosocial Profile, which includes one question that specifically concerns stress related to abuse. Substance use was measured by confidential self-report of tobacco, marijuana, alcohol, and illicit-drug use. Twenty-seven percent of the participants reported abuse, and 14% reported stress related to abuse. African-American women reported the highest rates of abuse but the lowest rates of stress related to the abuse. Abused white women were more likely to report smoking or alcohol/drug use (or both) than nonabused women, but there was no association between substance use and partner abuse for African-American, Hispanic, Asian, or "other" ethnicity women. Abused women from all ethnic groups reported significantly more stress overall, less social support, and lower self-esteem than did nonabused women ($p < .05$). This study differs from the findings of Campbell and her associates (1992), who found that violence during pregnancy was positively related to drug and alcohol abuse during pregnancy ($r = -.27$, $p = < .01$) in a post partum sample of 900 primarily poor African-American women in an urban area. Similarly, McFarlane, Parker, and Soeken (1996a) found that significantly more abused African-American and Caucasian pregnant women smoked and used alcohol/illicit drugs during pregnancy than nonabused women. They found that, as a triad, smoking, physical abuse, and alcohol/illicit drug use were significantly related to birth weight ($F[3,1040] = 30.19$, $p = <0.001$).

PRENATAL CARE

Early and consistent prenatal care allows ongoing assessment of maternal and fetal well-being, detection of actual or potential problems, and interventions to prevent, modify, or correct pregnancy complications. Absent or inadequate prenatal care may result in suboptimal management of preexisting or pregnancy-related conditions, such as hypertension, diabetes, and infections that could have a negative effect on pregnancy outcomes. Inadequate or absent prenatal care has been associated with PTB, although this relationship is less than clear (Goldenberg & Rouse, 1998).

Abused women, whose pregnancies may already be at risk because of trauma or substance use, could benefit from prenatal care. However, abuse survivors often do not receive adequate care. They may delay entry into care and miss scheduled appointments.

Conflicts with the father of the baby are frequently cited as one reason for delayed care among women entering prenatal care in the last month of pregnancy (McFarlane, Parker, & Soeken, 1996a). In some cases, women may delay care as they try to decide whether to continue or terminate the pregnancy. Ambivalence and denial may also play a role. In other cases, their partner may prevent them from seeking care. Abused women who use or abuse substances during pregnancy may avoid prenatal care because of shame, guilt, or fear of repercussions. Women may miss appointments because their abuser will not let them leave the house or because he denies them access to transportation. The abuser may also purposely detain women, making them late for prenatal appointments. The abused woman or her partner may decide she should miss an appointment if trauma injuries are evident. Finally, the woman may fear she could lose her children if the abuse becomes known.

A number of studies have repeatedly validated the relationship between abuse in pregnancy and delayed entry into prenatal care. McFarlane et al. (1996a) first documented that abused women were much more likely than nonabused women to delay prenatal care. In this study, abused African-American women were twice as likely to begin care during the third trimester, and abused Hispanic women were at a threefold risk of not starting care until the final trimester. Taggart and Mattson (1996) found an abuse rate during pregnancy of 21%. They also reported that abused women sought prenatal care 6.5 weeks later than the nonabused women. Almost 14% of these abused women stated that they had delayed care because of injuries. Long and Curry (1998) noted that Native-American women identified domestic violence as a significant impediment to obtaining prenatal care.

However, in Attala's (1994) survey of 400 women participating in the Women, Infants, and Children (WIC) supplemental food program, there was no relationship between a history of physical abuse and delay in seeking prenatal care. Thirty-one percent of her sample had experienced some physical abuse. Even though no relationship was found between abuse and delay in seeking prenatal care, only 25% of the participants had begun prenatal care after the first trimester.

In contrast with Attala's findings, Curry, Perrin, and Wall (1998) reported that abused adult women in their study were more likely to have unplanned pregnancies ($p < .001$) and to begin care after 20 weeks ($p < .01$) than nonabused women. Abused women were also more likely to have poorer past obstetric histories and to use tobacco, alcohol, and other drugs ($p < .05$).

RELATED HEALTH CONCERNS

In a focus group with sheltered women, Campbell, Pugh, Campbell, and Visscher (1995) described the relationship of abuse to pregnancy intention, pregnancy resolution (abortion, adoption, unwanted infant, wanted infant), and the decision-making process leading to the pregnancy and its resolution. Thematic analysis revealed five major themes: male-partner control, relentless abuse, lack of consistency and jealousy in the partner's relationship with the woman and with offspring, definition of manhood, and health problems. Although the generalizability of the findings is severely limited by the nonrepresentativeness of the sample (i.e., women in shelters), the findings suggest theoretical links between unintended pregnancy and abuse and deserve further investigation. The study findings also are consistent with those of another qualitative investigation (Campbell, Oliver, & Bullock, 1993), namely, that severe abuse during pregnancy can be motivated by the husband's (unfounded) suspicion that the baby does not belong to him. These and other studies further suggest that because of the abuser's common refusal to use condoms, abused women are at risk for sexually transmitted infections (Geilen, O'Campo, Faden, Kass, & Xue, 1994).

Campbell, Soeken, McFarlane, and Parker (1998) studied risk factors for femicide among an ethnically diverse sample ($n = 381$) of women who reported abuse. They found that regardless of ethnicity, women who were abused while pregnant were at a significantly greater risk for femicide than abused women who were not abused when they were pregnant, thus providing beginning evidence that abuse during pregnancy might be a predictor of potential lethal violence.

SPECIAL CONSIDERATIONS FOR WORKING WITH TEENS

If the pregnant woman is an adolescent, there are special considerations. Parents are often very influential in the decision-making of pregnant teens. On one hand, some teens feel pressured to stay in a relationship because their parents admire their boyfriend and encourage the relationship. Pregnant teens may feel further pressure to remain with an abuser in hopes that he will provide financial assistance for their baby. For example, one teen's parents discouraged her from ending her relationship with a violent man because her fiancé was wealthy and successful. On the other hand, for some teens becoming pregnant may be a last-resort strategy for getting out of an abusive family home environment.

In one study, 26% of pregnant teens reported being physically abused by their boyfriends, and half of them reported that the battering started or increased after the partner learned of the pregnancy (Brutin, 1995). In a study of rapid repeat pregnancy among adolescents, a sample of 100 young women, aged 13 to 21, who received prenatal care at a nonprofit health-care center were evaluated for abuse (Jacoby, Gorenflo, Black, Wunderlich, & Eyler, 1999). Experience with interpersonal violence correlated with rapid repeat pregnancy among this sample of low-income adolescents. Within 12 months of giving birth, 43.6% of the participants became pregnant. Within 18 months, 63.2% of participants had experienced at least one additional pregnancy. The participants also reported sexual abuse at some time in their lives, with 44% reporting experiences of physical abuse. Twenty-six percent of the participants reported abuse experiences during the study. The association between current abuse and the presence of at least one spontaneous abortion in the obstetrical history also was significant ($p = 0.007$), suggesting that these women may have been experiencing violence, with resultant pregnancy loss, over a long period of time.

THEORIES: WHY IS THERE ABUSE DURING PREGNANCY?

Theories of why some men abuse women during pregnancy vary widely. Early publications on abuse during pregnancy often noted that abuse began or escalated during pregnancy. Often this belief was a result of observations of the large numbers of pregnant women in shelters. Other observations noted the significant number of pregnant women coming to emergency departments following an abusive incident to "have the baby checked." Further explanations of abuse during pregnancy found that abuse might not actually begin in pregnancy; instead, the pregnant woman could be motivated to seek care and services regarding the abuse to protect her unborn child.

McFarlane, Parker, Soeken, Silva, and Reel (1999) found that in their sample of 199 abused pregnant women 18% were abused during pregnancy but not the year prior, 30% were abused the year before but not during their pregnancy, and 52% were abused both before and during the pregnancy. The timing of the abuse did not vary by ethnicity, and women who were abused both before and during the pregnancy reported greater severity on each of five severity measures than women abused only before or during the pregnancy.

The most commonly cited reason for abuse during pregnancy is jealousy. The abuser may view the fetus as a competitor for the woman's attention, or as an intruder in their relationship. The man's desire for power and control over the woman may be magnified by pregnancy, as the woman's attention is focused on her own health and on the developing fetus. He may resent the woman's increased contact with friends, family, and health-care providers during pregnancy. Many women report the abuser's response to the pregnancy is to deny paternity and to accuse her of infidelity (McFarlane, Parker, & Cross, 2001). In such cases, the abuse may reflect sexual jealousy, a hallmark of abusive men.

Stress is another commonly cited reason for abuse during pregnancy. The stress may derive from an unwanted or unplanned pregnancy or from marriage because of pregnancy. Increased gravidity may be a factor in abuse during pregnancy, perhaps because another child is unwanted or is perceived as a financial burden. Stress and conflict may also arise from discordance between the couple's feelings regarding the pregnancy.

Blows directed at the abdomen of a pregnant woman may represent a form of prenatal child abuse. The abuse may be a conscious or unconscious attempt to terminate the pregnancy or kill the fetus. A number of women in one study reported abdominal beatings that they believed were deliberate attempts to induce abortion because the abuser did not want the child to be born (Brendtro & Bowker, 1989). Abdominal trauma during pregnancy poses great risks for the woman and fetus/infant. Complications that have been associated with domestic abuse and other sources of abdominal trauma include vaginal bleeding, placental abruption, preterm labor and birth, uterine rupture, rupture of the membranes, abnormal fetal heart rate, and fetal and maternal death (Connolly, Katz, Bash, McMahon, & Hansen, 1997; Pak, Reece, Albert, & Chan, 1998; Williams, McClain, Rosemurgy, & Colorado, 1990).

Although each of the foregoing explanations of abuse during pregnancy may apply in any single abuse situation, none alone explains all cases of abuse during pregnancy. Campbell and Oliver (1992) questioned women about their perceptions of why the abuse occurred. Their replies varied. Twenty-percent reported the abuse was directed toward the baby, and another 20% believed that the abuse was pregnancy-related, resulting from her feeling ill or the stress of another child. This latter group thought the violence was directed at them, rather than at the baby. Another group of women cited jealousy as a factor. In the majority of cases, however, abuse during pregnancy was simply the continuation of ongoing violence and was unrelated to the pregnancy itself. In numerous studies, abuse before pregnancy seems to be the best predictor of abuse during pregnancy, occurring in 55% of all cases (McFarlane et al., 1999).

Physical abuse generally does not begin in a relationship until some level of commitment exists. In some cases, that commitment is symbolized by marriage. Pregnancy may also be perceived as a symbol of real or imagined commitment. As with marriage, pregnancy may precipitate abuse simply because the abuser believes he can abuse his partner with impunity and that the woman will not leave him because she is pregnant. It is possible that some men who do not abuse their partners during pregnancy have not yet established a pattern of violence and are therefore more easily held by societal condemnation of violence toward pregnant women. Over time, as the violence becomes a more integral part of the relationship, pregnancy may no longer be a deterrent.

Some abused women are never beaten when pregnant or experience decreased abuse when pregnant. McFarlane and colleagues (1999) and Campbell and others (1999) found rates of abuse to be lower in first-generation Hispanic women as compared to African-American or Caucasian women. Research to clarify which factors best predict and have a protective effect on abuse during pregnancy is still needed.

Ultimately, the abuser's desire for power and control and his belief that violence and coercion are legitimate means to achieve these ends prompt him to physically, sexually, or emotionally abuse his partner. This is true both during and outside of pregnancy. It is currently unclear how pregnancy affects the abuser's use of physical force to maintain his position of control. In some cases, there may be no relationship between pregnancy and abuse. How or why pregnancy affects violence against women in other situations may vary among and within abusive relationships.

A final explanation of why some women experience increased abuse during pregnancy has been noted in families with concurrent substance abuse. The explanation is particularly true for women who choose to abstain from drugs and alcohol during pregnancy while their partner continues to abuse those substances. These men often get high with their friends and are unhappy when they return home to a sober partner, particularly if she is perceived as critical of his intoxication (McFarlane, Parker, & Cross, 2001).

IMPLICATIONS FOR NURSING PRACTICE

The goal of nursing care is to promote health. Using a holistic perspective, this includes promoting physical, emotional, and psychosocial health. Nurses, nurse-midwives, and nurse practitioners who provide care to pregnant women are well aware of the need to attend to far more than just physical well-being to ensure an optimal pregnancy outcome. Because domestic violence impacts the lives and health of so many pregnant women, identification and assessment of and intervention with women experiencing abuse must become a routine part of prenatal care.

Before nurses can effectively assist battered women, they must examine their own beliefs and biases. Like many people outside the medical community, there are nurses who believe that domestic violence is a private affair to be managed within families and that in some instances violence against women may be justified or excused. For nurses to become effective agents in ending the cycle of violence in women's lives, they must accept two basic premises. First, domestic violence is a serious public-health problem, rather than a private problem, that therefore falls within the purview of nursing. Second, no woman, under any circumstances, deserves to be physically, sexually, or emotionally abused.

In addition to accepting these premises, nurses must become educated regarding the causes, characteristics, and health effects of abuse. Domestic violence, like any other specialty area or condition confronted by nurses, must be thoroughly understood before effective intervention can occur.

The nurse's tasks when dealing with battered women are to identify the presence of abuse; assess the nature, severity, and potential lethality of the abuse and the impact it has had on the woman's health; plan intervention strategies; intervene through referrals, information sharing, and support; and follow-up or assess the effectiveness of interventions. Throughout the nursing process, the primary role of the nurse is that of advocate. Advocacy includes assisting the battered woman to make informed decisions by information-sharing and providing continued support, regardless of the decisions and choices made.

Nurses often find their greatest rewards in the achievement of desired intervention outcomes. For this reason, nurses may try to "fix" things for battered women by giving advice and making elaborate arrangements to help them leave their abusers. It must be remembered that it is the abuse survivor's, not the nurses', choices and desires that must be followed. It can be very difficult and frustrating for nurses to understand and support the decisions of abused women when such decisions are contrary to their own beliefs. It is disheartening to witness the continued pain of battered women who choose to stay in abusive relationships. Effective advocacy requires understanding the difficulties involved in terminating any relationship and the knowledge that most women do eventually find a way to end the violence in their lives.

Identification

Three methods are useful in identifying battered women in a medical setting: chart reviews, direct questioning, and observing interaction between the woman and her partner. Chart reviews may only provide clues to past abuse (see the box that follows). Observation of the couple will probably reveal only emotional abuse. These methods must not be used to replace direct questioning but rather should be used in conjunction with it.

A number of possible "red flag" items in a woman's medical record strongly suggest abuse. These are listed in the Box 4-1. In addition, references to difficulty with vaginal examinations are frequently found in the charts of women with histories of child or adult sexual assault.

Observations of the woman and her partner during clinic visits, in childbirth classes, and during hospital stays for pregnancy complications or labor and delivery may also provide clues to the presence of abuse. Behaviors that suggest abuse are listed in the box.

Indicators of possible abuse in the woman's chart or those noted while observing interaction between the woman and her partner should prompt direct questions about abuse. The woman should be told what stimulated the question and why, for example, a history of preterm birth might be connected with abuse. In situations when the woman's partner is always present, it may be necessary to devise an excuse to reach her alone or to follow her into the bathroom to privately question her about abuse.

Certainly, not all survivors of domestic abuse have medical histories or have partners who behave in a way that raises nurses' suspicions about abuse. For this reason, all women must be assessed for abuse. This must be done by direct questioning, because the majority of women will not identify themselves as abuse survivors on self-completion history forms. Abuse assessment should not be limited to one question in a list of previous medical conditions. Assessment of abuse should be conducted separately. Multiple abuse-focused questions should be asked because women who deny abuse on the first question often answer positively to subsequent questions (Parker et al., 1994).

Clinical assessment for abuse, however, can be accomplished by a few abuse-focused questions asked in privacy and with concern for the woman. Soeken, McFarlane, Parker, and Lominak (1998) found that questions 2, 3, and 4 from the AAS (see Appendix A) clearly delineated between abused and nonabused women as defined by much longer instruments developed for research. The AAS developed by the Nursing Research Consortium on Violence and Abuse may be

---

BOX **4-1** **IDENTIFYING BATTERED WOMEN**

CHART REVIEW

- Assault, regardless of the assailant's stated identity
- Injuries inflicted by weapons
- Injuries consistent with assault, which are inadequately explained
- Multiple medical visits for injuries or anxiety symptoms
- Injury or assault during pregnancy
- History of depression, drug use, or suicide attempts
- Sex-specific or disfiguring injuries, such as to the face, breasts, or genitals
- Eating disorders
- Unexplained somatic symptoms, such as back, chest, or pelvic pain, or choking sensations
- Tranquilizer or sedative use

OBSTETRICAL/GYNECOLOGICAL HISTORY

- Spontaneous/elective abortions
- Sexually transmitted infections
- Sexual assault
- Late or inadequate prenatal care
- Substance use during pregnancy
- Preterm labor or preterm bleeding
- Low birth weight
- Unexplained fetal injuries, present at birth
- Unexplained intrauterine fetal demise
- Abruptio placentae
- Suicide attempts during pregnancy
- Poor weight gain during pregnancy
- Trauma injuries during pregnancy

OBSERVATIONS DURING CLINIC VISITS

- Partner is conspicuously unwilling to leave the woman's side
- Partner speaks for the woman or belittles what she says
- Partner makes derogatory comments about the woman's appearance or behavior
- Partner is oversolicitous with care providers
- Partner is emotionally absent or out of tune with the woman
- Woman is obviously afraid of her partner

---

useful for assessing abuse by a current partner. In obstetrical/gynecological settings, women should also be asked if they have ever been forced into sexual activities, either as a child or as an adult. Unresolved sexual-assault experiences may result in women having difficulty with pelvic examinations, intercourse, childbearing, and breast-feeding.

Some battered women may deny abuse during an initial assessment because of guilt, denial, shame, and the belief that the abuse is somehow her fault (Parker et al., 1994). Later in the woman's pregnancy, after rapport has been established with care providers, she may be more willing to reveal past or current abuse. Nurses must maintain an index of suspicion and ask additional abuse-focused questions after women's statements concerning relationship problems, or when evidence of trauma, drug use, and the like is present.

Early signs of abuse take many forms. These include warning signs like the partner being overly possessive and jealous, threatened by the woman's success or pregnancy, or cruel and violent in other relationships. Other behaviors include teasing or scaring the woman; for example, driving too fast is a warning sign. Nurses conducting childbirth-education classes may notice additional behaviors, such as men acting impatient with the woman, especially if she is having difficulty with certain instructions. Abusers often are rough with the woman—for example, pushing her into position for certain exercises. Often they act embarrassed by her behavior and appear more concerned with what the others in the class think about them than with the woman's comfort. Abusive men frequently "tease" the pregnant woman about being "so fat," "a cow," or "a blimp."

Assessment

After a woman has been identified as a survivor of domestic abuse, further assessment is needed. Assessment of the history and course of the abuse should include how long it has been occurring, the severity and frequency of the abuse, injuries and other health problems the woman believes have resulted from the abuse, and whether the abuse is escalating. When abuse episodes and resulting injuries are examined in chronological order, increasing severity and frequency may be noted.

Nonphysical and sexual abuse must also be explored. Most abusers use a number of nonviolent tactics to exert power and maintain control of the woman's thoughts, feelings, and actions. Power and control tactics include using intimidating words or gestures; abusing emotionally; isolating the woman from others; minimizing, denying, and blaming the woman for the abuse; using children as leverage; using male privilege, such as acting like the "master of the castle"; using economic abuse, such as controlling her access to money; and using coercion and threats. Knowledge of the degree of control the abuser exerts in the woman's life is useful in assessing the woman's current danger of harm and is also important when planning intervention strategies.

Assessment of the woman's current danger of serious injury or death is crucial. The Danger Assessment (see Appendix C) covers items believed to increase a woman's risk of homicide (Campbell, 1986). Questioning women about their perceptions of imminent danger is also useful because most abuse survivors are "tuned in" to their immediate risk of harm.

When assessing past abuse, women should be asked what resources (such as police, shelters, clergy, and family) they have used and how helpful these individuals or organizations have been. She should be questioned regarding the use of the court system and protective orders.

All assessments must be thoroughly documented. This can be a time-consuming process but may be helpful to the woman in future legal proceedings and may provide necessary communication for other health-care providers involved in the woman's care. Details should be documented in the woman's own words as much as possible. For example, instead of charting "G2P2, 16 weeks by dates, kicked in abdomen," write "42 y/o who states 'My husband punched me in the eye with his fist 2 mos. ago. Today, he kicked me in the stomach. He said he wanted to hurt the me and the baby.'" The latter note provides a much more vivid description of the woman's abuse.

Planning

Planning intervention strategies with survivors of domestic abuse consists of determining available options and the benefits and risks of each. Two factors are important in this phase of the nursing process: What does the woman want to do or have happen? What is her level of current danger?

Abused women essentially have three options: they can stay with the abuser, leave for a safe place, or have the abuser removed from the place of residence. In some cases, only the first two options are available. The role of the nurse in the planning phase of the nursing process is to provide the woman with the information necessary to make informed decisions.

Staying with the Abuser

Many if not most battered women prefer the option of staying in their current relationship provided the violence ends. However, opting to stay with the abuser generally means the violence will not only continue but also will likely worsen with time. In rare cases when the abuse is infrequent, minor, or relatively new in the relationship, the woman's partner may be assisted to end the violence while the relationship remains intact. He must be willing to accept responsibility for his actions and to seek counseling. If the couple cannot talk about the violence and the man is unwilling to accept responsibility, the violence will most likely continue. In many cases, even when the physical abuse ends, the use of other power and control tactics continues.

Throughout the process of providing information, it is appropriate for nurses to express their concerns, based on previous assessment, as long as this is done in a spirit of support rather than criticism. Gentle, sincere statements to the abuse survivor that she is a worthwhile person and does not deserve to be hurt can be very empowering. Her abuser has undoubtedly told her that she deserves the abuse, and she may have come to believe this.

A few hospitals and clinics have in-house family-violence counselors or advocates. If the abuse survivor is willing, have the advocate or counselor meet with the woman in the clinic or hospital at the time the abuse is revealed. If that is not possible, provide the woman with the advocate's phone number and encourage her to see or speak to him or her. Women who have not contacted referrals during their pregnancy may be willing to accept a visit from the advocate in the postpartum ward. Advocates from local battered women's services sometimes also visit clinics and hospitals to speak with battered women.

In hospital and clinic settings, it is often customary to refer patients with psychosocial issues to social workers, psychologists, or psychiatrists. Such referrals should never be made in place of referrals to battered women's services, and caution should be used in referring women to allied health professionals who may not have an adequate understanding of domestic violence. Referring abuse survivors to social workers, psychologists, or psychiatrists who have a poor knowledge or misunderstanding of domestic-violence issues may result in further emotional damage for the woman. It is also not in the woman's best interests to unnecessarily acquire a psychiatric diagnosis (a necessary part of reimbursement for services), because this could be used against her in child-custody cases.

Similar caution should be used when referring women to clergy or couples counseling. Well-meaning counselors sometimes encourage the woman to change her behavior to placate the abuser, thus reinforcing the view that the abuse is somehow her fault. Couples counseling may result in further abuse if it is attempted before the couple deals with their individual abuse issues separately. Similarly, chemical-dependency counseling should not be assumed to adequately deal with abuse issues.

A battered woman may choose to stay with or return to an abusive partner for many complex reasons. She stays or returns for many of the same reasons nonabusive but difficult relationships are maintained: financial constraints, societal and familial pressures, and because of children. Women are less likely to leave when they are pregnant. For many women, staying in the relationship may be preferable to single parenthood, inadequate housing, and financial deprivation.

If a woman chooses to stay with her partner, help her develop a safety or exit plan to be used if she feels in danger. She should have phone numbers, transportation plans, and knowledge of where to go. If possible, a bag with clothing, rent and utility receipts, birth certificates, toys, money, and extra car keys should be kept in a safe place. Encourage her to tell friends, family, and neighbors about the abuse so that they may be able to assist her in the future if necessary.

Encourage the abuse survivor to dial 911 if she is assaulted again. She should instruct her children to call if she is unable to do so herself. She should also be encouraged to attend battered-women's support groups or to seek counseling from someone sensitive to the issue of abuse. Provide her or her partner with referrals to groups for abusive men if the partner is willing to consider this option.

Finally, assure the battered woman that she will receive continued nursing support. A woman who feels criticized for her decisions may terminate her prenatal care or seek care elsewhere, where her abuse history is not known. For the battered woman, continued nursing support may be the key to ending the violence in her life at some point.

Leaving

If the abuse survivor chooses to leave her abuser, she must decide where she will go and have a clear idea of how safe she will be there. Women often choose to stay with family or friends. However, the welcome there may be short lived, and the woman may soon have to decide where to go next. Returning home to her abuser may become preferable to moving from one place to another. Or she may be forced to return if her abuser threatens or hurts her or her hosts.

The other option, although not always available, is to seek shelter at a battered-women's shelter or safe home. Shelters provide a level of safety and assistance in dealing with abuse issues that most friends and family cannot. Nurses may call the shelter to inquire about available space, but shelter workers will need to talk to the abuse survivor directly. If necessary, transportation to the shelter can be arranged.

Nurses should advise women to take their children with them when they leave. If they do not, they may have great difficulty obtaining legal custody in the future. Taking the children is even more crucial if the partner is also abusing them. Abused children are more likely to remain in their mother's custody if she removes them from the violent situation. Shelter workers can often arrange to have children brought to the shelter from school or elsewhere.

After she leaves, discourage the woman from having any contact with her partner, including phone contact. He will often make promises to change, plead for her return, or threaten suicide if she stays away. If contact does occur, the abuser will often "sweet-talk" or induce guilt or shame to get the woman to return home.

If the abuse survivor stays somewhere other than a shelter, she should have a plan of action should her partner locate her. She should consult a battered-woman's advocate regarding issues such as protecting her children from being abducted by the abuser and protecting herself at work and in the home.

Nurses should discuss financial issues with the battered woman. If she and her partner share bank accounts or credit cards, he can remove the money and cancel the accounts without notifying her. It is not unusual for this to occur. The woman may also do the same if she wishes.

Domestic-violence organizations provide group and individual counseling for battered women and their children and may provide counseling or educational sessions for male batterers. Battered-women's shelters also provide women and children with counseling and abuse education. Shelters provide safe lodging, clothing, food, and health-care access, as well as information concerning legal, economic, financial, employment, educational, and housing assistance. In planning to use a shelter, the nurse also needs to be aware of shelter limitations. Most shelters for abused women are overcrowded and may have a waiting list. It is preferable for the woman to contact the shelter prior to the next abusive episode and describe her situation. If her home is too dangerous, she might need to make temporary arrangements with a friend or relative or homeless shelter while calling the battered-women's shelter daily to determine space availability.

Although no shelter can guarantee complete safety for its occupants, every precaution is taken to ensure the safety and security of the women and children housed there. Most shelters will ask the woman to sign a confidentiality agreement that she will not reveal the location of the shelter to anyone. If this agreement is not kept, she endangers not only her life but also the lives of other residents and shelter staff. It is for this reason that most women are not allowed visitors or to receive phone calls. Women are not prisoners in the shelter and are free to meet with friends at another location. Most shelters exist in communities throughout the United States, and residents do not know that they are there. For more information on shelters and victim services, visit the website of the National Victim Services (http://www.dvsheltertour.org).

When discussing leaving the abuser, abuse survivors should be informed that they may be at increased risk of serious harm or death if they leave. If the woman has scored high on the Danger Assessment, her risk may be especially great. In extreme circumstances, battered-women's shelters may help the woman relocate to another state or country.

Removing the Abuser from the Home

The woman's partner may move out willingly or may be forced to leave by a vacate order or protective order. This is generally a temporary order, and it is most likely to be granted if the woman's name is on the lease or title for the residence or if the woman is unable to enter a shelter because it is full. If the partner leaves, safety issues should be discussed. The woman should have all locks changed and obtain an order for protection if she has not already done so. In many cases, pressing assault charges or obtaining protective orders can be a powerful deterrent to future violence. Most often, unless the woman's partner is on probation or has had previous charges against him, he will only spend a few hours or one night in jail if arrested on assault charges. If convicted, his sentence for a first offense is generally a fine and probation. In some states, assault convictions or protective orders may force the abuser to obtain chemical-dependency or male-batterer's counseling sessions. Women who are aware of these options are more likely to pursue legal remedies, knowing their partner may be helped to deal with his problems.

For nurses to provide accurate information to battered women, they must become familiar with state laws concerning domestic violence, sexual assault, and protective orders, as well as what domestic-violence resources are available in their community. Representatives from battered-women's shelters are willing to provide such education personally and often also have written material available. Although laws vary from state to state, domestic violence is illegal nationwide and can be (although it is not always) prosecuted in the same way as assault by a stranger. Many battered women are not aware of this. Marital rape is illegal in most states, and rape outside of marriage is illegal in all.

The abuse survivor is often the best judge of her own safety. She should plan what she would do if her partner comes to her door. She or her children should call 911 and report "some man" is at the door or trying to break in. If she reports that the man is her husband or boyfriend, police response time may be longer.

A Tested Nursing Intervention

Building on previous research documenting the relationship between abuse and low birth weight, Parker et al. (1999) tested an intervention to prevent further abuse to pregnant women. This prospective, ethnically stratified cohort design included 199 pregnant African-American, Hispanic, and Caucasian women who presented for care in prenatal public-health clinics in Virginia and Texas. All the women had experienced abuse within the prior 12 months, according to the AAS, and were still in a relationship with the abuser. Because assessment for abuse begins a process of intervention, it was impossible to randomly assign abused pregnant women into the treatment or control group. Therefore, a nonequivalent comparison group was used; it was composed of women who had recently delivered a baby and reported that they had been abused the year before they became pregnant or while they were pregnant. Only abused women who considered themselves still in a relationship (primarily because the abuser was the father of the baby) were eligible.

Women who received, in an empowering manner, a nursing intervention designed to provide them with information on the cycle of violence, a danger assessment, information on the options available to them, safety planning, and resource referrals had significantly lower scores ($p = .007$) for both physical and nonphysical abuse (as measured by the Index of Spouse Abuse) at 6 and 12 months after intervention. The difference in scores remained significant when ethnicity ($p = 0.007$) and age (teen versus adult, $p < 0.05$) were included in the analysis. Additionally, women in the intervention group used significantly more safety behaviors than did the comparison group ($p < 0.0001$). Safety behaviors included such actions as hiding money or keys, asking a neighbor to call the police, and gathering important papers. Eleven of the fifteen behaviors showed a significant change from visit one to visit two ($p < 0.0001$). Three additional behaviors changed significantly by visit three, and the fourth behavior (removing weapons from the home) increased significantly by visit four. There was no significant difference between ethnic groups.

The intervention protocol was administered to each woman in the intervention group three times during the pregnancy: at entry into the study (usually at the first prenatal visit) and in two additional sessions evenly spaced over the remaining weeks of pregnancy. The intervention was a one-to-one interview conducted in the prenatal clinics during regularly scheduled appointments. The intervention was based on the McFarlane and Parker (1994) abuse-prevention protocol developed from the Dutton (1992) empowerment model. The intervention was "brochure based"; that is, a brochure covering the topics was used at each meeting to assure that the content was consistently covered by all investigators and at all sites. The brochure was available in English and Spanish (Appendix A) and is at the website of the Nursing Network on Violence Against Women, International (http://www.nnvawi.org).

The specific topics covered during the intervention included information on the cycle of violence, information on applying for legal protection orders and filing criminal charges, and community-resource phone numbers such as those for shelters, hot lines, and law enforcement.

The intervention began with a discussion of the cycle of violence (Walker, 1979), which is a way of describing intimate partner violence that recognizes that women in abusive relationships are not being constantly abused and that the abuse is not inflicted at random times. The cycle explains how women become victimized and why extricating themselves from the relationship is so difficult. There are three phases in the cycle that vary in time and intensity for each couple.

During Phase 1, tension building, the tension within the relationship increases, and the woman, consciously or unconsciously, works to decrease the tension. This may be in the form of placating; anticipating her partner's every whim, keeping her and the children out of his way, or whatever she believes will avoid the violence. Langford (1998, 1996; Langford, Issac, & Kabat, 1998) describes this as "predicting the unpredictable." When minor incidents happen in phase 1, the woman is relieved and grateful that it was not more severe. For the abuser, of course, this behavior reinforces the legitimacy of his violence to her. By the end of phase 1, the woman is exhausted from the constant stress of anticipating the abuser's behavior, and she begins to withdraw from the relationship, fearing she will inadvertently set off an incident. The abuser, threatened by her withdrawal, becomes violent, and phase 2 begins.

Phase 2, the violent episode, is the acute battering incident that may last for minutes, hours, or days. Phase 2 is when the police, neighbors, or other family members are involved.

Phase 3, loving reconciliation, is often called the honeymoon stage, as it is a time of loving, tender, and remorseful behavior by the abuser. The abuser will buy gifts for the woman and her children, beg for forgiveness, and be a model loving husband or partner. These gestures make it more difficult for women to take action against the abuser. Their relationship during this phase is the woman's vision of the ideal relationship, and she believes that if she is just good enough or smart enough to keep her partner placated they will live happily ever after. Eventually, however, this phase ends, and once again tension begins building in the dyad.

The cycle is often different for each woman, and some women do not report a pattern or cycle to the abuse. For example, it is common for the calm phase of the cycle to stop and the abuser to go between phases one and two only. In using the cycle of violence as an intervention, allow the woman to describe her relationship, and look for the patterns that can be used to form a safety plan to protect the woman and children. Describing the pattern of violence will also allow the woman to gain a sense of control over the situation.

Each intervention session also included the following safety components: development of a safety plan, including securing and copying important papers; making copies of house and car keys; establishing a code with family and friends; hiding extra clothes, should a quick exit become necessary; identifying behaviors of the abuser indicating increased danger, such as threats of murder or suicide.

Discussions with each woman included suggestions on where to hide money, such as in an empty tampon container, as well as the hiding of important documents, again possibly with sanitary products or with a relative or trusted friend. The women were encouraged to mentally plan an escape, for example using a window if the abuser blocked the door, as well as avoiding rooms like the kitchen and bathroom where objects that can be used as a weapon, such as razors and knives, are frequently kept. Stressed throughout the intervention sessions was the woman's appraisal of the "safety" of adopting each behavior.

Frequently, other prenatal brochures, such as those dealing with breast-feeding or nutrition, were given to make the abuse brochure less conspicuous. If it was determined that it would not be safe for the woman to keep the brochure, interviewers assisted her in concealing the telephone number of the women's shelter by giving it as the number of a girlfriend or a local business. The intervention also included offering assistance with telephone calls to appropriate agencies and acting as advocates with other health-care personnel and the police. (It should be emphasized here that the abused woman must never tell the abuser of her intention to leave. Instead, she must leave in secret and only go back to get her belongings when accompanied by police, family, or friends so that she is not alone with the abuser, especially if the Danger Assessment score is high.)

The results of this study document that an intervention protocol for pregnant abused women that includes specific information on safety behaviors resulted in a significant increase in these behaviors adopted, with most safety behaviors adopted after the first intervention session. Clearly, routine screening for abuse and immediate implementation of a clinical intervention can possibly prevent future abuse and associated complications for mother and child. A clinical protocol to prevent abuse begins with assessment (Parker et al., 1999).

Follow-Up and Evaluation

In some cases, there will be no further contact between the nurse and the abuse survivor after intervention. This may occur if the intervention takes place postpartum in the hospital, if the woman changes location, or if she does not return to the clinic. In such cases, nurses receive no feedback on their interventions. A phone call to the woman inquiring about her welfare is often welcomed.

When there is further contact, nurses should provide continued support and encouragement. The nurse should let the abused woman know she is still willing to discuss this issue by asking the woman how things are going. Praise her accomplishments, no matter how small. Continue to encourage her to obtain counseling or join a support group if she has not done so already.

For women who leave their abusers, much grieving must be done. The woman may have lost a husband, a father for her children, her home, friends, and family. It may take time for her to work through the grief process and to begin making concrete future plans. For many women, it takes years before they fully realize the impact of the abuse on their lives.

Abuse during pregnancy poses an additional set of health risks for the abused woman. Her fetus may also be at risk. Because women have frequent, ongoing contact with nurses, nurse-midwives, or nurse practitioners during pregnancy, a level of rapport is often established that enhances the nurse's ability to identify and intervene with survivors of domestic abuse.

SUMMARY

Nurses encounter many abuse survivors in their clinic, hospital, and public-health practices. It is important to identify abused women so that they may be assisted in ending the violence. Nurses must acquire a working knowledge of abusive relationships, the health effects of violence against women, and the resources and options available to survivors of domestic violence, if they are to intervene effectively.

Violence against women is a serious public-health problem that must be addressed by all health-care professionals. Because nurses are trained in a holistic approach to health care, they are perhaps best suited to the task of providing an effective health-care response to domestic violence. By working closely with abused-women's services outside of the medical community, nurses can help end the violence in the lives of the women they serve.

References

Amaro, H., Fried, L., Cabral, H., & Zuckerman, B. (1990). Violence during pregnancy and substance use. *American Journal of Public Health, 80,* 575–579.

Attala, J. M., & Summers, S. M. (1991). A comparative study of health, developmental, and behaviorial factors in preschool children of battered and nonbattered women. *Children's Health Care, 28,* 189–200.

Bohn, D. K. (2002). Lifetime and current abuse, pregnancy risks, and outcomes among Native American women. *Journal of Health Care for the Poor and Underserved, 13*(2), 184–198.

Brady, J. P., Posner, M., Lang, C., & Rosati, M. J. (1994). *Risk and reality: The implications of prenatal exposure to alcohol and other drugs* [Online]. Available: http://www.aspe.hhs.gov/hsp/cyp/drugkids.htm.

Brutin, S. (1995). Legal response to teen dating violence. *Family Law Quarterly, 29*(2), 331–334.

Brendtro, M., & Bowker, L. H. (1989). Battered women: How can nurses help? *Issues in Mental Health Nursing, 10,* 169–180.

Bullock, L., & McFarlane, J. (1989). Higher prevalence of low birthweight infants born to battered women. *American Journal of Nursing, 89*(9), 47–51.

Campbell, J. (1986). Nursing assessment for risk of homicide with battered women. *Advances in Nursing Science, 8,* 36–51.

Campbell, J., Poland, M., Walker, J., & Ager, J. (1992). Correlates of battering during pregnancy. *Research in Nursing and Health, 15,* 219–226.

Campbell, J., Pugh, L. C., Campbell, D., & Visscher, M. (1995). The influence of abuse on pregnancy intention. *Women's Health Issues, 5*(4), 214–223.

Campbell, J., Soeken, K., McFarlane, J., & Parker, B. (1998). Risk factors for femicide among pregnant and non-pregnant battered women. In J. Campbell (Ed.), *Empowering survivors of abuse: Health care for battered women and their children.* Thousand Oaks, CA: Sage.

Campbell, J. C. (1989). A test of two explanatory models of women's response to battering. *Nursing Research, 38,* 18–24.

Campbell, J. C., & Alford, P. (1989). The dark consequences of marital rape. *American Journal Nursing, 89,* 946–949.

Campbell, J. C., & Oliver, C. (1992). *Why battering during pregnancy?* Unpublished manuscript.

Campbell, J. C., Oliver, C., & Bullock, L. (1993). Why battering during pregnancy? *AWHONN's Clinical Issues in Women's Health and Perinatal Nursing, 4,* 343–349.

Campbell, J. C., Ryan, J., Campbell, D. W., Torres, S., King, C., Stallings, R., & Fuchs, S. (1999). Physical and nonphysical abuse and other risk factors for low birthweight among term and preterm babies: A multiethnic case control study. *American Journal of Epidemiology, 150,* 714–726.

Chasnoff, I. J., Neuman, K., Thornton, C., Callaghan, M. A., & Angela, A. (2001). Screening for substance use in pregnancy: A practical approach for the primary care physician. *American Journal of Obstetrics & Gynecology, 184*(4), 752–758.

Connolly, A. M., Katz, V. L., Bash, K. L., McMahon, M. J., & Hansen, W. F. (1997). Trauma and pregnancy. *American Journal of Perinatology, 14*(6), 331–336.

Curry, M. A., Doyle, B. A., & Gilhooley, J. (1998). Abuse among pregnant adolescents: Differences by developmental age. *MCN: American Journal of Maternal Child Nursing, 23,* 144–150.

Curry, M.A., Perrin, N., & Wall, E. (1998). Effects of abuse on maternal complications and birth weight in adult and adolescent women. *Obstetrics and Gynecology, 92*(4 Pt 1), 530–534.

Delaney-Black, V. (2000). Alcohol consumption assessed across pregnancy adversely affects child behavior at school age. *American Journal of Obstetrics & Gynecology, 182*(1, part 2), S66.

Delaney-Black, V., Nordstrom-Klee, B., Covington, C., Templin, T., Ager, J., & Sokol, R. (2001). Prenatal drug exposure and growth to age 7. *American Journal of Obstetrics & Gynecology, 184*(1), S169.

Dutton, M. (1992). *Empowering and healing the battered woman.* New York: Springer.

Fried, P. A., Watkinson, B., & Gray, R. (1998). Differential effects on cognitive functioning in 9-12 year olds prenatally exposed to cigarettes and marijuana. *Neurotoxicology & Teratology, 20*(3), 293–306.

Frank, D. A., Augustyn, M., Knight, W. G., Pell, T., & Zuckerman, B. (2001). Growth, development, and behavior in early childhood following prenatal cocaine exposure: A systematic review. *Journal of the American Medical Association, 285*(12), 1613–1625.

Gazmarian, J., Petersen, R., Spitz, A., Goodwin, M., Saltzman, L., & Marks, J. (2000). Violence and reproductive health: Current knowledge and future research directions. *Maternal and Child Health Journal, 4*(2), 79–84.

Gielen, A. D., O'Campo, P. J., Faden, R. R., Kass, N. E., & Xue, X. (1994). Interpersonal conflict and physical violence during the childbearing year. *Social Science and Medicine, 39,* 781–787.

Goldenberg, R. L., & Rouse, D. J. (1998). Medical progress: Prevention of premature birth. *New England Journal of Medicine, 339*(5), 313–320.

Griesler, P. C., Kandel, D. B., & Davies, M. (1998). Maternal smoking in pregnancy, child behavior problems, and adolescent smoking. *Journal of Research on Adolescence, 8*(1), 159–185.

Hillard, P.J. (1985). Physical abuse in pregnancy. *Obstetrics & Gynecology, 66,* 185–190.

Institute of Medicine. (1985). *Preventing low birthweight.* Washington, DC: National Academy Press.

Jacobs, E. A. (2000). Fetal alcohol syndrome and alcohol-related neurodevelopment disorders. *Pediatrics, 106*(2), 358–361.

Jacoby, M., Gorenflo, D., Black, E., Wunderlich, C., & Eyler, A. E. (1999). Rapid repeat pregnancy and experiences of interpersonal violence among low-income adolescents. *American Journal of Preventative Medicine, 16*(4), 318–321.

Kershner, M., Long, D., & Anderson, J. E. (1998). Abuse against women in rural Minnesota. *Public Health Nursing, 15*(6), 422–431.

Langford, D. R. (1996). Predicting unpredictability: A model of women's processes of predicting battering men's violence. *Scholarly Inquiry for Nursing Practice, 10*(4), 371–385.

Langford, L., Issac, N. E., & Kabat, S. (1998). Homicides related to intimate partner violence in Massachusetts. *Homicide Studies, 2,* 353–377.

Lipscomb, L. E., et al. (2000). *PRAMS 1998 surveillance report.* Atlanta, GA: Division of Reproductive Health, National Center for Chronic Disease Prevention and Health Promotion, Centers for Disease Control and Prevention.

Mattson, S., & Rodriguez, E. (1999). Battering in pregnant Latinas. Issues in Mental Health Nursing, 20, 405–422.

McFarlane, J. (1993). Abuse during pregnancy: The horror and the hope. *AWHONN's Clinical Issues in Perinatal and Women's Health Nursing, 4,* 350–362.

McFarlane, J., & Parker, B. (1994). Preventing abuse during pregnancy: An assessment and intervention protocol. Maternal Child Nursing, 19(6), 321–324.

McFarlane, J., Parker, B., & Cross, B. (2001). Abuse during pregnancy: Prevention and intervention, 2nd ed. White Plains, NY: March of Dimes Education Foundation.

McFarlane, J., Parker, B., & Soeken, K. (1995). Abuse during pregnancy: Frequency, severity, perpetrator and risk factors of homicide. *Public Health Nursing, 12*(5), 284–289.

McFarlane, J., Parker, B., & Soeken, K. (1995). Abuse during pregnancy: Frequency, severity, perpetrator and risk factors of homicide. *Public Health Nursing, 12*(5), 284–289.

McFarlane, J., Parker, B., & Soeken, K. (1996a). Abuse during pregnancy: Associations with maternal health and infant birthweight. *Nursing Research, 45*(1), 37–42.

McFarlane, J., Parker, B., & Soeken, K. (1996b). Physical abuse, smoking, and substance use during pregnancy: Prevalence, interrelationships, and effects on birth weight. *Journal of Obstetric, Gynecological and Neo-Natal Nursing, 25*(4), 313–320.

McFarlane, J., Parker, B., Soeken, K., & Bullock, L. (1992). Assessing for abuse during pregnancy: Frequency and extent of injuries and entry into prenatal care. *Journal of American Medical Association, 267*(23), 3176–3178.

McFarlane, J., Parker, B., Soeken, K., Silva, C., & Reel, S. (1998). Safety behaviors of abused women following an intervention program offered during pregnancy. *Journal of Obstetric, Gynecologic, and Neonatal Nursing, 27*(1), 64–69.

McFarlane, J., Parker, B., Soeken, K., Silva, C., & Reel, S. (1999). Severity of abuse before and during pregnancy for African-American, Hispanic, and Anglo women. *Journal of Nurse Midwifery, 44*(2), 139–144.

McFarlane, J., Soeken, K., Reel, S., Parker, B., & Silva, C. (1997). Resource use of abused women following an intervention program: Associated severity of abuse and reports of the abuse ending. *Public Health Nursing, 14*(4), 244–250.

Murphy, C., Schei, B., Myhr, T., & Mont, J. (2001). Abuse: A risk factor for low birth weight? A systematic review and meta-analysis. *CMAJ-JAMC, 164*(11), 1567–1572.

Pak, L. L., Reece, E. A., Albert, R., & Chan, L. (1998). Is adverse pregnancy outcome predictable after blunt abdominal trauma? *American Journal of Obstetrics & Gynecology, 179*(5), 1140–1144.

Parker, B., McFarlane, J., & Soeken, K. (1994). Abuse during pregnancy: Effects on maternal complications and birthweight in adult and teenage women. *Obstetrics and Gynecology, 84*(3), 323–328.

Parker, B., McFarlane, J., Soeken, K., Silva, C., & Reel, S. (1999). Testing an intervention to prevent further abuse to pregnant woman. *Research in Nursing and Health, 22*, 59–66.

Pollack, H. A. (2001). Sudden infant death syndrome, maternal smoking during pregnancy, and the cost-effectiveness of smoking cessation intervention. *American Journal of Public Health, 91*(3), 432–436.

Sampselle, C. M., Petersen, B. A., Murtland, T. L., & Oakley, D. J. (1992). Prevalence of abuse among pregnant women choosing certified nurse-midwife or physician providers. *Journal of Nurse-Midwifery, 37*(4), 269–273.

Shu, X. O., Hatch, M. C., Mills, J., Clemens, J., & Susser, M. (1995). Maternal smoking, alcohol drinking, caffeine consumption, and fetal growth: Results from a prospective study. *Epidemiology, 6*(2), 115–120.

Soeken, K., McFarlane, J., Parker, B., & Lominak, M. (1998). The Abuse Assessment Screen: A clinical instrument to measure frequency, severity, and perpetrator of abuse against women. In J. Campbell (Ed.), *Empowering survivors of abuse: Health care for battered women and their children* (pp. 195–203). Thousand Oaks, CA: Sage.

Taggart, L., & Mattson, S. (1996). Delay in prenatal care as a result of battering in pregnancy: Cross-cultural implications. *Health Care for Women International, 17*, 25–34.

Thomas, J. (2001). Maternal smoking during pregnancy associated with negative toddler behavior and early smoking experimentation. *NIDA Notes, 16*(1) [Online]. Available: http://165.112.78.61/NIDA_Notes/NNVol16N1/Maternal.html.

Torres, S., Campbell, J. C., Campbell, D. W., Ryan, J., King, C., Price, P., Stallings, R., Fuchs, S., & Laude, M. (2000). Abuse during pregnancy: Prevalence and cultural correlates. *Violence and Victims, 15*(3), 303–322.

Varisco, R. (2001). Drug abuse and conduct disorder linked to maternal smoking during pregnancy. *NIDA Notes, 15*(5) [Online]. Available: http://165.112.78.61/NIDA_Notes/NNVol15N5/Drug.html.

Walker, L.E., (1979). *The battered woman.* New York: Harper & Row.

Wilbourne, P. I., Dorato, V., Yeo, R., & Curet, L. B. (2000). Relationship of social, medical, and substance use characteristics to gestational age in poly-substance using women. *American Journal of Obstetrics & Gynecology, 182*(1, part 2), S156.

Williams, J. K., McClain, L., Rosemurgy, A. S., & Colorado, N. M. (1990). Evaluation of blunt abdominal trauma in the third trimester of pregnancy: Maternal and fetal considerations. *Obstetrics & Gynecology, 75*(1), 33–37.

Young, C., McMann, J., Bowman, V., & Thompson, D. (1989). Maternal reasons for delayed prenatal care. *Nursing Research, 38*, 242–243.

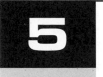

CHAPTER

5

Abuse and Neglect of the Elderly in Family Settings

- Mary Cay Sengstock, Yvonne Campbell Ulrich, and Sara A. Barrett

There has been a long-standing debate among professionals working with the elderly as to whether elder abuse and neglect should be viewed as a special type of family violence or as a particular problem of old age. The recognition that some abuse of the elderly includes the types of physical assaults that occur in other types of family violence supports the former position. Accordingly, elder abuse, along with child abuse and neglect and spouse abuse, has generally appeared in textbooks on family violence (Barnett, Miller-Perrin, and Perrin, 1997; Pagelow, 1984). Furthermore, theoretical models for abuse of the elderly are often derived from general family-violence theories, focusing on such factors as the psychopathology of abusers; situational issues, such as general family stress; or the specific stress involved in care of dependent family members (Barnett et al., 1997; Galbraith, 1989).

From a public-policy standpoint, management of elder abuse tends to follow the model of general family abuse, making use of such procedures as mandatory reporting statutes, originally developed for use with child abuse (Rinkle, 1989; Roby & Sullivan, 2000; Thobaben & Anderson, 1985). Techniques for identifying elder abuse are often borrowed from child-abuse-identification techniques (Sengstock & Hwalek, 1985-1986; Wolf, 1996a). And elder abuse is categorized as a criminal act, requiring that penalties be imposed on those responsible for the abuse (Blakely and Dolon, 2000; Quinn and Tomita, 1997; Roby and Sullivan, 2000; Thobaben, 1989).

The debate is not an insignificant issue, since it has profound consequences for the types of services to be provided to elderly victims, as well as the manner in which funding resources should be allocated. (See Box 5-1.)

The presence of this chapter in this volume reflects our own characterization of elder abuse as pertinent to a discussion of family violence. However, throughout the chapter we will also review the alternative concept, as well as other theories and research related to elder abuse and neglect.

Five major topics are considered:

- Characteristics and frequency of family abuse and neglect of the aged, including its manifestation in special categories of the elderly population
- Characteristics of the abused and abuser
- Proposed causes of elder abuse and neglect
- Means used by agencies to identify and serve abused and neglected elderly
- Suggested nursing care for elderly victims

The authors would like to express their deep appreciation to Ms. Sonya Berkley, M.A., of the Wayne State University Sociology Department, for her diligent bibliographic assistance.

BOX 5-1   **AN ONGOING DEBATE: IS IT ELDER ABUSE OR POOR CASE MANAGEMENT?**

Some suggest that the concern for elder abuse is largely an issue created by professional service providers and believe that the perception of elder abuse as a problem might not be shared by the general public or, in particular, by the elderly themselves, because an incapacitated, abused elder is not a positive image of old age (Harbison & Morrow, 1998). Early on, some specialists suggested that elder abuse is "the wrong issue" (O'Malley, 1986). The debate centers around the most frequent type of abuse of the elderly and the identity and intentions of the alleged "perpetrator."

THE CASE-MANAGEMENT MODEL

Those who object to the term "elder abuse" suggest that, unlike the beaten spouse or child, most elders are not injured by deliberate physical assaults but by the nondeliberate actions of inept or inadequate caregivers. They refer to several studies that have indicated the major category of elder abuse to be neglect directed against a dependent elder (Douglass, 1988; Fulmer & Ashley, 1989). The National Elder Abuse Incidence Study (NEAIS) findings showing neglect and self-neglect to be the overwhelming majority of elder abuse cases provided further support to this argument (Callaghan, 2000; Fulmer, 2000; NCEA, 1998; Phillipson, 2000). According to the case-management experts, the focus on abuse, with its assumption of deliberate action and the correlative need for legal action, diverts attention from the major problem, that is, the need for more social services directed toward the infirm aged (Callaghan, 1986, 1988, 2000; Douglass, 1988).

The fact that a considerable amount of elder "abuse" is actually neglect suggests the need to consider the identity and intentions of the alleged abuser. Who is the individual responsible for the alleged "abuse" of the elder? What are his or her intentions? Is the action deliberate or not?

Clearly, the intention of the alleged abuser is an important factor used to justify separating elder abuse from other forms of domestic abuse. Case-management proponents who argue that much of elder abuse is not deliberate do not deal with the issue that similar factors—inadequate preparation for caregiving and the lack of a deliberate intention to injure—are often raised with regard to child abusers as well; yet child abuse continues to be considered a category of domestic abuse.

Case-management experts also point out that an examination of cases, particularly of elder neglect, often reveals that no single individual can be clearly identified as the "abuser." Many dependent elderly persons, particularly older women who have never married, have no close relatives to care for them (Grambs, 1989). Even in cases in which offspring or other relatives could provide assistance, elder care is not like child care. Although parents are required to care for their children and can be charged with neglect for failing to do so, there is still considerable debate about whether family members, even sons and daughters, should be forced to assume the care of an aged relative, and clear public policy in this area is lacking (Verma & Haviland, 1988). In addition, some elder-neglect cases are actually cases of self-neglect (O'Brien, Thibault, Turner, and Laird-Fick, 1999; Quinn and Tomita, 1997). These are not elders living at the mercy of others, but persons who have chosen to not provide themselves with sufficient food, clothing, or medicine.

Therefore, many elder abuse cases clearly are different from both child and spouse abuse and cannot be included in a typology of family violence. Some argue further that only those cases of abuse or neglect that have originated in old age should be included in the category of elder abuse. For example, Douglass (1988) excluded cases of spouse abuse that had existed for many years, contending that long-term abusive patterns were not amenable to the types of remedies that would be used with abuse originating during old age.

An advantage of the case-management approach is that it excludes those cases most likely to be problematic for the theoretical model. This model of elder abuse is largely based on those cases that constitute neglect of a dependent elder. Cases of direct, intentional assault or cases in which violent behavior patterns are a long-standing family norm obviously do not fit this model. Defining them out of the universe is a convenient way of strengthening the case-management model.

(continued)

BOX	5-1	AN ONGOING DEBATE: IS IT ELDER ABUSE OR POOR CASE MANAGEMENT? *(Continued)*

THE DOMESTIC-ABUSE MODEL

Unlike proponents of the case-management approach, who tend to focus on the most frequent types of maltreatment in cases of elder abuse, proponents of the domestic-assault model of elder abuse are more likely to focus on the wide variety of mistreatment, including direct physical assault (Quinn & Tomita, 1997). Focusing on the needs of the victims of passive neglect, even if it is assumed they are the most numerous of the victims of elder abuse, fails to deal with the needs of those elders who are victims of other types of elder abuse and neglect.

Proponents of the domestic-violence model are also more likely to focus on identifying elderly victims of abuse, a process that uses symptoms that do not always point to specific abuse types early in the identification process. They also point out that it is difficult to determine at an early point whether the abuser's behavior, be it neglect or direct assault, is deliberate or not. Such questions must be answered later. Hence it is important not to jump to conclusions about the nature of the elder's situation until a thorough assessment has been made. It is also true that elderly victims of all types of abuse and neglect may require some of the same types of services, including those available only through agencies developed in response to the needs of family-violence victims. In short, they contend that elderly abuse victims are best served if it is initially assumed that they are victims of family abuse rather than of simple errors in case management (Hwalek, Neale, Goodrich, and Quinn, 1996; Hwalek and Sengstock, 1986; Neale, Hwalek, Goodrich, and Quinn, 1996; 1997; Quinn and Tomita, 1997).

CONSEQUENCES OF THE CONTROVERSY

The pragmatic consequences of this debate are not insignificant. On its outcome rests the nature—even the existence—of services to aged victims of maltreatment, by whatever name it is called (Callaghan, 1986, 2000). Services for elderly abuse victims are in short supply and needs are likely to increase (Wolf, 1996a). Needs and demands for assistance always exceed the supply, especially in times of budget-cutting fervor (Cravedi, 1986). Politicians have more demands for public services than they can supply. Hence they are only too ready to cut programs that can be shown to be unnecessary. This is more likely when the supposed "experts" present contradictory views.

The disagreements and conflicts between professionals and agencies concerning the definition and conceptualization of elder abuse also do considerable harm to elders and their families. They have consequences, not only in the manner in which the problem is viewed by researchers but also in its perception by policy makers, who are annoyed by the absence of clear terminology and program perspectives (Callaghan, 1986). There are long-term consequences for the many competing programs that serve victims of elder abuse.

If viewed as an "abuse" problem, then legal- and victim-assistance agencies may receive additional resources to assist elders; if viewed as a problem of "care management," then health and home-service agencies can claim the need for added resources to deal with the problem. Consequently, there is likely to be considerable competition among agencies to claim expertise in the definition of the problem. This is particularly true in light of the controversy between the case-management and domestic-violence models of elder abuse.

The status quo in social services for elderly abuse victims tends to be a family-violence model. If this model continues to prevail, it is likely that social services for aged victims will remain in much the same form as at present. Adult Protective Services (APS) would continue to remain a central focus of a service plan. The likelihood of hidden abuse and the need to develop methods of identifying victims would continue to be an important part of the assistance process. Services would largely be channeled through APS, with referrals to a variety of agencies and service types, including legal assistance, police involvement, and the possibility of shelter, as well as more

(continued)

BOX	5-1	AN ONGOING DEBATE: IS IT ELDER ABUSE OR POOR CASE MANAGEMENT? *(Continued)*

traditional medical and social services. The services required in every elder abuse case would vary considerably, depending on such factors as the type of abuse, the identity of the abuser, and the degree of intentionality.

If the care-management model should replace the existing approach, drastic changes in services for the aged would be likely. Adult Protective Services would be deemphasized, as the care-management model does not assume an adversarial relationship between victim and abuser. So-called abusers are actually well-meaning caregivers who will be quite willing—even anxious—to learn and adopt more effective methods of providing care. Consequently, there would be no need for such programs as legal assistance, protective intervention, or temporary shelter.

The case-management model has an obvious advantage. Under this approach, services to assist caregivers in managing their roles more effectively would predominate. The services it would emphasize are sorely needed by many elderly victims and their caregivers, particularly victims of passive neglect, on which the model is based. Examples are training programs for caregivers, in-home assistance programs to supervise the care process and monitor the patients' progress, and programs to provide respite for overburdened caregivers. Indeed, removal of the stigma of "abuser" might make it easier for the stressed-out caregiver to accept assistance. Because neglected aged are a major, if not *the* major category of elderly victims of abuse, the model would encourage the establishment of the most effective services to a category of victims now being inadequately served. (Also see Box 5-5 for a discussion of the problems of service provision to abused and neglected elders.)

The disadvantage of the model is also obvious. By its unitary focus on a single type of elder abuse, albeit a common one, the model would eliminate services to elderly victims of abuse that are not included in the model of inadequate but well-meaning care. Because these victims, however few in number, may be in mortal danger and in greatest need of intervention, the omission would portend dire and formidable consequences. At the present time, there is considerable dependence on services provided in the APS model, so it appears likely that this will be the model followed for the foreseeable future.

CHARACTERISTICS OF DOMESTIC ABUSE OF THE AGED

Types of Elder Abuse

Previous research has indicated that "elder abuse" actually constitutes a variety of behaviors, all of which threaten the health, comfort, and possibly the lives of elderly people. However, the nature of the threat and its effect on aged persons' health and comfort may take different forms. From its first observation as a social problem to the present, elder abuse has focused on a broader range of behaviors than other family abuse, including the six major categories of abuse and neglect subsequently listed (Block & Sinnott, 1979; Douglass, Hickey, and Noel, 1980; Harbison and Morrow, 1998; Kransnow and Fleshner, 1979; Lau & Kosberg, 1979; Nerenberg, 2000; Roby & Sullivan, 2000; Teaster, Roberto, Duke, & Kim, 2000; Wolf, 1996a). Indeed, some authorities prefer the generic term "elder mistreatment" rather than "elder abuse" to signify this broader range of offensive actions (Daniels, Baumhover, and Formby, 1999; Hudson, 1997; Le, 1997; Quinn & Tomita, 1997; Tomita, 2000).

Research and training on elder abuse and neglect have been plagued by inadequate and conflicting definitions (Goodrich, 1997). Our categorization follows closely the guidelines of the American Medical Association (AMA; 1992), with the exception noted later. Other categorizations tend to include the same types of behaviors but may also include or emphasize different types. The six categories are:

- Psychological or emotional neglect includes isolating or ignoring the elder.
- Psychological or emotional abuse involves assault or the infliction of pain through verbal or emotional rather than physical means. Examples are verbal assault (screaming, yelling, berating) and threats that induce fear; these do not involve use of a weapon.
- Violation of personal rights includes acts that deprive an older adult of the right to make his or her own choices and to act on his or her own behalf. Examples are forcing a person to move into a nursing home against his or her will, prohibiting him or her from marrying, or preventing free use of the elder's own money. Violation of personal rights, together with financial abuse (listed next), are often characterized as "exploitation" of the elderly.
- Financial abuse includes the theft or misuse of an aged individual's money or property. Examples are taking money from a bank account without the elder's consent, selling a home without knowledge or permission, cashing a Social Security check and not returning the money to the recipient, and failure to use financial resources for the elder's benefit. The AMA guidelines single out this last type, financial neglect, as a separate category (AMA, 1992).
- Physical neglect includes the failure to provide an aged and dependent individual with the necessities of life: food, shelter, clothing, and medical care. In fact, such neglect may be as injurious and life-threatening as a direct attack. Abandonment, an extreme form of neglect in which a caregiver simply leaves and refuses to provide care any longer, is also included here, although some states consider it a separate category (Neale, Hwalek, Goodrich, and Quinn, 1996; Thomas, 2000; Wolf, 1996a).
- Physical abuse means apparently deliberate direct attacks that can cause physical injury. Included in this category are slaps, punches, beatings, and pushes, as well as threats in which a weapon, such as a knife or gun, is directly involved. Sexual assault is also included here, although some experts prefer to view this as a separate category, and the Older Americans Act does not define it as a type of abuse (Fulmer, 1989; Roby & Sullivan, 2000; Teaster et al., 2000).

Some categorizations distinguish between "active neglect" and "passive neglect," with the former being a deliberate act and the latter resulting from inadequate knowledge of the elder's needs or from the stresses of long-term caregiving (Douglass, 1988; Wolf, 1996a; Wolf, Halas, Green, & McNiff, 1985-1986). Elder abuse includes several categories that are not part of most conceptualizations of spouse abuse. Psychological abuse and neglect, for example, are not usually considered a part of the definition of spouse abuse, which is usually confined to direct physical assault (Barnett, et al, 1997; Pagelow, 1984). Similarly, concerns about spouse abuse do not usually focus on the theft or misuse of the victim's property or the violation of the victim's rights, although both might often occur with spouse abuse. Regardless of the terminology, the elder abuse clearly refers to a wider range of behaviors than either spouse abuse or child abuse (Pollick, 1987; Roby & Sullivan, 2000; Wolf, 1996a).

Because both elder abuse and child abuse include neglect, elder abuse is in some ways more similar to child abuse than to spouse abuse (Pagelow, 1984; Wolf, 1996a). However, there are some major differences between elder abuse and child abuse. Whereas parents are almost universally held responsible for care of their children, the same obligation for adult offspring to care for their parents does not apply (Pollack, 1995). Although financial abuse of the elderly is a common problem, reference to financial abuse of children is rare because they are unlikely to have substantial amounts of money or property.

Perhaps the most significant difference between abuse of children and of the elderly, however, is that the elderly are adults and entitled to adult rights. Unless mentally impaired, they are entitled to make choices with regard to their lives and cannot be forced to alter their life-styles without their consent. Elders, therefore, unlike children, cannot simply be removed from a dangerous home situation if it is one in which they choose to remain (Quinn & Tomita, 1997; Phillipson, 2000).

Because of the wide variety of types of behaviors included in the concept of elder abuse, recent research has focused on the manner in which these various types are viewed. For example, it is fairly clear that direct physical assaults can cause serious injury, but does the general public see psychological or financial abuse as being a serious form of abuse? How serious is physical neglect? To what extent should extenuating circumstances, such as an overstressed caregiver, be considered? Research suggests that elder abuse of all types is considered unacceptable, both by professionals who deal with the elderly and by the community. Although there might be some disagreement regarding fine distinctions (e.g., whether a specific statement constituted verbal abuse), most respondents considered psychological, social, or financial abuse to be as harmful as physical abuse or neglect (Hudson & Carlson, 1998; Moon, 2000). Furthermore, respondents in a sample of persons aged 40 and over did not believe that abuse had to be repeated in order to be unacceptable (Hudson & Carlson, 1998; Tatara, 1997).

In sum, the categories of behavior included in definitions of elder abuse are considerably broader in scope than those included in either spouse or child abuse. Elder abuse may also differ from spouse or child abuse in that there is some question regarding whether the apparently similar categories are truly equivalent; for example, neglect is a different type of behavior when directed against a child than against a dependent adult.

Frequency of Elder Abuse

It has long been realized that establishing the frequency of elder abuse was a daunting task. In the past, many studies have had small sample sizes (Block & Sinnott, 1979; Lau and Kosberg, 1979), and most were analyses of whatever cases the researchers were able to uncover rather than being representative of the aged population (Sengstock & Liang, 1982; 1983). Furthermore, some early studies did not examine case-related data but relied on service providers' general impressions of the nature of the problem (Douglass et al., 1980; Hickey & Douglass, 1981a,

1981b). These early studies resulted in a number of estimates of the frequency of elder abuse. Steinmetz (1981) suggested that approximately 11% of the elderly population might be vulnerable to elder abuse, and Block and Sinnott (1979) estimated that abuse is a problem for at least 4% of the elderly population.

Not until the mid-1980s was there an attempt to estimate the rate of elder abuse using a systematic sample. This research studied 2,020 community-dwelling elderly in Boston and revealed a rate of 3.2 %, or 32 cases of elder abuse per 1,000 older persons (Pillemer & Finkelhor, 1988). Three types of elder abuse and neglect were included: physical abuse, physical neglect, and psychological abuse. Several types were not included, and it is questionable whether the Boston-area elderly population could be considered representative of the elderly population as a whole.

A decade later, more effective measures of elder-abuse frequency were developed. A frequency study in the Netherlands found elder abuse to have a prevalence rate of 5.6%; however, since this involved prevalence rather than incidence (i.e., the number of continuing cases, rather than the number of specific incidents of abuse in a given time frame), it could be expected to be higher (Comijs, Pot, Smit, Bouter, & Jonker, 1998).

About the same time, the Administration on Aging and the Administration for Children and Families sponsored a joint project, the National Elder Abuse Incidence Study (NEAIS) to estimate the incidence of elder abuse (Mixon, 2000; National Center on Elder Abuse [NCEA], 1998; Thomas, 2000). This study obtained data from a scientifically selected sample of 20 counties in 15 states, used a definition of abuse that included all the types previously listed here, and included persons 60 years of age and older. The NEAIS uncovered an estimated rate of 1.2%, or approximately 12 cases per 1,000 older persons (Thomas, 2000).

Hence the 1.2% figure is the most appropriate estimate of the incidence of elder abuse to date. In all studies, however, the figures represent abuse that has been observed and reported. Even when special care is taken, it is unknown how many cases go unobserved and unreported. Indeed, the NEAIS cautions that up to five times as many cases of elder abuse may exist as are reported to Adult Protective Services (APS); this reference to the large number of unreported cases has been referred to as the "iceberg theory" (NCEA, 1998).

Frequency of Various Abuse Types and the Importance of the Clinical Setting

In the NEAIS, nearly half of the cases uncovered were neglect (NCEA, 1998; Phillipson, 2000), with all other categories constituting the remainder. This confirms the belief expressed by many service providers. In other research, however, the frequency of each type of elder abuse differs. In Illinois, financial abuse was the largest category (nearly half), with emotional abuse and neglect about one-third each (Neale et al., 1996). The Netherlands study found verbal aggression (what we have called psychological abuse) to be most common, followed by financial abuse and physical abuse (Comijs et al., 1998).

In early studies, the type of abuse appeared to vary by the professional background of the identifying worker. Social workers, for example, were more likely to observe psychological abuse, health-care workers to uncover physical abuse or neglect, and workers for legal-aid agencies to recognize financial abuse (Block &

Sinnott, 1979; Lau & Kosberg, 1979; Sengstock & Liang, 1983). This was largely because agencies tended to identify forms of abuse that most closely corresponded to the forms of treatment that they offered (Sengstock & Barrett, 1981). Research, as well as the experience of professionals, has also found that the different types of abuse rarely occur in isolation; it is common for elderly abuse victims to suffer from multiple types, as well as to be victims of multiple incidents (Comijs et al., 1998; Sengstock & Liang, 1983).

This reflects a problem in the identification and treatment of elder abuse. Because most elderly are seen by only one of these agencies, professionals must become aware of the many different types of abuse or neglect, including those not normally seen in their professional activities, and also be able to identify and refer cases for appropriate assistance. Furthermore, they must recognize that single incidents or types of abuse are rare; the presence of one type of incident is a strong indication that other incidents or types may also have occurred.

The enduring character of abuse becomes more evident when the length of time over which the abuse has occurred is considered. Reporters indicate that abuse continues over a substantial period of time (Sengstock & Liang, 1982). If it is assumed that "a long time" probably indicates at least one year, then apparently half or more of victims have endured abusive family situations for a period of one year or longer.

Finally, some categories of abuse or neglect of elderly persons appear to require special attention and approaches. Three such types deserve mention: elderly women who are victims of spouse abuse, victims of abuse or neglect who are in institutions for the elderly, and persons who engage in self-neglect.

For example, the elderly battered woman may have the same need for physical treatment and protection as the younger woman, but because of her age and health status she is more often seen by agencies for the elderly and may not be eligible to stay in most shelters. Institutional abuse or neglect usually occurs in isolated settings and is not visible to outsiders; hence it presents special problems of identification and treatment. The elderly victim who freely chooses to neglect his or her health or safety must clearly be handled in a different manner than would the elderly person who is victimized by someone else. Throughout the chapter, special boxed sections will detail the special characteristics and needs of each of these three types.

CHARACTERISTICS OF ABUSED AND ABUSERS

Who is a likely victim of elder abuse? Who is most likely to be an abuser? This section discusses the demographic characteristics associated with abuse and neglect of the aged by their families. The characteristics of the victim will be considered first. For this section we rely on a wide variety of studies, including one in which we were involved.

Demographic Characteristics of Victims

Not surprisingly, the majority of elder-abuse victims are women (Block & Sinnott, 1979; Neale, Hwalek, Goodrich, and Quinn, 1997; Phillipson, 2000; Sengstock & Liang, 1983). Because the majority of the elderly population is female, this is to be expected. However, it has been suggested that the rate of abuse of elderly males may be higher than the rate of abuse of elderly females (Dimah & Dimah, 2002; Pillemer & Finkelhor, 1988).

Most experts have noted that the oldest old (aged 80 and above) and those with some type of impairment are the most frequent victims of abuse (Neale et al., 1997; Phillipson, 2000; Sengstock & Liang, 1983). The NEAIS study confirmed the greater risk of impaired elderly (NCEA, 1998; Phillipson, 2000). Among the disabilities observed are some degree of mental or emotional impairment and the inability to prepare food, perform personal hygiene, or take medicine. Medication may itself be a means of abuse, because some elders are given excessive doses of drugs by their doctors or families to make them more manageable. It is also true, however, that the physically and mentally healthy elderly may also be the victims of abuse (Sengstock & Liang, 1982; 1983).

The socioeconomic level of victims is somewhat of an enigma. The NEAIS study found that two-thirds of the neglected elderly had annual incomes under $10,000 (NCEA, 1998). It is easy to see why such individuals would feel dependent on their families and unable to escape the abusive situation. The middle class and even the wealthy are not immune to the problems of domestic abuse, however, although they may be better able to hide these problems from authorities (Barnett et al., 1997; Sengstock & Liang, 1983). The elderly may be prone to abuse because of their financial resources (Quinn & Tomita, 1997). Contrary to customary belief, some abusers are financially dependent on their elderly victims, who were the major source of income for their families (Greenberg, McKibben, & Raymond, 1990; Neale et al., 1997; Wolf, Godkin, & Pillemer, 1984).

There is no clear pattern of living arrangements for elder abuse victims. Some live alone; others live with spouses or children (Neale et al., 1997). Living alone does not preclude abuse by family members, who may abuse the aged person during visits or subject them to neglect or isolation. One study suggested that elderly-abuse victims had few friends, and contact with family consisted mainly of a visit or phone call every week or less (Sengstock & Liang, 1982). This finding is similar to that found in a number of studies of domestic violence, that is, abusive families have very little contact outside the family, making it impossible for members to obtain outside support in times of trouble and leaving no one to intervene if abuse occurs (Barnett et al., 1997).

Abused and Neglected Elders in Ethnic Communities

One neglected dimension of research on elder abuse is its characteristics in different racial and cultural populations (Griffin, 1994; Hudson, Armachain, Beasley, & Carlson, 1998; Phillips, deArdon, & Briones, 2000). Early studies found a majority of victims to be white, but this was largely due to a bias in the sample studied (Block & Sinnott, 1979). When agencies serving minority populations are included in a study, it becomes clear that minority aged are also at risk (Neale et al., 1997; Sengstock & Liang, 1983). That such research is critical is indicated by the few facts that are known about minority abuse patterns.

In the Hispanic population, for example, little is known about caregiving and interpersonal violence. However, the life expectancy of Hispanics is shorter, with earlier onset of the chronic diseases of old age, so caregiving may be required for persons at younger ages. It has also been found that Hispanic caregivers may have less social support than Anglo caregivers—contrary to the often-heard assumption that ethnic groups take care of their own (Gelfand, 1994; Phillips et al., 2000). Power imbalance in families has also been associated with caregiving problems (specifically abuse directed toward the caregiver); because power imbalance is more common in Hispanic families, this suggests that family caregiving may be more problematic in this group (Phillips et al., 2000). Elders in this community also define neglect and financial exploitation differently than most Americans do; for example, some define the refusal of children to provide a home for their parents as abuse (Moon, 2000; Sanchez, 1996). This definition may apply to other groups as well. The Hispanic population is also quite heterogeneous, including a wide variety of national origins and various levels of assimilation to the United States. Hence, it cannot be concluded that all these people have similar cultural patterns (Montoya, 1997; NCEA, 1998).

Among African-American elders, financial abuse and deliberately inflicted physical neglect have been found to be common. It is also suggested that African-American males are at particularly high risk for mistreatment and that female children are more likely to be abusive (Dimah & Dimah, 2002). It has also been noted that the long history of violence and discrimination directed against members of the community may result in their having learned such behavior, which may then be directed against their own members (Griffin, 1994). With African Americans, as with other ethnic groups, care should be taken not to assume that all members of the group are alike. For example, the problems of rural African-Americans are distinctly different from those of urban dwellers (Griffin, 1994).

Native-American populations also exhibit patterns that suggest the possibility of higher rates of abuse. For example, researchers have found that Native Americans had higher rates of prior abuse, such as having been abused as children (Baldridge, 2001; Hudson et al., 1998). If, as some suggest, prior abuse makes one more likely to abuse or be abused later in life, then the possibility of elder abuse in Native-American communities may be high, in spite of the fact that Native Americans hold elders in high regard and have strong values condemning elder abuse (Hudson et al., 1998).

Even the definition of unacceptable behavior varies from one cultural group to another. For example, Korean-American elders in one study viewed the unrestricted use of elders' money by their children as appropriate, a situation that could lead to severe financial exploitation; indeed, several incidents of financial abuse have been discovered in this group. In contrast, Native-American elders were highly disapproving of financial exploitation (Moon, 2000). Research has also found that variability within an ethnic group is quite common, particularly if one compares recent immigrants to more assimilated elders (Moon, 2000; Nagpaul, 1997; Pablo & Braun, 1997). Consequently, firm generalizations on the basis of a person's ethnic origins are inappropriate. It has also been suggested that there may be differences in rates of elder abuse by religion (Anetzberger, 1987).

Clearly, there is a great need for further study on the special manifestations of elder abuse and neglect in different segments of the population, as well as a determined effort to identify and manage problemmatic situations in minority communities. Probably the most important conclusions to be drawn from the data to date are that elder abuse and neglect can occur with all types of older persons, including those of different racial and ethnic groups, income levels, and religions, and that special efforts are necessary to identify and assist these elderly victims. Particular efforts may be necessary to reach persons from various minority communities who may be unaware of the resources available and reluctant to reveal their plight to outsiders. Later, we suggest some of the problems in these areas, as well as techniques for providing this special care.

Portrait of the Abuser

The national-incidence study found that the abusers were usually the elders' children or spouses (Phillipson, 2000). This has been found in other studies as well (Dimah and Dimah, 2002; Hwalek, Neale, Goodrich, & Quinn, 1996; Neale et al., 1997). Studies have also found the most frequent abuser to be a member of the victim's household, 40 years of age or older, and female, a situation that may reflect the fact that women are more frequently the caregivers in constant contact with the incapacitated elderly (Block & Sinnott, 1979; Lau & Kosberg, 1979; Sengstock & Liang, 1983). However, it has also been found that abusive children were almost evenly divided between sons and daughters (Sengstock & Liang, 1983).

Although, as noted, spouse abuse is not unknown among the aged (Hwalek et al., 1996; Neale et al., 1997; Sengstock and Liang, 1983), some experts do not believe that it should be included as a type of elder abuse (Douglass, 1988). The special problem of intimate violence in old age is discussed in Box 5-2.

Abusers other than the spouse can be grandchildren, siblings, nieces, nephews, and cousins. Sometimes the abuser is not a relative; these abusers can be friends, roomers, and landlords. In one study, more than one-fourth of the abusers were more than 60 years old; they were themselves well into the category of being elderly (Sengstock & Liang, 1983).

One issue that should be considered is the relationship between the types of abuse and the abuser. Some evidence shows that certain types of abuse are more likely to be inflicted by specific types of abusers. Thus, physical abuse may be more likely to be inflicted by sons; physical neglect is likely to be perpetrated either by sons or siblings (Sengstock & Liang, 1983), although differences and sample sizes are small. In some cases of neglect, the "abuser" is actually the elder him- or herself. (For a discussion of self neglect, see Box 5-3.)

The abusers most likely to be involved in emotional neglect or deprivation of rights were daughters (nearly half) and sisters (one-third) (Sengstock & Liang, 1983). An interesting aspect of this study is that no sons or unrelated persons were implicated in cases of emotional neglect. It might be suggested that the persons accused in these situations—daughters and sisters—were persons from whom the elderly, and service providers who consult with them, would most likely expect emotional support (Sengstock, 1991). The expectation of emotional support would particularly apply to daughters. Emotional support is not usually thought to be the responsibility of men, so parents would not be likely to express disappointment if their sons failed to provide such support. Neither would they be likely to expect such help from unrelated persons. Gender-related factors in elder abuse have been mentioned by others as well (Aitken & Griffin, 1996; Dimah and Dimah, 2002; Quinn & Tomita, 1997; Teaster et al., 2000).

Direct emotional abuse may be more characteristic of sons because this type of abuse includes more direct action—such as verbal assaults and creating fear—which many people might consider to be more appropriate masculine behavior (Sengstock, 1991). This might account for the greater representation of sons in

(text continues on page 112)

BOX 5-2 **INTIMATE PARTNER ABUSE AGAINST OLDER WOMEN AND MEN**
by Yvonne Ulrich

The recognition of domestic violence as a distinct aspect of elder abuse carries important implications for prevention of situations that can even become lethal. Both the fields of elder abuse and of domestic violence have knowledge, experience, and methods that together can offer more effective care to older women and men who are simultaneously experiencing aging and an abusive or dangerous intimate partner relationship.

As noted, past formulations have sometimes seen abuse by intimate partners as not belonging under the category of elder abuse (Douglass, 1988). A 1992 forum held by the Women's Initiative of the American Association of Retired Persons and 1993 hearings of the U.S. Senate Special Committee on Aging resulted in recognition of domestic violence as a distinct aspect of elder abuse (Anetzberger, 2001; Brandl & Raymond, 1997a; Ogg & Munn-Giddings, 1993; Wolf, 1996b).

What is it like to be aging and experiencing abuse from an intimate partner? Like other abuse, intimate partner abuse may take the form of physical abuse, verbal abuse, financial deprivation, neglect, or even sexual abuse. Abuse may be considered high-severity if she or he experiences being hit, slapped, kicked, or otherwise physically hurt or being forced to engage in sexual activities. Low-severity abuse can be defined as being pushed or grabbed or threatened.

Studies of incidence of intimate partner abuse tend to include all ages and are not limited to abuse of older women. Pillemer & Finkelhor (1988), extrapolating from their stratified random urban sample of community-dwelling elders who lived with others, estimate a national number of 406,000 elders experiencing spouse abuse within the past year. Examining their total group of abuse victims ($n = 63$), the researchers reported wife-to-husband violence as 36% and husband-to-wife as 22%. These patterns of conflict are reported by abuser or abused in spouse-abuse situations. Yet the National Center on Elder Abuse in 1994 received reports that 61.4% of all victims of domestic elder abuse were women and in 13.8% of all elder abuse the perpetrator was the spouse (Tatara, 1998). Hudson (1997), in her review of the incidence of mistreatment, observed that in cases reported to authorities a disproportionate number of women are victims; that is not the case, however, in self-reported intimate partner-abuse situations.

Older women who are experiencing abusive relationships from spouses or intimate partners may have lived in abusive intimate relationships for 30 to 50 years or more. In another pattern, the abuse may have begun recently from a partner who had previously been nonviolent or from a new marriage (Brandl & Raymond, 1997b; Phillips, 2000).

Researchers know little about what it is like to be aging and experiencing abuse because studies focused on any aspect of older-women partner abuse are hard to find (Grunfeld, Larsson, Mackay, & Hotch, 1996; Ogg, 1993; Phillips, 2000; Wolf, 1996b). The fact that a few studies interviewed the victim of intimate partner abuse in-depth make these works particularly valuable. In a grounded-theory approach, four English-speaking working-class women, 63 to 73 years old, expressed how they made sense of their experiences of battering. The women had been contacted as part of a routine follow-up of the Vancouver Hospital Domestic Violence Program. These women had histories of ulcer, hemorrhage, multiple surgeries, chest pain, heart disease, and multiple facial injuries. Themes not characterized by previously reported interviews with younger battered women were survival concerns in long-term coping with serious abuse, memories linked to children's ages, community support, and turning points (Grunfeld, Larsson, Mackay, and Hotch, 1996). A second study that completed in-depth interviews with 10 abused wives 50 years of age or older found some of the same themes as the Canadian study and echoed the significance of children and the pressure that was stimulated by guilt when the woman faced the idea of children being raised without a father (Phillips, 2000).

(continued)

BOX	5-2	**INTIMATE PARTNER ABUSE AGAINST OLDER WOMEN AND MEN (Continued)**

Three other case studies developed from observations of care providers show patterns of nondisclosure over the lifetime of the couples and the women's adaptations to the situations. The cases are followed by a discussion of the decision-making of the care teams. Gesino, Smith, & Keckich (1982) describe the mental-health problems of two older women who had experienced abuse over a lifetime and their depression at a sudden change in their role provided by death or the suddenly declining health of their spouse. Mitchell and Smyth (1994) describe spouse abuse and childhood sexual abuse over a lifetime in a three-generational family. Bergeron (2001) describes a case where there is a lifetime history of physical abuse that in later years became verbal abuse from an increasingly agitated spouse then diagnosed with Alzheimer's Disease. These cases illustrate the power relations, gender effects, and long-term nature that can characterize abuse between intimate partners as compared with abuse from a caregiver. Excerpts from these cases are woven into the following discussion of intervention.

EFFECTS OF PARTNER ABUSE ON OLDER WOMEN'S HEALTH

It seems reasonable that abuse will have a negative effect on the health of older women in abusive intimate relationships. Although most studies focus on maltreatment and may hide effects particular to spouse abuse, a few studies approach documentation of these women's health problems. McCauley, Kern, Kolodner, Derogatis, & Bass (1998) studied violence toward women from anyone. Women completing surveys in four community-based, primary-care, internal-medicine practices self-reported violence within the past year. Those women who were 46 years and older (51.8%, $n = 1,257$) and who experienced high-severity violence (15.4%, $n = 79$) reported more symptoms and higher levels of psychological distress than those who experienced low-severity violence or no violence (26.7%, $n = 47$).

Mouton studied older women who had experienced abuse from their spouse "or someone important to them" (Mouton, Rovi, Furniss, and Lasser, 1999). In a cross-sectional survey of 257 women aged 50 to 79 ($n = 63$), the investigator measured overall self-reported health status in women who had experienced domestic violence sometime during their life or during the past year. Women volunteers for interviews were recruited from those women who came for screening visits to the Women's Health Initiative site in Newark, NJ. The Medical Outcomes Study Short Form consisted of ratings for components of physical health and mental health. Women who had experienced physical assault and women who had experienced threat had lower scores on physical and significantly lower scores on mental components than women who did not have those experiences of abuse.

HOMICIDES OF OLDER WIVES

Health problems are not the only problems associated with intimate partner abuse in older women. As with younger women, death can be the outcome. More recent studies have begun to document the incidence of homicide, as well as suicide, involving older women and their intimate partners. As in the area of health problems, intimate partner homicide studies rarely focus only on older women. This omission is important because the relationship of the offending party to the woman may help understand risk factors for homicide.

Malphurs & Cohen (2002) studied spousal-consortial murder–suicides among persons 55 years or older identified from medical examiner records; cases were those reported from January 1, 1998 through December 31, 1999 in which there was no evidence of a suicide pact (i.e., a note signed by both persons). The investigators found that 25% of the 20 homicide–suicides had a history of domestic violence, compared with 5% of the suicide controls ($p = .04$). The relationships

(continued)

BOX 5-2 **INTIMATE PARTNER ABUSE AGAINST OLDER WOMEN AND MEN *(Continued)***

between older husbands and wives who had a history of domestic violence may have been one of dominance, dependency, and submission (Berman, 1996; Cohen, 2000). Female victims were thought to be unknowing or unwilling partners in the homicide–suicide. Other studies have characterized such marital relationships as extremely close, deeply attached, or stable when compared to suicide-only relationships (Brown & Barraclough, 1999; Morton, Runyan, Moracco, & Butts, 1998).

NURSING CARE OF OLDER WOMEN AND MEN ABUSED BY INTIMATE PARTNERS

Nursing care for older women or men in abusive intimate relationships requires a knowledge of aging issues and approaches to intimate partner domestic violence. Here, I suggest interventions specific to this population, gleaned from reports in the literature, experience of clinicians, research teams, and case studies. The assumption is that every general type of intervention suggested here is based on interventions that took place, generally, with victims of intimate partner abuse; the specific circumstances need not be repeated here. Interventions include both those for the individual and for the community (Nerenberg, 1997; Phillips, 2000).

OLDER WOMEN'S VALUES

Seaver (1996) reminds us that the moral imperative for older women is to "care." In addition, the values of older women may be those of an earlier generation. Older women may have a "til death do us part" philosophy and may have no intention of ever leaving the relationship (Phillips, 2000). Besides the stigma of divorce that exists in many areas, older women may feel that it is their responsibility to stay and make the marriage work or to fulfill her husband's demands (Gesino, Smith, & Keckich, 1982) or that sex is her duty regardless of how she feels (Mitchell & Smyth, 1994).

DISCLOSURE

Because of the number of these women who need medical care, either in primary-care settings or in an emergency department, standard practice should be to ask questions about lifetime and current abuse. Phillips (2000) reported that her research team had success as they asked older women: "Has ___ ever hit you?" or "Has ___ even threatened you?" or "What happens when you and ___ disagree?" These strategies might open the discussion to explore for abuse (Neufeld, 1996). It will be important to ask her these questions when she is alone and not in the presence of her partner, who may be her abuser. As C. R. Block has pointed out based on her research team's experience with older women (personal communication, January 2000), it may be more difficult for an older woman to answer questions or fill out surveys simply because her dependence on public transportation does not allow for time variations.

The importance of lifetime assessment for all types of abuse is reinforced by case studies that show that answering questions about abuse during the past year is not adequate to women's experience (Bergeron, 2001; Gesino, Smith, and Keckich, 1982; Grunfeld et al., 1996). Many older women do not experience physical hitting but instead are the recipients of verbal abuse (Harris, 1996). As the case studies illustrate, the physical abuse may become verbal in later years, or perhaps verbal abuse precedes serious abuse. In these situations, as in physical abuse, the woman is encouraged to seek support appropriate for older women. Clinicians as well as researchers remind us that cases of older women abused by intimate partners are complex; there may be multiple forms of abuse (Penhale, 1999). The cycle of violence so familiar to many clinicians and to the general public seems less prominent for older women and their partners. Most older women report there are few apologies from the abuser (Brandl & Raymond, 1997a).

(continued)

BOX	5-2	INTIMATE PARTNER ABUSE AGAINST OLDER WOMEN AND MEN *(Continued)*

The case studies of Grunfeld, Larsson, Mackay, & Hotch (1996) suggest helping the woman frame her experience in the context of what is and what is not acceptable treatment from another person. Helping her find a word that she is comfortable with using may facilitate her talking about her experience (Phillips, 2000). As an advocate, showing your compassion and making her aware of resources appropriate for older women abused by intimate partners can make a difference (Brandl & Raymond, 1997a). It is important to work alongside her, toward her goals, rather than to adopt confrontational techniques that may actually be counterproductive for older abused women (Seaver, 1996).

SUPPORT GROUPS

Nerenberg (1997) suggests that support groups be facilitated by persons who are knowledgeable about the process of aging as well as domestic violence. At the very least, one facilitator should be an older woman. Facilitators and counselors without this knowledge may actually endanger older women who are in abusive intimate relationships. It is critical that the older abused woman is accurately perceived as experiencing all of the unique problems of being older as well as being battered so that there can be interventions that are effective (Seaver, 1997).

COMMUNITY LEVEL

Interventions for older women must take place within existing structures and laws. There is agreement that the "system" may not be prepared to deal effectively with the older abused woman. There may be no shelter geared for the needs of older women; police may be less than sympathetic with older women who have been abused for years; or judges may make inappropriate decisions (Nexus, 1995; Vinton, Altholz, & Lobell-Boesch, 1997). Often, the abuser of an older woman is a likable person even respected in the community, and authorities may react in disbelief (Brandl & Raymond, 1997a). Home-support services may not be appropriate for an older woman, especially if she fears for her safety or is socially isolated (Vinton, Altholz, & Lobell-Boesch, 1997). Older women may be trapped in relationships by intervention and policies that do not allow care for both parties, unless services are reflective of needs of both parties (Bergeron, 2001).

Phillips (2000) encourages nurses to engage at the community level in a number of practical ways. Acknowledging the strength of nurses for storytelling, Phillips suggests educating the public, their own social groups, families, and church groups about how domestic violence affects older women. Nurses, because of their training and experience, are further challenged to provide testimony to community leaders.

PROBLEMS PRACTITIONERS FACE

Although abuse incidence "during the past year" in older women and men is negatively related to age, we do not yet understand what happens in a long-term relationship when hitting stops, nor for that matter do we understand what happens when it has been continuous over the long term. Women may be hidden in abusive relationships by a society that does not recognize that older women may be abused even by spouses that they have lived with for years. Unless women over 50 are accurately perceived, they will not be adequately helped (Seaver, 1996).

The fields of elder abuse and domestic violence have each developed knowledge, experience, and methods that, if integrated, can address some of the identified gaps in both systems. It is important for nurses and caregivers to recognize the similarities and differences between the family-violence paradigm and that of elder abuse to be able to determine appropriate intervention so that victims will benefit (Phillips, 1988; Vinton, 1991; Brandl & Raymond, 1997a; Anetzberger, 2001; Bergeron, 2001).

(continued)

BOX 5-2	INTIMATE PARTNER ABUSE AGAINST OLDER WOMEN AND MEN *(Continued)*

In summary, recommendations include:

- View the problem of domestic violence against older women as a function of an elder's met or unmet needs; the key is knowing the appropriate applications of the elder-abuse and family-violence paradigms (Phillips, 1988, 2000).
- View physically abused elder women as battered women who can be empowered by connecting with shelters and support services (Vinton; 1991).
- Use referral protocols that differentiate between domestic violence and elder abuse, in order to develop effective treatment (Anetzberger, 2001).
- Identify the theory or theories guiding their decisions and actions, and evaluate "fit" as the case develops. Theories such as caregiver-stress theory and domestic-violence theory may guide the practitioner to reflect on the needs of both partners. This approach will potentially affect laws, and policies, as well as practice. Using and evaluating theory to tailor interventions is important because it can point to erroneous decisions of the practitioner or it can strengthen the position taken by the professional (Bergeron, 2001). Consistent with Bergeron, Phillips (1988) points out that these issues are critical for providers to be aware of because it places responsibility for treatment on the knowledge base where it belongs.

emotional abuse than in the more passive emotional neglect. However, daughters were almost as likely to engage in direct emotional abuse as their brothers, and unrelated persons and other relatives also appeared in considerable numbers. Sons and daughters were also the most likely to engage in financial abuse, each representing about one-fourth of the cases. Other relatives and unrelated persons were also found in these categories (Sengstock & Liang, 1983).

Thus, the data suggests that sons and daughters are the major perpetrators of most types of elder abuse, with sons more likely to engage in active, direct abuse. Daughters are more likely to be accused of indirect emotional neglect. Other relatives and unrelated persons tend to be suspected abusers primarily in instances of direct abuse. They are less likely to be implicated in neglect, probably because aged victims do not depend on them for help and would not recognize its absence as neglect.

PROPOSED CAUSES OF ELDER ABUSE

There are many theories explaining the existence of family violence and abuse. Theories that explain why parents abuse their children and husbands beat their wives abound. As interest in elder abuse has increased, so also have the number of theories that explain why adults abuse their aging parents. Unfortunately, most of these explanations remain untested; some are backed by research, but others are simply assertions of variables that appear to be important. One study listed 12 different explanations of factors that are thought to be related to elder abuse, including economic conditions and dependency, as well as substance abuse, inadequate housing, and family violence (Kosberg & Garcia, 1995).

In this section, we examine some of the proposed explanations for elder abuse, together with references to available research data. However, we must emphasize that none of these theories can be considered well-established, accurate

BOX	5-3	A SPECIAL CATEGORY OF ELDER MISTREATMENT: SELF-NEGLECT

References to self-neglect appeared in the medical literature in the 1960s, when it was referred to as senile breakdown (MacMillan & Shaw, 1966) or recluse behavior (Granik & Zeman, 1960). Later, the term "Diogenes Syndrome" was introduced (Clark, Manikar, & Gray, 1975). In general, these terms refer to an extreme failure on the part of older persons to perform the activities necessary to maintain normal life and health. Examples are the failure to eat or dress properly or take prescribed medications; at its extreme, elders have been found living in squalor in a rat- or roach-infested house or apartment, with papers and other inflammable debris piled four- to five-feet high throughout. Some have suggested that self-neglect is the most recent official term for a pattern of community deviance or "nonconformity" that is as old as the world (Bozinovski, 2000).

Attention was brought to self-neglect in the 1990s, when a survey of state agencies revealed that it was the form of elder abuse and neglect most commonly seen by state agencies (National Center on Elder Abuse [NCEA], 1998). Thus, self-neglect cases in the United States were estimated at 1.15 million, while all other forms of elder abuse and neglect combined numbered 1.1 million (Tatara & Kuzmeskus, 1997). Many experts long believed that this was the case (Callaghan, 2000). Because it is so common, it is surprising so little has been done to describe and deal with the problem (Bozinovski, 2000).

There is serious question as to whether self-neglect should be included as a category of elder abuse and neglect. However, it is likely to remain so for a variety of reasons. Most obvious is that most states include self-neglect within the elder-abuse statutes; hence, agencies that confront self-neglect are required to report it (Duke, 1991). Because it is assigned to Adult Protective Services, no other agencies are officially assigned to deal with the problem. The fact that it is the most common form of abuse or neglect that agencies observe is another reason. Self-neglect is difficult to identify in the abstract; that is, it is a conclusion drawn after initial observation of an apparently neglected elder. Only later is it learned that the neglect is self-inflicted. Consequently, it is usually recognized in the general process of identification of elder abuse and neglect, and nurses must be aware of the problem and alert to its characteristics.

Most people engage in some self-neglectful activities, such as smoking or not following medical advice (O'Brien et al., 1999). However, self-neglect refers to such behavior in the extreme. Definitions of self-neglect vary. Some define self-neglect in relation to health care only and would exclude behavior that is not damaging to health, such as hoarding (Reed & Leonard, 1989). The National Association of Adult Protective Services Administrators, on the other hand, takes a broad view and includes the failure to provide oneself with such necessities as shelter, food, and appropriate clothing, as well as other resources for physical, mental, and emotional health (Duke, 1991).

Several different reasons for self-neglect have been delineated. In some cases, this behavior is part of a long-standing pattern; in others, it is a dramatic change from previous activities. It is commonly suggested that people who engage in self-neglect are mentally or physically incapable of caring for themselves, due to dementia, alcoholism, confusion, and the like, whereas others—perhaps as many as half—appear to have no major physical or mental impairments (O'Brien et al., 1999).

In interviews with self-neglecters, Bozinovski (2000) found that they tended to be persons who had suffered many losses and they were attempting to maintain their self-identity in the face of a threatening world; consequently, they were distrusting of others, including service providers. Their isolation makes them unlikely to come to the attention of professional agencies and creates special problems for detection (O'Brien et al., 1999).

Once identified, serious ethical issues arise concerning the appropriateness of intervention in cases of self-neglect. Should medical and social agencies intervene in cases in which an elderly person chooses to neglect him- or herself? Are not adults free to make such choices if they wish? Are agency professionals simply imposing their own views of proper behavior on others who may prefer a different life-style?

(continued)

BOX 5-3
A SPECIAL CATEGORY OF ELDER MISTREATMENT: SELF-NEGLECT *(Continued)*

Even though most states include self-neglect among the types of abuse and neglect that must be reported, most jurisdictions also accord mentally competent individuals the right to make choices about health care and other aspects of their lives, provided their behavior is not injurious to others (Benton & Marshall, 1991; Skelley-Walley, 1995). Consequently, a thorough assessment of the elder's mental and physical status, together with the situation as a whole, is essential. Such assessment is not always easy.

Assessment of mental competency, for example, may need to take into account the fact that competency is a complex issue, that some patients are capable of appearing competent for limited periods of time, or that persons may be competent in one area but not in others. For example, a generally competent individual may be capable of handling financial decisions but incapable of understanding the long-term impact of a medical condition, or vice versa (Simmons and O'Brien, 1999; Skelley-Walley, 1995). In some cases, self-neglect may be part of a long-term suicidal pattern or may coexist with other types of abuse or neglect, and workers should be alert to this possibility. Self-neglect may be part of a broad-ranging continuum: Family members who care for an aged relative may become discouraged with his or her self-neglectful behavior and be careless in providing care. Conversely, an elder may become depressed at a lack of concern on the part of the family and begin to neglect him- or herself. Indeed, self-neglect has also been associated with depression.

Assessing the threat to others is difficult, particularly if the self-neglectful individual's living arrangements are in close proximity to others. Piles of inflammable debris or vermin-infected garbage are a greater threat to the community if one lives in an apartment complex than an isolated cabin, for example (Sengstock, Thibault, & Zaranek, 1999).

On one hand, people who are found to be mentally incompetent or incapable of self-care due to physical incapacitation are clearly in need of assistance. Once referred for psychiatric treatment, the outcome in these cases is still unclear; some studies report marked improvement in some cases, and others suggest much more bleak outcomes (O'Brien et al., 1999).

On the other hand, if elders are found to be mentally competent and still choose to follow their aberrant life-style, provided the behavior is not threatening to others, then the choice should be theirs to make. Health-care professionals should insure, however, that the elder is indeed competent to make a decision and that the decision is a free one, not generated either by fear or a lack of understanding of the resources available. They should also take care to insure that they have complied with any and all legal requirements of the state in which the patient resides, including any reporting requirements.

When mentally competent elders persist in the behavior and community health-safety issues are involved, city or state health and safety laws may have to be invoked. For example, an apartment-dwelling elder who threatens other residents and his visiting nurse by continuing to smoke near his oxygen supply may be warned that his oxygen may not be delivered, his nurse may no longer visit, or his lease may be terminated. Or an elder whose garbage-infested house is drawing rats to the neighborhood may be given notice that the city may force clean up of the property at the owner's expense (Sengstock et al., 1999).

explanations of the problem. Certainly, no single theory yet developed is adequate to explain the existence and nature of elder abuse. Nonetheless, the theories can provide professionals with valuable indicators of the probability of abuse.

Most theories of domestic abuse have been developed by associating specific instances of known abuse with other factors in the victim's social-psychological environment. Such theories suggest the types of factors that may be related to abuse and that should be viewed as "danger signals" by nurses and other persons who work with elderly persons. Therefore, they suggest the need for further inquiry by concerned professionals. We examine two categories of theories: general theories of family violence and explanations of abuse relating directly to the aging process.

General Theories of Family Violence

One point that has been stressed regarding characteristics of the elderly is the continuity of personality and behavior throughout life (Back, 1976; Gelfand, 1994; Neugarten, Havighurst, & Tobin, 1968). Gerontologists who espouse this point emphasize the fact that most individuals exhibit a constant pattern of personality characteristics and behavior patterns from youth through their middle years and into old age. Radical changes, either in personality or behavior, are rare once one reaches old age, absent a discernable mental impairment. This theory suggests that the family problems of the aged, including potentially abusive behavior, may be similar to those of younger persons. Consequently, theories of family violence that have been useful in analyzing child and spouse abuse should be examined to determine if they apply to elderly abuse. We consider three types of general theories of domestic abuse: abuser-focused theories, situational stress theories, and theories focusing on the nature of family relationships.

Abuser-Focused Theories

Domestic abuse has often been explained in relation to the psychopathological state of the abuser. In essence, theories that take this approach suggest that the abusive individual is mentally ill and that the abusive behavior is the result of this mental illness. A closely related theory associates domestic abuse with the misuse of alcohol or other substances. This approach is often taken by people with a serious concern about substance abuse. They suggest that alcoholics or drug addicts are highly likely to engage in abusive behavior. In contrast, some theorists suggest that the alcohol or drug is not the basic cause of the abusive behavior; rather, the abuser uses substance abuse as a "cover-up" for abusive tendencies already present. In either instance, the cause of the abuse is thought to be in the psychological state of the abuser. Whether mentally ill or under the influence of alcohol or drugs, the abuser is therefore incapable of controlling behavior. This approach is tempting because it provides an obvious factor that is responsible for the abuse and an equally obvious solution: cure the psychopathological problem, and the abuse will cease (Eigenberg, 2001; Mignon, Larson, & Holmes, 2002).

Unfortunately, studies of domestic abuse rarely have access to independent evidence of mental illness and substance abuse. Hence it is difficult to ascertain the percentage of cases in which either or both of these factors exist. In the study by Sengstock and Liang (1982), for example, case workers were asked whether they had noted the presence of these factors in each instance of abuse reported. Workers noted the presence of mental illness, substance abuse, or both in a relatively small percentage of the cases. A total of only nine, or 12% of the cases, involved abusers who were alcoholics, drug abusers, or diagnosed mentally ill and who therefore had a psychic state that made behavior control difficult or impossible. It appears that the psychopathological state of the abuser is responsible in relatively few cases of elder abuse.

The failure of such causal factors to appear in studies of abuse may be related, however, to the inability of the researchers to uncover the evidence. Either the data-collection instruments may fail to elicit this information from the professional workers, or, in some cases, undiagnosed mental illness, alcoholism, or drug abuse may be present with agency workers unaware of it.

Those cases of elder abuse in which mental illness or substance abuse is present often appear particularly serious or difficult to control. It has been suggested, for example, that substance abuse puts the victim at higher risk for further abuse (Hwalek et al., 1996). In some cases, there is a greater chance that services will be refused, probably because of fear of the abuser (Neale et al., 1997).

Case studies are illustrative. In one instance, an alcoholic daughter subjected her recently widowed mother, who had a heart condition, to constant verbal abuse. She also depended on her mother to care for her three active children because her alcoholism had forced her to relinquish custody. Another woman was subjected to constant threats and emotional abuse by her elderly alcoholic husband. Still another woman had an alcoholic grandson who constantly stole money she had given him to pay her bills.

Even more serious abuse occurs in cases in which mental or emotional illness is present. One aged woman had been severely beaten by her schizophrenic son who lived with her. She was also deprived of the companionship of her daughter; the daughter had been beaten by the brother and was therefore afraid of visiting. In another case, the aged victim had evicted her emotionally ill son from her home, yet the son continued to return home, often breaking into the home while the mother was at work. The victim had sought legal assistance from a legal-aid agency and the county prosecutor to protect herself from her son's abusive behavior.

In terms of providing service to victims, it appears inadvisable to rely heavily on the notion that abuse is caused by such factors as mental illness or substance abuse. If an agency finds such problems in an instance of elder abuse, it is imperative that these problems be treated as a part of the entire family problem. However, an assumption that such factors must be involved would prevent workers from looking for other relevant factors. Such other factors can be valuable "danger signals."

Elder abuse may occur in many cases where mental illness or drug or alcohol abuse is not present, and these factors may not always lead to abuse of aged family members. But because the risk of abuse in such cases is sufficiently high, agency workers should make inquiries to determine the possible presence of abusive behavior. This would be necessary even if the alcoholic, drug addict, or mentally ill individual was an aged person, because such patterns can be associated with abuse in a variety of ways. The psychologically disturbed individual may abuse others, or an elderly addict or mentally ill person may be abused by others as a reaction to the disturbing behavior patterns. As noted, some elder abuse is actually elder–elder abuse.

Situational-Stress Theories

One of the factors frequently cited as a cause of family abuse is stress in the environment. Proponents of the stress-as-cause view indicate that situational factors such as poverty, isolation, or occupational stress may cause people to abuse members of their families. Child and spouse abuse consistently occurs more frequently, although not exclusively, in lower class groups, which are presumed to experience greater stress because of economic deprivation (Barnett et al., 1997; Eigenberg, 2001; Mignon et al., 2002).

Perhaps the primary proponent of the situational-stress model was Gil (1971), who believed that there would be no child abuse if it were not for such factors as poverty or job stress. Expanding on this approach to child abuse, Justice and Justice (1976) noted that families who have a considerable number of other problems were more likely to abuse their children. In their cases of abusive parents, they found an unusually high frequency of persons who had undergone a "prolonged series of changes"—economic crises, illnesses, deaths, and accidents. They emphasized that the prolonged series of stressful situations, rather than a single stressful event, promotes violence. It has also been noted that abusive families are socially isolated and unlikely to have social resources to call on when stressful situations occur (Barnett et al., 1997; Eigenberg, 2001; Mignon et al. 2002).

No definitive studies support the view that situational-stress factors play a role in abuse of the aged. However, professionals who work with the elderly and their caregivers suggest that the problems associated with care of an aged person may create stress and promote abuse. Such age-specific problems are discussed in a later section. In this section, we discuss some more general, non-age-related stress factors that may tend to promote elder abuse.

Similar to the theory promoted by Justice and Justice (1976) that a family is more likely to abuse children when confronted with a multitude of problems is the notion that abuse of the elderly may exist in families plagued with many problems, serious and otherwise. Sengstock and Liang (1982) found that elder-abuse victims reported an exceptionally large number of problems they or their families had experienced. These are clearly "multiproblem" families, and it is probable that the elder abuse could not have been corrected until the accompanying problems and tensions had been alleviated. As with other types of domestic violence, treatment of the entire family and its problems is necessary (Sengstock, Barrett, & Graham, 1984).

The situational-stress theory of domestic abuse has been severely criticized. It has often been noted that situational stress is inadequate in explaining child abuse because it fails to show why some families react to stress and frustration by abusing their children or spouses, whereas others, subjected to the same stress, do not. Similarly, a stress model does not totally explain why some adults, when faced with severe family stress, would react by abusing an aged member while others would not (Eigenberg, 2001; Mignon et al., 2002).

However, the stress model does call attention to the fact that outside factors must be considered in explaining the abusive behavior. If the abuser is an individual with serious personal problems, these problems must be dealt with sympathetically before the relationship with others can be rebuilt on a nonviolent basis. Furthermore, the family has to be dealt with as a unit, lest the abuser return to his or her abusive behavior when family problems and the interactions of other family members reassert themselves.

Theories Focusing on the Nature of Family Relationships

Another approach to family violence that has received considerable support is a model that views domestic abuse in the context of general family relationships. This approach suggests that a well-established pattern of violent behavior on the part of an individual need not necessarily suggest the existence of a situational or psychopathological state. Rather, such behavior, like nonviolent behavior, can be learned early in life (Barnett et al., 1997; Eigenberg, 2001; Mignon et al., 2002). Evidence indicates that elderly victims, as well as the members of their families, may indeed have learned abusive behavior as an appropriate approach to solving life's problems (Sengstock & Liang, 1982).

Normative Violence. It has been suggested by some authors that domestic abuse is part of a general pattern of "normative violence," in which violent behavior is accepted, even approved, as a normal part of family life (Gelles, 1993; United Nations, 2001). One study of elderly victims asked respondents if they were ever punched or hit or threatened with a knife or gun, whether as part of the reported abuse or not (Sengstock & Liang, 1982). Nearly one half of these elderly people reported that they had been punched or hit; 10% had been threatened by another person wielding a knife; and 35% of these aged persons had been threatened with a gun. In contrast, a study of domestic violence using a national random sample found that 10% of persons had been hit or kicked sometime during their marriages and that 4% had been threatened with a knife or gun (Straus, Gelles, & Steinmetz, 1980). Although the studies are not totally comparable, the national data does suggest that this group of aged victims had considerably more violence in their backgrounds. These people appeared to be part of a "subculture of violence," and may have come to accept violent action as "normative" or appropriate.

In the first national survey of family violence, a large majority (greater than 70%) of the respondents expressed their belief that physical punishment of children was appropriate and necessary (Gelles & Straus, 1988; Straus et al., 1980). This belief may cause children to grow up with the idea that physical responses are appropriate for a larger, stronger person who has his or her will thwarted by a smaller, weaker person. It would not be surprising if child-abuse victims learned that such behavior was appropriate when and if they should move into such a position in reference to their parents.

So the aged parents may have taught the behavior that was later used against them. It was also noted that the abusive behavior is closely related to the social role generally associated with certain types of abusers. Sons were more likely to engage in direct abuse, whereas daughters were more likely to be responsible for emotional abuse or neglectful behavior. Such differences suggest that abuse may be learned as a part of normal sex-role patterns, in which men are expected to react in a direct, physical manner, and women are expected to react with emotional outbursts and to withhold affection and support (Sengstock, 1991). Hence the data provides some support for the learning theory of domestic abuse.

Long-Standing Patterns of Family Violence. When attitudes and behaviors that support the use of violence and force are firmly established in a family, it is likely that violence and force will be directed toward those family members least able to defend themselves. These victims are more likely to include children or the aged. Often, the most tragic cases are those showing evidence of a long-term abusive pattern in the family. In these cases, abusive behavior may continue for the entire duration of a marriage, or the victims of abuse may alternate between one generation and another. Abusive behavior patterns are highly likely to be passed from parents to children (Straus et al., 1980).

Several cases illustrate this type of pattern. A stroke victim with partial paralysis was hospitalized following an "accident" in which she had allegedly fallen down the stairs. Actually, her husband, who had abused her for most of their married life, had pushed her down the stairs. As a child, she had also been abused by her mother. In planning for her release from the hospital, the hospital staff arranged for this victim to live with her daughter instead of returning to her abusive husband. However, it was found that the daughter's husband was also abusive (Sengstock & Liang, 1982). So this family is now in its third generation of abuse and is rearing a fourth generation of young people who view abuse as a well-established and seemingly appropriate dimension of family life.

In another case, a woman's children were removed from her custody because she had abused them. Subsequent to the removal of her children, she assumed a role in the care of her invalid father. This case was discovered when the daughter poured boiling water over her father, scalding him badly. Cases such as these suggest that the common pattern of removing a victim from an abusive situation often does little to resolve the situation. Although it may protect the specific individual victimized at a given time, it does nothing to assist the abuser in controlling his or her behavior. As a result, the abuse may simply be transferred to another likely victim: from child to aged parent, from aged parent to spouse, or from one intimate partner to another.

Although abuse by children seems more likely, elder abuse can also appear in marital or pseudomarital relationships (Sengstock, 1991; Sengstock & Liang, 1982; Vinton, 1991), an issue not recognized as elder abuse by some authors (Douglass, 1988). This type of abuse may be more common when one partner is either considerably older or more infirm than the other. The previous case of an aged woman whose husband pushed her down the stairs is an example.

In several cases, the usual domestic-violence sex roles were reversed, with the woman being the abuser and the man, the victim. In two separate cases, children removed an infirm father from the home because they saw evidence that their mother was abusing their father, physically, emotionally, or both. In both instances, the mother claimed that her children were abusing her because they had deprived her of her husband's presence in the home; yet in one instance a medical examination showed clear evidence of malnutrition in the father, whose condition improved greatly after being removed from his wife's care. A case worker reported that one of these women had stated that her husband had made her suffer for most of her life, and it was now his turn to suffer. In a third case, the wife and children together took the husband's money and abandoned him. (Additional information on elderly spouse abuse may be found in Box 5-2.)

Victim Precipitation Among the Elderly. A common explanation for domestic abuse is victim precipitation: the victim "asked for it." That is, through his or her own misbehavior or goading, the victim "forced" the offender to take revenge. This view is found often with regard to spouse abuse (United Nations, 2001). Evidence of this pattern has also been found in some cases of elder abuse (Sengstock and Liang, 1982). Some service providers believed abuse was precipitated by the victim, at least in part, when an aged parent attempted to retain more control over his or her children than most young adults were likely to allow. Examples were cases in which a parent, usually a mother, opposed a child's marriage or religious choice or considered aspects of a child's behavior to be inappropriate. Agency workers suggested that the abuse would probably not have occurred, or would not have been so severe, if the elders had not engaged in the provocative behavior. Although most domestic-violence authorities do not accept the notion of victim precipitation, it is clear that the abuse is not likely to cease unless the elderly person can be induced to give up, at least to a degree, the behavior that provokes the abuse.

Family Financial Issues. It has been suggested that abuse of elderly may be provoked by financial difficulties on the part of one or more members of the family (Greenberg et al., 1990; Neale et al., 1997; Wolf et al., 1984). Abusers may include siblings, spouses, grandchildren, children, as well as unrelated persons, but children are probably the most frequent (Hwalek et al., 1996; Sengstock & Liang, 1982). For example, a son took $80,000 from his father's bank account while his widowed father was in a nursing home and also attempted to block his father's remarriage to protect any remaining property. Another man who spoke only Spanish was tricked into signing over his home to his son, who then mortgaged the home and forced his father to make the payments. In a third case, the abuser was a 20-year-old woman who made frequent visits to her great-grandmother; during the visits she stole the lady's bank books and emptied the accounts.

In some cases, the family member appears to be in true financial need and therefore is tempted to take money from the aged person, who is probably seen as having little use for it. As noted, this may be particularly characteristic of some ethnic communities. In many instances, however, it is difficult to avoid the conclusion that greed motivates the actions. Recognition of this is an important part of clinical assessment. Clinical personnel should investigate the possibility of abuse in cases in which family members appear inordinately concerned about the financial assets of an elder or their possible depletion through medical expenses.

Explanations of Abuse Relating to the Aging Process

Normal family relations can by their nature be tense and stressful. However, the aging process creates additional stress and tension in a family. Below we discuss several aging-related factors that may be possible causes of elder abuse.

Demographic and Economic Changes

There are no data that clearly indicates whether the incidence of elder abuse is on the rise. Current statistics are largely based on reports to official agencies or observations by reporters (Hwalek et al., 1996; Neale et al., 1997; Phillipson, 2000; Thomas, 2000). Consequently, they are likely to increase with the number and skill of the reporters and observers, as well as with the resources of the agencies involved. Furthermore, statistics on elder abuse in past decades are impossible to reconstruct. Thus, any comparison with past data is likely to note an increase in frequency, but this is largely an artifact of the available data.

It has frequently been suggested, however, that the demographic and economic patterns in place today promote the likelihood of elder abuse due to the increasing number of elderly and the correlative difficulty for adult children to provide necessary care for aged parents (Quinn & Tomita, 1997; Weith, 1994). In the past, families were considerably larger, and the life expectancy of the elderly was substantially shorter. Consequently, there were several children in a family who could share the responsibilities of caring for an aged parent, and the caregiving period was likely to be only a few years, perhaps a decade at most.

Changes in the medical care available to the aged have greatly increased their life span, with the result that many elderly may live two or more decades during which they require constantly increasing assistance from their children. The trend toward smaller families means that this increased responsibility falls on the shoulders of fewer and fewer children. So even the best-intentioned children may find it difficult to care adequately for their aged parents. The increased life span has been accomplished largely as a result of modem medicine with all of its attendant costs. In families already burdened by the high cost of living, the cost of medical care for an aged parent can overextend the available resources. Such factors probably account, in large part, for the frequency of abuse among the infirm aged. Therefore, elder abuse might be decreased by a greater availability of services to assist families in the care of their aged members.

Changes in the Elderly Person's Life

The debilitating process of aging compounds the difficulties of care of an aged parent (Quinn & Tomita, 1997). Many people look forward to retirement as a time of increased freedom and opportunity. However, many factors may intervene to thwart these plans. Old age can be a time of decreasing physical and mental capacity, increasing dependence on others, loss of independence, and loss of social relationships and status (Gelfand, 1994). Thus aged persons often find that the activities they were formerly able to perform for themselves—personal care, care of the home, meal preparation—are now beyond their capacity. Former social roles, such as caring for children or grandchildren or holding valued positions in business or community, are no longer theirs. They may have lost valued relatives or friends through illness or death. Thus they suffer great loss of self-esteem as they see themselves becoming progressively less capable.

They simultaneously become increasingly dependent on their children, not only for personal care and assistance with normal household tasks but also for most of their social needs. Dependence on children for personal care is particularly embarrassing, because most families have strong taboos against parents and children seeing each other naked.

Changes in the Lives of Adult Offspring

The increased care required by an aging parent comes at a highly inopportune time in the lives of many adult offspring. Most caretaking offspring are in middle age, a time that presents its own difficulties (Sengstock & Liang, 1982; 1983). Men may face retirement and look forward to a more leisurely life-style. Children may have left the home or at least have reached an age when they no longer need constant care. Middle-aged adults often reach the point where they no longer need to obtain sitters for their children, only to discover that their mobility is then limited by having to find someone to care for an aged parent in their absence.

With normal child care, parents can look forward to a not-too-distant day when the child will be independent. With care of an aged parent, however, caregivers must face ever-increasing dependence for periods of indeterminable duration.

Caretaking has usually fallen to women, who mostly stayed at home. In recent years, however, the increased number of women who work outside the home, particularly after their children are in school, reduces the possibility of available middle-aged caregivers. This caretaking period is also likely to fall at a time when the adult offspring are themselves aging and may be in poor health (Block and Sinnott, 1979; Sengstock, 1991; Sengstock & Liang, 1983).

For many middle-aged women, the pressures of parent care may place them in a no-win situation. They are caught between the needs of their aged parents and in-laws and those of their husbands and children. Their husbands may demand more adult time alone; their children may be reaching the difficult teen years. Conversely, their time and energies are increasingly sapped by the growing needs of their aged parents. They may often be emotionally and physically unable to cope with both.

It is tempting to criticize middle-aged offspring for being thoughtless and unloving when they resist caring for an aged parent or, even worse, when the person under their care suffers neglect or abuse. These problems in the caregivers' lives are very real, however, and the problem of elder abuse is not likely to be resolved as long as there are inadequate supports for families dealing with such stresses (Sengstock, Barrett, & Graham, 1984).

Problems of Intergenerational Living

If the needs of an elderly person are such that he or she can no longer live alone, relocation with other family members can create stress that may precipitate abuse. Even families maintaining positive relationships may undergo severe stress from the problems of constant daily contact. Adding an additional person to a household may create problems of crowding. Adult offspring and grandchildren may be forced to give up their privacy and alter their life-styles to accommodate an aged person's needs. Often, the caretaking child feels that he or she was forced into having the aged parent in the home, particularly if siblings are not subjected to the same responsibility. Power conflicts are also likely to occur, as the members of each generation, with their differing views, express conflicting opinions over household maintenance, child care, and family activities.

It is tempting to suggest that a middle-aged offspring or grandchild who would resent making such adjustments in deference to a beloved parent or grandparent is thoughtless and unfeeling. However, no one can maintain a totally selfless demeanor for an extended period of time. The needs of all persons in a multigenerational household must be accommodated for such a pattern to be successful on a long-term basis. Too often the supports necessary for such accommodations are unavailable to the families who require them. Such supports might include day-care centers for the aged, provisions for short-term respite care to afford a family an occasional vacation, as well as financial supports for families who assume the responsibility of in-home care.

Aging and Long-Standing Family Relationships

All the factors previously mentioned can create serious difficulties even for the most loving children who are anxious to provide the best care for their aged relatives. However, family-violence experts have noted for some time that many families do not resemble the image of the loving, harmonious family (Barnett et al., 1997). Not only can elder abuse be an extension of existing violent family patterns, but also families that have contained conflict may be unable to continue to do so when confronted with elder care. Children who have never had a good relationship with their parents may be able to avoid open conflict by maintaining a degree of social distance between the generations. The constant contact required by a caretaking relationship may destroy this fragile peace.

It has been noted that some offspring are unable to accept the new relationship in which their parents are no longer all-powerful and are instead increasingly dependent on their children (Block & Sinnott, 1979). The aged parent may also be unable to accept the adult status of their children; may make constant, unreasonable demands; and may interfere with their adult children's lives and decisions. Such parent–adult child relationships appear most likely to be involved in elder abuse.

For elder abuse from spouses, cases already discussed demonstrate a continuation of an extended abusive pattern. In some instances, however, the abuse may be precipitated by problems of aging. For example, a fragile marital relationship may be unable to survive the increased contact that accompanies retirement. Couples may also find that role reversal accompanies old age. Thus a husband who is accustomed to his wife handling all household tasks may be unable to deal with her becoming an invalid. Our study uncovered one case of severe neglect that involved a frail but proud old man whose invalid wife badly needed health-care assistance; he insisted they could care for themselves (Sengstock & Liang, 1982).

Such cases may be common, as the caregivers may be aged and frail. It is not unknown for 80- or 90-year-old parents to depend totally on their 60- or 70-year-old offspring, who may be incapable of performing elder-care tasks. To accuse a 70-year-old caregiver of neglect for failing to provide bedside assistance needed by a bedridden parent or spouse may be highly unreasonable. Hence, nursing interventions for an aged person must be planned with assurance that the family is capable of carrying out the plans without undue stress.

Loneliness of the Single Aged as a Cause of Abuse

When family abuse is discussed, the usual patterns include traditional family relationships: spouses, children, or, less frequently, grandchildren, siblings, nieces, and nephews. However, this pattern does not always apply to the elderly, many of whom either live alone or with a spouse who is also elderly. Although most have relatives nearby to help, some do not. Hence they may be willing to trust a friendly outsider who offers assistance, perhaps more willing than might be prudent. One assumes the elderly would be extremely cautious in admitting unknown persons into their homes. On occasion, however, aged persons may be less cautious, often with sad results.

In the study by Sengstock and Liang (1982), one case involved a stroke victim who was unable to remain alone after her return from the hospital. Because of the cost of a homemaking service, she and her family accepted the offer of a distant relative to come into the home and provide care. Unknown to the family, the willing housekeeper was a drug addict and was extremely abusive to the aged lady, screaming at her and refusing to assist her in going to the bathroom, even attacking her physically. Another aged woman took in a boarder who was presumed to be a good risk; however, she kept late hours and was loud, making it difficult for the elderly landlady to sleep. After being asked to move, she refused, and the lady had to seek legal assistance to remove the boarder from the house.

Another situation that portends abuse is the life-style of the aged single male. Whether widowed, divorced, or never married, these men often find that their ability to attract women has drastically decreased; yet they still have the same sexual needs and desire for female companionship. As a result, they often place themselves in situations in which they can easily be taken advantage of by younger women, who promise companionship and sexual favors and then abuse them, usually by stealing money. Thus aged persons should exercise caution before taking anyone into their home or their confidence. With family and close friends, they are likely to have at least an inkling of the person's behavior patterns and the likelihood of risk. With strangers, they often know nothing about the risk until it is too late.

Theories of Elder Abuse as Clinical Indicators

No theory has clearly and indisputably been established as an explanation for elder abuse. The proposed theoretical positions remain largely hypotheses. The theories, however, may be valuable indicators of the likelihood of abuse. Aged persons who exhibit, or whose families exhibit, any of the relevant characteristics are in considerable danger of being physically or emotionally abused, severely neglected, or placed in a position of extreme financial disadvantage. They may also be unaware of an alternative to their present situation. Because of the greater health needs of the aged, they may have contact with nurses more than with most other professionals; the nurses can help in providing assistance.

Because the same family patterns affect young and old alike, some explanations of domestic violence in general are equally applicable to elder abuse. Hence some aged appear to be abused because they have the misfortune to be associated with family members who have severe psychological or emotional problems, lending support to abuser-focused theories. The situational stress theory appears promising because a substantial number of aged abuse victims come from families that have an unusually large number of serious family problems. Support can also be found for the view that elder abuse occurs in families having a long-term, well-established behavior pattern in which violence and abuse play an accepted role.

Finally, certain social correlates of the aging process play a special role in the development of the types of family tension that may lead to elder abuse. The increased life expectancy of the aged, with its escalating years of dependency and burgeoning health care costs, places an ever-increasing burden on fewer and fewer children for a longer period of time. Such tensions often place severe stress on families already strained by crises of middle age or tenuous family ties. Steps in preventing elder abuse must recognize the legitimacy of such family needs. Proposed solutions should include the means to relieve the tensions of the caregiving family if elder abuse is to be halted or avoided.

MEANS USED BY AGENCIES IN IDENTIFYING AND SERVING ABUSED ELDERLY

Assisting abused and neglected elderly is a two-part process. People who are victims of elder abuse or neglect must first be identified, which can be daunting. Once elder abuse has been identified, the services required to assist the elderly person and prevent further abuse must be found. In this section we focus on both of these problems.

Difficulties of Identifying Elder Abuse and Neglect

Abused elders, like other victims of family abuse, are very difficult to identify. It has long been recognized that abuse of the elderly is probably greatly underreported (NCEA, 1998; O'Brien, Thibault, Turner, & Laird-Fick, 1999).

The unclear and conflicting definitions of elder abuse provide little guidance to agencies (Goodrich, 1997). Some suggest that financial abuse and sexual abuse are particularly difficult to identify and substantiate (Nerenberg, 2000;

Teaster et al., 2000). Like other victims of family violence, abused elders are often reluctant to report their abuse. Conversely, official agencies are reluctant to invade the privacy of the home. People are embarrassed to admit that their own families depart from the presumed norm of family harmony and love and wish to maintain the family's reputation; they may fear the loss of the relationship with the abuser, who may be a beloved child and perhaps their closest remaining relative (Quinn & Tomita, 1997). Elderly victims may fail to report out of fear of the abuser, who may threaten further violence, loss of support, or other reprisals. Many elderly victims are also reluctant to turn to professional agencies because they lack knowledge or have fear of the agencies (Gelfand, 1994).

Abuse and neglect are particularly difficult to identify in certain cultural groups (Carson, 1995; Tomita, 1998). Many state definitions and reporting requirements ignore cultural differences that exist among these groups (Griffin, 1994). Researchers also suggest that identification in such groups is complicated by a strong belief that such problems should remain within the family, as well as by family members' reluctance to confide such information to outsiders, accept outside intervention, and even speak openly about problems of any type (Davidhizar, Dowd, Giger, and Newman, 1998; Le, 1997; Moon and Benton, 2000; NCEA, 1998; Tomita, 1998, 2000). This has been found to be true among Asians, Hispanics, and Native Americans, among others. It has also been found that some ethnic communities, particularly Hispanics and Asians, tend to define abuse solely in a family context; consequently, they are unlikely to report abuse by outsiders (Moon, 2000).

Disorientation, senility, or a simple lack of knowledge concerning available services may also render a victim incapable of reporting his or her abuse. Those victims who are aware of available resources may still resist reporting because they feel incapable of coping with the ensuing responsibilities. Possible court appearances or conversations with the police can be difficult and fear-provoking experiences (Reulbach & Tewksbury, 1994; Sengstock and Hwalek, 1986c).

There is great variability among agencies and workers in their ability to identify abuse. That is partly because agencies are more likely to observe abuse in the area they are accustomed to treating (Douglass et al., 1980; Hickey & Douglass, 1981a, 1981b; Sengstock & Liang, 1982; 1983). However, even within the same agency, there may be variability between workers in their knowledge and concern about elder abuse. Some astute professionals, realizing that effective service is often worker dependent, have learned to inquire as to which worker is on call before reporting a case. Hence recognition of elder abuse is quite dependent on two factors: the nature of the agency and the interest of the individual worker (Sengstock and Barrett, 1982, 1986; Sengstock & Liang, 1983).

Many agencies have developed their own techniques for the identification of elderly victims of abuse, including clinical techniques for use in hospitals and agencies, procedures for use in state protective-service departments, and measures for use in research (Neale et al., 1996; Sengstock & Hwalek, 1985-1986, 1987; Sengstock, Hwalek, & Moshier, 1986). Early measures had numerous flaws, such as the inclusion of items that measured more than one type of abuse, requiring observers to make multiple judgments, like determining the presence of abuse as well as the deliberateness of the act, and the omission of some types of abuse, particularly sexual assault (Sengstock & Hwalek, 1985-1986). Measures include short protocols to identify persons at risk (Hwalek & Sengstock, 1986), as well as comprehensive measures designed to document symptoms of various types of abuse, the degree of intentionality of the abuser, and possible service needs of victims (Sengstock & Hwalek, 1986a, 1986b). The validity and effectiveness of such measures is still under study (Neale, Hwalek, Scott, Sengstock, & Stahl, 1991).

The abuse of elders confined to institutions, such as nursing homes and long-term-care facilities, is also an area of concern (Pillemer and Moore, 1990; U.S. House Select Committee on Aging, 1985). Although this is a widely discussed problem, empirical research on the subject is limited and frequently low in quality (Himmelstein, Jones, & Woolhandler, 1983; Kimsey, Tarbox, & Bragg, 1981; Shaw, 1998). Identification is a particularly critical problem with this population because the abused often are fearful of retaliation if they report abuse. They may also be unaware of their rights or physically or mentally incapable of protecting themselves (Hodge, 1998; Kimsey et al., 1981). One measure has been adapted for use with this population (Sengstock & Hwalek, 1986a; Sengstock, McFarland, & Hwalek, 1990). See Box 5-4 for further discussion of institutional abuse.

Services Provided to Elderly Victims of Abuse and Neglect

Even if an elderly abused person decides to report the experience or is recognized by some agency, it is not clear that he or she will receive appropriate assistance in dealing with the matter. The tendency to "accept and hide" that appears with most domestic abuse occurs with elder abuse as well. Hence, the services vary from state to state and tend to be uneven in type and quality (Goodrich, 1997). This situation engenders a serious dilemma for service providers seeking the best outcomes for their clients, as we discuss in Box 5-5.

Physicians, who are most likely to see the physical evidence of serious violence, have a long-standing reputation for trying to avoid dealing with domestic abuse of all types, including the elderly. Efforts to alter this pattern have occurred in recent years, however (Haviland & O'Brien, 1989; Vernon & Bennett, 1995). Police and the courts, normally the avenue of redress for the victim of criminal assault or civil injury, have largely ignored domestic assaults, including those involving the elderly (Blakely & Dolon, 2000).

The lack of attention to elder abuse in the legal sphere has been attributed to a variety of reasons, including a lack of training, lack of police resources, and a number of beliefs held by the police, including the beliefs that such things are best left a private matter, that little can be done for such cases, and that domestic disturbance calls can be dangerous for the police (Blakely and Dolon, 2000; Calvert, 1974; Daniels et al., 1999; Straus et al., 1980). Prosecutors are often reluctant to prosecute because many elders are incapable of providing good evidence (Stiegel, 2000). There is some indication, however, that the police and courts are becoming more helpful in elder-abuse cases (Blakely & Dolon, 2000; Heisler, 2000; Quinn and Tomita, 1997; Ruelbach & Tewksbury, 1994; Stiegel, 2000).

Research has suggested that a wide variety of services are needed by elderly victims of abuse or neglect, and that close collaboration among agencies providing these services is necessary (Quinn & Tomita, 1997). Noncriminal approaches to such domestic problems are usually recommended; these may consist of such varied assistance as in-home social work (Kinderknect, 1986); legal assistance (Heisler and Quinn, 1995; Sengstock & Barrett, 1986); and crisis intervention,

BOX	5-4	THE SPECIAL PROBLEM OF INSTITUTIONAL ABUSE

Institutional abuse is included with no other type of domestic abuse, which further differentiates elder abuse from other categories of domestic violence.The increased number of elderly who live in institutional settings, such as nursing homes, homes for the aged, senior citizen complexes, board-and-care homes, and the like, necessitates the subcategorization of this abuse. There is a great deal of public concern over the safety of patients in these settings (Pillemer & Moore, 1990).

This concern has translated into legislation aimed at protecting residents in such facilities, as well as prosecuting the perpetrators of the abuse. In 1978, the U.S. Congress introduced the Long-Term Care Ombudsman program in the various states and charged those programs with receiving and investigating complaints of abuse or neglect in long-term-care facilities (Hodge, 1998; Nelson, Huber, & Walter, 1995; Skelley-Walley, 1995). Prior to that time, such cases were largely handled at the local level, with a high degree of variability in the effectiveness of managing the complaints. Congress also charged Medicaid Fraud Units with the responsibility of checking into abuse of patients, as well as fraud against the health-care system, in institutions receiving Medicaid payments. Laws on institutional abuse, like those in the domestic violence area, vary from state to state but generally include the same major types of mistreatment reported in community settings: physical abuse, sexual abuse, emotional or psychological abuse, neglect, and financial exploitation (Hodge, 1998).

Although there is little data on elder abuse and neglect in general, this is particularly so with elders living in institutions (Shaw, 1998). However, there is little question that this concern is well placed. Reported cases are appalling. In the area of physical abuse, examples include kicking patients in the face and body, dragging them down the hall, rape, and threats to give patients lethal doses of medication or to attack family members. Patients were not taken to the bathroom and were then ridiculed when they soiled their beds. Aides have washed patients with filthy rags soiled with urine or feces. Neglect cases have included malnutrition, dehydration, untreated decubiti, and leaving patients in rooms littered with feces, vomit, blood, or urine. Patients requiring a two-person transfer have been moved alone, resulting in fractures or other injuries. Prescribed medications were given late or not at all, and records were falsified to hide the failure. Patients' pensions and personal-needs accounts have been stolen or misappropriated (Hodge, 1998). The impact on patients can be immense. One patient went blind from the injuries; another became so withdrawn she could no longer communicate with her family (Payne & Cikovic, 1995). Some patients were too frightened to eat or drink, and some died (Hodge, 1998).

There is no clear definition as to what is meant by "institutions for the elderly." A wide variety of facilities come under this category, from those providing skilled nursing care to those that provide only shared living facilities (Pillemer & Moore, 1990). Long-term-care ombudsmen have the responsibility of overseeing all these types of facilities—an enormous task to be accomplished with relatively slim resources (Netting, Huber, Paton, & Kautz, 1995). One reason for the high level of concern about institutional abuse is that conditions in such settings are conducive to the perpetration of abuse and neglect, for a variety of reasons.

One such condition is the wide range of potential abusers in these settings. Whereas the typical community-dwelling elder commonly comes into contact only with family and friends, institutionalized elders may be at risk of abuse by dozens of people everyday: staff members; other residents; visitors, both their own and those of other patients; vendors who may come into the facility; intruders; and the like (AMA, 1992; Hodge, 1998; Pillemer & Moore, 1990).

Another condition is the high percentage of institutional residents who have some type of impairment, including visual or hearing problems, as well as dementia. It has been estimated that as many as half of institutional elderly suffer from some type of dementia (AMA, 1992). This makes institutional abuse particularly difficult to prosecute, and the outcomes are uncertain because the victims' limited capacity makes them poor witnesses. Besides the dementia issue, most are fearful,

(continued)

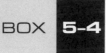

BOX 5-4   THE SPECIAL PROBLEM OF INSTITUTIONAL ABUSE *(Continued)*

and some will have died before a case can come to court (Hodge, 1998). When cases do go to court, results are apparently better if a witness observes the abusive act. Sexual offenders are most likely to receive a prison sentence, but few other offenders do (Payne & Cikovic, 1995).

The abuse of patients by staff members is a particular concern. It is widely recognized that institutional staff may be inadequate in number, poorly trained, and have little background in the care of the elderly. This is especially true in facilities, such as boarding homes, that do not provide skilled nursing care (AMA, 1992; Pillemer & Moore, 1990). This lack of training is complicated by the difficult job staff are required to perform. The jobs are very stressful, and there is little time allotted for workers to provide high-quality personal care to their patients (Pillemer & Moore, 1990; Shaw, 1998).

It has been found that workers in these settings tend to view the patients in a negative light—as being feeble, incompetent, and requiring discipline. Because so many patients are demented, it is not surprising that staff are also likely to report numerous conflicts with patients, many of them initiated by the patients. And many staff members have never been taught how to deal appropriately with patient aggression (Pillemer & Moore, 1990; Shaw, 1998).

All types of nursing-home employees have been found to commit patient abuse, but the most common abusers were nurses' aides, who make up the largest category of employees in nursing homes. A gender-related pattern also appeared in the reports. Male workers were more likely to commit such offenses, even though more women work in such jobs. It was also noted that male patients appeared to be at greater risk of abuse and that abusive workers were more likely to attack persons of the same sex (Payne & Cikovic, 1995).

One study interviewed nursing-home staff members about the abuse they had observed. More than one-third of the respondents reported having observed at least one incident of physical abuse, and more than three-fourths observed an incident of psychological abuse or neglect in the previous year (Pillemer & Moore, 1990). Of these, approximately 20% saw improper restraints; 17% saw such behavior as pushing or shoving a patient; half to two-thirds observed workers yelling or swearing at patients; and one-fourth saw patients isolated inappropriately. Also observed were threats to hit or throw something at patients, and denying patients food or privileges (Pillemer & Moore, 1990).

The possibilities and resources for abuse are also different in institutional facilities. The disabilities of institutionalized elderly may require the use of various restraints; the improper use of such restraints offer opportunities for abuse. For example, patients may be left restrained in chairs or beds for long periods or restraints may be improperly applied so that they may cause injury. The use of chemical restraints—overmedication for the convenience of staff members—is often noted (AMA, 1992; Sengstock, McFarland, & Hwalek, 1990). Theft or misuse of patient property may seem to be a minor problem, but in light of the fact that the institution is the elder's home and personal property and rights have been reduced to a minimum, the loss of any single item may loom large in the patient's mind (Sengstock et al., 1990).

ASSESSMENT AND MANAGEMENT

Identification of abuse or neglect is particularly important in institutional facilities because of the nature of the residential population. Many institutionalized elderly are incapable of taking care of themselves and are dependent upon others for their safety. They therefore are unable to recognize and report abusive actions on their own. Furthermore, those who are mentally alert may be afraid to report for fear of later retaliation from the abuser or other staff (Sengstock et al., 1990).

Nurses who work in hospitals or doctors' offices may come into contact with such patients when they appear for treatment of other ailments. Hence there is a particular need to be alert to

(continued)

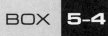

THE SPECIAL PROBLEM OF INSTITUTIONAL ABUSE *(Continued)*

the presence of suspicious symptoms when patients from such settings come in for care. The same techniques for identification that have been presented elsewhere in this chapter may be used, with the special provision that additional types of abuse, such as chemical restraints, may be present (Sengstock et al., 1990). Although identification of the abuser is problematic, this is usually not the responsibility of the nurse but of the agency responsible for receiving reports of abuse. Nurses should be aware that the guidelines and reporting mechanisms for abuse and neglect in institutional settings may be different from those that apply to community-dwelling elderly (AMA, 1992). Nurses should learn the proper reporting agency for the different types of settings in the state in which they work.

Nurses in residential institutions for the elderly whose positions place them in authority bear particular responsibilities. They must be aware of the wide variety of types of abuse and neglect, particularly those that are most common in institutional facilities, as prevously indicated. They must remain alert to the wide variety of people who come and go and may perpetrate abuse against residents. Providing effective training and supervision of staff in these facilities is critical, especially in regard to the psychosocial aspects of nursing-home care, the stress that accompanies these positions, and the difficult patient behaviors that staff will inevitably encounter (Hodge, 1998; Pillemer & Moore, 1990).

In a study of nursing-home employees, it was noted that certain types of people seemed more able to handle the problems of these highly stressful jobs. These were people who derived satisfaction from the work, were able to separate stresses of job and home, had positive experiences with elderly people, and had long-term values of respect and caring. Staff had to learn to become immune to the patients' aggressive behaviors. Poor pay, working double shifts, and insufficient time to do the required tasks, however, increased the employees' stress levels and, therefore, their likelihood of committing abusive acts (Shaw, 1998).

In the end, nursing-home workers should never be allowed to forget that, for these patients, the nursing home is their home (Hodge, 1998). And they are entitled to the security, protection, and comfort that the term implies.

counseling, and support services for both the victim and the family (Kinney, Wendt, & Hurst, 1986; Quinn & Tomita, 1997). Services through religious groups are also suggested, particularly for certain populations (Johnson, 1995). Many of these services available are general services to the elderly and are also available to elders who are not members of the religious group. Services may vary depending on the type of abuse and other characteristics of the victims (Duke, 1997; Quinn and Tomita, 1997; Sengstock, Hwalek, & Stahl, 1991).

When legal recourse is chosen, civil rather than criminal means are often more appropriate for dealing with elder abuse because of the lesser stigma attached to such a judgment, allowing both offender and victim to deal with the problem more easily. In some cases, however, criminal remedies may be the only effective alternative (Quinn and Tomita, 1997).

Provision of services is complicated by disagreements as to the types of services needed and their effectiveness. For example, the appropriate role for legal interventions has been debated (Reulbach & Tewskbury, 1994; Hodge, 1998). The appropriateness of intervention in cases in which an elder refuses services and the competency of an elder to make such decisions are also controversial

BOX 5-5 A DILEMMA OF SERVICE PROVISION FOR ELDERLY VICTIMS OF ABUSE AND NEGLECT

The lack of most services required by abused or neglected elders presents a serious dilemma for the concerned professional. On one hand, by state law, they have a professional responsibility to report suspected abuse or neglect that they observe. On the other hand, they are aware of the dearth of services available to resolve the problem once it is reported. What is to be gained by reporting an abused or neglected client if it does not bring about positive change in the situation?

Providing for the needs of abused or neglected elders may involve complicated medical procedures, include physically demanding work, or be expensive to provide. (See Box 5-1.) Medications required by many elderly can cost hundreds of dollars per month and may not be covered by insurance. Patients may not have received the required medications or prosthetic devices through no fault of their own or their caregivers but through a lack of resources to obtain them.

Time and energy for caregiving are not limitless. If an elder is cared for by a single caregiver, many of the required treatments may be beyond the ability of the individual to provide. Turning a patient multiple times a day to prevent decubiti is exhausting work. Hospital and nursing personnel do this on 8- or 12-hour shifts and return home at the end of the day. A family caregiver must continue this process 24 hours a day, 7 days a week, week after week, often without respite. The assigned caregiver, perhaps an unemployed son or alcoholic daughter, often is not the best person for the task.

As noted throughout this chapter, for many families few options are available to care for their elderly relatives. One reason is the enormous cost associated with health care for the elderly. The cost of institutional placement is usually prohibitive. Even respite care may cost $50 or more for just half a day. Working families cannot afford these expenses, but they often fall above the appropriate income level for government services. If a caregiver must leave an elder alone for a few hours to go to the grocery store or pharmacy to pick up food or medicine, is this neglect? If an unfortunate incident occurs—if the elder should fall or a fire breaks out—is the caregiver culpable?

Another problem involves the technological skill associated with care of an infirm older person. Spouses and many children charged with the care of an elderly relative are often relatively uneducated. Nurses have spent many years learning the technological skills required to manage modern medically advanced care. It is virtually impossible for a lay caregiver to develop that same level of knowledge and skill in the short time allotted for most discharge planning. If the caregiver is not up to the task or makes mistakes, whose fault is it?

Political leaders, agencies who assist the elderly, and the general public are united in their concern for the welfare of the aged and united in their belief that elder abuse and neglect are serious problems, greatly in need of attention (Hudson & Carlson, 1998; Moon, 2000; Tatara, 1997). This has resulted in the proliferation of laws required the reporting of abuse, with sanctions for professionals who do not report.

Remedies for elder abuse and neglect largely remain in the realm of punitive action, in spite of much literature indicating that the bulk of elder abuse is actually benign neglect. (See Box 5-1 for a discussion of the case-management model of elder-abuse prevention.) Precious little attention has been paid to the problem of elder care in general, which has been left largely in the hands of the family. Needed services for caregiving families are often limited or unavailable (Neale et al., 1997; Quinn and Tomita, 1997).

What should be done in the case of a well-intentioned caregiver who is doing the best job possible, given the limited resources? Should the case be reported? If it is, the caregiver may be faced with criminal action and the family disrupted. But little may be done for the elder's problem, and considerable trouble may ensue for the family as a whole. The professional reporter may also be faced with court appearances and required documentation, only to learn several months later that the elder is in little better shape—perhaps worse—than was originally observed. It is little wonder, then, that some astute professionals admit not reporting elder abuse or neglect—even if required by mandatory reporting statutes—if, in their professional judgement, they are fairly certain that no effective assistance will ensue. Nurses and other health professionals understand these issues better than most and should make efforts to inform the public and government officials about their existence.

(Duke, 1997). See also Boxes 5-1, 5-3, and 5-5, in which the controversies over the types of services and the management of self-neglect cases are discussed.

Moreover, many services are unavailable in certain areas, particularly rural communities (Griffin, 1994). Funding mechanisms often exclude certain types of services or make them available only after a determination of need. Service provision is often complicated by agency fragmentation. Many service providers, originally trained before recognition of the problem, still lack relevant training or experience. Handling elder abuse is especially difficult for new workers or those who handle only an occasional case of this type. In some ethnic communities, notably Native-American and African-Americans ethnic groups, fewer health and social services are available (Carson, 1995; Gelfand, 1994; Griffin, 1994; John, Hennessy, Dyeson, & Garrett, 2001).

Service providers should distinguish between short-term services that must be provided immediately and those that should be provided on a longer-term basis. The former category includes obtaining treatment for injuries and removing the victim and his or her assets from the control of the abuser (Quinn & Tomita, 1997). Experienced professionals suggest that long-term-care management or monitoring is particularly useful in abuse cases, as are strategies to reduce caregiver stress; it may also be necessary to alter the living arrangements of the victim (Haviland & O'Brien, 1989; Quinn & Tomita, 1997). In general, treatment for abuse victims should be integrated into a comprehensive, unified whole (Goodrich, 1997; Sengstock, Hwalek, & Petrone, 1989; Wolf, Halas, Green, & McNiff, 1985-1986; Wolf, Strugnell, & Godkin, 1982).

All types of services, from identification to amelioration, are subject to the financial resources of the sponsoring agencies. As agencies, both public and private, suffer funding deficits, services are likely to be limited or cut altogether, even though the number of abuse cases is rising (Quinn & Tomita, 1997). Some states, for example, are known to limit the number of services victims may receive, or the period of time over which they are eligible (Neale et al., 1997). One clear problem is the uneven quality of services provided to abuse victims by different agencies (Sengstock & Liang, 1982). For example, some medical institutions are quite effective in observing abuse whereas others avoid the problem. Religious institutions are mentioned by some victims as being unsympathetic, yet some churches exhibit considerable concern.

Impact of the Individual Professional

Because some abuse victims are so reluctant to deal with the abuse, they refuse professional help even if it is offered. Hence, dealing with elder abuse is a task that requires great care and tact. Clearly a major factor in generating effective service for abused elders is a high degree of personal concern and interest on the part of the specific professional assigned to the case. It is not enough for an agency to have a general policy of helping abused victims, because individual professionals can often avoid such cases if they wish.

Because many health and social-service professionals tend to view elder abuse as a private matter, some service providers hesitate to suggest alternate living arrangements or services, fearing they will intrude into the elder's personal affairs. This is particularly common with elder abuse because adults are seen to have the right to make decisions on their own (Quinn and Tomita, 1997). The result, however, is that providers feel no obligation to suggest alternatives of which aged victims may be unaware. Therefore, the abuse victim sees no alternative to accepting the abuse.

Conversely, some providers in agencies with little commitment to dealing with elder abuse can be extremely helpful, spending much time and effort unraveling the bureaucratic red tape (Sengstock & Liang, 1982; Quinn & Tomita, 1997). One might say these professionals have had their "consciousness raised." They inquire about the family situation and are more likely to learn of abuse if it exists. Because of the nature of elder abuse, a substantial number of visits and a considerable rapport must be developed with most clients before they are willing to discuss family abuse.

There is no replacement for careful and conscientious concern on the part of each individual professional in dealing with the complex problems of an abused or neglected elder. All professionals must be knowledgeable about the problem of elder abuse and neglect and be aware of the types and definitions of abuse in their particular state. They must be capable of identifying victims within their patient or client caseload. They must be aware of the services available in the community to serve the needs of these patients. And finally, they must be thorough and compassionate in working with elders and their families in order to sort out the difficult issues.

Need for Further Research and Planning

In summary, domestic abuse of all types, including abuse of the elderly, has been greatly neglected by service providers. The increasing number of aged is likely to be accompanied by an increase in the problems related to their care and, consequently, an increase in the number of abused and neglected elderly (NCEA, 1998; Quinn & Tomita, 1997). The emotional, physical, and financial resources of caregiving in families are likely to be depleted quickly, leading to resentment against the aged. In such settings, the elderly are more likely to be abused. Increased support for elders and their caretaking families is necessary if such abuse is to be avoided. Some agencies have developed alternative programs for providing services, with varying degees of success (Kallen, 1984; Sengstock, Hwalek, & Stahl, 1991).

Strategies of intervention must be developed, not only to end the abuse but also to help in establishing the physical and mental well-being of the entire family. For most abused elders, severance of the abusive relationship is not viewed as a desirable alternative. Further research and planning, as well as interagency collaboration, is necessary to determine the needs of aged abuse victims and the most appropriate ways to provide for them (Quinn & Tomita, 1997).

SUGGESTED NURSING CARE FOR ELDER-ABUSE VICTIMS

Because of the problems previously mentioned regarding identification and testing of elder abuse and verification of hypotheses, the suggestions made in this section must be viewed as tentative. It is fairly certain that the description of possible symptomatology is representative of elder abuse cases studied to date. The presented at-risk indicators may require revision, however, when more knowledge has been accumulated in this area.

Assessment

Obtaining an accurate assessment of abuse in an elderly client requires that the nurse overcome a number of formidable obstacles (Fulmer & Cahill, 1984;

Phillips & Rempusheski, 1985; Wolfe, 1998). These include the reluctance of the victim to reveal an abusive experience; the necessity of developing a strong, trusting relationship before abuse can be identified; the absence of clearly defined symptomatology for elder abuse; the difficulty of distinguishing symptoms of elder abuse from the normal symptoms of aging; and the values held by the health-care provider regarding abuse. In this section, these difficulties, together with possible remedies, are discussed.

Reluctance of Victims to Report

The reluctance of abuse victims to report abuse and the reasons for this reluctance have been noted previously. Victims often fear retaliation from the abuser, loss of support, or loss of their relationship with loved ones. They may also feel guilt or shame if they have raised children who are abusive or have maintained close social or familial ties with abusive relatives. They are unwilling to admit the presence of an abusive situation to someone perceived to be an authority because they fear the possible consequences. Some elderly victims of rather severe abuse cannot admit even to themselves that a beloved relative would abuse them. Such victims are therefore incapable of reporting the abuse, as they are not really aware that abuse is occurring.

Developing Trust

Such reluctance to admit abuse must be overcome before a client is likely to admit abuse. Development of a trusting relationship with the client is essential to his or her eventual acceptance of services (Montoya, 1997). A client is not likely to admit abuse unless he or she feels that the nurse is accepting and does not present a threat to the client's well-being. A victim must believe that the nurse does not judge him or her for being in or remaining in an abusive situation. The abused person must also believe that the nurse has a genuine desire to help and will not reveal the difficulty to authorities without permission. Consequently, any aged patient with a possible vulnerability toward abuse must be approached by the nurse in a holistic and nonthreatening manner. In addition, it is preferable that the same nurse care for the patient to facilitate the development of such a relationship. Box 5-6 provides some suggestions for establishing an atmosphere that may promote trust in a patient.

Particularly with short-term clients, it may be difficult to develop the degree of trust necessary in the nurse-client relationship to obtain an accurate patient assessment. Professionals interviewed by Sengstock and Barrett (1982) often stated that an abusive situation was not uncovered until the professional and client had established a long-term, trusting relationship. Many of the service providers expressed concern that abuse might be overlooked when the client required only short-term intervention or presented at-risk indicators that were unfamiliar to the practitioner.

This raises questions about whether high-risk versus low-risk victim profiles can accurately assess the presence or absence of abuse, based on short-term intervention (i.e., one or two visits). Although there is urgency to assess abuse at an early state, abuse victims may not readily offer information concerning the abuse until the latter part of a lengthy assessment (Wolfe, 1998).

As previously noted, it may be particularly difficult to obtain information from those of certain cultural groups. Furthermore, the problem may be even more complicated by a language barrier. In some instances, translation may be

BOX 5-6	**HINTS FOR INTERVIEWING ELDER ABUSE VICTIMS AND CAREGIVERS/ALLEGED ABUSERS**

FOR BOTH VICTIMS AND CAREGIVERS/ALLEGED ABUSERS

- Always separate the victim from the caregiver, alleged abuser, and other family members.
- Provide a confidential setting.
- Establish rapport (i.e., be friendly, shake hands, and so forth).
- Allow the respondent to maintain his or her defenses.

FOR VICTIMS

- Provide a framework within which the respondent can talk (i.e., "describe a typical day").
- Ask direct questions. (Do not be afraid to ask if anyone has hit or otherwise hurt the respondent.)
- Indicate the range of options that the alleged victim has. (For example, let him or her know what examinations, tests, and such you plan to perform, places he or she could get help, and other places he or she could live.)
- Make sure that a thorough physical exam is performed on the alleged victim.

FOR CAREGIVERS/ALLEGED ABUSERS

- Indicate the requirement to report the case and its symptoms to the Adult Protective Services (APS) unit.
- Refer to APS as a resource for the victim and family.
- Do not use APS as a threat or oversell the power of APS. (Don't say, for example, "They'll do whatever they have to do.")
- Do not accuse or confront the caregiver or alleged abuser. You are not a police officer or a judge.

necessary; this can present a problem, however. Having a family member translate, for example, may involve the perpetrator or others involved in the abuse. And some ethnic clients may be even more unwilling to reveal their problems to persons acquainted with their own family and community. It is best, therefore, to involve someone who knows the language and culture but is sufficiently detached from the community so that the patient need not be concerned about a breach of confidentiality.

Identification of Abuse as a Two-Step Process

Because of the difficulty in obtaining an admission of abuse, it is often the nurse's responsibility to identify a victim of elder abuse by observing presenting at-risk findings. Unfortunately, the identification of abuse is still uncertain. Existing procedures are still in the process of being verified (Hwalek & Sengstock, 1986; Neale et al., 1991). Although lists of indicators have been developed, no set of factors can clearly identify elder abuse in the absence of other verifying evidence. So the identification of elderly abuse victims should be a two-step process in which at-risk individuals are first identified for special attention and then the abuse or neglect is verified through a more intensive examination of symptoms and case history.

Identifying At-Risk Elders. The first step in the identification of abused elders is distinguishing elders who are at greatest risk of being abused (Jones, Dougherty, Scheible, & Cunningham, 1988). Here, the nurse should be inclusive rather than risk eliminating any possible victims. Although no measure has yet been proven successful in establishing at-risk factors, two points may be made in this regard.

First, certain characteristics of the elderly place them in a situation of extreme dependence on others (Dunlop, Rothman, Condon, Hebert, & Martinez, 2000). Any elder who is incapable of providing for his or her own daily needs and is dependent on another person or persons for assistance is automatically in an at-risk situation. Persons who are mentally or physically incapacitated should always be considered at high risk. As indicated previously, this is only an indication of risk, not abuse; care should be taken to ensure that a premature diagnosis of abuse not be imputed, to the embarrassment of all.

Second, elders who are fully competent and exhibit no signs of abuse should be questioned to determine whether they too may be at risk. Nurses must develop an ability to question clients about issues such as abuse or neglect in a open and accepting manner, so that the client may feel free to indicate the existence of activities about which he or she might otherwise feel embarrassment or shame (Wolfe, 1998). Only the nurse's accepting demeanor can indicate that she or he has heard of such cases in the past and will not be shocked by the revelation. For example, the nurse may ask an elderly client to "describe a typical day" in his or her life. In the process of describing such a day, the client may reveal that he or she is left alone for long periods or is fearful of the behaviors of other family members. (See Box 5-6 for additional suggestions.)

Direct questioning is also important (Wolfe, 1998). Clients should be asked if they have been struck, ridiculed, or had money stolen from them. If the nurse is open and accepting of the responses, elders will feel free to answer such questions. Nurses should become comfortable asking such questions, practicing the process on a friend if necessary. If the nurse appears the least bit uncomfortable with the questions and possible responses, the patient will sense this and be reluctant to respond candidly.

The Hwalek-Sengstock Elder Abuse Screening Test (H-S/EAST) has been developed to assist in screening elders for at-risk responses (Hwalek & Sengstock, 1986; Neale et al., 1991). This instrument is still in the process of testing and cannot be depended on as the only screening instrument, but it does provide a useful set of questions. The complete H-S/EAST consists of 15 items, with two subsets consisting of nine and six items, being tested separately. Table 5-1 provides a list of the six-item subset, together with an indication of the at-risk response for each. These items are examples of questions that might be used in interviewing elders to determine their risk for abuse or neglect.

Verification of Abuse. Clients believed to be at risk should be further observed for other possible indicators of abuse. This is the second step in the process, in which the nurse should verify the existence of abuse through the documentation of specific symptoms as well as the collection of other evidence. The symptoms can be determined by an examination of the patient, and characteristics can be identified by judicious questioning in obtaining a client's case history.

Table 5-2 provides an outline for a patient examination and lists a number of indicators through the examination that may suggest abuse. Caution must still be exercised at this point, however, since any single factor may not support the suspicion that the client is being victimized by family, friends, or both (Wolfe, 1998). For example, absence of a prosthetic device or inappropriate dress may indicate

Table 5–1 • **Sample Questions From the Six-Item Hwalek-Sengstock Elder Abuse Screening Test (H-S/EAST)**

H-S/EAST ITEM	AT-RISK RESPONSE
4. "Decisions" Who makes decisions about your life, for example, how you should live or where you should live?	"Someone else"
5. "Uncomfortable" Do you feel uncomfortable with anyone in your family?	"Yes"
7. "Unwanted" Do you feel that nobody wants you around?	"Yes"
10. "Being Forced" Has anyone forced you to do things you didn't want to do?	"Yes"
13. "Annoyance" Does anyone tell you that you give them too much trouble?	"Yes"
15. "Hurt/Harmed" Has anyone close to you tried to hurt you or harm you recently?	"Yes"

Hwalek, M. A., and Sengstock, M. C. (1986). Assessing the probability of abuse of the elderly: Toward the development of a clinical screening instrument. *Journal of Applied Gerontology, 5*, 169; and Neale, A. V., Hwalek, M., Scott, R.O., Sengstock, M.C., & Stahl, C., 1991. Validation of the Hwalek-Sengstock Elder Abuse Screening Test. *Journal of Applied Gerontology, 10*(4), 409, 415.

a problem in care of the elder; such a factor alone, however, does not verify the existence of abuse. Even fractures or extensive bruising, taken alone, may not be clear indicators of abuse.

Because there are no clear physical indicators of elder abuse, the nurse may often find that a victim of abuse must be identified on the basis of a configuration of symptoms, derived from the physical examination as well as the client's case history (Fulmer & Wetle, 1986; Jones, Dougherty, Scheible, & Cunningham, 1988). Hence, extensive bruising or an appearance of malnourishment, when coupled with the nurse's observation of other indicators, such as overt antagonism between the client and family or friends, may warrant suspicion of abuse.

It is therefore imperative that the nurse obtain a thorough case history of a client when abuse is a possible cause of the findings. A thorough assessment includes an overview of the physical, social, and psychological characteristics of the elder and his or her significant others, especially those on whom the supposed victim is dependent. Relevant factors in the case history are outlined in Table 5-3. Because this depth of information is often impossible to obtain, the nurse must be prepared to obtain much of the assessment data from objective observations of the client and the client's family, social network, and environment. A summary of indicators of abuse, available from combined information obtained in both the examination and history, may also be found in Box 5-7.

Differentiating Abuse from the Normal Aging Process

Although physical indicators appear to be among the most valid symptoms of abuse or neglect in the child or middle-aged person, apparent symptoms of abuse in an elderly person may in fact be related to the aging process (Ham,

Table 5-2 • **Physical Examination of the Elderly: Indicators of Potential or Actual Elder Abuse or Neglect**

AREA OF ASSESSMENT	SYMPTOMS OF POSSIBLE ABUSE/NEGLECT*
General appearance	Fearful, anxious
	Marked passivity
	Appears malnourished
	Poor hygiene
	Inappropriate dress in relation to weather conditions
	Physical handicap
	Antagonism and/or detachment between elder and caregiver
Vital statistics	
Height	
Weight	Underweight
Head circumference	
Skin	Excessive or unexplainable bruises, welts, or scars, possibly in various stages of healing
	Decubitus ulcers
	Burns
	Infected or untreated wound
Head	
Eyes	No prosthetic device to accommodate poor eyesight
Ears	No prosthetic device to accommodate poor hearing
Nose	
Neck	
Chest	
Abdomen	Abdominal distention
Genital/urinary	Vaginal lacerations
	Vaginal infection
	Urinary-tract infection
Rectal	
Musculoskeletal	Skull/facial fractures
	Fractured femur
	Fractures of other parts of the body
Neurological	Limited motion of extremities
	Difficulty with speech
	Difficulty with swallowing

* Symptoms listed may be symptoms of normal aging. Therefore, physical symptoms must be assessed in conjunction with the patient's personal history.

1981; Sengstock & Barrett, 1981; Wolfe, 1998). The physiological processes that govern normal aging lead to physiological changes such as increased capillary fragility, osteoporosis, poor balance, poor vision, mental confusion, and musculoskeletal stiffness. Hence the elderly may be more likely to lose their balance and fall. Because they are more likely to suffer from skeletal fractures and bleed, a relatively minor fall may result in numerous fractures and extensive bruising, subdural hematomas, and possibly fatal hemorrhages. In addition, elderly clients who suffer from senile dementia may develop delusions concerning the treatment they receive from others. Thus physiological aging may generate complaints of mistreatment.

Because such findings may mimic abuse, some have warned against falsely diagnosing abuse as the cause of suspicious physical and psychological symptoma-

Table 5–3 • **History of Elder: Possible Indicators of Potential or Actual Elder Abuse**

AREA OF ASSESSMENT	AT-RISK RESPONSES OR INDICATORS OF POSSIBLE ABUSE/NEGLECT
Primary concern/reason for visit	Historical data that conflicts with physical findings
	Acute or chronic psychological and/or physical disability
	Inability to participate independently in activities of daily living
	Inappropriate delay in bringing elder to health-care facility
	Reluctance on the part of caregiver to give information on elder's condition
	Inappropriate caregiver reaction to nurse's concern (overreacts, underreacts)
Family health	
Elder	Substance abuse
	Grew up in a violent home (abused as child, spouse; abused children)
	Excessive dependence of elder on child(ren)
Child(ren) of elder	Were abused by parents
	Antagonistic relationship with elder
	Excessive dependence on elder
	Substance abuse
	History of violent relationship with other siblings and/or spouse
Siblings	Antagonistic relationship between siblings
	Excessive dependence of one or more siblings on another or each other
Other family members and family relations	Other history of abuse and/or neglect or violent death
Household	Violence and aggression used to resolve conflicts and solve problems
	Past history of abuse and/or neglect among family members
	Poverty
	Few or no friends or neighbors or other support systems available
	Excessive number of stressful situations encountered during a short period of time (such as unemployment, death of a relative or significant other)
Health history of elder	
Childhood	History of chronic physical and/or psychological disability
Midlife	History of chronic physical and/or psychological disability
Nutrition	History of feeding problems (GI disease, food preference idiosyncrasies)
	Inappropriate food or drink
	Dietary intake that does not fit with findings
	Inadequate food or fluid intake
Drugs/medications	Drugs/medications not indicated by physical condition
	Overdose of drugs or medications (prescribed or over-the-counter)
	Medications not taken as prescribed
Personal/social	Caregiver has unrealistic expectations of elder
	Social isolation (little or no contact with friends, neighbors, or relatives; lack of outside activity)
	Substance abuse
	History of spouse abuse (as victim and/or abuser)
	History of antagonistic relationships among family members (between family members in general, including elder)
	Large age difference between elder and spouse
	Large number of family problems
	Excessive dependence on spouse, children, or significant others

(continued)

Table 5-3 • History of Elder: Possible Indicators of Potential or Actual Elder Abuse (Continued)

AREA OF ASSESSMENT	AT-RISK RESPONSES OR INDICATORS OF POSSIBLE ABUSE/NEGLECT
Discipline	
Physical	Belief that the use of physical punishment is appropriate
	Threats with an instrument as a means to punish
	Use of an instrument to administer physical punishment
	Excessive, inappropriate, or inconsistent physical punishment
	History of caregiver and/or others "losing control" and/or "hitting too hard"
Emotional/violation of rights	Fear-provoking threats
	Infantilization
	Berating
	Screaming
	Forced move out of home
	Forced institutionalization
	Prohibiting marriage
	Prevention of free use of money
	Isolation
Sleep	
Elimination	
Illness	Chronic illness or handicap
	Disability requiring special treatment from caregiver and others
Operations/hospitalizations	Operations or illness that required extended and/or repeated hospitalizations
	Caregiver's refusal to have elder hospitalized
	Caregiver overanxious to have elder hospitalized
Diagnostic tests	Caregiver's refusal for further diagnostic tests
	Caregiver's overreaction or underreaction to diagnostic findings
Accidents	Repeated
	History of preceding events that do not support injuries
Safety	Appropriate safety precautions not taken, especially in elders known to be confused, disoriented, and/or with physical disabilities restricting mobility
Health-care utilization	Infrequent
	Caregiver overanxious to have elder hospitalized
	Health-care "shopping"
Review of body systems	

tology (Ham, 1981). Though such warnings may be well-founded, professionals must not prematurely dismiss the possibility of abuse in the face of suspicious findings. Professionals tend to notice abuse only when actively looking for the problem.

Careful questioning by the nurse when collecting historical data may determine such things as whether a client who complains of mistreatment is exhibiting symptoms of confusion or dementia or is expressing a valid complaint of abuse. Thus, the importance of obtaining a thorough, objective history on elderly clients cannot be overemphasized.

BOX 5-7 MAJOR SIGNS AND SYMPTOMS OF ABUSE AND NEGLECT OF OLDER ADULTS

What follows is a list of major symptoms that might indicate that an older adult is abused or neglected. The list is not intended to be exhaustive. Nor is the presence of any or several symptoms conclusive proof that abuse or neglect has occurred.

PHYSICAL SYMPTOMS OF ABUSE

- Injuries that show the form of common objects (e.g., bruises in the shape of a hand, coat hanger, or cord; burns in the shape of an iron or cigarette)
- Delay in seeking care; that is, indications that the injury has been in existence for several days or weeks
- Bruises or other injuries at different stages of healing; they may indicate delay in seeking care (Red, blue, and purple bruises signify 0 to 48 hours; green, 5 to 8 days; yellow, 1 to 2 weeks; and brown, 2 to 4 weeks.)
- Bruises on inner places of the body (e.g., inner thigh or arm) that are unlikely to have been caused by a bump or fall. (Bruises on the inner thigh near the genital area may also be an indication of sexual abuse; a genital exam and tests for sexually transmitted diseases should be conducted.)

PHYSICAL SYMPTOMS OF NEGLECT

- Presence of decubiti
- Malnutrition without a medical reason*
- Sudden or unexplained weight loss*
- Patient not taking medications as prescribed*

GENERAL INDICATIONS OF ABUSE, NEGLECT, OR MALTREATMENT

- Symptoms don't match explanation (For example, x-rays show a spiral fracture, indicating a twisting injury, but the caregiver says the patient fell.)
- "Doctor/hospital hopping" (That is, the patient is seen by a variety of different doctors or hospitals—this may be an attempt to prevent discovery of abuse or neglect.)
- Patient not allowed by family member to talk or be alone with the doctor or nurse
- Patient fear of caregiver or family member
- Major changes in the patient's pattern (For example, not paying bills as usual suggests that someone may be stealing patient's funds.)

---

*These may also be an indication of financial abuse.

See also: Sengstock, M. C., & Hwalek, M. (1986a). *The Sengstock-Hwalek Comprehensive Index of Elder Abuse* (2nd ed.). Detroit, MI: SPEC Associates; and Sengstock, M. C., & Hwalek, M. (1986b). *The Sengstock-Hwalek Comprehensive Index of Elder Abuse: Instruction manual.* Detroit, MI: SPEC Associates.

Values of Health-Care Providers

The beliefs of the health-care provider may have a significant impact on whether an abusive situation is recognized and then treated as such. In describing the process health-care providers use in identifying abuse and determining subsequent intervention strategies, Phillips and Rempusheski (1985) describe four decision outcomes. The first focuses on the resources that the caregiver possesses. For example, if the caregiver is poor, has failing health, or lacks knowledge regarding the needs of the elder, the health-care provider may attribute the problem to the situation, rather than to a deliberate attempt of the caregiver to neglect the elder.

The second decision outcome considers the attributes of the elder in relation to the diagnosis of abuse. Thus, if the elder is difficult to get along with or exhibits confused and combative behavior, the health-care provider may attribute possible abuse symptoms to the character of the elder rather than to the behavior of the caregiver. Conversely, an elderly patient with possible abuse symptoms who is good-natured and coherent may be further examined regarding the existence of abuse.

The third decision process observes that an assessment of abuse or neglect is affected by the worker's perception of caregiver effort. If the health-care provider believes that the caregiver is doing his or her best to meet the elder's needs, a diagnosis of abuse is less likely to occur, even if symptoms point to its presence.

The fourth decision process refers to the relationship between the health-care provider and the caregiver. A health-care worker who experiences a positive relationship with the caregiver is less likely to identify abuse as the source of the elder's problems. Similarly, a poor relationship between the health-care provider and the caregiver may be projected onto the relationship between the caregiver and the elder, leading to a diagnosis of abuse that may not be accurate.

Intervention

An elderly client may be reluctant to admit the existence of abuse even though a number of historical and physical findings point to its presence. It would be wise, therefore, for the nurse to proceed as if the client is at risk, until abuse has been ruled out as a possible contributor to an elderly patient's problem. This is particularly appropriate because all states now have elder abuse laws; though laws very greatly from state to state, the reporting of elder abuse is almost always required (Heisler, 2000; Mixon, 2000; Stiegel, 2000; Wolf, 1996a). Three factors appear to be important in the development of an adequate program of intervention: the establishment of a strong trusting relationship with the client, maintenance of a single individual as primary-care provider, and the development of a comprehensive plan that can be followed by and coordinated with all caregivers.

Trust as a Major Component of Care

Besides being critically important during assessment, a trusting relationship appears to be the most critical component in the provision of adequate care to aged abuse victims. Clients, especially those who have experienced the trauma of domestic violence, are not likely to accept assistance from nurses or other outsiders unless they believe the care provider is deserving of their trust. Such trust can be fostered by the nurse's attitudes toward the elderly client. Exhibiting sympathetic concern for the client and his or her feelings, understanding the problems the client is experiencing, taking an interest in his or her well-being, and being willing to expend effort in the client's behalf can encourage trust. Such concern is particularly evident in the nurse's nonjudgmental demeanor. Elderly abuse victims frequently become quite defensive of their loved ones, even if they are abusive. It is crucial that the nurse allow them to maintain this defensiveness. Abuse victims are not likely to accept care if they feel that the nurse is critical either of them or of their loved ones.

Unfortunately, establishing a trusting relationship is particularly difficult in elder-abuse cases, because of the barrier abuse victims typically have to the development of a trusting relationship, and because of the lengthy time span required for the development of trust.

Many elder-abuse victims have had little opportunity to maintain trusting relationships with others, as those closest to them are the same persons who abuse them. They are often unable to confide in family members because the relatives may have difficulty relating both to the abuser and the victim. As a result, abused elders often lack the ability to trust and confide in anyone. The concerned nurse must overcome this barrier before a trusting relationship can be established with the victim.

Developing a trusting relationship in itself is a time-consuming process, as previously discussed. The compassionate demeanor of the nurse is the critical component in this process.

Importance of a Primary-Care Provider

The role of a primary-care nurse is a critical factor, both in promoting continuity of care and in developing trust. This person must be sympathetic to the problem of abuse and be someone with whom the client is able to communicate. She or he should also be aware of assessment, supportive, and legal information regarding elder abuse (Fulmer, Street, & Carr, 1984; Hackbarth, Andreson, & Konestabo, 1989). The role of the primary-care nurse can be particularly important in dealing with abuse cases because both victim and family are usually reluctant to accept outside help. Professionals who have had little contact with such persons may find them uncooperative and unwilling to accept help. The nurse who is knowledgeable about elder abuse and has established a trusting relationship with the client can be a liaison between the victim and professionals from other areas.

An example is the common situation in which the nurse refers a client to social services. In such a situation, the nurse should provide the social worker with a detailed history of the client, explaining why abuse is suspected and discussing all factors contributing to the abusive situation. The nurse should also prepare the client and preferably be present during the social worker's initial visit. Although these measures might appear time-consuming and unnecessary under normal circumstances, in the case of the abused elder they are critical factors. Abused elders are more likely to accept outside assistance if it is encouraged and supported by a professional whom the victim already trusts.

Persons who belong to ethnic or cultural minority groups are more reticent to trust outsiders. Often they have had little experience outside their own communities, and outside relationships they have had may have been intimidating. Even members of their own community, or persons who speak their language, may be distrusted, if the patient fears they will disclose their family business to others in the community. In such cases, the best alternative may be to provide a contact who understands the language and culture, but is sufficiently removed from the local community as to ensure confidentiality.

Development of a Comprehensive Plan

The importance of a comprehensive plan cannot be overemphasized. Such interventions must be the result of an ongoing process that is originally based on an accurate assessment of the client's condition and developed as much as possible in collaboration with the victim and family and that undergoes constant reassessment and alteration as new observations about the client's needs become evident. Such a plan should prove to be an effective method in the establishment of a trusting relationship as well as in the provision of high-quality care to the elder-abuse patient.

The plan is particularly important when only short-term care is to be provided or when the client is to be assisted by a number of care providers. Other nurses and professionals involved in the elder's care should be fully familiarized with the plan of care for the client and should be observant of other at-risk findings that the client and situation exhibit. These observations should be continually added to the initial assessment of the client to maintain an accurate record concerning the client's overall situation.

Evaluation of Nursing Intervention

Evaluating the effectiveness of nursing intervention in elder-abuse cases is another challenging problem. Particularly in cases in which nursing intervention is short-term in nature, nurses may be unable to ascertain whether they had an enduring effect on the well-being of an abused elderly patient. However, some outcomes help determine whether the assistance has been of value, including the client's acknowledgment of the abuse; willingness of the victim, abuser, and family to accept outside help; and removal of the victim from the abusive situation.

Victim's Acknowledgment of Abuse

Because of the previously discussed reluctance to admit abuse, an admission by the victim that abuse exists should be considered an important sign that the client has made progress. Remedying an abusive situation often requires years of diligent assistance by numerous dedicated professionals. If the nurse's work leads the client to begin this process, this is a major accomplishment.

Willingness to Accept Intervention

As noted earlier, research suggests that much elder abuse is actually neglect and is caused by the stress of caring for an elderly, dependent relative. In such cases, day care, meal services, and other assistance with activities of daily living can be of great benefit in alleviating the stress in the family and the resulting abuse. Hence the willingness of abuser, victim, or other family members to see a counselor, reorganize family activities, or accept day care or housekeeping services is an indication that the abuse may be on the road to resolution.

Removal of the Victim from the Abusive Situation

When elder abuse is the result of a long-standing pattern of abuse, even long-term nursing intervention will likely not have a substantial impact on the abusive pattern. The only likely solution is the separation of the abuser and the abused (Quinn & Tomita, 1997), and this should thus be seen as a positive step. The victim could be moved to a nursing home or a senior citizens' residence. Placement with another relative may not be a positive step because a habitually abusive family tends to foster abuse in all members.

PROSPECTS FOR THE FUTURE

Abuse of the elderly has been neglected by both professionals and the public. Although the past decade has seen a dramatic increase in attention to this problem, many service providers are still unable to deal with elder abuse in an adequate manner. Existing research provides some basis for clinical practice, but considerable need remains for development of theory and methodology.

In the area of diagnosis, promising efforts have been undertaken to develop clear statements of case-history characteristics and physical symptoms that can be used to identify the presence of elder abuse or neglect (Fulmer & Wetle, 1986; Hwalek & Sengstock, 1986; Neale et al., 1991). However, further refinement in this area is an ongoing need.

In large part, education of the public and of those providing health, social, and psychological intervention will facilitate the process of building trust between the primary-care provider and victim.

Other care providers should work through the trusted primary-care professional. All components of the care must be recorded so that all professionals can follow the progress of the client and achieve continuity in care. It is hoped that the element of trust will grow as the client becomes aware of a sincere concern on the part of the nurses who provide care.

In turn, such measures will enable the client to be more open with the nurse and will lead to greater insight into the elderly individual's physical, psychological, and social situations, resulting in more appropriate measures in the client's care. It should be recognized that diagnosis and treatment of this problem requires patience, and in many cases long-term intervention, before the victim will acknowledge his or her predicament and discuss it with a professional willing to help.

As noted, it can therefore be difficult for the nurse to evaluate the effectiveness of the intervention. But nurses can gain satisfaction from knowing that they have helped a patient begin to deal with the problem and that they are forerunners in the development of methods of assistance to elderly abuse victims who have heretofore been neglected by other professionals in the health-care arena.

References

Aitken, L., & Griffin, G. (1996). *Gender issues in elder abuse.* Thousand Oaks, CA: Sage.

American Medical Association. (1992). *Diagnostic and treatment guidelines on elder abuse and neglect.* Chicago: American Medical Association.

Anetzberger, G. J. (1987). *The etiology of elder abuse by adult offspring.* Springfield, IL: Charles C. Thomas.

Anetzberger, G. J. (2001). Elder abuse identification and referral: The importance of screening tools and referral protocols. *Journal of Elder Abuse & Neglect, 13*(2), 3–22.

Back, K. W. (1976). Personal characteristics and social behavior: Theory and method. In R. H. Binstock & E. Shanas (Eds.), *Handbook of aging and the social sciences.* New York: Van Nostrand Reinhold.

Baldridge, D. (2001). Indian elders: Family traditions in crisis. *The American Behavioral Scientist, 44*(9), 1515–1517.

Barnett, O.W., Miller-Perrin, C. L., & Perrin, R. D. (1997). *Family violence across the lifespan: An introduction.* Thousand Oaks, CA: Sage.

Benton, D., & Marshall, C. (1991). Elder abuse. *Clinics in Geriatric Medicine 7,* 831–845.

Bergeron, L. R. (2001). An elder abuse case study: Caregiver stress or domestic violence? You decide. *Journal of Gerontological Social Work, 34*(4), 47–63.

Berman, A. L. (1996). Dyadic death: A typology. *Suicide and Life Threat Behavior, 26,* 342–350.

Blakely, B. E., & Dolon, R. (2000). Perceptions of adult protective services workers of the support provided by criminal justice professionals in a case of elder abuse. *Journal of Elder Abuse and Neglect, 12*(3/4), 72–94.

Block, M. R., & Sinnott, J. D. (1979). *The battered elder syndrome: An exploratory study.* College Park, MD: Center on Aging.

Bozinovski, S. D. (2000). Older self-neglecters: Interpersonal problems and the maintenance of self-continuity. *Journal of Elder Abuse and Neglect, 12*(1), 37–56.

Brandl, B., & Raymond, J. (1997a). *Developing services for older abused women: A guide for domestic abuse programs.* Madison, WI: Wisconsin Coalition Against Domestic Violence.

Brandl, B., & Raymond, J. (1997b). Unrecognized elder abuse victims: Older abused women. *Journal of Case Management, 6*(2), 62–68.

Brown, M., & Barraclough, B. (1999). Partners in life and death: The suicide pact in England and Wales 1988–1992. *Psychological Medicine*, 29, 1299–1306.

Callaghan, J. J. (1986). Guest editor's perspective. *Pride Institute of Long Term Health Care*, 5(4), 2–3.

Callaghan, J. J. (1988). Elder abuse: Some questions for policy-makers. *The Gerontologist*, 27, 453–458.

Callaghan, J. J (2000). Elder abuse revisited. *Journal of Elder Abuse and Neglect*, 12(1) 33–36.

Calvert, R. (1974). Criminal and civil liability in husband–wife assaults. In S. Steinmetz & M. Straus (Eds.), *Violence in the Family*. (pp. 88–91). New York: Harper & Row.

Carson, D. K. (1995). American Indian elder abuse: Risk and protective factors among the oldest Americans. *Journal of Elder Abuse and Neglect*, 7(1), 17–39.

Clark, A., Manikar, G., & Gray, I. (1975). Diogenese syndrome: A clinical study of gross self-neglect in old age. *Lancet*, (7903), 366–368.

Cohen, D. (2000). Homicide-suicide in older people. *Psychiatric Times*, 17(1), 49–52.

Comijs, H. C., Pot, A. M., Smit, J. H., Bouter, L. M., & Jonker, C. (1998). Elder abuse in the community: Prevalence and consequences. *Journal of the American Geriatrics Society*, 46(7), 885–888.

Cravedi, K.G. (1986). Elder abuse: The evolution of federal and state policy reform. *Pride Institute Journal of Long Term Health Care*, 5(4), 4–9.

Daniels, R. S., Baumhover, L. A., & Formby, W. A. (1999). Police discretion and elder mistreatment: A nested model of observation, reporting, and satisfaction. *Journal of Criminal Justice*, 27(3), 209–225.

Davidhizar, R., Dowd, S., Newman-Giger, J. (1998). Recognizing abuse in culturally diverse clients. *The Health Care Supervisor*, 17(2), 10–20.

Dimah, A., & Dimah, K. P. (2002). Gender differences among abused older African Americans and African American abusers in an elder abuse provider agency. *Journal of Black Studies*, 32(5), 557–573.

Douglass, R. L. (1988). Domestic mistreatment of the elderly: Toward prevention. Washington, DC: American Association of Retired Persons.

Douglass, R. L., Hickey, T., & Noel, C. (1980). *A study of maltreatment of the elderly and other vulnerable adults*. Ann Arbor, MI: University of Michigan Institute of Gerontology.

Duke, J. (1991). A national study of self-neglecting APS clients. In T. Tatara & M. Rittman (Eds.), *Findings of elder abuse studies* (pp. 25–53). Washington, DC: National Aging Resource Center on Elder Abuse.

Duke, J. (1997). A national study of involuntary protective services to adult protective services clients. *Journal of Elder Abuse and Neglect*, 9(1), 51–86.

Dunlop, B. D., Rothman, M. B., Condon, K. M., Hebert, K. S., & Martinez, I. L. (2000). Elder abuse: Risk factors and use of case data to improve policy and practice. *Journal of Elder Abuse and Neglect*, 12(3/4), 95–122.

Eigenberg, H. M. (2001). *Women battering in the United States: Till death do us part*. Prospect Heights, IL: Waveland.

Fulmer, T. (1989). Mistreatment of elders: Assessment, diagnosis, and intervention. *Nursing Clinics of North America*, 24(3), 707–716.

Fulmer, T. (2000). The first national study of elder abuse and neglect: Contrast with results from other studies. *Journal of Elder Abuse and Neglect*, 12(1), 15–17.

Fulmer, T., & Ashley, J. (1989). Clinical indicators of elder neglect. *Applied Nursing Research*, 2(4), 161–167.

Fulmer, T., & Cahill, V. M. (1984). Assessing elder abuse: A study. *Journal of Gerontological Nursing*, 10(12), 16–20.

Fulmer, T., Street, S., & Carr, K. (1984). Abuse of the elderly: Screening and detection. *Journal of Emergency Nursing*, 10(3), 131–140.

Fulmer, T., & Wetle, T. (1986). Elder abuse screening and intervention. *Nurse Practitioner*, 11(5), 33–38.

Galbraith, M. W. (1989). A critical examination of the definitional, methodological, and theoretical problems of elder abuse. In R. Filinson & S. R. Ingman (Eds.), *Elder abuse: Practice and policy* (pp. 35–42). New York: Human Sciences Press.

Gelfand, D. E. (1994). *Aging and ethnicity: Knowledge and services*. New York: Springer.

Gelles, R. J. (1993). Through a sociological lens: Social structure and family violence. In R. J. Gelles & D. R. Loeske (Eds.), *Current controversies on family violence* (pp. 31–62). Newbury Park, CA: Sage.

Gelles, R. J., & Straus, M. A. (1988). *Intimate violence*. New York: Simon and Schuster.

Gesino, J. P., Smith, H. H., & Keckich, W. A. (1982). The battered woman grows old. *Clinical Gerontologist*, 1(1), 49–67.

Gil, D. (1971). Violence against children. *Journal of Marriage and the Family*, 33(4), 637–648.

Goodrich, C. S. (1997). Results of a national survey of state protective services programs: Assessing risk and defining victim outcomes. *Journal of Elder Abuse and Neglect*, 9(1), 69–86.

Grambs, J. D. (1989). *Women over forty*. New York: Springer.

Granik, R., & Zeman, F. (1960). The aged recluse: An exploratory study with particular reference to community responsibility. *Journal of Chronic Disease*, 12, 639–653.

Greenberg, J. R., McKibben, M., & Raymond, J. A. (1990). Dependent adult children and elder abuse. *Journal of Elder Abuse & Neglect*, 2(1/2), 73–86.

Griffin, L. W. (1994). Elder maltreatment among rural African Americans. *Journal of Elder Abuse and Neglect*, 6(1), 1–27.

Grunfeld, A. E., Larsson, D. M., Mackay, K., & Hotch, D. (1996). Domestic violence against elderly women. *Canadian Family Physician*, 42, 1485–1493.

Hackbarth, D., Andreson, P., & Konestabo, B. (1989). Maltreatment of the elderly in the home: A framework for prevention and intervention. *Journal of Home Health Care Practice*, 2(1), 43–56.

Ham, R. (1981). Pitfalls in the diagnosis of abuse of the elderly. In B. B. Harris (Ed.), *Abuse and neglect of the elderly in Illinois: Incidence and characteristics, legislation and policy recommendations* (pp. B-1-B-7). Springfield, IL: State of Illinois.

Harbison, J., & Morrow, M. (1998). Re-examining the social construction of "elder abuse and neglect": A Canadian perspective. *Ageing and Society, 18,* 691–711.

Harris, S. H. (1996). For better or for worse: Spouse abuse grown old. *Journal of Elder Abuse & Neglect, 8*(1), 1–34.

Haviland, S. & O'Brien, J. (1989). Physical abuse and neglect of the elderly: Assessment and intervention. *Orthopaedic Nursing, 8*(4), 11–19.

Heisler, C. J. (2000). Elder abuse and the criminal justice system: New awareness, new responses. *Generations, 24*(2), 52–58.

Heisler, C. J., & Quinn, M. J. (1995). A legal perspective. *Journal of Elder Abuse and Neglect, 7*(2/3), 131–156.

Hickey, T., & Douglass, R. L. (1981a). Mistreatment of the elderly in the domestic setting: An exploratory study. *American Journal of Public Health, 71,* 500–507.

Hickey, T., & Douglass, R. L. (1981b). Neglect and abuse of older family members: Professionals' perspectives and case experiences. *The Gerontologist, 21,* 171–176.

Himmelstein, D. U., Jones, A. A., & Woolhandler, S. (1983). Hypernatremia dehydration in nursing home patients: An indicator of neglect. *Journal of the American Geriatrics Society, XXXI,* 466–471.

Hodge, P. D. (1998). National law enforcement programs to prevent, detect, investigate, and prosecute elder abuse and neglect in health care facilities. *Journal of Elder Abuse and Neglect, 9*(4), 23–41.

Hudson, M. F. (1997). Elder mistreatment: Its relevance to older women. *Journal of the American Medical Women's Association, 52*(3), 142–158.

Hudson, M. F., & Carlson, J. R. (1998). Elder abuse: Expert and public perspectives on its meaning. *Journal of Elder Abuse and Neglect, 9*(7), 77–97.

Hudson, M. F., Armachain, W. D., Beasley, C. M., & Carlson, J. R. (1998). Elder abuse: Two Native American views. *The Gerontologist, 38*(5), 538–548.

Hwalek, M. A., Neale, A. V., Goodrich, C. S., & Quinn, K. M. (1996). The association of elder abuse and substance abuse in the Illinois elder abuse system. *The Gerontologist, 36,*(5), 694–700.

Hwalek, M. A., & Sengstock, M. C. (1986). Assessing the probability of abuse of the elderly: Toward the development of a clinical screening instrument. *Journal of Applied Gerontology, 5,* 153–173.

John, R., Hennessy, C. H., Dyeson, T. B., & Garrett, M. D. (2001). Toward the conceptualization and measurement of caregiver burden among Pueblo Indian family caregivers. *The Gerontologist, 41*(2), 210–219.

Johnson, R. E. (1995). A religious perspective. *Journal of Elder Abuse and Neglect, 7*(2-3), 157–167.

Jones, J., Dougherty, J., Scheible, D., & Cunningham, W. (1988). Emergency department protocol for the diagnosis and evaluation of geriatric abuse. *Annals of Emergency Medicine, 17*(10), 1006–1015.

Justice, B., & Justice, R. (1976). *The abusing family.* New York: Human Sciences Press.

Kallen, D. J. (1984). Clinical sociology and adolescent medicine: The design of a program. *Clinical Sociology Review, 2,* 78–93.

Kimsey, L. R., Tarbox, A. R., & Bragg, D. F. (1981). Abuse of the elderly—the hidden agenda: I. The caretakers and the categories of abuse. *Journal of the American Geriatrics Society, XXIX,* 465–472.

Kinderknecht, C. H. (1986). In-home social work with abused or neglected elderly: An experiential guide to assessment and treatment. *Journal of Gerontological Social Work, 9,* 29–42.

Kinney, M. B., Wendt, R., & Hurst, J. (1986). Elder abuse: Techniques for effective resolution. In M. W. Galbraith (Ed.), *Convergence in aging: Vol. 3. Elder abuse: Perspectives on an emerging crisis* (pp. 110–124). Kansas City, KS: Mid-America Congress on Aging.

Kosberg, J. I., & Garcia, J. L. (1995). Common and unique themes on elder abuse from a world-wide perspective. Part of a symposium: Elder abuse: International and cross-cultural perspectives. *Journal of Elder Abuse and Neglect, 6*(3/4), 183–197.

Kransnow, M., & Fleshner, E. (1979, November). Parental abuse. Paper presented at the 23rd Annual Gerontological Society Meeting, Washington, DC.

Lau, E., & Kosberg, J. (1979). Abuse of the elderly by informal care providers. *Aging,* (September-October), 10–15.

Le, Q. K. (1997). Mistreatment of Vietnamese elderly by their families in the United States. *Journal of Elder Abuse and Neglect, 9*(2), 51–62.

MacMillan, D., & Shaw, P. (1966). Senile breakdown in standards of personal and environmental cleanliness. *British Medical Journal, 2,* 227–229.

Malphurs, J. E., & Cohen, D. *A newspaper surveillance study of homicide-suicide in the United States.* Tampa, FL: Department of Aging & Mental Health, University of South Florida.

McCauley, J., Kern, D. E., Kolodner, K. K., Derogatis, L. R., & Bass, E. B. (1998). Relation of low-severity violence to women's health. *Journal General Internal Medicine, 13,* 687–691.

Midwest Research Institute. (1977). *Crimes against the aging: Patterns and prevention.* Kansas City, MO: Midwest Research Institute.

Mignon, S. I., Larson, C. J., & Holmes, W. M. (2002). *Family abuse: Consequences, theories, and responses.* Boston: Allyn and Bacon.

Mitchell, C. A., & Smyth, C. (1994). A case study of an abused older woman. *Health Care for Women International, 15,* 521–535.

Mixon, P. M. (2000). Counterparts across time: Comparing the National Elder Abuse Incidence Study and the National Incidence Study of Child Abuse and Neglect. *Journal of Elder Abuse and Neglect, 12*(3/4), 19–27.

Montoya, V. (1997). Understanding and combating elder abuse in Hispanic communities. *Journal of Elder Abuse and Neglect, 9*(2), 5–17.

Moon, A. (2000). Perceptions of elder abuse among various cultural groups: Similarities and differences. *Generations, 24*(2), 75–80.

Moon, A., & Benton, D. (2000). Tolerance of elder abuse and attitudes toward third-party intervention among African American, Korean American, and white elderly. *Journal of Elder Abuse and Neglect, 12*(3/4), 283–303.

Morton, E., Runyan, C. W., Moracco, K. E., & Butts, J. (1998). Partner homicide-suicide involving female homicide victims: A population-based study in North Carolina, 1988–1992. *Violence & Victims, 13,* 91–106.

Mouton, C. P., Rovi, S., Furniss, K., & Lasser, N. L. (1999). The associations between health and domestic violence in older women: Results of a pilot study. *Journal of Women's Health & Gender-Based Medicine, 8*(9), 1173–1179.

Nagpaul, K. (1997). Elder abuse among Asian Indians' traditional versus modern perspectives. *Journal of Elder Abuse and Neglect, 9*(2), 77–92.

Nahmiash, D., & Reis, M. (2000). Most successful intervention strategies for abused older adults. *Journal of Elder Abuse and Neglect, 12*(3/4), 53–70.

National Center on Elder Abuse. (1998). National elder abuse incidence study: Final report. Washington, DC: Author.

Neale, A. V., Hwalek, M. A., Goodrich, C. S., & Quinn, K. M. (1996). The Illinois elder abuse system: Program description and administrative findings. *The Gerontologist, 36*(4), 502–511.

Neale, A. V., Hwalek, M. A., Goodrich, C. S., & Quinn, K. M. (1997). Reason for case closure among substantiated reports of elder abuse. *Journal of Applied Gerontology, 16*(4), 442–458.

Neale, A. V., Hwalek, M., Scott, R. O., Sengstock, M. C., & Stahl, C. (1991). Validation of the Hwalek-Sengstock Elder Abuse Screening Test. *Journal of Applied Gerontology, 10*(4), 417–429.

Nelson, H. W., Huber, R., Walter, K. L. (1995). The relationship between volunteer long-term care ombudsmen and regulatory nursing home actions. *The Gerontologist, 35*(4), 509–517.

Nerenberg, L. (1997). *Final report to the Administration on Aging for restructuring aging and domestic violence services.* Washington, DC: National Center on Elder Abuse.

Nerenberg, L. (1997). Foreward to the second edition. In M. J. Quinn & S. K. Tomita (Eds.), *Elder abuse and neglect: Causes, diagnosis, and intervention strategies* (2nd ed., pp. xi–xv). New York: Springer.

Nerenberg, L. (2000). Forgotten victims of financial crime and abuse: Facing the challenge. *Journal of Elder Abuse and Neglect, 12*(2), 49–73.

Netting, F. E., Huber, R., Paton, R. N., & Kautz, J. R. (1995). *Social Work, 40*(3), 351–357.

Neufeld, B. (1996). SAFE questions: Overcoming barriers to the detection of domestic violence. *American Family Physician, 53,* 2575–2580.

Neugarten, B. L., Havighurst, R. J., & Tobin, S. S. (1968). Personality and patterns of aging. In B. L. Neugarten (Ed.), *Middle age and aging.* Chicago: University of Chicago Press.

Nexus. (1995). Moving towards a peaceful life: Carole Seaver talks about the Milwaukee women's center and its older battered women's program. In L. Nerenberg (Ed.), *Final report to the Administration on Aging for Restructuring Aging and Domestic Violence Services.*

O'Brien, J. G., Thibault, J. M., Turner, L. C., & Laird-Fick, H. S. (1999). Self neglect: An overview. *Journal of Elder Abuse and Neglect, 11*(2), 1–19.

O'Malley, T. A. (1986). Abuse and neglect of the elderly: The wrong issue? *Pride Institute Journal of Long Term Home Health Care, 5*(4), 25–28.

Ogg, J. (1993). Researching elder abuse in Britain. *Journal of Elder Abuse & Neglect, 5*(2), 37–54.

Ogg, J., & Munn-Giddings, C. (1993). Researching elder abuse. *Aging and Society, 13,* 389–413.

Pablo, S., & Braun, K. L. (1997). Perceptions of elder abuse and neglect and help-seeking patterns among Filipino and Korean elderly women in Honolulu. *Journal of Elder Abuse and Neglect, 9*(2), 63–76.

Pagelow, M. D. (1984). *Family violence.* New York: Praeger.

Payne, B. K., & Cikovic, R. (1995). An empirical examination of the characteristics, consequences, and causes of elder abuse in nursing homes. *Journal of Elder Abuse and Neglect, 7*(4), 61–74.

Penhale, B. (1999). Bruises on the soul: Older women, domestic violence and elder abuse. *Journal of Elder Abuse and Neglect, 11*(1), 1–22.

Phillips, L. R. (1988). The fit of elder abuse with the family violence paradigm, and the implications of a paradigm shift for clinical practice. *Public Health Nursing, 5*(4), 222–229.

Phillips, L. R. (2000). Domestic violence and aging women. *Geriatric Nursing, 21*(4), 188–193.

Phillips, L., deArdon, E. T., & Briones, G. S. (2000). Abuse of female caregivers by care recipients: Another form of elder abuse. *Journal of Elder Abuse and Neglect, 12*(3/4), 123–143

Phillips, L., & Rempusheski, V. (1985). A decision-making model for diagnosing and intervening in elder abuse and neglect. *Nursing Research, 34,* 134–139.

Phillipson, C. (2000). National elder abuse incidence study. *Journal of Elder Abuse and Neglect, 12*(1), 29–32.

Pillemer, K., & Finkelhor, D. (1988). The prevalence of elder abuse: A random sample survey. *The Gerontologist, 28*(1), 51–57.

Pillemer, K., & Moore, D. W. (1990). Highlights from a study of abuse of patients in nursing homes. *Journal of Elder Abuse and Neglect, 2*(1/2), 5–29.

Pollack, D. (1995). Elder abuse and neglect cases reviewed by family courts. *Journal of Family Violence, 10,* 413–424.

Pollick, M. (1987) Abuse of the elderly: A review. *Holistic Nursing Practice, 1*(2), 43–53.

Quinn, M. J., & Tomita, S. K. (1997). Elder abuse and neglect: Causes, diagnosis, and intervention strategies (2nd ed.). New York: Springer.

Reed, P., & Leonard, V. (1989). An analysis of the concept of self-neglect. *Advanced Nursing Science, 12,* 39–53.

Reulbach, D. M., & Tewksbury, J. (1994). Collaboration between protective services and law enforcement: the Massachusetts model. *Journal of Elder Abuse and Neglect, 6*(2), 9–21.

Rinkle, V. (1989). Federal initiatives. In R. Filinson & S. R. Ingman (Eds.), *Elder abuse: Practice and policy* (pp. 129–137). New York: Human Sciences Press.

Roby, J. L., & Sullivan, R. (2000). Adult protective service laws: A comparison of state statutes from definition to case closure. *Journal of Elder Abuse and Neglect, 12*(3/4), 17–51.

Sanchez, Y. M. (1996). Distinguishing cultural expectations in assessment of financial exploitation. *Journal of Elder Abuse and Neglect, 8*(2), 49–59.

Seaver, C. (1996). Muted lives: Older battered women. *Journal of Elder Abuse & Neglect, 8*(2), 3–21.

Sengstock, M. C. (1991). Sex and gender implications in cases of elder abuse. *Journal of Women and Aging, 3*(2), 25–43.

Sengstock, M. C., & Barrett, S. (1981, July). *Techniques of identifying abused elders.* Hamburg, Germany: Twelfth International Congress of Gerontology.

Sengstock, M. C., & Barrett, S. (1982, November). *Legal services for aged victims of domestic abuse: The experience of one legal aid agency.* Toronto, Ontario: American Society of Criminology.

Sengstock, M. C., & Barrett, S. (1986). Elderly victims of family abuse, neglect, and maltreatment: Can legal assistance help? *Journal of Gerontological Social Work, 9*(3), 43–61.

Sengstock, M. C., Barrett, S., & Graham, R. (1984). Abused elders: Victims of villains or of circumstances? *Journal of Gerontological Social Work, 8*(1,2), 101–111.

Sengstock, M. C., Hwalek, M. (1985-1986). A critical analysis of measures for the identification of physical abuse and neglect of the elderly. *Home Health Care Services Quarterly, 6*(4), 27–39.

Sengstock, M. C., & Hwalek, M. (1986a). *The Sengstock-Hwalek Comprehensive Index of Elder Abuse* (2nd ed.). Detroit, MI: SPEC Associates.

Sengstock, M. C., & Hwalek, M. (1986b). *The Sengstock-Hwalek Comprehensive Index of Elder Abuse: Instruction manual.* Detroit, MI: SPEC Associates.

Sengstock, M. C., & Hwalek, M. (1986c). Domestic abuse of the elderly: Which cases involve the police? *Journal of Interpersonal Violence, 1*(3), 335–349.

Sengstock, M. C., & Hwalek, M. (1987). A review and analysis of measures for the identification of elder abuse. *Journal of Gerontological Social Work, 9,* 21–36.

Sengstock, M. C., Hwalek, M., & Moshier, S. (1986). A comprehensive index for assessing abuse and neglect of the elderly. In M. W. Galbraith (Ed.), *Elder abuse: Perspectives on an emerging crisis: Vol. 3. Convergence in aging* (pp. 41–64). Kansas City, MO: Mid-America Conference on Aging.

Sengstock, M. C., Hwalek, M., & Petrone, S. (1989). Services for aged abuse victims: Service types and related factors. *Journal of Elder Abuse and Neglect, 1*(4), 37–56.

Sengstock, M. C., Hwalek, M., & Stahl, C. (1991). Developing new models of service delivery to aged abuse victims: Does it matter? *Clinical Sociology Review, 9,* 142–161.

Sengstock, M. C., & Liang, J. (1982). *Identifying and characterizing elder abuse.* Detroit, MI: Wayne State University Institute of Gerontology.

Sengstock, M. C., & Liang, J. (1983). Domestic abuse of the aged: Assessing some dimensions of the problem. In *Interdisciplinary topics in gerontology: Vol. 17. Social gerontology.* Basel, Switzerland and New York: S. Karger.

Sengstock, M. C., McFarland, M. R., & Hwalek, M. (1990). Identification of elder abuse in institutional settings: Required changes in existing protocols. *Journal of Elder Abuse and Neglect, 2*(1/2), 31–50.

Sengstock, M. C., Thibault, J. M., & Zaranek, R. (1999). Community dimensions of elderly self-neglect. *Journal of Elder Abuse and Neglect, 11*(2), 77–93.

Shaw, M. M. C. (1998). Nursing home resident abuse by staff: Exploring the dynamics. *Journal of Elder Abuse and Neglect, 9*(4), 1–21.

Simmons, P. D., & O'Brien, J. G. (1999). Ethics and aging: Confronting abuse and self-neglect. *Journal of Elder Abuse and Neglect, 11*(2), 33–54.

Skelley-Walley, J. E. (1995). An ombudsman perspective. *Journal of Elder Abuse and Neglect, 7*(2-3), 89–113.

Steinmetz, S. (1981). Elder abuse. *Aging,* (January/February), 6–10.

Stiegel, L. (2000). The changing role of the courts in elder abuse cases. *Generations, 24*(2), 59–64.

Straus, M. A., Gelles, R. J., & Steinmetz, S. K. (1980). *Behind closed doors.* New York: Anchor Books.

Tatara, T. (1997, November). *Attitudes toward elder mistreatment and reporting: A multicultural study.* Paper presented at the meeting of the Gerontological Society of America, Cincinnati, OH.

Tatara, T., & Kuzmeskus, L. (1997). *Summaries of the statistical data on elder abuse in domestic settings for FY 95 and FY 96.* Washington, DC: National Center on Elder Abuse.

Tatara, T. (1998). Elder abuse information series #1: Elder abuse in domestic settings. *National Elder Abuse Incidence Study.* Washington, DC: National Center on Elder Abuse.

Teaster, P. B., Roberto, K. A., Duke, J. O., & Kim, M. (2000). Sexual abuse of older adults: Preliminary findings of cases in Virginia. *Journal of Elder Abuse and Neglect, 12*(3/4), 1–16.

Thobaben, M. (1989). State elder/adult abuse and protection laws. In R. Filinson & S. R. Ingman (Eds.), *Elder abuse: Practice and policy* (pp. 138–152). New York: Human Sciences Press.

Thobaben, M. & Anderson, L. (1985). Reporting elder abuse: It's the law. *American Journal of Nursing, 85,* 371–374.

Thomas, C. (2000). The first national study of elder abuse and neglect: Contrast with results from other studies. *Journal of Elder Abuse and Neglect, 12*(3/4), 1–14.

Tomita, S. K. (1998). The consequences of belonging: Conflict management techniques among Japanese Americans. *Journal of Elder Abuse and Neglect, 9*(3), 41–68.

Tomita, S. K. (2000). Elder mistreatment: Practice modifications to accommodate cultural differences. *Journal of Elder Abuse and Neglect, 12*(3/4), 305–326.

U.S. House Select Committee on Aging. (1985). *The rights of America's institutionalized aged: Lost in confinement* (Committee Publication No. 99-543). Washington, DC: U.S. Government Printing Office.

United Nations. (2001). Violence against women in the family: What causes violence against women in the home? In H. M. Eigenberg (Ed.), *Women battering in the United States: Till death do us part* (pp. 147–160). Prospect Heights, IL: Waveland.

Verma, S., & Haviland, S. (1988). Ethical issues related to institutionalization. In J. G. O'Brien (Ed.), *Ethical and legal issues in care of the elderly* (pp. 44–56). East Lansing, MI: Department of Family Practice, Michigan State University.

Vernon, M., & Bennett, G. (1995). "Elder abuse": The case for greater involvement of geriatricians. *Age and Aging, 24*(May), 177–179.

Vinton, L. (1991). Abused older women: Battered women or abused elders? *Journal of Women & Aging, 3*(1), 5–19.

Vinton, L., Altholz, J. A. S., & Lobell-Boesch, T. (1997). A five-year follow-up study of domestic violence programming for older battered women. *Journal of Women & Aging, 9*(1/2), 3–15.

Weith, M. E. (1994). Elder abuse: A national tragedy. *FBI Law Enforcement Bulletin, 63*(February), 24–26.

Wolf, R. S. (1996a). Understanding elder abuse and neglect. *Aging, 397,* 1–5.

Wolf, R. S. (1996b). Elder abuse and family violence: Testimony presented before the U.S. Senate Special Committee on Aging. *Journal of Women & Aging, 13*(4), 71–83.

Wolf, R. S., Godkin, M. A., & Pillemer, K. A. (1984). Final report from three model projects. Worcester, MA: University of Massachusetts Medical Center, Center on Aging.

Wolf, R. S., Halas, K. T. Green, L. B., & McNiff, M. L. (1985-1986). A model for the integration of community-based health and social services. *Home Health Care Services Quarterly, 6,* 41–57.

Wolf, R. S., Strugnell, C. P., & Godkin, M. A. (1982). *Preliminary findings from three model projects on elderly abuse.* Worcester, MA: University of Massachusetts Medical Center, Center on Aging.

Wolfe, S. (1998). Look for signs of abuse. *Medical Economics, 61*(8), 48–51.

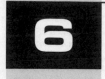

CHAPTER

6 Children of Abused Women

• Helene Berman, Jennifer Hardesty, and Janice Humphreys

Shelter

big old house
creaks and moans
til mothers come
and children's sounds
fill its empty rooms
little families
with shattered dreams
and broken hearts
run from daddy's fist
to this
a shelter home
refuge from
sweet love
gone amiss

Susan Venters

Reprinted from *Every Twelve Seconds*, compiled by Susan Venters
(Hillsboro, Oregon: Shelter, 1981) by permission of the author.

Children throughout the world have many opportunities to encounter violence. They may experience it directly or indirectly, as the intended "targets" or as witnesses, in their homes, in their schools, in their neighborhoods, through the media, or in the context of war. Until recently, only those who were the direct recipients of violence, and thus bore the physical scars of abuse, were deemed worthy of research or programmatic attention. During the past 15 years, however, a growing body of scholarly work has reversed this trend and provided ample evidence that children who witness violence endure many of the same outcomes as those who are abused directly.

Typically, children who witness violence in their homes do so during their growth years, during the phase of life when they are learning about themselves, their relationships with others, and the world around them. Although childhood is most commonly thought to be a time of innocence and predictability, this depiction is by no means the reality for large numbers of children who grow up amid violence. Instead, children exposed to the abuse of their mother experience the world as a place where adults in intimate relationships hurt each other and sometimes other people around them. Children who live in homes where women are subject to beatings see homes as places where women are subordinate to men and where men assert their power with their fists. For these young people, the world is experienced as a place where violence is an integral part of everyday life, where danger is commonplace, and where interactions are chaotic and unpredictable.

In this chapter, we focus on children who have been exposed to violence in their homes, and more specifically, those who have been exposed to the abuse of their mothers by intimate male partners. Although it is acknowledged that both mothers and fathers may be perpetrators and/or recipients of violence, available statistics support the notion that women are by far the recipients while men are the perpetrators. We present information on the estimated number of children exposed to the abuse of their mothers; theoretical frameworks that attempt to explain children's experiences; current knowledge regarding the physical, mental, cognitive, and social effects of witnessing violence; and proposed nursing care, with emphasis on primary, secondary, and tertiary prevention. Although research with child witnesses to violence has increased exponentially in the past decade, as has other family-violence research, this body of knowledge has its limitations. Nevertheless, a growing awareness of the problems and strengths of the children who are exposed to violence in their homes is manifest. A critical examination of this literature can foster insight and understanding regarding the needs for nursing exhibited by these children and their families.

SCOPE OF THE PROBLEM

Determining how many children are exposed to violence in their homes is a complex and controversial undertaking for a variety of conceptual and procedural reasons. Although an in-depth discussion of these is beyond the scope of this chapter, several relevant issues will be briefly highlighted to demonstrate the inherent difficulties in ascertaining the prevalence of the problem. Most significant is that, currently, no national prevalence studies in either Canada or the United States directly measure the number of children who are exposed to violence in their homes. Thus, estimates have been projected from available family-violence surveys, with adjustments made for the number of families with children and the average number of children in each household. For example, Carlson (1984) used figures from the first National Family Violence Survey to estimate that, based on an average of two children in 55% of violent households, at least 3.3 million children in the United States between the ages of 3 and 17 were at risk for exposure to parental violence every year. Similar calculations based on the second National Survey led Straus (1992) to postulate that as many as 10 million children are exposed to violence in their homes each year.

In a recent national survey of child development in Canada, parents were asked how often their children, ages 2 to 11, observed violence carried out in the home by older siblings or parents. Based on data from the 1996 National Survey in Canada, 8.6% of children, or approximately 330,000, were reported by a parent to have witnessed some form of violence in the home. Rodgers (1994) reported that Canadian children were present during almost 40% of wife-assault cases, that women feared for their lives in approximately 52% of these cases, and that 61% of the attacks witnessed by children had resulted in serious injury to the women.

Though these figures lend strong support to the assertion that large numbers of children are exposed to violence each year, a number of constraints remain. Whether the focus should be on children who witness all forms of violence between intimate partners or solely on those who witness violence against women has been a source of contention among researchers (Jouriles, McDonald, Norwood, & Ezell, 2001). Whereas children are likely to be affected by their exposure to any form of violence, there is compelling evidence that male-to-female violence is qualitatively different from female-to-male violence.

Another thorny area concerns the nature of the sample used in prevalence surveys. More specifically, there is little consensus for whether the surveys should utilize samples of couples or samples of individuals. Surveys that include data from individuals who are not part of an intimate relationship are necessarily going to yield much lower findings of intimate partner violence than those surveys that are limited to couples. For example, analyses of data from both the National Crime Victimization Survey (Greenfield et al., 1998) and the National Violence Against Women Survey (Tjaden & Thoennes, 1998) revealed surprisingly low rates of violence against women, 0.75% and 1.50%, respectively. It is particularly noteworthy, however, that in both of these national surveys, the findings were based on data from individual respondents. In contrast to these results, family-violence researchers have reported much higher estimates of violence against women using data from couples, with estimates ranging from 16% (Straus & Gelles, 1990) to 21% (Shafer, Caetano, & Clark, 1998).

How violence is defined presents further challenges. Much of the research to date has utilized narrow conceptualizations of violence, with physical acts of aggression as measured by the Conflict Tactics Scale (Straus, 1979) being the most commonly used indicator of violence. Other researchers have argued for the use of broader definitions that encompass physical, emotional, and sexual dimensions of violence. The use of divergent definitions of violence results in markedly inconsistent estimates that, in turn, have enormous implications for reported estimations of the number of children who are exposed to violence in the home. Further, whether children respond differently to different forms of violence exposure is not well understood. In view of the multitude of ways women are abused, and the recognition that children are affected by their exposure to multiple forms of violence, it is critical that definitions be sufficiently broad to capture the full range of children's exposure.

Understanding what is meant by "witnessing violence" presents another challenge to researchers in this field. As used throughout this chapter, the terms "witnessing violence" and "violence exposure" are used interchangeably and are defined broadly to include acts that are both directly observed and heard. Alternatively, children may neither see nor hear the violence but will see bruises on their mothers in the aftermath of a violent episode. Consistent with the general trend in the literature, we include the many ways in which children may be exposed to the abuse of their mothers in the home in our understanding of what it means to witness violence.

A final noteworthy issue concerns the reliance on parent reports regarding what their children have seen or been exposed to. This "adultcentric" bias, or tendency to examine the worlds of children from the vantage point of the adults in their lives, may contribute to an inaccurate portrayal of children's experiences. There is some evidence that children often see more than their parents think they see, and that they are, in fact, much more aware of the violence in their homes than their parents realize or acknowledge (Osofsky, 1997; Richters & Martinez, 1993). Consequently, parents may unknowingly underreport what their children have seen. Published estimates based solely on parent reports may not fully reflect the extent to which children are exposed to violence in their homes. Given the many challenges implicit in this focus of study and the lack of consensus regarding relevant definitions and constructs arriving at agreed-upon estimates is a daunting, but necessary, task.

RELATIONSHIP TO OTHER TYPES OF ABUSE

The impact of children's exposure to the abuse of their mothers is unclear. In general, it is agreed that a supportive and nurturing family environment, in conjunction with opportunities to interact with peers and others outside the home, is necessary for children to grow and thrive. Further, it is widely acknowledged that when violence and aggression are common features of family and community life, the child's capacity for growth is significantly impaired. Less well understood, however, is the precise nature and extent to which such violence exposure is harmful and the role that this exposure plays in the development of subsequent violence exposure and experiences (Graham-Bermann & Levendosky, 1998).

The early research on child witnesses to the abuse of their mothers offers convincing evidence that many, though not all, of these children are at risk for emotional and behavioral problems during childhood and adolescence (Jaffe, Wolfe, & Wilson, 1990; Wolfe, Wekerle, Reitzel, & Gough, 1995). Several authors have stated that children who come from violent homes are likely to experience violence in future adult relationships. In one of the earlier studies examining this relationship, Kalmuss (1984) used survey data from adults and found that observing aggression and violence between parents was more strongly related to involvement in severe marital violence than was being a victim of abuse during adolescence. More recent studies support this general pattern. According to Doumas, Margolin, and John (1994), male abusers consistently reported that they had witnessed violence in their families of origin. These researchers also noted that this finding was much more apparent among males than among females.

In a comprehensive review of the long-term effects of childhood exposure to domestic violence, Rossman (2001) examined retrospective and prospective studies of children who had been exposed to violence. Although many studies included in this review used samples of individuals who had experienced various forms of childhood abuse, not solely those who were exposed to abuse of their mothers, findings demonstrated a clear relationship between childhood exposure to domestic violence and later participation in criminal and violent behavior. Witnessing violence in the home was associated with violence in later interpersonal relationships as well.

Few prospective studies have been conducted. However, based on what is known to date, there appears to be a reasonably strong link between victimization during childhood and subsequent aggression during adulthood. Over a five-year period, Widom (1998) followed a group of individuals who had experienced childhood physical abuse, neglect, or sexual abuse. Those who had been abused and neglected had significantly lower IQ scores than the control group, higher rates of unemployment, a higher number of divorces and separations, more suicidal attempts, and higher rates of antisocial personality disorder, which is generally associated with more criminal behavior. However, as Rossman (2001) noted, understandings regarding the impact of exposure of children to parental violence are limited by the small number of long-term prospective studies.

Many authors have also noted a significant overlap between abuse of women and child abuse (Jouriles, Barling, & O'Leary, 1987; Lisak, Hopper, & Song,

1996). According to Lisak and others, one-third of 595 college men in their sample had been physically abused before the age of 16, and 37% admitted to physically abusing a child or adult. The risk of exposure to abuse begins before the child is born. There is a growing awareness that pregnancy may trigger battering or significantly increase its severity. See Chapter 4 for a more detailed discussion of the dynamics of this phenomenon.

Early exposure to violence in the home has important implications for the establishment of intimate relationships during adolescence. Of particular concern is the growing evidence that violence in dating relationships strongly correlates with childhood exposure to violence between parents (Carr & VanDeusen, 2002; Reitzel-Jaffe & Wolfe, 2001; Tjaden & Thoennes, 1998; Wolfe, Wekerle, Reitzel, & Gough, 1995). Further, there is evidence that the effects of this relationship are more harmful to females than to males. According to Harned (2001), the physical and psychological outcomes for women who had been victimized in the context of dating violence were significantly more detrimental than those observed in victimized men. In a recent report by Silverman, Raj, Mucci, and Hathaway (2001), approximately one in five young women, grades 9 through 12, reported having experienced dating violence. Reported outcomes for this group included a range of health problems such as substance abuse, pregnancy, unhealthy weight-control patterns (e.g., use of laxatives and vomiting), and suicidal thoughts and attempts.

Clearly, many children who grow up amid violence in their homes are routinely exposed to a multitude of other forms of violence through the media and in their communities, neighborhoods, and schools (Osofsky, 1997). In research on violence in the lives of girls, Berman and her colleagues (Berman et al., 2000; Berman & Jiwani, 2002) documented the occurrence of sexual harassment as a common feature of everyday life for girls as young as eight years of age. According to these researchers, sexual harassment is one of the most pervasive, pernicious, and highly public forms of violence that girls encounter. Further, efforts to stop it are often met by dismissive attitudes on the part of adults in trusted positions.

Garbarino, Kostelny, and Dubrow (1991) studied the dangers that children face in the war zones throughout the world and the "smaller" war zones of the inner cities in the United States. These researchers traveled to Mozambique, Cambodia, Nicaragua, Palestine, and Chicago. Based on extensive interviews with children, Garbarino and his associates concluded that the environmental hazards confronting children in large American cities are comparable only to the dangers experienced by children living in situations of armed conflict. Untangling the unique effects of the multiple forms of violence poses a significant challenge to researchers interested in understanding the effects of violence on children, but doing so is critical.

THEORETICAL PERSPECTIVES

Various theoretical and conceptual models of children's responses to the abuse of their mothers have been described in the literature. Together, these offer a contextual framework for greater understanding of the needs and issues faced by this population and provide some general direction for further research. Social learning theory and trauma theory have informed much of the published research in this field and collectively provide a framework for examining individual children's responses to violence exposure. Critical/feminist theory has received less attention but is included here because of its potential to contribute important knowledge and understandings and its insistence that individual responses to violence be considered within their broader social, political, and cultural contexts.

Social Learning Theory

One of the widely held theories about aggressive behavior in children and adults is the belief that "violence begets violence" (Widom, 1989) and the intergenerational transmission of violence theory. Derived in part from social learning theory, the essence of the intergenerational-transmission-of-violence perspective is that children who learn violent behavior patterns in the home are more likely to engage in similar patterns later in life (Straus, Gelles, & Steinmetz, 1980). The belief that victims of violence grow up to become perpetrators of violence has contributed to the fear often expressed by young males that they will some day become like their abusive fathers. Given the high rates of aggressive and violent behavior often described among children from violent families, their concerns are not unwarranted (Widom, 1989).

Varying degrees of support for the social learning perspective have been described in the literature. The early research related to children exposed to the abuse of their mothers documented a multitude of behavioral and emotional problems (Holden & Ritchie, 1991; Hughes, 1988; Jaffe, Wolfe, Wilson, & Zak, 1986). Most of these studies used the Achenbach Child Behavior Checklist (CBCL) and revealed the presence of internalizing behaviors, primarily among girls, and externalizing behaviors, more evident in boys. Although not a direct test of social learning theory, the occurrence of aggressive behaviors in child witnesses lends support to the notion that such behaviors are learned in the home, at least in part through observations of their parents. Jouriles and his colleagues (Jouriles, Murphy, & O'Leary, 1989; Jouriles, Spiller, Stephens, McDonald, & Swank, 2000) have demonstrated that marital aggression is a strong predictor of child misconduct and personality problems. Further support comes from a study of 46 preschool-age children. In this research, Graham-Bermann and Levendosky (1998) found that children who were exposed to violence in the home had significantly more internalizing and externalizing problems than comparison children had. Exposed children also showed more negative affect; used power, control, and bullying tactics in interactions with their peers; were more aggressive; and had more ambivalent relations with their caregivers.

Although the social learning perspective has some merits as well as considerable intuitive appeal, findings from a number of studies have led researchers to question its relevance, at least as the sole explanatory framework. Kaufman and Zigler (1987) raised important criticisms of the intergenerational-transmission-of-violence hypothesis when they drew attention to the fact that not all children who experience violence go on to become abusers themselves. These authors conducted a review of the research on adults who grew up amid violence but were not abusive with their own children and concluded that no more than 30% of those who experienced or witnessed violence as children were currently abusive. Kaufman and Zigler identified a variety of mitigating factors that contributed to the cluster of protective factors, including lack of parental ambivalence about their children, healthy children, few life stressors, ability to openly express anger about their own abuse, abusive behavior by only one parent, a supportive relationship with the nonabusive parent, and a determination not to perpetuate the cycle of violence. The role of protective factors and resilience is discussed later in this chapter.

The best conclusion that can be drawn from these findings is that a history of violence in the family of origin can, indeed, seriously affect children, but exposure to violence does not automatically result in serious behavioral problems and a certainty of violence in future relationships. More important, the findings of these studies imply that the trajectory from violence exposure to violence perpetration is neither simple nor linear and that a more complex constellation of factors, including type and duration of violence exposure, as well as environmental and structural factors, must be brought to bear when seeking to understand what happens when children are exposed to violence directed toward their mothers.

Posttraumatic Stress Theory

During the past ten years, a number of investigators have examined the relevance of posttraumatic stress disorder (PTSD) for an understanding of the consequences of children's exposure to violence or trauma. The primary symptoms of PTSD are intense fear, helplessness, or horror; young children may exhibit disorganized or agitated behavior. The remaining symptoms of PTSD are reexperiencing phenomena, avoidant symptoms, and autonomic hyperarousal (American Psychiatric Association [APA], 1987). The body of research on PTSD includes studies of children who have grown up in various war zones around the world (Arroyo & Eth, 1985; Berman, 1999; Garbarino et al., 1991; Kinzie, Sack, Angell, Manson, & Rath, 1986; Saigh, 1991), who had been kidnapped (Terr, 1990), and who had witnessed the murder of a parent (Pynoos & Eth, 1984). Although first conceptualized with respect to adults and, more specifically, Vietnam veterans, the PTSD symptomatology in these children suggests it may have relevance to children and adolescents.

Building upon this literature, more studies have been conducted that reveal traumatic responses among children who had been exposed to violence in their homes (Berman, 1999; Graham-Bermann & Levendosky, 1998; Lehmann, 1997; Rossman & Ho, 2000; Silvern & Kaersvang, 1989). Silvern and Kaersvang (1989) have suggested that observing violence between parents traumatizes children. They further suggest that trauma can result from perceived endangerment, even if no physical harm actually occurs. This idea is consistent with Saigh's (1991) finding with respect to children in Beirut that traumatic responses may result in response to direct encounters with traumatic events or to the awareness that such events have occurred.

Although trauma theory likely has some relevance and contributes to a general understanding of the stressful nature of early exposure to violence, the use of PTSD as an organizing construct for understanding children's responses to violence exposure has some important constraints. As first articulated by the APA (1987), traumatic events were defined as those events that were "outside the range of usual human experience." Several writers have challenged this definition (Brown, 1991; Herman, 1992). The essence of the criticisms is that, because violence is such a common part of the everyday lives of many women and children, it cannot be construed as being outside the range of normal.

For many children who grow up amid violence in their homes, trauma is not a single, isolated event. When children are forced to confront violence repeatedly, the trauma becomes a central condition of their lives; there is no "post" trauma period. Even if they are fortunate enough to escape from immediate harm, the task goes beyond "getting over" a horrible experience. Rather, the challenge is to find ways to make sense of their lives and their families when terrifying experiences are a part of everyday reality and traumatic stress is chronic and enduring. Herman (1992) has persuasively argued for the need to recognize "complex PTSD" to reflect this more chronic form of trauma. In response to this concern, the revised DSM-IV criteria no longer includes the original "outside the range of usual experience" proviso.

Though this change represents a significant improvement, other limitations remain. By focusing on a set of symptoms as the primary determination of children's responses, it is easy to pathologize and individualize the problem of violence. Similarly, the current emphasis on identification of a "disorder" effectively discourages investigators from examining the strengths and resources that enable children to grow and thrive in the face of seemingly overwhelming challenges. Concerns regarding the cultural relevance of PTSD across diverse settings also warrant consideration. Although many of the same signs and symptoms may be evident among individuals exposed to trauma in differing cultural groups and societies, these do not necessarily mean the same thing across the varied contexts.

Finally, PTSD was first conceptualized in relation to adults. Whether a similar construct can capture the experience of children, or whether their responses are qualitatively different from those observed in adults, is not yet well understood. However, some beginning research in this area suggests that children's posttraumatic responses are distinctly different from those observed among adults (Pynoos & Nader, 1993; Terr, 1990). Despite limitations inherent in the conceptualization of posttraumatic stress, its potential relevance for understanding the meaning of growing up amid violence is clear and convincing. The literature discussed thus far demonstrates that many of children's responses to overwhelming life events fall under the broad category of trauma responses and result in significant effects upon health.

Critical and Feminist Theory

The African-American socialist and feminist writer bell hooks (1984) observed that violence directed against women and children is an expression of male domination, but she cogently argued that an analysis of violence must be more comprehensive than that which focuses solely on male domination over women. Instead, violence must be conceptualized as a means of social control that is manifested in many ways, and at many different levels, throughout society. Further, such an analysis must take into consideration other sources of oppression, including that based on race and class.

The violence that children witness in their homes, typically perpetrated by their fathers against their mothers, is influenced and shaped by social, economic, cultural, and ideological structural processes. These processes are woven deeply into the fabric of the modern family and the larger society. Thus, the violence in children's lives is not purely spontaneous, made under conditions freely chosen. Rather, it is socially produced and experienced in situations that have been handed down from countless generations. From a critical feminist framework, it becomes possible to conceptualize children's exposure to violence not as a private or individual problem but as a public issue demanding social change.

Much of the research in the broad area of violence against women has been explicitly conducted from a critical or feminist perspective. With respect to research related to child witnesses, this is not the case. Most of this research has been conducted using theoretical models linked to social learning theory, trauma theory, or developmental theory. Although each of these perspectives has contributed to a substantial body of knowledge regarding this group of children, a number of limitations are noteworthy. The emphasis of the research on children exposed to violence has been on individual responses and patterns of behavior, devoid of gender analyses regarding the issue. In the context of violence against women and children, gender-neutral descriptions obscure the root causes of violence and leave the underlying gender-related dynamics unnamed and invisible. Instead, structured and systemic social problems appear as random, unpatterned, and individualized.

In recent years, a number of explicitly critical and feminist studies have been conducted, many by nurse researchers (Berman, 1999, 2000; Ericksen & Henderson, 1998; Humphreys, 1995, 2001a). Berman's research was a "critical narrative analysis" designed to examine the experiences of two groups of children who had grown up amid violence, namely children of war and children of battered women. An assumption underlying this research was that the contextual dimensions of children's experiences are valued and inseparable from the way in which children strive to bring a sense of coherence into their lives. Thus, by listening to the stories children told, this research sought to give voice to individual experiences and meanings but placed them in a broader context and thereby examined the social and political connectedness of those experiences. Although the critical and feminist theoretical perspectives have informed much of the research on violence against women, we believe it also holds considerable promise for those committed to an understanding of the needs of children who are exposed to violence.

HEALTH EFFECTS OF EXPOSURE TO VIOLENCE IN THE HOME

In the last decade, researchers have become more aware that children's exposure to domestic violence is a significant public-health problem and, as a result, children of abused women have received increased attention in the literature. Approaches to studying these children have become more sophisticated, as researchers attempt to untangle the complex relationships between domestic-violence exposure and child health outcomes. Despite a variety of methodologies, instruments, and samples, the research consistently shows that exposure to violence is associated with negative health effects for children (Onyskiw, 2002a). Still, not all children exposed to the abuse of their mothers exhibit negative effects, leading some researchers to examine factors that contribute to resiliency in this group of children.

In this section, we summarize the current knowledge of the health effects on children of exposure to domestic violence. We organize research findings by categories consistent with the literature: physical health effects, mental health effects, cognitive effects, and social effects. Although discussed separately, these categories overlap, and difficulties in one area can create challenges in other areas. For example, a child's depressive symptoms (mental health effect) can affect school performance (cognitive effect) as well as the ability to make friends (social effect). In each section, we identify short- and long-term effects of violence exposure, factors that may influence these effects, and relevant research limitations. Then we summarize the literature on behavioral responses of children exposed to domestic violence and discuss the influence of cultural diversity. Finally, we present factors associated with resiliency.

Physical Health Effects

Physical health effects on children exposed to domestic violence have received limited attention in the literature (Onyskiw, 2002a). Existing knowledge suggests the need to further explore this area. Some common physical health effects include allergies; respiratory-tract infections; somatic complaints, such as headaches; gastrointestinal disorders, for example, nausea and diarrhea; and sleep difficulties, such as nightmares and bedwetting (Berman, 1999; Campbell & Lewandowski, 1997; Davis & Carlson, 1987; Kerouac, Taggart, Lescop, & Fortin, 1986; Lemmey, McFarlane, Wilson, & Malecha, 2001; Wildin, Williamson, & Wilson, 1991). Attala and McSweeney (1997) reported speech, hearing, and visual problems, as well as delays in immunizations.

Growing up in a violent home also affects children's use of health services. In a health maintenance organization studied by Rath and colleagues (1989), children of abused women used health services six to eight times more often than children in the comparison group did. Onyskiw (2002a) examined the health status and use of health services in children exposed to domestic violence in a representative sample of Canadian children. Exposed children had lower general health status and more health problems than comparison children had, which limited their participation in age-appropriate activities. However, exposed children had no more contact with family practitioners and less contact with pediatricians than comparison children had. Instead, they reported more contact with other medical doctors, public-health nurses, child-welfare workers, and therapists. They also reported more use of prescription medications than nonexposed children reported.

Kerouac and colleagues (1986) reported that Canadian children growing up in violent homes missed school for health-related problems more often than the national average. Hurt, Malmud, Brodsky, and Giannetta (2001) similarly found an association between higher exposure to violence and more days of school absence, although they did not distinguish between exposure to family violence and to community violence. Other risk factors, such as social and economic disadvantage, are likely to compound the physical health effects on children from witnessing violence.

Mental Health Effects

Children of abused women tend to have higher rates of depressive symptoms; higher levels of anxiety, worry, and frustration; lower self-esteem; and more stress-related disorders than other children do (Ericksen & Henderson, 1992, 1998; Fantuzzo et al., 1991; Graham-Bermann & Levendosky, 1998; Humphreys, 1991; Hurt et al., 2001; Moore & Pepler, 1998). A significant number of exposed children have scores in the clinical ranges for depression, on standardized measures (Davis & Carlson, 1987). According to the National Longitudinal Survey of Children and Youth (Dauvergne & Johnson, 2002), Canadian children exposed to physical fighting at home are significantly more likely than children in nonviolent homes to exhibit hyperactivity and emotional/anxiety disorders. Exposed children also show elevated rates of posttraumatic stress symptoms (Boney-McCoy & Finklehor, 1995; McCloskey, Figueredo, & Koss, 1995), with some meeting the diagnostic criteria for PTSD (Graham-Bermann & Levendosky, 1998; McCloskey & Walker, 2000; Silva et al., 2000).

Early exposure to domestic violence may result in long-term mental health effects. Studies indicate that exposure to domestic violence during childhood is associated with higher adulthood reports of depression, stress symptoms, and low self-esteem (Forsstrom-Cohen & Rosenbaum, 1985; Henning, Leitenberg, Coffey, Turner, and Bennett, 1996; Silvern et al., 1995; Straus, 1992). However, Langhinrichsen-Rohling and colleagues (1998) did not find a relationship between depression, hopelessness, and suicidal behaviors of college students and their childhood exposure to domestic violence. Other factors, such as severity of the violence witnessed, are likely to play a role in increasing or decreasing the likelihood that child witnesses will experience mental-health problems in adulthood (Maker, Kemmelmeir, & Peterson, 1998).

Social Effects

Exposure to domestic violence is associated with lower levels of social competence in children (Adamson & Thompson, 1998; Fantuzzo et al., 1991; Graham-Bermann & Levendosky, 1998; Moore & Pepler, 1998), lower levels of prosocial behaviors (Onyskiw & Hayduk, 2001), and less positive and less effective interactions with other children (Dauvergne & Johnson, 2002). The behavioral responses of these children are likely to contribute to their social-adjustment difficulties (Rossman, 2001). For example, children with high levels of externalizing behaviors may act aggressively toward peers, which may lead to peer rejection. Exposed children tend to have greater expectations of aggressive or hostile intent in social interactions than do nonexposed children (Pollak & Kistler, 2002), which may interfere with their ability to appropriately respond to peers. Children with high levels of internalizing problems may appear shy and withdrawn and have difficulty initiating social interactions. Exposed children also have difficulty developing empathy and perspective-taking skills necessary for forming positive peer relationships (Rossman, 2001).

Violence exposure also affects social relationships through its effect on attachment security. Greater exposure to violence is associated with less secure attachment in children, especially in girls (Posada, Waters, Liu, & Johnson, in press). Less secure attachment can lead to difficulty establishing close interpersonal relationships. A study of high school students found that abuse in the family of origin and early attachment problems were associated with a higher risk of dating violence (McGee, Wolfe, & Wilson, 1997), and Henning and others (1996) found that early exposure to violence was associated with poorer social adjustment in adulthood.

Cognitive Effects

Research on exposure to domestic violence and cognitive effects reports mixed results. Some researchers have used standardized measures of intelligence or intellectual functioning and concluded either no significant difference between exposed and nonexposed children (Christopoulous et al., 1987) or lower scores on cognitive tests for exposed children (Moore & Pepler, 1998). Moore and Pepler found that cognitive test scores for children residing in a shelter for battered women were similar to children residing in homeless shelters and to children living in one-parent families. All three groups scored lower than children residing in two-parent families. Their findings suggest that shared risk factors, such as socioeconomic status and parental stress, may account for differences in cognitive responses.

After controlling for socioeconomic status, Rossman (1998) found no significant differences in verbal scores between exposed and nonexposed children. However, in a study of preschool children, Huth-Bocks, Levendosky, and Semel (2001) found that exposed children had significantly poorer verbal abilities, even when controlling for socioeconomic status and child abuse. Violence exposure affected verbal abilities and visual–spatial abilities through its effect on maternal depression and quality of the home environment. Thus, domestic violence may disrupt maternal functioning and other family processes, which in turn affects children's intellectual development (Jaffe, Wolfe, & Wilson, 1990).

Others have used measures of academic performance, such as learning problems or grade-point average, to assess cognitive effects. A study of inner-city children found that higher exposure to family and community violence was correlated with lower grade-point average and lower school competency. Child gender, child IQ, caregiver IQ, caregiver self-esteem, caregiver cocaine use, or the quality of the home environment did not account for the associations (Hurt et al., 2001). In contrast, Mathias, Mertin, and Murray (1995) found no differences in academic abilities between exposed and nonexposed children. Clearly, more research is needed to delineate the complex relationships among violence exposure, cognitive functioning, and other risk factors.

BEHAVIORAL RESPONSES TO DOMESTIC-VIOLENCE EXPOSURE

The Child Behavior Checklist (Achenbach & Edelbrock, 1978), CBCL, is most frequently used to rate the behaviors of children exposed to domestic violence (Onyskiw, 2002a). The CBCL assesses children's adjustment in two domains: internalizing behaviors (e.g., anxiety, inhibited behavior) and externalizing behaviors (aggression, delinquent behavior).

Compared to children in nonviolent homes, exposed children exhibit higher levels of both internalizing and externalizing behaviors (Edleson, 1999a). For a significant number of children, scores on internalizing and externalizing behaviors are high enough to warrant clinical intervention (Onyskiw, 2002a). Internalizing and externalizing behaviors are common initial responses to traumatic experiences. Over time, the behaviors tend to decrease if exposure to violence ends (Holden, Stein, Ritchie, Harris, & Jouriles, 1998; Rossman, 2001). Behavioral responses may vary by gender, with boys exhibiting more externalizing behaviors and girls more internalizing behaviors (Carlson, 1991; Jaffe et al., 1986; Kerig, 1998). Carlson (1991) found that male adolescents exposed to violence were significantly more likely to have run away and to report suicidal thoughts and were more than twice as likely to have hit their mothers, as compared to nonexposed adolescents. Witnessing domestic violence was unrelated to female adolescents' behavior or emotional functioning. Similarly, Onyskiw and Hayduk (2001) found that boys exhibited more externalizing behaviors than girls did but found no sex differences for internalizing behaviors. Others have found girls to show more externalizing and internalizing problems and depressive symptoms or more problems in the clinical range, compared to boys, or they have found no significant differences in boys and girls (Hughes, Vargo, Ito, & Skinner, 1991; Sternberg et al., 1993).

Kerig's (1997) study of gender, appraisals, and children's response to violence suggests different pathways to the development of maladjustment in girls and boys. For girls, as exposure to violence increases and as their parents' arguments become more frequent, intense, and unresolved, so does their tendency to blame themselves for their parents' arguments, which may lead to internalizing problems, such as hopelessness, anxiety, and depression. Boys feel increasingly threatened as exposure to violence increases and as the arguments become more frequent, intense, and unresolved. Kerig suggests that the pathways to maladjustment for boys may be a mismatch between their belief that they should be able to do something to stop the violence and the ineffectiveness of doing so. The resulting frustration from this situation may result in boys feeling anxiety and behaving aggressively. Further research is needed to understand how children's responses to violence exposure differ by gender (Edleson, 1999a).

A child's age or stage of development is another potential influence. Behavioral changes in infants and preschool children include sleep disturbances, somatic complaints, and regression in toilet training and language. School-age children may demonstrate behavior problems specific to the school environment and to peer relationships. Adolescents may act out with substance abuse and delinquency. Boys in particular may try to intervene in violent episodes to protect their mothers, placing themselves at risk for injury (Margolin & Gordis, 2000). Mohr, Lutz, Fantuzzo, and Perry (2000) encourage researchers to use a developmental perspective in their theoretical and methodological approaches to understanding the effects of domestic-violence exposure on children. Other factors to consider include social and economic disadvantage, parental separation, repeated moves, maternal depression, proximity to violent events, frequency and severity of violence, mothers' responses to violence, child strengths, and social and cultural supports (Campbell & Lewandowski, 1997; Onyskiw, 2002a).

A criticism of the research on children's behavioral responses to violence exposure is the overuse of samples from battered-women's shelters. In Onyskiw's (2002a) review of 47 studies, 70% included children residing with their mothers in shelters for battered women. Women who seek shelter differ from those who do not in terms of socioeconomic status, severity and duration of abuse, and access to social support (Johnson, 1996; Jouriles et al., 1998; Trainor, 1999). Time spent in shelter residence is typically that of stress and crisis; thus, children's behaviors at that time may reflect the stress of change more than the effects of violence exposure. Because mothers' reports are most frequently used, reports of externalizing behaviors may be elevated or more negatively skewed due to the distress of staying at a shelter.

Ware and colleagues (2001) attempted to address this criticism in their study of 68 children who scored at clinical levels of conduct problems during shelter residence. On one hand, follow-up assessment indicated that although mothers' distress levels decreased after leaving the shelter, their reports of their child's conduct problems remained high. On the other hand, mothers' reports of children's internalizing behaviors decreased over time, suggesting that mothers' distress may impact their reports of child internalizing problems. Their findings support the notion that children who reside in shelters are a high-risk group for aggressive and defiant behavior. Studies indicate that about one-third of children in shelters demonstrate such conduct problems at clinical levels, in contrast to about 2% to 15% in community samples (Ware et al., 2001).

Domestic violence may indirectly affect children's adjustment through its effect on mothers' parenting abilities. Abused women experience high levels of psychological distress, including heightened levels of fear, anxiety, and depression, and lower self-esteem. Each of these conditions can negatively affect parenting by decreasing emotional availability and responsiveness (Cascardi & O'Leary, 1992). For example, Onyskiw and Hayduk (2001) found that exposure to family aggression increased preschool and young school-age children's use of physical and indirect aggression through its disruption of maternal responsiveness. Also, maternal depression directly increased children's internalizing behaviors, which in turn influenced externalizing behaviors (e.g., child depression contributed to aggressive behavior). In contrast, Levendosky and Graham-Bermann (2001) found that mothers' psychological functioning had direct effects on children not solely mediated through its effects on parenting. Thus, even if abused mothers are able to effectively parent, their depressed mood may still affect children, particularly because children worry about their mothers and may be sensitive to variability in parental functioning.

Several researchers have challenged the assumption that abuse compromises mothers' parenting abilities. According to Ford-Gilboe, Wuest, Merritt-Gray, and Berman (2001), both mothers and children reported that abused women are nurturing parents who are emotionally available to their children and who care for their children in diverse and creative ways. According to adult daughters of abused women, mothers are essential to the ability to overcome the challenges of growing up in a violent home (Humphreys, 2001a). Furthermore, Sullivan, Nguyen, and colleagues (2000) found no evidence that abuse increased mothers' parenting stress or use of discipline. Instead, abuse directly affected children's adjustment and, in turn, children's heightened adjustment problems affected mothers' parenting stress.

In response to the abuse of their mothers, children may exhibit caring and protective behaviors. Humphreys (1989, 1990) found that children of abused women demonstrated deliberate, creative, and diverse caring behaviors. Through these behaviors, children attempted to protect (e.g., intervening to stop abuse, calling the police) and support their mothers. Supportive behaviors included instrumental assistance in the home to alleviate the general burden to the mothers. Children's supportive behaviors also enhanced the relationship between the abused mother and child, a relationship that may have mediated the long-term effects of violence on the children. Although children take protective and supportive actions, exposure to violence cannot be viewed as beneficial to children.

Noticeably absent from the literature is attention to the influence of fathers on children's adjustment (Levendosky & Graham-Bermann, 2001). Ericksen and Henderson (1998) report the strong connection children feel to their fathers despite the violence; thus, children are likely to be sensitive to the quality of their fathers' parenting. The abuser's relationship to the child is important to consider. In the study of Sullivan, Juras, and colleagues (2000), children's reports of their competency and self-worth were related to their relationship to the mother's abuser. Children of biological and stepfather abusers scored lower on all measures of child adjustment (behavior problems, self-perception, and depression), compared to children of those who were not father figures (i.e., partners or former partners who did not play a significant role in the child's life). Stepfathers and non–father figures were more emotionally abusive to children and created more fear for the children. Although biological fathers were more available, children were more likely to witness abuse from biological fathers. Witnessing this violence may be particularly painful for children and may contribute to more negative effects.

CULTURAL EFFECTS ON RESPONSES TO VIOLENCE IN THE HOME

Few researchers have examined the cultural effects on responses to domestic violence. O'Keefe (1994) examined white, Latina, and African-American abused women's reports of their children's adjustment and noted that their children had serious behavioral and emotional problems; however, African-American mothers rated their children more competent compared to the other mothers. Edleson (1999b) reported that race does not appear to be associated with different outcomes for children who witness domestic violence. Nonetheless, lack of attention to issues of cultural diversity is a limitation of the literature. Many studies on children exposed to domestic violence have included ethnically diverse samples. Researchers report ethnicity in their sample descriptions but few include ethnicity in their analyses (Campbell & Lewandowski, 1997). Differences across ethnic groups may play a role in the prevalence of domestic violence, family members' perceptions of violence, and the willingness of family members to disclose or report domestic violence. Ethnicity also relates to other factors such as economic status, which in combination may affect child outcomes in unique ways (Jouriles et al., 2001).

RESILIENCY OF CHILDREN EXPOSED TO DOMESTIC VIOLENCE

Although exposure to domestic violence is associated with myriad negative health effects, some reports indicate that 50 to 70% of children go on to productive lives and successful relationships as adults (Wolfe & Korsch, 1994). Resilience, a pattern of successful adaptation in individuals despite challenging or threatening circumstances, is thought to explain this phenomenon (Garmezy, 1981). Three areas contribute to resiliency: dispositional attributes in the child (e.g., temperament, personality, physical health, and appearance), family factors (e.g., family warmth, support, and organization), and extrafamilial support factors (e.g., a supportive network and success in school). More researchers have turned their attention to understanding the interaction of risk and protective factors that contribute to resiliency.

Using the life-history method, Humphreys (2001a, 2001b) conducted in-depth interviews with 10 resilient adult daughters who had grown up in violent homes. The process that contributed to resiliency for these women was dynamic and involved characteristics of the child, supportive aspects of the family, and external forces. Child characteristics included physical attractiveness, intelligence, and a cognitive style that allowed them to remain optimistic and persevere. Family factors included supportive relationships with a caring adult, especially a mother or grandmother. External support came from friends, school, and the media. Through external relationships, the women learned that the violence in their homes was not a normal part of family life. Despite being resilient, the women were not completely protected from suffering. In young adulthood, some experienced weight problems and periods of depression. Nonetheless, the combination of risk and protective factors in these women's lives contributed to successful and productive adult lives.

ASSESSMENT

Every child should be assessed for her or his exposure to violence. With respect to children who are potential witnesses to violence, the imperative to assess is particularly important because the signs are often subtle and easy to overlook. The indicators of potential or actual intimate partner abuse of women from both a health history and physical examination, listed in Chapter 11, can be used to identify battered women (see Tables 11-1 and 11-2). Even if clients deny exposure to family violence, the nonjudgmental approach of nurses indicates that violence is an acceptable topic to discuss. Furthermore, nurses who ask all clients the following questions (or similar ones) educate them in the importance of problems in these areas: "Has anyone ever hurt you?" "Has anyone ever forced you to do something that made you uncomfortable?" "How are conflicts resolved at your house?" "How do decisions get made at your house?" The nurse who never assesses for family violence is likely to never "see" it in the clients she or he serves.

INTERVENTION

Interventions with children who have been exposed to the abuse of their mothers cover a broad spectrum. The nurse is concerned about the inadvertently injured child of an abused woman, as well as the adolescent who has questions about violence in adult relationships. The following discussion describes general areas of intervention according to the level of prevention. Box 6-1 summarizes primary, secondary, and tertiary interventions.

Primary Prevention

Primary prevention includes all interventions that prevent violence against women and the primary prevention strategies discussed for child abuse (see Chapter 9). Prevention of woman abuse is discussed at length in Chapter 11. Primary prevention includes child and family health-promotion activities with both well and at-risk populations. The type of nursing intervention at this level varies with the location and nature of practice. We begin this section by presenting a framework, or guiding principles, for the development and implementation of primary-prevention programs. We then describe primary-prevention initiatives that may be implemented in a wide array of settings, including schools, health settings, or community organizations.

Principles of Primary Prevention

In a review of the research related to antiviolence programs, Haskell (1998) identified four key elements necessary for an effective framework: The framework must explicitly state the normative assumptions that are used to inform

BOX **6-1** INTERVENTIONS

PRIMARY PREVENTION

- Prevention of violence against women and children
- Decreased societal tolerance for violence (within families and without)

COMMUNITY-BASED INTERVENTIONS AND PROGRAMS

- Family-life classes in schools that provide experience with child-rearing and adult-relationship dilemmas
- Big Brothers and Big Sisters programs
- Education in schools on family violence and violence in dating relationships
- Nonviolent conflict-resolution programs for children

SECONDARY PREVENTION

- Development and implementation of protocols to routinely identify, treat, and refer survivors of family violence
- Developmentally appropriate support and encouragement to discuss worries and concerns
- Health screening for women and children on entry
- Crisis intervention
- Academic programs for shelter children
- Structured, developmentally appropriate daily programs for children
- Therapy and counseling as needed
- Parent-child programs that enhance child-rearing
- Follow-up to evaluate the effectiveness of programs and services

TERTIARY PREVENTION

- Public-health or visiting-nurse referrals for rehabilitation services
- Support and services to assist in marital disputes or child-custody disputes

policies and programs. Violence must be examined using both individual and social explanations. A gendered analysis must be used to situate violence in social relations of inequality. Lastly, the framework must assist young people to address, and end, violence and sexism in their personal lives.

Many examples of exemplary educational programs have been developed. Based on the collective knowledge gleaned from these programs, and building upon Haskell's framework, we suggest five interrelated principles as necessary core components of effective school-based antiviolence education.

First, programs need to be appropriately tailored to the unique developmental needs of each age group.

Second, effective antiviolence programs must incorporate recognition of the multiple realities and positions of privilege that influence how violence is understood and experienced. In particular, attention to social identities based on age, race, class, ability, or sexual orientation are essential aspects of any effective programming initiative. Programs must address how to act not only as individuals but also as groups witnessing or participating in violence. Further, programming must incorporate a recognition of the multiple ways that violence is enacted, including physical, emotional, verbal, or sexual ways, and provide personal and hypothetical examples of the various forms of violence.

Third, prevention programs that address the root causes of violence, and that are sufficiently broad in scope and analysis, are needed. Too often, programs are directly aimed at increasing individual awareness, assertiveness, and self-esteem or focus on conflict resolution. According to Olweus (1993), however, most bullies score average or above average on standard self-esteem measures. The implicit assumption of assertiveness programs is that violence occurs because of problems in self-esteem, communication, or conflicts "gone awry." It is further assumed that it is the responsibility of the individual on the receiving end of violence to stop it. The fundamental problem with such programs is that they tend to ignore unequal power relations and imply a level playing field. In effect, this approach fosters a "blame-the-victim" attitude and decreases the understanding of how gendered violence is experienced. Instead of becoming more visible, the manifestations of violence are camouflaged, further obscuring the potential for children to name, negotiate, and resist the violence in their lives.

Closely related to the third principle, we propose a fourth: gender-neutral teaching strategies that ignore the social context in which violence is perpetuated should be eliminated. Gender-neutral strategies overlook or minimize the importance of deconstructing traditional notions of femininity. As a result, conflict resolution and empathy-building programs based on gender-neutral policies fail to recognize that girls are likely to be over-socialized toward an empathic role in relationships and, thus, tend to reinforce the traditional notions.

The fifth principle is that the content of antiviolence programs should be made more relevant and that a gender analysis should become the organizing principle for all support programs for children and youth. This approach will encourage girls and boys to think critically about gender and to examine the effects of gender socialization on their lives. Such programming should begin with elementary school children. We recommend that a gender-based curriculum be located within a primary-prevention framework with committed government funding and attention focused on the function that sexual aggression serves for males. The goal is to establish interventions that build male and female self-esteem without invoking perpetrator/victim identification.

Community-Based Interventions

All types of abuse of family members occur in a society that condones violence within the context of the family. Implicit and explicit approval of the use of violence contributes to its occurrence within families. Frequently, such approval is manifested in the perpetuation of unequal power relationships based on gender inequality. Therefore, interventions at the societal level that diminish tolerance for violence and that challenge gender inequality are primary preventions for all types of violence. When violence against family members, including corporal punishment as a means of discipline for children, is no longer tolerated under any circumstances, much will have been accomplished toward diminishing the incidence of violence of all types.

Because violence in the home does not occur in isolation, efforts aimed at the prevention of violence in the lives of children must simultaneously focus on the home and the community and should ideally involve every realm of social and cultural life. It is therefore critical that primary-prevention programs be conceptualized as collaborative initiatives and that such programs be developed in partnership with schools, parents, counselors, community agencies, and health professionals. Although not generally mentioned in the literature, we believe that children and youth should also have a voice in the development of programs intended to be of benefit to them.

For programs to be effective, they need to be appropriate to the child's developmental needs. At the level of primary prevention, programs for infants and preschool children should include provisions for home visitation by public-health nurses or specially trained paraprofessionals for all new parents. Because of the large number of women who have experienced violence, it is important that such initiatives be geared to all new families, not only those traditionally considered to be at risk. Consistent with this notion, a growing number of programs have incorporated screening for woman abuse as a routine, universal component of the family assessment. Although the mandate of home-visitation programs varies considerably, most afford excellent opportunities for public-health nurses to engage in dialogue about the child's developmental needs and the challenges of parenting faced by new mothers. At the same time, home visits are an ideal way to gain insight into family relationships and the potential for violence. Despite the effectiveness of home visitation programs, current political and economic priorities in Canada and the United States have resulted in a reduction of many excellent programs, and those that are offered tend to be limited to designated at-risk groups (Olds et al., 1998; Wolfe & Jaffe, 2001).

Programs such as Big Brothers and Big Sisters can assist school-age children and adolescents to develop significant, supportive relationships outside their immediate families. When children lack frequent contact with one parent, most often fathers, such community-based programs can provide positive experiences and role modeling that can enhance children's resilience to potential and actual stressors.

Adolescence is a critical phase during which young people experiment with different roles, develop an expanded repertoire of problem-solving skills, become increasingly able to think abstractly, begin to comprehend more fully the consequences of their actions, and contemplate possibilities for the future. The influence of parents is at least partially replaced by influence from peers. For many youth, adolescence is a time for experimentation with, and initiation of, intimate relationships. Primary-prevention programs most likely to succeed are those that incorporate a recognition of the issues that are of importance to this group and that are presented in a nonjudgmental manner.

Providing a safe space in which teens can openly discuss their thoughts regarding relationships, the choices and responsibilities that accompany dating, what it means to engage in healthy relationships, and the multiple meanings that abuse has for young men and women is critical in raising awareness of the potential for dating violence (Gray & Foshee, 1997).

School-Based Interventions

Antiviolence education should be an integral component of the curriculum in every primary and secondary educational institution. Gamache and Snapp (1995) have described five strategies for violence prevention that are applicable at the elementary school level. The first, called "peacemakers," encourages young children to think globally about world issues or about individuals who have helped to make the world a better place. This exercise provides a means for children to discuss values and responsibility but is most relevant when combined with other antiviolence approaches.

Effective education programs build on self-esteem. Several limitations to this approach were noted here, but it is appropriate when conducted in conjunction with other efforts. Skills education is a third approach suggested by Gamache and Snapp (1995). In general, this widely accepted strategy entails a combination of assertiveness training, self-control, problem-solving, and conflict resolution. Many schools have included aspects of some or all of these into their curricula for all children. An example of this approach is Second Step: Skill Training Curriculum to Prevent Youth Violence, a program developed in Seattle, Washington. Designed for preschool through grade eight, this program teaches empathy, impulse control, problem-solving, and anger management.

A final approach suggested by Gamache and Snapp (1995) is violence education; it is based upon a more direct approach, namely the explicit teaching of violence. Core messages in this approach are:

- Violence is a learned behavior and can be unlearned.
- There are alternatives to violence.
- Violence rarely solves problems and usually creates new ones.
- Violence hurts and is not entertaining, fun, or glamorous.

My Family and Me: Violence Free was one of the first programs developed for the primary prevention of family violence, and it continues to be widely used today (Petersen & Gamache, 1988). One version is intended for use with kindergarten through third grades and another for fourth through sixth grades. This curriculum may help children to identify abusive actions and, thus, can promote early intervention with students who are being physically abused or are witnessing violence in their homes. Under the guidance of their teachers, the curriculum helps children gain a sense of their own uniqueness and worth, learn assertiveness skills for nonviolent conflict resolution, and develop a personal safety plan to use in violent emergency situations. Although the evaluation of this program has been limited, there are indications that it has contributed to positive changes, including increased knowledge about domestic violence (Jones, 1991).

Family-life classes in schools provide school-age children and adolescents with opportunities to experiment with various child-rearing and adult-relationship quandaries under the supervision of experienced nurses, counselors, and teachers. Parental involvement in such programs further allows parents to become more knowledgeable and to guide their children toward greater understanding of the difficulties of adult relationships and parenting.

School-based initiatives for adolescents can be implemented in schools by nurses or teachers, and can be particularly influential and informative. During the past ten years, a number of programs have been developed and implemented for this age group. One example is A School-Based Anti-Violence Program (ASAP), developed in Canada for use in the schools as a means of assisting school personnel, parents, students, and the community to discuss domestic and school violence (Sudermann, Jaffe, & Shieck, 1996). This program consists of a manual and video and has three key components: educator and staff development awareness, community involvement, and student programs. Emphasis is placed on the promotion of nonviolent attitudes and behaviors, but one of the more unique aspects of the program is the integration of community members into the program. Evaluation of this program has revealed positive results for male and female junior (grades 9 and 10) students and for female senior students. One possible explanation for the less positive results among senior male students may be that violent patterns in dating relationships are already established, so participation in the program contributes to defensiveness and resistance (Sudermann, Jaffe, & Hastings, 1995). This finding lends support to the importance of implementing prevention programs during the primary school years.

Secondary Prevention

When children are exposed to the abuse of their mothers, nursing interventions are termed "secondary prevention." The goals of secondary prevention are early identification and intervention to prevent recurrence of violence. Nursing interventions are aimed at limiting the impact of battering on mothers and their children. Nurses clearly have an important role in identifying abused women and their children and are in a unique position to provide treatment and support services, document abuse, and advocate support for their clients.

During the past decade, the health-care system has adopted various protocols and implemented training to enable nurses to effectively identify and respond to abused women and their children. In 1992, the Joint Commission on Accreditation of Healthcare Organizations (JCAHO) added guidelines for domestic-violence victim identification and response to existing care standards for victims of physical and sexual abuse, child abuse, and rape (Scott & Matricciani, 1994). A number of professional organizations, such as the American Medical Association, have developed and distributed screening and identification guidelines, and some states mandate such protocols. Most hospitals and increasingly other health-care settings now have protocols in place (Culross, 1999). At minimum, such protocols should include guidelines for screening, assessment, planning, implementation, and evaluation.

Screening

Nurses should screen every client for domestic violence, just as they assess for other potential or actual health problems. Screening should occur at routine intervals or any time there are signs of domestic violence, such as maternal depression and anxiety, failure to keep appointments, reluctance to talk about home or family issues, internalizing or externalizing child behaviors, hypervigilance, and frequent complaints with no apparent medical basis (Socolar, 2000).

Before screening, nurses should inform their clients of any legal obligation to report abuse. Nurses are mandated reporters of child abuse. In states and provinces where witnessing domestic violence is considered child abuse, nurses are mandated reporters of this form of abuse. Except in those states or provinces and in cases of child abuse, nurses will keep information about violence in the home confidential. Edleson (1999a) warns against defining all exposure to domestic violence as child maltreatment because it denies that the majority of children in these situations show no negative development problems and show strong coping abilities, and it denies the women's efforts to provide safe environments for their children.

When children exposed to domestic violence are not identified in the health-care system, they have increased health problems that result in more frequent emergency department visits, other hospitalizations, and increased use of outpatient health care facilities (Campbell & Lewandowski, 1997). Abused women and their children most often visit the emergency department for medical complaints, not trauma, suggesting the need to intervene in other health-care settings. Primary-care settings are ideal for identification of and intervention with abused women and their children. A significant number of abused women have indicated they prefer to receive help in a health-care setting rather than in a shelter for battered women (Hadley, Short, Lesin, & Zook, 1995). Further, women in the early stages of battering may not identify themselves as abused nor associate their children's physical and mental health problems with domestic violence. Thus, for these women, a health-care setting may be an optimal location for early identification and intervention.

According to McFarlane, Parker, Soeken, and Bullock (1992), pregnancy offers an opportunity for abused women to be seen regularly by their health-care providers; the women can then receive assessment and intervention. Abuse during pregnancy can have serious consequences (e.g., low birth weight and death) for the mother and the fetus. The implications of abuse are as serious as any other potential problems during pregnancy and thus should be part of a routine assessment. Early intervention during pregnancy may prevent children's exposure to violence in the future (see Chapter 4 for further discussion).

A challenge of identifying children of abused women in adult health-care settings, however, is that the focus is often on treating the adult, so children's needs often remain unidentified or unmet. Greater recognition that the family may be the more appropriate unit of care would facilitate the inclusion of children in the screening process. Nonetheless, intervening on behalf of abused women has the potential to also help children. For example, when screening women for abuse, nurses should also ask about their children's exposure to violence and their responses. With increasing evidence of children's responses to violence, health-care professionals are recognizing the need to also screen and assess on behalf of children (Socolar, 2000). The American Medical Association's recommended intimate partner-violence screening questions could be asked with children age two or younger in the room. More general questions (e.g., "What happens in your house when people get angry?") could be asked with children of any age in the room (Zink, 2000).

An opportunity to screen children for violence exposure exists during routine child health examinations. Depending on the child's age, nurses may directly screen children for exposure to abuse. Humphreys (2001a) suggested that a simple question like "What is dinnertime like at your house?" may elicit information about the day-to-day life of children. When screening children, nurses need to be aware of children's fear of reprisals if they disclose information about abuse. She recommended prefacing questions with: "Because violence in families is so common, I routinely ask everyone I see about it." Nurses also can routinely screen mothers during child health visits to give them an additional opportunity to disclose abuse. In contrast to direct screening, nurses can also detect possible exposure to domestic violence by recognizing signs of distress, such as aggressive behavior, running away, or unexplained somatic complaints.

Until recently, screening for violence exposure was not a routine part of child health-care visits. Although pediatricians received training on the identification of child abuse and neglect, they often were not trained on the identification of adult domestic violence, nor did they consider it part of their role (Culross, 1999). The American Academy of Pediatrics (AAP) now recognizes the profound effects of domestic violence exposure on children (1998). Pediatricians are in a position to identify abused women, and intervention on their behalf is an effective way to prevent negative child outcomes. The AAP encourages pediatricians to be aware of the signs of abuse (e.g., facial bruising, depression, anxiety, failure to keep appointments, reluctance to answer questions about discipline) in the mothers of children they see and to intervene in a sympathetic way that assures confidentiality and prioritizes safety. Pediatricians can call on nurses to assist in screening and assisting abused women and their children.

Efforts to screen for domestic violence must extend beyond primary health-care settings. According to Onyskiw (2002b), children of abused women may be more likely to visit other health-care providers, which may include providers in walk-in clinics or emergency departments. Abused women may be reluctant to take their children to a family practitioner or pediatrician because abuse may be more likely detected. This is problematic because nurses in these other settings may have less opportunity to become familiar with the family's situation and thus may not attribute children's health problems to violence exposure.

Assessment

When children of abused women are identified, nurses should take a thorough history (abuse history and psychosocial history); assess the mental and physical health effects; take into account the total situation, including the psychosocial context; and instigate suitable interventions, including appropriate referrals and long-term follow-up. The safety of the children and their mothers, the mothers' desires and motivations to change or leave the abusive partner, and children's attachment to the abuser should be assessed. Even in the case of mandated reporting, a careful assessment of risk and protective factors is necessary before drawing conclusions about risk and harm to children (Edleson, 1999a).

One of the crucial areas of safety planning is an accurate and detailed assessment of degree of danger the woman is experiencing. The Danger Assessment (DA) is one of several risk-factor lists and instruments that have been developed over the past few years (Campbell, 1995; Campbell, Sharps, & Glass, 2001). This instrument is a short (17-item) yes/no risk-factor list designed to help women assess their own risk of homicide or serious abuse from a violent relationship. The higher the score, the more assertive nurses should be in safety planning. In prior studies, scores of eight or more were found in the groups at the highest risk (Campbell et al., in press; Campbell, Sharps, & Glass, 2001). See Appendix C for Danger Assessment.

In addition to assessing danger, nurses should assess mothers' perceptions of the children's involvement in and responses to violence. Even if mothers are not overwrought or overly depressed, they may be unaware of children's perceptions of parental conflict. In one study, neither parents nor teachers recognized the high anxiety in children exposed to family and community violence (Hurt et al., 2001). Ericksen and Henderson (1998) suggest that abused women and their children have divergent realities in terms of perceptions of violence in the home and of the children's needs. Through in-depth interviews, Ericksen and Henderson discovered that whereas mothers gave very vague descriptions of abuse and minimized the abuse their children were exposed to, children provided very explicit and clear descriptions of the violence they witnessed. For this reason, nurses should directly assess children in addition to assessing their mothers.

Nurses in primary care should continue to assess children over time, as the health effects of violence exposure may persist over time or surface later (Humphreys, 2001b). In Berman's (1999) study, children described numerous ways in which witnessing violence compromised their health (e.g., loss of sleep, eating disturbances, difficulty carrying on with daily routine, and lack of energy); the effects persisted over time. Screening and assessment should continue even if children have been removed from the violent situation. Abuse does not typically end when women leave abusive partners, and children often witness violence that occurs after separation. In one study, children were more likely to witness abuse if incidents occurred after separation (Hotton, 2002), possibly because violence occurs in the context of shared-custody tasks, such as exchanging the children for visitation. Several researchers have reported that women who shared custody with their abusers after divorce face continued abuse and make ongoing efforts to ensure their own and their children's safety (Hardesty & Ganong, 2002; Wuest, Berman, Ford-Gilboe, & Merritt-Gray, 2002).

Planning

After a thorough assessment, nurses can develop short- and long-term interventions. Planning for interventions should take into account personal, family, cultural, and environmental factors, as well as the potential risk to abused women and their children. Interventions should include appropriate referrals to community resources for safety, advocacy, and support.

Safety planning should be predicated on the degree of danger (Campbell, 1995; Hardesty & Campbell, in press) and should be a part of all interventions regardless of whether the mother is returning to or leaving the abusive partner. The risk of danger is particularly high when the woman has left or is planning to leave the abuser (Campbell et al., in press). As noted, shared-custody arrangements may provide opportunity for abuse (Ericksen & Henderson, 1998; Hardesty & Ganong, 2002). Some abused mothers are required by courts to maintain contact (Jaffe and Geffner, 1998). A key risk factor after separation is the abuser's access to the woman, making unsupervised visitations and exchanges a risky time for severe or lethal violence to the woman and her children (Sheeran & Hampton, 1999).

Many abused women want their children to maintain a relationship with their fathers after separation. They face a dilemma of balancing safety needs with the desire for their children to have contact with both parents (Hardesty & Ganong, 2002). They may also feel guilty for "breaking up" a two-parent family, and they may worry about their children's adjustment to separation or divorce. Nurses can acknowledge this dilemma and normalize mothers' worries. Nurses can encourage abused women to prioritize safety when making decisions about father–child contact after separation or divorce. For example, nurses can suggest to women that they create a parenting plan to be approved by the court that includes specific safety strategies, such as use of a third party to exchange children for visitation (Hardesty & Campbell, in press).

In many cases, the best way to protect the child is to protect the mother from the abuser. Safety planning with the mother will help the child, as the child's safety is intricately related to and dependent on the mother's safety (Culross, 1999). However, when possible, safety planning with mothers should include specific strategies for children (Hardesty & Campbell, in press). See Box 6-2.

Nurses, with the help of the mother, can bring children into the planning process. Safety planning can help empower children to identify safety issues and problem-solve in ways that will afford protection. It also can minimize risk and help reduce children's anxiety and fears. Nurses can encourage critical thinking by working collaboratively with children (Hart, 2001).

Specific safety strategies for children should be age appropriate, and the child must be capable and competent enough to carry them out. Development

BOX 6-2 SAFETY PLANNING WITH CHILDREN

QUESTIONS TO CONSIDER WHEN DEVELOPING A CHILD-SAFETY PLAN

- What is the degree of risk to the mother?
- What is degree of risk to the child (e.g., child abuse or death)?
- What are the child's individual needs (e.g., what is the child afraid of or worried about)?
- What are the child's abilities (e.g., age/developmental status, mental/physical health)?
- What are the child's feelings toward the abuser (e.g., conflicted, angry, ambivalent)?

POSSIBLE SAFETY STRATEGIES

- Avoid places, times, or circumstances that have been associated with prior violent incidences.
- Never intervene in a violent incident but instead escape to safety and call 911.
- Learn how to use the phone, including how to call long distance. Practice making calls.
- Know a way to reach your mother or a trusted adult at all times, and know how to call 911.
- Be familiar with any protective orders in place that may influence police response.
- Identify all ways of escape (windows, doors), and identify where all phones are located.
- Locate a safe place (e.g., church) or a trusted adult to go to if necessary.
- Create a contract to be approved by the court that outlines your rights, your father's responsibilities, and any consequences if the order is violated.
- Children must understand that a safety plan is not a guarantee for safety. Just as the child is not responsible for the violence, the child is also not responsible for the failure of any safety strategy.

Based on Hart, B. J. (2001). *Safety planning for children: Strategizing for unsupervised visits with batterers* [Online]. Available: http://www.mincava.umn.edu/hart/safetyp.htm.

also should be considered both in terms of understanding and responding to violence. For example, in planning for what to do if things get dangerous, an older child may be more able to dial 911, whereas it may be safer to instruct a younger child to go to the neighbor's house. It may be more important to advise older children to escape and not intervene than younger children who are less likely to intervene. It is also necessary to take into account the degree of attachment the child has to the abuser. It may be unreasonable to expect a boy strongly attached to his father to call the police on his dad. Nurses can assess the availability of social supports to assist the child in safety planning. A caring and trusted adult can provide the child with a safe place to go when necessary.

Direct interventions with a child depend on the timing of the encounter, age and responses of the child, and family circumstances. Even a child in battered-women's shelters requires different interventions. If the child is returning to the violent home, interventions may need to focus on the most basic safety needs. If the family is relocating, the nurse may have the opportunity to help the mother and child learn new ways of living and responding. Interventions in battered women's shelters are discussed next.

Battered Women's Shelters

Although there is some variability, battered women's shelters are generally emergency shelters for women and their children, where they are provided temporary safe haven within a communal shelter setting. Abused women and their children are allowed to stay at the shelter for a relatively short period of time (usually a maximum of 30 to 60 days), during which they are assisted in assessing their situation, gaining knowledge and insight about woman abuse, and obtaining social services. The women and their children may leave the shelter to relocate with family or friends or to their own new residence. Many women and their children return to their previous homes with the belief that their absence, and their new information and insight, will help stop the violence.

In recent years, attention to the needs of children who accompany their mothers to shelters has increased. Because of limited funds, however, resources have generally been directed toward assisting the mothers with counseling, social services, and relocation services, all of which indirectly benefit children. Even with limited funds, many shelters have always offered specialized services to children. Nurses involved with shelters can contribute to those services or assist in their development when such services are unavailable. As with every practice setting, certain aspects are constraining. For example, abused women and their children are often a transient population (length of shelter stay varies from a few days to months) and children vary widely by age range (from infants to teenagers) and developmental stage. Shelters face challenges such as limited availability of staff and limited privacy, space, and accessibility to provide services and treatment.

All children admitted to battered-women's shelters should have access to health screening and treatment. An individual health history and assessment of each child should be conducted to identify his or her experience and response. Health problems should receive immediate attention through nursing staff or community referral. Clinical experience with abused women and their children in shelters has revealed many more commonalities regarding the provision of maternal child care between these and other settings than might be expected. Children of abused women may have difficulties unique to their experience. Some may have been physically injured in an attack on their mothers immediately preceding admission to the shelter. But these injuries require the same attention as any other injury.

Mothers also have needs for information regarding their children's growth, development, state of health, and guidance. Nursing staff can develop with the mother and children a health plan with health-related goals to achieve while at the shelter. Nursing involvement is an obvious benefit and can provide an excellent opportunity for nursing-student clinical experiences (Urbancic, Campbell, & Humphreys, 1993).

Children commonly experience a variety of stress-related symptoms during their stays at shelters. They may return to behaviors, such as bedwetting, thumbsucking, and bottle-feeding, that previously had been abandoned. Nurses can assess children's stress and coping and discuss them with mothers. Mothers may lack knowledge of children's responses and should be reassured that these behaviors are normal and generally disappear once order has been established. Preliminary evaluation studies also suggest that the therapeutic environment of the battered-women's shelter can help to reduce children's symptoms (Graham-Bermann, 2001).

Battered-women's shelters that have children's services usually offer some structured programs for children. The form of these programs varies greatly. They generally include all or part of the following components: crisis-intervention activities, academic programs, daily programs, therapy/counseling, parent–child programs, and advocacy programs. These components are not mutually exclusive. Various approaches to these components have been reported and are presented in the following discussion.

Crisis Intervention. The difficulties that children often face in response to violence exposure may be further exacerbated when they are brought to shelters (Jaffe, Wolfe, & Wilson, 1990). The children may have experienced a complete disruption in their familiar support systems, particularly with school, friends, neighborhood, and, usually, the significant adult male in their lives.

Jaffe and colleagues (1990) have identified "subtle symptoms" in children of abused women. They described three areas that require careful investigation, especially in children who do not demonstrate pronounced reactions to observations of abuse: responses and attitudes about conflict resolution, assigning responsibility for violence, and knowledge and skills in dealing with violence incidents. According to Jaffe and colleagues, children often experience violence in ways that are not apparent. Within the category of responses and attitudes, they described children who concluded that violent conflict resolution was acceptable behavior, who learn to rationalize violence, and who blame their mothers for causing the violence. Other children assigned blame for the violence to their fathers but pursued strategies for resolution of the violence (e.g., poisoning father) that were clearly desperate. Some children assumed an exaggerated sense of responsibility for the violence in their family. This response was reported as typical of many young children. Finally, children often lacked basic knowledge of community resources to assist them with crises or basic skills for handling emergency situations.

Academic Program. Children in shelters frequently are unable to attend their regular schools for safety (fathers may attempt to find them) and other reasons (teasing or harassment by peers). Some shelters send children to local schools where the circumstances of children's attendance are understood. Others provide on-site educational services.

School nurses can make important contributions to specialized academic programs for children exposed to violence. Previously discussed approaches that encourage children and mothers to disclose their worries and fears help children in school settings as well. Often, nurses who are initially approached with some physical problem and perceived as being helpful will be sought out in the future for other less tangible difficulties. School nurses also can help teachers and other staff members understand why children sometimes return to the security of habits (e.g., thumb-sucking, special toys, and nail biting) during times of stress. Nursing assessments of children's physical complaints (e.g., stomach pains) can reassure everyone that the problem can be "cured" with attention, quiet time, and reassurance rather than a visit to the emergency room.

Daily Program. Daily programs for children in shelters vary greatly. Generally programs are structured to ensure that a similar schedule is followed most weekdays. At a minimum, routine child care allows mothers to attend to the many obligations associated with obtaining social services, hunting for an apartment, and finding employment. For children in shelters, structured time and activities provide organization and security in strange environments. If sufficiently qualified staff is available, routine play sessions can be educational and therapeutic, thereby enhancing individual counseling.

It is important for children of abused women to be exposed to adults, both female and male, who respect each other and work together. Early in the women's shelter movement, men were rarely seen inside shelters. Fortunately, many male staff and volunteers now provide positive role models for children.

Therapy/Counseling. Children need to talk about their experiences and their feelings. They may blame themselves for the violence in their homes, especially if abusive episodes were associated with parental conflicts over child-rearing. Children may also feel that they are responsible for their mother's decision to leave the home, return, or get a divorce. What appears to be an egocentric perception by children of abused women may be reality. The best interests of children are frequently central to women's decisions about the future. A mother may stay in an abusive relationship because she believes that her children will benefit from the ongoing presence of an adult male. Alternatively, women may ultimately decide to leave an abusive situation because the violence is affecting the children (Hardesty, 2001; Humphreys, 1998).

Children may have spent an inordinate amount of time trying to be "good" to prevent future episodes of violence. If children have intervened in attempts to stop violence between adults, they may have a false sense of confidence in their abilities to keep batterers from abusing again. If they were successful in the past at stopping abuse, children may feel personal failure if subsequent interventions were unsuccessful.

Many authors have described the valuable role of therapy for children. Therapy approaches vary and can include individualized approaches, such as trauma-focused therapy, or small-group therapy to help children express their emotions and feelings. Approaches may vary from Big Brother/Sister recreational-type approaches to play therapy to longer-term, more intensive contacts that more closely resemble traditional psychotherapy. Therapy with children can include the whole family, sibling groups, or the mother–child dyad. The type of intervention depends on the ages, developmental levels, and needs of the children. Individualized therapy can be particularly useful when cultural background or other characteristics are likely to influence children's responses to domestic violence.

Parent-Child Program. Some shelters provide services to abused women that are intended to enhance their relationships with their children and, if necessary, to teach nonviolent methods of child-rearing. Shelters do not allow the use of violent conflict-resolution tactics, including corporal punishment, by anyone. For some mothers, this necessitates learning new ways of disciplining their children. Nurses can take an active role in helping mothers develop a repertoire of disciplinary approaches, considering the most appropriate approaches for their children and circumstances and modeling the use of the different strategies. The goal is to improve children's adjustment by improving mothers' parenting competence.

Sullivan, Nguyen, and colleagues (2000) warn against assuming that all abused women are impaired in their ability to parent or that they are responsible for their children's adjustment problems. As these authors aptly note, it is men's use of violence that increases children's behavioral problems, which in turn increases mothers' parenting stress and need to use discipline. To reduce the negative affects of violence exposure on children, parenting classes must be mandated for abusive fathers, not the mothers whom they have abused. Women who want or need parenting classes should be able to access them but should not be required to attend classes just because they have been abused. Most mothers will want help understanding their children's behavioral problems and how they can appropriately respond to them. However, we should not assume that all abused mothers want or need help. Women are active agents who, despite abuse, nurture their children in diverse and creative ways. Any assistance should be driven by what these women request and should acknowledge their strengths and capabilities.

Advocacy Program. Abused women and their children need follow-up services after they leave shelters. At a minimum, shelter staff can connect women and children to appropriate community services. Nurses can help them develop goals and objectives for maintaining and improving their well-being after leaving the shelter. Some shelters provide outreach services, such as therapy/counseling, information, or education programs, that women and their children can take advantage of after leaving.

Children of abused women are often victimized by prolonged legal disputes over custody and visitation issues. The legal battle can be a prolonged affair, involving years of threats and conflicts, which many children discover continues long after the separation and any court decisions. Some shelters provide legal-advocacy programs that provide information and support related to custody and visitation.

Tertiary Prevention

Ideally, abuse of women is never allowed to progress to this stage of intervention; however, this is often not the case. Tertiary prevention is required when children of abused women have experienced irreversible effects from the violence. The goal of tertiary prevention is rehabilitation and healing of the children to the maximum level of functioning possible with the limitations of any negative effects. Many of the secondary-prevention strategies apply to tertiary prevention. One difference is that a goal of tertiary prevention is to establish long-term comprehensive services for women and children.

Home-visitation programs are one option for long-term services. When physical injuries have resulted in disability, women and their children may be eligible for a visiting-nurse program. Home-visiting nurses can provide assistance with actively finding community support. Home-visiting programs also can be educational interventions. For example, in Sullivan and colleagues' (1998) home-visitation advocacy program, advocates support mothers in solving problems, such as finding jobs, arranging transportation, getting information about educational opportunities, and communicating with the school system. The goal is to reduce mothers' frustrations and improve parenting.

A coordinated community response (CCR) involving the health-care system, legal system (including those who work with divorce and custody issues), domestic-violence advocates, and child-welfare workers is important at any level of intervention but may be particularly useful at the tertiary level. A CCR seeks to integrate the variety of resources from which abused women and their children are likely to require services (Sullivan & Allen, 2001). An integrated effort increases the availability and accessibility of resources, advocacy, and support to women and their children. A CCR also increases the communication within and among organizations, promotes exchange of resources, and helps in development of shared goals. In addition, a CCR may decrease revictimization, the amount of time families are involved in the system, and the number of families who return to system. It can encourage batterer accountability. Unfortunately, child-welfare workers and abused-women's advocates often find themselves at odds with each other while working with families. They share similar interests in stopping violence; however, their perspectives and approaches differ. Nurses are in an excellent position to collaborate with both groups of professionals to work toward a common goal.

IMPLEMENTATION

Most abused women care about their children's safety and want to protect them. Their worrying affects how they respond to battering, which in turn affects their children (Humphreys, 1995). Nurses can help battered women and indirectly help their children by easing the worrying. One way to do this is by encouraging a discussion of worries. Clients may benefit by actively discussing their thinking and responses. Nurses can tell battered women that by helping themselves they are helping their children. This may free battered women to focus on themselves without feeling that they are neglecting their children. Humphreys (1995) indicates that nurses should use both "worry" and "fears" when initiating such discussions, as these terms mean different things to battered women. She also suggests open discussion of worries and fears in both private and group settings so that women can share their common experiences, learn and critique responses, and be reassured that they are not alone in their worrying.

Nurses also can help women recognize their children's needs and the ways in which they might support them. For example, the women in Ericksen and Henderson's (1998) study indicated that they did not know how to talk to their children or what questions to ask them. They reported that their children had enormous unmet needs and that they felt inadequate in helping their children. Nurses can educate mothers about the health effects of exposure to domestic violence to help them understand their children's reactions and how to respond to them.

Particularly during separation/divorce, mothers may have difficulty being emotionally available to their children, as much of their energy is expended negotiating the various systems (e.g., the legal system), making custody and visitation decisions, and, for many, managing continued harassment and control (Ericksen & Henderson, 1998; Ford-Gilboe, Wuest, Merritt-Gray, & Berman, 2001; Hardesty, 2002). They also may feel ambivalent about what is best for themselves and their children because, while they want to move on, they are tied to their former partners through the children.

During this time, children need their mothers (Ericksen & Henderson, 1998). They are likely to feel sad over their parents' separation, miss their father, and be concerned about the future. They may worry that their mothers will leave them, too. Children of abused women, like all children, need to express their worries and concerns, but because children are often protective of their mothers, they may be reluctant to express their own feelings. They also may feel loyalty conflicts, wanting to meet the emotional needs of both parents. Nurses can ask children about their worries or fears, and with their permission, share them with their mothers. Nurses also can educate children about domestic violence and dispel any beliefs that violence is a routine part of normal family life (Humphreys, 2001a). Finally, nurses can assess the availability of social supports that can provide valuable opportunities for children to share their conflicting feelings without getting "caught in the middle" by confiding in a parent.

From research on children of domestic violence and children of war, Berman (1999) offers several guiding principles that should apply to all interventions with children exposed to violence. The practitioner should:

- Listen to children in a sincere and nonjudgmental manner.
- Respect the child and recognize his or her strengths.
- Be willing to try nontraditional approaches with children from diverse cultural backgrounds.
- Be aware of the political dimension of violence, with a view toward enabling the child to develop age-appropriate understandings of political and social contexts
- Develop strategies to help children find health.

EVALUATION

Evaluation is an ongoing process through which the nurse reviews the changes made in terms of the identified goals. Long-term follow-up is necessary as situations and needs change. In terms of evaluating the effectiveness of intervention programs, existing research is in its early stages (Graham-Bermann, 2001). At present, intervention programs tend to use a "one-size-fits-all" approach; thus, they work for some children but not others. Children have different responses to witnessing domestic violence; some are negatively affected while others appear to manage well. Different responses to violence exposure require intervention programs targeted to children's specific needs. Controlled-outcome studies comparing the effectiveness of different interventions are clearly needed to guide nurses in choosing programs that work.

Evaluation studies with abused women and their children are challenging for several reasons. Abused women may not stay in shelters long enough to complete an evaluation. Although evaluations with women and children residing in shelters are convenient, they are limited because only a small number of women seek shelter. Tracking is a problem when doing evaluations with women and children in the community. Women may relocate, or batterers may keep women and children isolated. Furthermore, evaluations of children after they leave shelters must account for where they go. Some children return to the home with the abuser, others relocate, and some children have continued contact with abusers through custody or visitation arrangements. These children are likely to demonstrate different outcomes after leaving the shelter.

Based on a review of existing evaluation research, Graham-Bermann offers the following suggestions for designing more effective interventions:

- Target intervention efforts to groups of children with similar profiles, violence experiences, and exposures.
- Compare the same program with different populations of exposed children (e.g., shelter versus community population).
- Compare different treatment approaches in systematically controlled studies.
- Evaluate interventions designed for children with different symptoms (e.g., internalizing versus externalizing symptoms).
- Identify features of interventions that are effective (e.g., therapist characteristics, setting, techniques).
- Extend the follow-up period to track program effects over time and identify which children improve, worsen, or stay the same.
- Adopt minimum standards and criteria for evaluating the effectiveness of interventions.

SUMMARY

Children exposed to the abuse of their mothers are at risk for a variety of emotional, cognitive, and behavioral difficulties. However, research has described the important mediating effects on children of even one positive relationship with a significant person. Nurses should be aware of family violence and assess every client and family for this problem. Early identification and intervention can stem detrimental effects and help individuals and families toward recovery.

References

Achenbach, T. M., & Edelbrock, C. S. (1978). The classification of child psychopathology: A review and analysis of empirical efforts. *Psychological Bulletin, 85,* 1275–1301.

Adamson, L. A., & Thompson, R. A. (1998). Coping with interparental verbal conflict by children exposed to spouse abuse and children from nonviolent homes. *Journal of Family Violence, 13,* 213–232.

American Academy of Pediatrics. (1998). The role of the pediatrician in recognizing and intervening on behalf of abused women. *Pediatrics, 101*(6), 1091–1092.

American Psychiatric Association. (1987). *Diagnostic and statistical manual of mental disorders* (3rd. ed., rev.). Washington, DC: Author.

Arroyo, W., & Eth, S. (1985). Children traumatized by Central American warfare. In S. Eth & R. S. Pynoos (Eds.), *Post-traumatic stress disorder in children* (pp. 103–120). Washington, DC: American Psychiatric Press.

Attala, J., & McSweeney, M. (1997). Preschool children of battered women identified in a community setting. *Issues in Comprehensive Pediatric Nursing, 20,* 217–225.

Berman, H. (1999). Health in the aftermath of violence: A critical narrative study of children of war and children of battered women. *Canadian Journal of Nursing Research, 31*(3), 89–109.

Berman, H. (2000). The relevance of narrative research with children who witness war and children who witness woman abuse. *Journal of Aggression, Maltreatment and Trauma, 3*(1), 107–125.

Berman, H., & Jiwani, Y. (Eds.) (2002). *In the best interests of the girl child.* London, Ontario: Centre for Research on Violence Against Women and Children.

Berman, H., McKenna, K., Traher, C., Taylor, G., & MacQuarrie, B. (2000). Sexual harassment: Everyday violence in the lives of girls and women. *Advances in Nursing Science, 22*(4), 32–46.

Boney-McCoy, S., & Finklehor, D. (1995). Psychosocial sequelae of violent victimization in a national youth sample. *Journal of Consulting and Clinical Psychology, 63,* 726–736.

Brown, L. S. (1991). Not outside the range: One feminist perspective on psychic trauma. *American Imago, 46,* 119–133.

Campbell, J. C. (1995). Assessing dangerousness. Newbury Park, CA: Sage.

Campbell, J. C., Koziol-McLain, J., Glass, N. E., Webster, D., Block, R., McFarlane, J., & Campbell, D. W. (in press). Validation of the danger assessment: Results from the 12 city femicide study. *National Institute of Justice Briefs.*

Campbell, J. C., & Lewandowski, L. A. (1997). Mental and physical health effects of intimate partner violence on women and children. *Anger, Aggression, and Violence, 20*(2), 353–374.

Campbell, J. C., Sharps, P. W., & Glass, N. E. (2001). Risk assessment for intimate partner homicide. In G. F. Pinard & L. Pagani (Eds.), *Clinical assessment of dangerousness: Empirical contributions* (pp. 136–157). New York: Cambridge University Press.

Carlson, B. E. (1984). Children's observations of interparental violence. In A. R. Roberts (Ed.), *Battered women and their families: Intervention strategies and treatment programs* (pp. 147–167). New York: Springer.

Carlson, B. E. (1991). Outcomes of physical abuse and observation of marital violence among adolescents in placement. *Journal of Interpersonal Violence, 6,* 526–534.

Carr, J. L., & VanDeusen, K. M. (2002). The relationship between family of origin violence and dating violence in college men. *Journal of Interpersonal Violence, 17,* 630–646.

Cascardi, M., & O'Leary, K. D. (1992). Depressive symptomatology, self-esteem and self-blame in battered women. *Journal of Family Violence, 7*(4), 249–259.

Christopoulous, C., Cohn, D. A., Shaw, D. S., Joyce, S., Sullivan-Hanson, J., Kraft, S. P., & Emery, R. E. (1987). Children of abused women: Adjustment at time of shelter residence. *Journal of Marriage and the Family, 49,* 611–619.

Culross, P. L. (1999). Health care system responses to children exposed to domestic violence. *The Future of Children: Domestic Violence and Children, 9*(3), 111–121.

Dauvergne, M., & Johnson, H. (2002). Children witnessing family violence. *Juristat: Canadian Centre for Justice Statistics* (Statistics Canada, Catalogue No. 85-002-XPE), 21*(6), 1–13.

Davis, L. V., & Carlson, B. E. (1987). Observations of spouse abuse: What happens to the children. *Journal of Interpersonal Violence, 2*(3), 278–291.

Doumas, D., Margolin, G., & John, R. S. (1994). The intergenerational transmission of aggression across three generations. *Journal of Family Violence, 9*(2), 157–175.

Edleson, J. L. (1999a). Children's witnessing of adult domestic violence. *Journal of Interpersonal Violence, 14,* 839–870.

Edleson, J. L. (1999b). *Problems associated with children's witnessing domestic violence.* [Online]. Available: http://www.vawnet.org.

Ericksen, J. R., & Henderson, A. D. (1992). Witnessing family violence: The children's experience. *Journal of Advanced Nursing, 17,* 1200–1209.

Ericksen, J. R., & Henderson, A. D. (1998). Diverging realities: Abused women and their children. In J. C. Campbell (Ed.), *Empowering survivors of abuse: Health care for battered women and their children* (pp. 138–155). Thousand Oaks, CA: Sage.

Fantuzzo, J. W., DePaola, L. M., Lambert, L., Matino, T., Anderson, G., & Sutton, S. (1991). Effects of interparental violence on the psychological adjustment and competencies of young children. *Journal of Consulting and Clinical Psychology, 59,* 258–265.

Ford-Gilboe, M., Wuest, J., Merritt-Gray, M., & Berman, H. (2001, September). *Beyond leaving: Understanding health promotion processes of single mothers and their children.* Paper presented at the Eleventh International Conference of the Nursing Network on Violence Against Women, Madison, WI.

Forsstrom-Cohen, B., & Rosenbaum, A. (1985). The effects of parental marital violence on young adults: An exploratory investigation. *Journal of Marriage and the Family, 47,* 467–472.

Gamache, D., & Snapp, S. (1995). Teach your children well: Elementary schools and violence prevention. In E. Peled, P. Jaffe, & J. Edelson (Eds.), *Ending the cycle of violence: Community responses to children of battered women* (pp. 209–231). Thousand Oaks, CA: Sage.

Garbarino, J., Kostelny, K., & Dubrow, N. (1991). *No place to be a child: Growing up in a war zone.* Lexington, MA: D. C. Heath & Co.

Garmezy, N. (1981). Children under stress: Perspectives on antecedents and correlates of vulnerability and resistance to psychopathology. In A. I. Rabin, J. Arnoff, A. M. Barclay & R. A. Zucker (Eds), *Further explorations in personality* (pp. 70–81). New York: Wiley Interscience.

Graham-Bermann, S. A. (2001). Designing intervention evaluations for children exposed to domestic violence: Applications of research and theory. In S. A. Graham-Bermann & J. L. Edleson (Eds.), *Domestic violence in the lives of children: The future of research, intervention, and social policy* (pp. 237–267). Washington, DC: American Psychological Association.

Graham-Bermann, S. A., & Levendosky, A. A. (1998). Traumatic stress symptoms in children of battered women. *Journal of Interpersonal Violence, 14,* 111–128.

Gray, H., & Foshee, V. (1997). Adolescent dating violence: Differences between one-sided and mutually violent profiles. *Journal of Interpersonal Violence, 12,* 126–141.

Greenfield, L. A., Rand, M., Craven, D., Klaus, P. A., Perkins, C. A., Ringel, C., Warchol, G., Maston, C., & Fox, J. A. (1998). *Violence by intimates: Analysis of data on crimes by current or former spouses, boyfriends, and girlfriends.* Washington, DC: U.S. Department of Justice, Bureau of Statistics.

Hadley, S., Short, L., Lesin, N., & Zook, E. (1995). Women kind: An innovative model of health care response to domestic abuse. *Women's Health Issues, 5,* 189–198.

Hardesty, J. L. (2001). *"I just can't get him out of my life!" Co-parenting after divorce with an abusive former husband.* Unpublished doctoral dissertation, University of Missouri, Columbia.

Hardesty, J. L. (2002). Separation assault in the context of post-divorce parenting: An integrative review of the literature. *Violence Against Women, 8*(5), 593–621.

Hardesty, J. L., & Campbell, J. C. (in press). "He still controls me through the children": Post-separation safety planning for battered women and their children. In P. G. Jaffe (Ed.), *Ending domestic violence in the lives of children and parents: Promising practices for safety, healing and prevention.* Toronto, Canada: University of Toronto Press.

Hardesty, J. L., & Ganong, L. H. (2002). *A grounded theory model of negotiating co-parenting with an abusive former husband.* Manuscript submitted for publication, Johns Hopkins University, Baltimore.

Harned, M. (2001). Abused women or abused men? An examination of the context and outcomes of dating violence. *Violence & Victims, 16,* 269–285.

Hart, B. J. (2001). *Safety planning for children: Strategizing for unsupervised visits with batterers* [Online]. Available: http://www.mincava.umn.edu/hart/safetyp.htm.

Haskell, L. (1998). *Violence prevention education in schools: A critical literature review.* Unpublished manuscript.

Henning, K., Leitenberg, H., Coffey, P., Turner, T., & Bennett, R. T. (1996). Long-term psychological and social impact of witnessing physical conflict between parents. *Journal of Interpersonal Violence, 11,* 35–51.

Herman, J. L. (1992). *Trauma and recovery.* New York: Basic Books.

Holden, G. W., & Ritchie, K. (1991). Linking extreme marital discord, child rearing, and child behavior problems: Evidence from battered women. *Child Development, 62,* 311–327.

Holden, G. W., Stein, J. D., Ritchie, K. L., Harris, S. D., & Jouriles, E. N. (1998). Parenting behaviors and beliefs of battered women. In G. W. Holden, R. Geffner, & E. N. Jouriles (Eds.), *Children exposed to marital violence: Theory, research, and applied issues* (pp. 289–334). Washington, DC: American Psychological Association.

hooks, b. (1984). *Feminist theory from margin to center.* Boston, MA: South End Press.

Hotton, T. (2002). Spousal violence after marital separation. Juristat Service Bulletin: Canadian Centre for Justice Statistics (Catalogue 85-002 ISSN 0715-271X). Ottawa, Canada: Statistics Canada.

Hughes, H. M. (1988). Psychological and behavioral correlates of family violence in child witness and victims. *American Journal of Orthopsychiatry, 58,* 77–90.

Hughes, H. M., Vargo, M. C., Ito, E. S., & Skinner, L. K. (1991). Psychological adjustment of children of battered women: Influences of gender. *Family Violence Bulletin, 7,* 15–17.

Humphreys, J. C. (1989). *Dependent-care directed toward the prevention of hazards to life, health, and well-being in mothers and children who experience family violence.* Unpublished doctoral dissertation, Wayne State University, Detroit.

Humphreys, J. C. (1990). Dependent-care directed toward the prevention of hazards to life, health, and well-being in mothers and children who experience family violence. *MAINlines, 11*(1), 6–7.

Humphreys, J. C. (1991). Children of battered women: Worries about their mothers. *Pediatric Nursing, 17*, 342–345.

Humphreys, J. C. (1995). The work of worrying: Battered women and their children. *Scholarly Inquiry for Nursing Practice: An International Journal, 9*(2), 127–145.

Humphreys, J. (1998). Helping battered women take care of their children. In J. C. Campbell (Ed.), *Empowering survivors of abuse: Health care for battered women and their children* (pp. 103–115). Thousand Oaks, CA: Sage.

Humphreys, J. C. (2001a). Growing up in a violent home: The lived experience of daughters of battered women. *Journal of Family Nursing, 7*(3), 244–260.

Humphreys, J. C. (2001b). Turnings and adaptations in resilient daughters of battered women. *Journal of Nursing Scholarship, 33*(3), 245–251.

Hurt, H., Malmud, E., Brodsky, N. L., & Giannetta, J. (2001). Exposure to violence: Psychological and academic correlates in child witnesses. *Archives of Pediatric Adolescent Medicine, 155*(12), 1351–1356.

Huth-Bocks, A. C., Levendosky, A. A., & Semel, M. A. (2001). The direct and indirect effects of domestic violence on young children's intellectual functioning. *Journal of Family Violence, 16*(3), 269–290.

Jaffe, P. G., & Geffner, R. (1998). Child custody disputes and domestic violence: Critical issues for mental health, social service, and legal professionals. In G. W. Holden, R. Geffner, & E. N. Jouriles (Eds.), *Children exposed to marital violence: Theory, research, and applied issues* (pp. 371–408). Washington, DC: American Psychological Association.

Jaffe, P. G., Wolfe, D. A., & Wilson, S. K. (1990). *Children of battered women*. Newbury Park, CA: Sage.

Jaffe, P. G., Wolfe, D. A., Wilson, S. K., & Zak, L. (1986). Family violence and child adjustment: A comparative analysis of girls' and boys' behavioral symptoms. *American Journal of Psychiatry, 143*(1), 74–77.

Johnson, H. (1996). *Dangerous domains: Violence against women in Canada*. Toronto, Canada: Nelson Canada.

Jones, L. (1991). The Minnesota School Curriculum Project: A statewide domestic violence prevention project in secondary schools. In B. Levy (Ed.), *Dating violence: Young women in danger* (pp. 258–266). Seattle, WA: Seal Press.

Jouriles, E. N., Barling, J., & O'Leary, K. D. (1987). Predicting child behavior problems in maritally violent families. *Journal of Abnormal Child Psychology, 15*, 165–173.

Jouriles, E. N., McDonald, R., Norwood, W. D., & Ezell, E. (2001). Issues and controversies in documenting the prevalence of children's exposure to domestic violence. In S. A. Graham-Bermann & J. L. Edleson (Eds.), *Domestic violence in the lives of children: The future of research, intervention, and social policy* (pp. 13–34). Washington, DC: American Psychological Association.

Jouriles, E. N., McDonald, R., Norwood, W. D., Ware, S. H., Spiller, L. C., & Swank, P. R. (1998). Knives, guns, and interparent violence: Relations with child behavior problems. *Journal of Family Psychology, 12*(2), 178–194.

Jouriles, E. N., Murphy, C. M., & O'Leary, K. D. (1989). Interspousal aggression, marital discord, and child problems. *Journal of Consulting and Clinical Psychology, 57*, 453–455.

Jouriles, E. N., Spiller, L. C., Stephens, N., McDonald, R., & Swank, P. (2000). Variability in adjustment of children of battered women: The role of child appraisals of interparent conflict. *Cognitive Therapy and Research, 24*, 233–249.

Kalmuss, D. (1984). The intergenerational transmission of marital aggression. *Journal of Marriage and the Family, 46*, 11–19.

Kaufman, J., & Zigler, E. (1987). Do abused children become abusive parents? *American Journal of Orthopsychiatry, 57*, 186–193.

Kerig, P. K. (1997). Gender issues in the effects of exposure to violence on children. In B. B. R. Rossman (Chair), *Assessing the impact of exposure to violence on children: Risk and protective factors in children, families, and communities*. Keynote panel presented at the Second International Conference on Children Exposed to Violence, London, Ontario, Canada.

Kerig, P. K. (1998). Gender and appraisals as mediators of adjustment in children exposed to interparental violence. *Developmental Psychology, 29*(6), 931–939.

Kerouac, S., Taggart, M., Lescop, J., & Fortin, M. (1986). Dimensions of health in violent families. *Health Care for Women International, 7*, 423–426.

Kinzie, J. D., Sack, W. H., Angell, R., Manson, S. M., & Rath, B. (1986). The psychiatric effects of massive trauma on Cambodian children: I. The children. *Journal of the American Academy of Child Psychiatry, 25*, 370–376.

Langhinrichsen-Rohling, J., Monson, C. M., Meyer, K. A., Caster, J., & Sanders, A. (1998). The associations among family-of-origin violence and young adults' current depressed, hopeless, suicidal, and life-threatening behavior. *Journal of Family Violence, 13*, 243–261.

Lehmann, P. (1997). The development of posttraumatic stress disorder (PTSD) in a sample of child witnesses to mother assault. *Journal of Family Violence, 12*, 241–257.

Lemmey, D., McFarlane, J., Wilson, P., & Malecha, A. (2001). Intimate partner violence: Mother's perspective of effects on their children. *Maternal Child Nursing, 26*(2), 98–103.

Levendosky, A. A., & Graham-Bermann, S. A. (2001). Parenting in battered women: The effects of domestic violence on women and their children. *Journal of Family Violence, 16*(2), 171–192.

Lisak, D., Hopper, J., & Song, P. (1996). Factors in the cycle of violence: Gender rigidity and emotional constriction. *Journal of Traumatic Stress, 9*, 721–743.

Maker, A. H., Kemmelmeier, M., & Peterson, C. (1998). Long-term psychological consequences in women of witnessing parental physical conflict and experiencing abuse in childhood. *Journal of Interpersonal Violence, 13*, 574–589.

Margolin, G., & Gordis, E. B. (2000). The effects of family and community violence on children. *Annual Reviews Psychology, 51,* 445–479.

Mathias, J. L., Mertin, P., & Murray, A. (1995). The psychological functioning of children from backgrounds of domestic violence. *Australian Psychologist, 30,* 47–56.

McCloskey, L. A., Figueredo, A. J., & Koss, M. P. (1995). The effects of systematic family violence on children's mental health. *Child Development, 66,* 1239–1261.

McCloskey, L. A., & Walker, M. (2000). Posttraumatic stress in children exposed to family violence and single-event trauma. *Journal of the American Academy of Child and Adolescent Psychiatry, 38*(1), 108–115.

McFarlane, J., Parker, B., Soeken, L., & Bullock, L. (1992). Assessing for abuse during pregnancy: Severity and frequency of injuries and associated entry into prenatal care. *Journal of the American Medical Association, 267,* 2370–2372.

McGee, R. A., Wolfe, D. A., & Wilson, S. K. (1997). Multiple maltreatment experiences and adolescent behavior problems: Adolescents' perspectives. *Development and Psychopathology, 9,* 131–149.

Mohr, W. K., Lutz, M. J. N., Fantuzzo, J. W., & Perry, M. A. (2000). Children exposed to family violence: A review of empirical research from a developmental-ecological perspective. *Trauma, Violence, & Abuse, 1*(3), 264–283.

Moore, T. E., & Pepler, D. J. (1998). Correlates of adjustment in children at risk. In G. W. Holden, R. Geffner, & E. Jouriles (Eds.), *Children exposed to marital violence: Theory, research, and intervention* (pp. 157–184). Washington DC: American Psychological Association.

O'Keefe, M. (1994). Racial/ethnic differences among battered women and their children. *Journal of Child and Family Studies, 3,* 285–305.

Olds, D., Henderson, C., Cole, R., Eckenrode, J., Kitzman, H., Luckey, D., Pettitt, L., Sidora, K., Morris, P., & Powers, J. (1998). Long-term effects of nurse home visitation on children's criminal and antisocial behavior: 15-year follow-up of a randomized trial. *Journal of the American Medical Association, 280,* 1238–1244.

Olweus, D. (1993). *Bullying at school: What we know and what we can do.* Cambridge, MA: Blackwell.

Onyskiw, J. E. (2002a). Domestic violence and children's adjustment: A review of research. *Journal of Emotional Abuse, 3*(1–2).

Onyskiw, J. E. (2002b). Health and use of health services of children exposed to violence in their families. *Canadian Journal of Public Health, 93*(6), 416–420.

Onyskiw, J. E., & Hayduk, L. A. (2001). Processes underlying children's adjustment in families characterized by physical aggression. *Family Relations, 50,* 376–385.

Osofsky, J. D. (1997). The violence intervention project for children and families. In J. D. Osofsky (Ed.), *Children in a violent society* (pp. 256–260). New York: Guilford Press.

Petersen, K., & Gamache, D. (1988). *Family and me: Violence free: A domestic violence prevention curriculum.* St. Paul, MN: Minnesota Coalition for Battered Women.

Pollak, S. D., & Kistler, D. J. (2002). Early experience is associated with the development of categorical representations for facial expressions of emotion. *Proceedings of the National Academy of Sciences, 99*(13), 9072–9076.

Posada, G., Waters, E., Liu, X. D., & Johnson, S. (in press). Specific domains of marital discord and attachment security: Girls and boys. In E. Waters, B. Vaughn, G. Posada, & D. Teti (Eds.), *Patterns of secure base behavior: Q-sort perspectives on attachment and caregiving in infancy and childhood.* Hillsdale, NJ: Erlbaum.

Pynoos, R. S., & Eth, S. (1984). The child as witness to homicide. *Journal of Social Issues, 40,* 269–290.

Pynoos, R. S., & Nader, K. (1993). Issues in the treatment of post-traumatic stress in children and adolescents. In J. P. Wilson & B. Raphael (Eds.), *The international handbook of traumatic stress syndromes* (pp. 535–549). New York: Plenum.

Rath, G. D., Jaratt, L. G., & Leonardson, G. (1989). Rates of domestic violence against adult women by men partners. *Journal of American Board of Family Practitioners, 227,* 227–233.

Reitzel-Jaffe, D., & Wolfe, D. A. (2001). Predictors of relationship abuse among young men. *Journal of Interpersonal Violence, 16*(2), 99–115.

Richters, J. E., & Martinez, P. (1993). The NIMH Community Violence Project: I. Children as victims of and witnesses to violence. In D. Reiss, J. E. Richters, M. Radke-Yarrow, & D. Scharff (Eds.), *Children and violence* (pp. 7–21). New York: Guilford Press.

Rodgers, K. (1994). Wife assault: The findings of a national survey. Juristat Service Bulletin: Canadian Centre for Justice Statistics (Catalogue 85-002 ISSN 0715-271X). Ottawa, Canada: Statistics Canada.

Rossman, B. B. R. (1998). Descartes' error and posttraumatic stress disorder: Cognition and emotion in children who are exposed to parental violence. In G. W. Holden, R. Geffner & E. Jouriles (Eds.), *Children exposed to marital violence: Theory, research, and intervention* (pp. 223–256). Washington, DC: American Psychological Association.

Rossman, B. B. R. (2001). Longer term effects of children's exposure to domestic violence. In S.A. Graham-Bermann & J. L. Edleson (Eds.), *Domestic violence in the lives of children: The future of research, intervention, and social policy* (pp. 35–65). Washington, DC: American Psychological Association.

Rossman, B. B. R., & Ho, J. (2000). Posttraumatic response and children exposed to parental violence. In R. A. Geffner, P. Jaffe & M. Sudermann (Eds.), *Children exposed to domestic violence: Current issues in research, intervention, prevention, and policy development* (pp. 85–106). Binghamton, NY: Howarth Press.

Saigh, P. A. (1991). The development of posttraumatic stress disorder following four different types of traumatization. *Behavioral Research Therapy, 29,* 213–216.

Scott, C. J., & Matricciani, R. M. (1994). Joint Commission on Accreditation of Healthcare Organizations standards to improve care for victims of abuse. *Maryland Medical Journal, 43,* 891–898.

Shafer, J., Caetano, R., & Clark, C. (1998). Rates of intimate partner violence in the United States. *American Journal of Public Health, 88,* 1701–1704.

Sheeran, M., & Hampton, S. (1999). Supervised visitation in cases of domestic violence. *Juvenile and Family Court Journal, 50*(2), 13–26.

Silva, R. R., Alpert, M., Munoz, D. M., Singh, S., Matzner, F., & Dummit, S. (2000). Stress and vulnerability to posttraumatic stress disorder in children and adolescents. *American Journal of Psychiatry, 157*(8), 1229–1235.

Silverman, J. G., Raj, A., Mucci, L. A., & Hathaway, J. E. (2001). Dating violence against adolescent girls and associated substance use, unhealthy weight control, sexual risk behavior, pregnancy, and suicidality. *Journal of the American Medical Association, 286*, 572–579.

Silvern, L., & Kaersvang, L. (1989). The traumatized children of violent marriages. *Child Welfare, 68*, 421–436.

Silvern, L., Karyl, J., Waelde, L., Hodges, W. F., Starek, J., Heidt, E., & Min, K. (1995). Retrospective reports of parental partner abuse: Relationships to depression, trauma symptoms and self-esteem among college students. *Journal of Family Violence, 10*, 177–202.

Socolar, R. R. S. (2000). Domestic violence and children: A review. *North Carolina Medical Journal, 61*(5), 279–283.

Sternberg, K. J., Lamb, M. E., Greenbaum, C., Cicchetti, D., Dawud, S., Cortes, R. M., Krispin, O., & Lorey, F. (1993). Effects of domestic violence on children's behavior problems and depression. *Developmental Psychology, 29*, 44–52.

Straus, M. A. (1979). Measuring intrafamily conflict and violence: The Conflict Tactics (CT) Scales. *Journal of Marriage and the Family, 41*, 75–88.

Straus, M. A. (1992). Children as witnesses to marital violence: A risk factor for lifelong problems among a nationally representative sample of American men and women. In D. F. Scwarz (Ed.), *Children and violence: Report on the 23rd Ross roundtable on critical approaches to common pediatric problems* (pp. 98–104). Columbus, OH: Ross Laboratories.

Straus, M. A., & Gelles, R. J. (1990). *Physical violence in American families: Risk factors and adaptations to violence in 8,145 families.* New Brunswick, NJ: Transaction.

Straus, M. A., Gelles, R. J., & Steinmetz, S. K. (1980). *Behind closed doors: A survey of family violence in America.* New York: Doubleday.

Sudermann, M., Jaffe, E., & Hastings, E. (1995). Violence prevention programs in secondary (high) schools. In E. Peled, P. Jaffe, & J. Edleson (Eds.), *Ending the cycle of violence: Community responses to children of battered women* (pp. 232–254). Thousand Oaks, CA: Sage.

Sudermann, M., Jaffe, P., & Schieck, E. (1996). *A.S.A.P.: A school-based anti-violence program.* London, Ontario, Canada: London Family Court Clinic.

Sullivan, C. M., & Allen, N. E. (2001). Evaluating coordinated community responses for abused women and their children. In S. A. Graham-Bermann & J. L. Edleson (Eds.), *Domestic violence in the lives of children: The future of research, intervention, and social policy* (pp. 269–282). Washington, DC: American Psychological Association.

Sullivan, C., Allen, N., Nguyen, H., Gauthier, L., Shpungin, E., Bybee, D., & Baker, C. (1998). *Beyond blaming mom: Evidence for viewing mothers as nurturing parents of children exposed to domestic violence.* Manuscript under review, Michigan State University, East Lansing.

Sullivan, C. M., Juras, J., Bybee, D., Nguyen, H., & Allen, N. (2000). How children's adjustment is affected by their relationships to their mothers' abusers. *Journal of Interpersonal Violence, 15*, 587–602.

Sullivan, C. M., Nguyen, H., Allen, N., Bybee, D., & Juras, J. (2000). Beyond searching for deficits: Evidence that physically and emotionally abused women are nurturing parents. *Journal of Emotional Abuse, 2*(1), 51–71.

Terr, L. (1990). *Too scared to cry.* New York: Harper Collins.

Tjaden, P., & Thoennes, N. (1998). *Prevalence, incidence, and consequences of violence against women: Findings from the National Violence Against Women Survey* [Research in brief]. Washington, DC: National Institutes of Justice and Centers for Disease Control and Prevention.

Trainor, C. (1999). *Canada's shelters for abused women.* Juristat: Canadian Centre for Justice Statistics (Statistics Canada, Catalogue No. 85-002-XPE), *19*(6), 1–10.

Urbancic, J., Campbell, J. C., & Humphreys, J. (1993). Student clinical experiences in shelters for battered women. *Journal of Nursing Education, 32*, 341–346.

Ware, H. S., Jouriles, E. N., Spiller, L. C., McDonald, R., Swank, P. R., & Norwood, W. D. (2001). Conduct problems among children at battered women's shelters: Prevalence and stability of maternal reports. *Journal of Family Violence, 16*(3), 291–307.

Widom, C. S. (1989). Does violence beget violence? A critical examination of the literature. *Psychological Bulletin, 106*, 3–28.

Widom, C. S. (1998). Childhood victimization: Early adversity and subsequent psychopathology. In B. P. Dohrenwend (Ed.), *Adversity, stress, and psychopathology* (pp. 81–95). New York: Oxford University Press.

Wildin, S. R., Williamson, W. D., & Wilson, G. S. (1991). Children of battered women: Developmental and learning profiles. *Clinical Pediatrics, 30*(5), 299–304.

Wolfe, D. A., & Jaffe, P. (2001). Prevention of domestic violence: Emerging initiatives. In S. Graham-Bermann & J. L. Edleson (Eds.), *Domestic violence in the lives of children: The future of research, intervention, and social policy* (pp. 283–298). Washington, DC: American Psychological Association.

Wolfe, D. A., & Korsch, B. (1994). Witnessing domestic violence during childhood and adolescence: Implications for pediatric practice. *Pediatrics, 94*, 594–599.

Wolfe, D. A., Wekerle, C., Reitzel, D., & Gough, R. (1995). Strategies to address violence in the lives of high-risk youth. In E. Peled, P. G. Jaffe, & J. Edleson (Eds.), *Ending the cycle of violence: Community response to children of battered women* (pp. 255–274). Newbury Park, CA: Sage.

Wuest, J., Berman, H., Ford-Gilboe, M., & Merritt-Gray, M. (2002). Illuminating social determinants of women's health using grounded theory. *Health Care for Women International, 23*, 794–809.

Zink, T. (2000). Should children be in the room when the mother is screened for partner violence? *The Journal of Family Practice, 49*(2), 130–136.

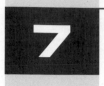

Sexual Abuse in Families

• Joan C. Urbancic

The media has focused on recent cases of children who have been abducted by strangers, sexually abused, and then brutally murdered. Horrendous as such events are, the kidnapped, sexually abused child is the rare exception; the child who is sexually abused by someone he or she knows and trusts is not. Indeed, one of the most notorious scandals in recent years is the disclosure about sexual abuse of children by Catholic priests. For many of us who work with survivors of sexual abuse, the abuse by priests and other clergy is viewed as incestuous because of the profound betrayal of trust by a person who is expected to protect, teach, and guide children and to be a role model. The same dynamics are involved as when so much trauma and suffering is caused by sexual abuse from a child's relative or close family caregiver.

It reminds us that children have been victims of sexual exploitation from earliest times and continue to be victims as society often turns away from this painful reality. This chapter addresses childhood sexual abuse, with a focus on incest. Because of the betrayal of trust, confusion, sense of helplessness, and secrecy associated with the abuse, it is generally recognized that the potential for psychological trauma is greater than if the perpetrator were a stranger (Kendall-Tackett, Williams, & Finkelhor, 1993). Most children and adults do not disclose their abuse, or if they do they are often disbelieved and blamed by those from whom they seek consolation and protection.

Although nurses are frequently in key positions to identify and provide therapeutic involvement with adult and child victims, they are often uncomfortable and reluctant to address the issue. Consequently, victims may interpret the nurse's avoidance as further evidence of their shame, self-blame, and worthlessness, so their distorted self-image is reinforced. Therefore, it is imperative that every nurse be knowledgeable about childhood abuse and become proficient in encouraging their patients to disclose their abusive experiences and share their feelings about them. Disclosing experiences and sharing feelings may be the first step for victims in resolving their sexual-abuse trauma.

Before nurses can effectively engage in therapeutic involvement with adult or child victims of sexual abuse, they must first become aware of their own attitudes about sexual abuse and incest. If a nurse has a history of childhood abuse, she will need to resolve her own issues before becoming effective in assisting others to do so. Otherwise, the nurse's unconscious and unintentional response to the victim may be one of avoidance. After teaching a nursing class for a number of years with a heavy focus on family violence, it has become clear to me that it is very traumatic for many nursing students to read and discuss chapters on family violence. This underscored need for most of the students to address these issues, and most did seek counseling or some resolution of their own trauma.

DEFINITION OF SEXUAL ABUSE AND INCEST

The Child Abuse Prevention and Treatment Act (CAPTA) uses the following definition for child abuse: "the employment, use, persuasion, inducement, enticement, or coercion of any child to engage in, or assist any other person to engage in, any sexually explicit conduct or simulation of such conduct for the purpose of producing a visual depiction of such conduct" (Legal Information Institute, 1995). This definition is quite broad, and it reflects the growing concern about exploitation of children through pornography, which has become more widespread through the Internet. The definition also applies to incest, with the additional specification that the perpetrator is a relative or surrogate relative who exploits the child for his or her sexual gratification, before the child reaches 18 years of age. Exploitation involves a wide variety of behaviors, including disrobing; masturbation; voyeurism; fondling; digital or object penetration; anal, oral, or vaginal penetration; and using the child for pornographic purposes. The most common scenario for incest is a gradual evolution of sexual activity by the abuser that is shrouded in secrecy and leaves the child feeling confused, helpless, guilty, and ashamed.

The definition assumes a power imbalance between the child and the offender so that the child or adolescent is unable to give true consent because of physical, cognitive, and psychological immaturity. This is the case even though the child may believe she consented and may have sought the sexual activity. Consequently, it is widely accepted that the child is always a "victim" in incestuous relationships because a child is never in a position to give informed consent. The adult always assumes a power position and pressures or forces the child in various ways to cooperate. These pressures as perceived by the child may be fear of punishment, rejection, or abandonment by the adult, as well as promises of material goods and special favors or privileges. Because the sexual activity usually begins with fondling and rarely involves violence, it may be pleasurable and sexually stimulating for the child. Because "children are children," it is natural for them to seek pleasure. For the adult survivor who believes that she voluntarily participated in the incest, guilt, shame, and self-blame may be more of an issue. Sometimes, the sexual exploitation that begins in childhood continues into adulthood, and the woman functions as a psychologically helpless child who is unable to extricate herself from her abuser. Nevertheless, the adult is always responsible and must nurture, protect, and guide the child; set limits on inappropriate behaviors; and teach age-appropriate behaviors.

Although it may seem clear that the adult is always the responsible person, earlier writers blamed the child and reported seductive behaviors and active participation by the children (Bender & Blau, 1937; Henderson, 1972). Current investigators and clinicians maintain that flirtatious behavior is an attempt for nurturance, not sexual gratification. If the child is seductive, it is because she has been taught that sexual contact is an effective means to gain attention, affection, and special favors.

If the incest has continued for years, it is common to progress to oral sex, mutual masturbation, and even vaginal intercourse. The pressure on the child to cooperate and to maintain the relationship is the most crucial issue to assess in incest experiences. Many children have severe guilt, feelings of helplessness, and shame, but they continue to maintain the secrecy because of domination by the adult and fear that disclosure will lead to punishment, greater shame, rejection, and disbelief by the social network. Although a variety of psychological and physical symptoms are likely to develop when the incestuous relationship becomes protracted, only a minority of children self-disclose even if the relationship is ended (Faller, 2002; Smith et al., 2000).

Researchers have debated the significance of false positives (children who claim to be abused and were not) versus false negatives (children who fail to disclose abuse when they were abusd). According to Faller (2002), research agendas and practice guidelines assume false positives to be the greater problem. But in a review of eight studies, she reported that false negatives are the greater risk. Children may not disclose abuse because of fear, shame, or guilt. Many times, young children have no concept of sexual abuse and do not understand they have been abused. Sometimes, so many traumatic events happen to the child that the sexual abuse may not be a salient issue at that time. Or, communication problems between the interviewer and the child preclude an effective interview. For example, interviewers are taught to use open-ended questions, but the child may not have sufficient understanding of what is being asked. Finally, some children recant previously disclosed sexual abuse. Faller states that no empirical method can distinguish the retraction of a false disclosure from the recantation of a true one.

Although it is widely accepted that cross-generational incest should be defined as abusive, it is less clear when making a determination about same-age peers. Russell (1986) used an age differential of five years to qualify sexual activity between siblings as abusive. However, Urbancic (1992), in her clinical practice and research, identified frequent cases of females who were coerced into sexual activity by brothers of similar age to the victim. However, incest can be considered nonabusive when it occurs between brothers, sisters, cousins, or other relatives who are close in age and when it is mutually desired and without coercion. Wilson, Friedman, and Lindy (2001) used a constructionist approach to explain the psychological trauma of sexual abuse. According to these researchers, individuals "construct and construe" their own meaning of the abuse, and the meaning is different for each person. Therefore, therapists must enter the world of the survivor to understand how the sexual abuse affected her and what aspects were the most troubling.

Male children are also the victims of childhood sexual abuse, and the caseloads of therapists are beginning to support the belief that male child sexual abuse is underreported and more prevalent than statistics indicate. Nevertheless, research (Finkelhor, 1994; Herman, 2000) indicates that female children are sexually abused more frequently than male children, and most of the literature relates to the female child victim. For that reason, the female rather than the male pronoun is used throughout this chapter. Because sexual abuse is a criminal offense with mandatory reporting, the perpetrator will most commonly be referred to as the "offender" and the object of his abuse as the "victim." Because the majority of offenders are male, the pronoun "he" is used when discussing the offender.

PREVALENCE OF INCEST

Incest occurs more frequently than people care to recognize. Some argue that the increasing incidence is related to a growing awareness by the public and skillful assessment by professionals. However, some who argue against this thought point to the weakening of the family in terms of divorce, stepfamilies, and single families. Classic studies with adults (Finkelhor, 1994; Russell, 1986) indicate that stepfathers are eight times more likely to abuse their stepdaughters, use force, and engage in more protracted and severe abuse than biological fathers. These studies support the belief that because the biological fathers generally have more involvement in the early socialization of the daughters than stepfathers, they have stronger parent–child bonding, which is a strong deterrent to incest. Only one child out of seven children is abused by strangers (American Psychiatric Association, 1999).

In addition to the weakening of parent–child bonding, another important factor contributing to the increasing incidence of childhood sexual abuse is the deterioration of sexual mores and the widespread acceptance of "sexual liberation" for everyone. Television, movies, and videos promote "doing whatever feels good," and females are depicted as seductive or insatiable sexual objects. Although condoms are crucial for "safe sex" in the age of AIDS, the possibility that abstinence is the "safest sex" is rarely considered in a society that values individualism and unfettered sexual gratification more than self-discipline and responsibility.

In determining the prevalence rates of childhood sexual abuse, data is derived either from official records of child-abuse reports or from surveys conducted with adults who disclose their abuse retrospectively. There is general agreement that regardless of the outcomes, the rates are highly underreported. Although there is agreement that reports of incest are increasing, incidence and prevalence studies with adults (Finkelhor, 1994; Russell, 1986; Wyatt & Powell, 1988) for childhood sexual abuse have reported a range of figures, primarily because of the differences in definition and methodology. Most studies indicate that approximately one-third of women and one-sixth of men in North America have reported sexual victimization that occurred during their preteen years or younger. The most valid study in terms of sample and methodology appears to be Russell's (1986) large study (n = 953) of a randomly selected sample of women from the San Francisco area. Russell identified 16% of the sample as being sexually abused by a relative before the age of 18; 4.5% of the victims in the sexually abused subsample were abused by their fathers. A larger percentage of women were sexually abused by nonfamily members (approximately 33%). Wyatt's (1985) prior random-sample study of 248 women reported similar findings.

The best figures based on official child-abuse reports are derived from the Third National Incidence Study of Child Abuse and Neglect, orNIS-3 (Sedlak & Broadhurst, 1996). Congress mandated three such studies with results published in 1981, 1988, and 1996. The purpose of these studies was to provide updated estimates of child abuse and neglect for Congress and the nation. All three of the NIS studies used two standards of abuse, and data was gathered according to both standards. Under the more stringent, the harm standard, the incidence of childhood sexual abuse increased from 119,200 cases in 1988 to 217,700 in 1996 (an 83% increase). The second and less stringent endangerment standard indicated an increase in incidence of sexual abuse from 133,600 in 1988 to 300,200 in 1996 (a 125% increase). Most authorities believe the increase in incidence is due, in part, to professionals becoming more adept at identifying and reporting abuse. Across the three studies using both standards, female children were sexually abused three times more often than boys were.

Because the NIS studies are based on reported cases of abuse, they are believed to be gross underestimates. Retrospective research with adults indicate that only 6% to 12% of cases are reported to authorities (Berliner & Elliiott, 2002). Child as well as adult victims are more likely to disclose if asked directly about the abuse. In one study, the rate of child sexual abuse in adult female psychiatric patients increased from 6% to 70% when clinicians began to ask directly. (Briere & Zaidi, 1989). Contrary to the NIS studies, Jones and Finkelhor (2001) noted that in recent years the reporting of childhood sexual abuse has declined in a majority of states. Their claim seems to contradict the NIS studies. However, the data from the latest NIS was collected in 1994. Data collection over an extended period of time is needed to determine if rates are indeed declining.

Jacobson and Herald (1990) reported a prevalence of one in six males and one in five females who disclosed a history of major childhood sexual abuse on admission to a psychiatric inpatient setting. In addition, 56% of those who reported being abused had not disclosed this abuse to previous therapists. Other studies have identified a higher incidence of 34% to 53% (Briere, 1992; Eilenberg, 1996; Greenfield, Strakowski, Tohen, Batson, & Kolbrener, 1994; Henley & Kristiansen, 1997; Mueser et al., 1998). It is unclear why such a high prevalence of sexual abuse exists among psychiatric patients. Although it is true that many victims come from severely dysfunctional families, others come from families that do not appear overtly dysfunctional. A reluctance by mental-health professionals to accept that childhood sexual abuse can be a core factor in adult mental-health illness reflects the continuing adherence to Freudian oedipal theory in which the victim is blamed and the abuse is minimized.

Despite many studies, no evidence indicates that childhood sexual abuse is more common among lower socioeconomic groups or among black or white populations. Children who live with a stepfather are at risk, especially if the mother is employed outside the home. In addition, children from socially isolated, dysfunctional, or abusive families are at risk. Unavailability of parents and families in which parents were abused are other risk factors.

HISTORICAL AND THEORETICAL PERSPECTIVES

Although the theme of incest has been prevalent in art and literature since ancient times, research has not been extensive until the last 20 years. The earliest research focused primarily on the characteristics of the offender and the family dynamics. Few studies examined the effects of incest on the child, and those that did were limited by sample size, control, and methodology. Nevertheless, these researchers claimed that the child often initiated and enjoyed the incestuous relationship and that trauma to the child (usually a female) was rare. In addition to the belief of questionable trauma, many clinicians did not think incest was a significant issue because of its rare occurrence. As late as 1972, the prominent psychiatrist Henderson insisted that incest was an uncommon event and therefore of little concern.

Herman (1997) claimed that the history of psychological trauma is characterized by episodic amnesia. By this, she means that several times over the last 100 years the study of psychological trauma has been initiated, abandoned, and then resumed again. This episodic and amnesiac history occurred because the reality of interpersonal trauma is so revolting, controversial, and unthinkable that it became an anathema. It is difficult to accept both the vulnerability as well as capacity for evil in human nature. The key to public acceptance of psychological trauma is support from political movements that gives victims "voice." According to Herman, the three main traumas of the 20th century were those of hysteria in women, shell shock or combat neurosis, and, most recently, sexual abuse and domestic violence. Because of the societal tendency to deny, victims have historically been discredited, disbelieved, or rendered invisible. This phenomenon is clearly illustrated in the false-memory movement of the 1990s in which alleged sexual offenders claimed that they were unjustly accused of abuse and that the false memories of victims were implanted by incompetent therapists.

Herman (1997) noted that the psychological traumas could not have invaded societal consciousness without the support of a political movement at the time. The recognition of hysteria in women developed because of antichurch sentiment and a focus on scientific knowledge. Freud and Janet both studied under the eminent French neurologist Charcot, who described the archetypal hysterical woman with great scientific precision. Although Charcot was brilliant with his description of the condition and changed the societal attitude toward women, he was not concerned with the etiology of hysteria, which so many women presented. Freud and Janet, who were intense rivals, were determined to discover the etiology of hysteria, but to do so they were forced to question the affected women in-depth. Consequently, the women began to discuss the sexual trauma in their lives. Freud, in particular, began to probe the minds of his "hysterical" female patients and eventually came to the conclusion that the basis for their psychological trauma was sexual assault, abuse, and incest that they suffered at the hands of fathers. Based on his research, Freud published his paper, the "Aetiology of Hysteria" in 1896 but later repudiated it because of the scorn and revilement that he received from his peers over his claim that hysteria was due to intrafamilial sexual abuse. Eventually, he revised this theory to claim that hysteria was not due to actual abuse but to the " female fantasy" of a desire to possess her father. This belief became the basis for Freud's development of the oedipal complex and psychoanalysis. According to Herman, it is truly ironic that the dominant psychological theory of the 20th century was born out of the denial of women's reality.

Later, in letters to Wilhelm Fliess from 1887 to 1902 (published in 1954), Freud does admit that many of his female patients actually had been molested as children. Nevertheless, many writers claim that Freud's theory established the groundwork for the disregard of children's reports of sexual molestation and turned the focus on their supposed fantasies and seductive behavior. Freud's views continue to have a powerful impact on mental-health professionals, as shown by the disbelief and discomfort that many professionals feel when confronted by client's disclosures of incest (Courtois, 1999; Herman, 1997; Russell, 1986; Wyatt & Powell, 1988). Feminists (Herman, 2000; Rush, 1980; Russell, 1986) have viewed incest and family violence as extreme manifestations of the imbalance of power between men and women. Within this view, females are socialized to be devalued sexual objects. Herman (1997) maintained that only a feminist perspective can explain how sexual abuse can be so imbalanced, with most perpetrators men and most victims female children. She further stated that the feminist perspective makes the most sense in explaining the bitter conflict that results when perpetrators are expected to be accountable for their crimes.

In the late 1980s, researchers began documenting a large percentage of patients in psychiatric hospitals and outpatient clinics with histories of childhood physical and sexual abuse. As patients were encouraged to disclose and talk about their abuse, their mental health began to improve (Herman, 1992). From that time forward, the research on childhood sexual abuse exploded. Initial research focused on incidence and effects of the abuse and has now progressed to treatment outcomes. At the same time, the research on incest began to coalesce with that of traumatic stress, and it soon became clear that many sexual-abuse and domestic-violence victims, like combat veterans, suffered from posttraumatic stress disorder. Herman (2000) pointed out that because of the women's liberation movement of the 1970s, it became clear that women in civilian life accounted for more PTSD than men in combat. Thus, the hysteria of women and combat neurosis became one.

But acceptance of the reality of incest has not been a smooth road. Because of the increase in child-abuse reporting in the 1980s, criminal prosecution of offenders by adult victims also increased. Many of the court cases involved victims who experienced delayed or recovered memories of their childhood abuse in adulthood. Therefore, most states had passed legislation to extend the time limits for which a victim could prosecute her offender. In response, an aggressive organization, the False Memory Syndrome Foundation (FMSF), was mobilized to support the alleged and convicted perpetrators. Composed mainly of offenders and a few academics and defense attorneys, the FMSF conducted a highly publicized campaign in the media and courts to fight the incest allegations. FMSF Executive Director Pamela Freyd provided the leadership for the organization in an effort to clear her husband who was accused of incest by his daughters. The FMSF concluded that the memories of their daughters were false and implanted by feminist therapists who were determined to destroy the sanctity of the family. The FMSF was quite successful in mobilizing the press and public support for their claims and in winning several court cases. Thus, victims of childhood incest and sexual abuse were again revictimized by a society that doubted the validity of their claims and by therapists who became afraid to inquire about childhood sexual abuse for fear of being sued.

Since that time, a growing body of research has been emerging about the validity of recovered or delayed memories. The American Psychological Association, the American Psychiatric Association, and the American Medical Association have all issued formal documents recognizing the existence of "traumatic amnesia." The DSM-IV also recognizes the possibility of such memories. Most clinicians and researchers also acknowledge the possibility that a small number of patients may be vulnerable to suggestions by therapists and that a small percentage of reported false memories were indeed false.

Research studies indicate that many women who report childhood sexual abuse also report having only partial memories for their abuse. Although total repression happens less often, it does occur in a small percentage of women. Out of 147 women who participated in Urbancic's study (1992), 10% ($n = 14$) reported totally forgetting their abuse memories. In a recent study of college women (Epstein & Bottoms, 2002), 15% ($n = 14$) of the 104 women who identified themselves as experiencing childhood sexual abuse reported that they had a period of time in their lives when they could not remember the abuse. However, Epstein and Bottoms used multiple questions about the memories and concluded that only 4% of the sample really qualified for complete repression according to the Freudian definition. Elliot and Briere, in their nationally representative general-population study (1995), reported that 30% of women and 14% of men who identified themselves as having childhood sexual-abuse experiences reported a period of memory loss of their abuse. In a review of ten studies that reported on women's forgetting of the child sexual abuse, Epstein and Bottoms indicated a range of partial or total forgetting of 16% to 64%. Other researchers (Chu, Frey, Ganzel, & Matthews, 1999; Williams, 1994; Wilsnack, Wonderlich, Kristhanson, Vogeltanz-Holm, & Wilsnack, 2002) have also documented that forgetting and then subsequently remembering abuse is not uncommon among women who report childhood sexual experiences. Women who with a therapist remembered childhood sexual abuse ranged from 1.8% of women in the study by Wilsnack and others (2002) to 3% of women in a study by Polusny and Follette (1996).

Researchers have recognized the likelihood that some of the accused who FMSF supported were falsely accused (Briere, 1996; Chu, Frey, Ganzel, & Matthews, 1999; Courtois, 1999) and that overzealously attempting to uncover abuse can be as harmful as failing to identify it. A subset of adults who were severely abused as children may be more apt to dissociate, be highly imaginable, and be suggestible to false memories during psychotherapy. Briere points out that some therapists are guilty of bad therapy by being too authoritarian and trying to convince clients that they have been abused when there is no basis. However, Briere notes that bad therapy is not the same as recovering bad memories. He also asserts that those who have been falsely accused of being abusers are also victims and, thus, they have a right to legal and personal redress. However, these writers emphasize that the overwhelming majority of people who claim to have been sexually abused as children have, indeed, suffered those experiences.

Many frameworks attempt to explain the traumatic effects of childhood sexual abuse. One belief common to all frameworks is that a child is always a victim in incestuous relationships. Several researchers have espoused a cognitive model to explain how the child processes the abuse and tries to make sense out of his or her world (Burgess, Hartman, Wolbert, & Grant, 1987; Carmen & Rieker, 1989). Basically, a cognitive model maintains that if a traumatic experience has appropriate processing, it will become neutralized, resolved, and stored in distant memory. When traumatic experiences are not resolved, they remain in active memory or are defended by cognitive mechanisms, such as dissociation, repression, splitting, suppression, and compartmentalization. Because the sexual offender demands secrecy, the child is forced to develop defenses to prevent disclosure, and development proceeds for the child under the profound burden of trauma encapsulation. These researchers claim that childhood sexual-abuse experiences result in long-term effects of low self-worth, self-blame, a lack of self-efficacy, self-fragmentation, dissociations, and self-destructive behaviors.

Finkelhor and Browne (1986) explained the effects of incest with their four trauma-causing factors called traumagenic dynamics. Finkelhor and Browne maintained that some of these four factors occur in all types of psychologically traumatic situations, but only in the incest experience do all four occur together. The four factors are the following:

- "Traumatic sexualization refers to a process in which a child's sexuality (including both sexual feelings and sexual attitudes) is shaped in a developmentally inappropriate and interpersonally dysfunctional fashion as a result of the sexual abuse" (p.181). An example of traumatic sexualization is rewarding a child for the sexual behavior, which in turn teaches the child that sexual behavior can be used as a means to meet one's needs.

Finkelhor and Browne have claimed that children with incest experiences develop inappropriate repertoires of sexual behavior, are confused about sexual self-concepts, and have unusual emotional associations to sexual activities.

- "Betrayal refers to the dynamic in which children discover that someone on whom they are vitally dependent has caused them harm" (p. 182). The child may experience betrayal by the actions of the abuser, as well as from the nonoffending parent and other adults from whom they seek protection.
- "Powerlessness—or what might also be called 'disempowerment,' the dynamic of rendering the victim powerless—refers to the process in which the child's will, desires, and sense of efficacy are continually contravened" (p. 183). Powerlessness occurs when a child is repeatedly used sexually against her will and is unable to disclose the activity because of a fear of the consequences.
- "Stigmatization, the final dynamic, refers to the negative connotations— for example, badness, shame, and guilt—that are communicated to the child about the experiences and that then become incorporated into the child's self-image" (p. 184). The stigmatization may develop during the abuse itself or after disclosure when adults react with shock, horror, and blame of the child.

Kendall-Tackett (2002) described another model of childhood trauma that focuses on four pathways that can influence the health of adult survivors: behavioral, social, cognitive, and emotional pathways. Although her research examined child abuse in general, she reported that many of the outcomes indicated greater adverse effects for survivors of childhood sexual abuse than of other forms of abuse and neglect.

The most recent and dramatic shift in theoretical explanations for the effects of childhood sexual abuse, and incest in particular, came with the explosion of studies on traumatic stress and the psychobiological model. With these studies, awareness emerged that many survivors of childhood trauma are similar to other people who have experienced long-term and severe trauma, such as concentration-camp survivors or political prisoners who are abused and tortured repeatedly over many years. The common presentations of these survivors of psychological trauma led to the new diagnostic category of complex posttraumatic stress disorder (PTSD). Despite the worldwide database of approximately 20,000 annotated and indexed articles on traumatic stress and PTSD, scientists have more questions than answers about this phenomenon. Wilson, Friedman, and Lindy (2001) claimed that PTSD is a complex shift in the steady state of an organism that may have profound and permanent psychobiological effects. Thus, researchers and clinicians are expressing increasing concern about PTSD because of its significance for human evolution and the survival of humankind.

Today, most researchers and clinicians recognize a spectrum of PTSD, with chronic and severe experiencing of childhood trauma, such as incest, often earning the diagnosis of complex PTSD. Wilson and colleagues (2001) described the psychobiology of stress as involving a process, unlike homeostasis, called allostasis. It refers to the body's efforts to maintain stability under various types of stressors on the normal levels of adaptive biological functioning. Under typical stress exposure, the hypothalamic-pituitary-adrenal (HPA) axis is stimulated to produce catecholamines and cortisol that eventually return to baseline once the threat is gone. However, with chronic severe stressors, these hormones remain high and result in a state of allostatic load with pathophysiologic consequences (McEwen, 1998).

Thus, a critical challenge for therapists working with incest survivors who are experiencing allostatic load is to assist them in normalizing their stress response and reducing their hyperarousal, mood instability, cognitive distortions, anger, and other maladaptive psychobiological functioning. Because many children who have been traumatized by childhood incest have been diagnosed with PTSD or some of its components, it is helpful to examine the treatment model of Wilson and others (2001). These researchers view PTSD as a psychobiological stress-response syndrome and claim that traumatic life events impact the potential for coping and may produce acute, chronic, delayed, and complex forms of PTSD. The foundation of the Wilson model is the relationship between the core PTSD symptoms and their synergistic impact on ego states, self structure, and identity configuration. The core triad of PTSD symptoms are the target of treatment for both adults and children, and they consist of traumatic intrusive memories and stressful reexperiencing of the traumatic events; behavior that includes avoidance, numbing, depression, and coping adaptations; and psychobiological alterations in behavior.

The reexperiencing of memories, which is the hallmark of PTSD, can take many forms, including emotional flooding without visual imagery, nightmares, flashbacks, dissociative episodes, and unconscious reenactments with trauma-specific significance. For treatment to be effective, it must integrate the traumatic experiences into the cognitive schema of the survivor so that it becomes only a part of her life history and one that the survivor can discuss without being emotionally retraumatized.

The second target symptom of PTSD are behaviors by the survivor that deal with the trauma of reexperiencing. The survivor uses a variety of strategies, including withdrawal and avoidance of anything that might trigger the memories of the trauma. The person may become emotionally constricted and alienated from others, have amnesia for trauma-related events, develop compulsive overactivity, and use of alcohol or drugs excessively.

The third symptom of psychobiological changes in behavior is expressed through sleep disturbances, inability to modulate affect, cognitive deficits, hypervigilance and hyperarousal, chronic fatigue, somatic symptoms, and high-risk behaviors (Wilson et al., 2001).

Besides the target symptoms, PTSD affects interpersonal relations (i.e., attachment and intimacy) and self (i.e., identity and life-course development). When the trauma occurs in childhood, such as with incest, then personality may be affected, and permanent features of PTSD may become part of the person's character structure. Such features can include self-destructive tendencies, shame, self-doubt, guilt, loss of self-esteem, narcissism, depression, and a sense of futility in living (Wilson et al., 2001).

According to Wilson and others (2001), the three PTSD target symptoms and the two target symptoms relating to intimacy and self comprise the five portals of treatment of persons with PTSD. Once entry is gained, the process of healing becomes a collaborative relationship between therapist and survivor.

Briere (2002) integrated most of the previously described theories. His theory, the self-trauma model, combines trauma theories with cognitive psychology, behavioral psychology, and self-psychology. In particular, Briere incorporated the most recent neurophysiological research with early attachment and memory work and emphasizes that implicit memories and emotions are critical components in understanding and treating the traumas of childhood. He maintained that postabuse symptoms reflect an effort by the survivor to process and integrate overwhelming trauma from the past. It is the therapist's responsibility "to help the client to do better what he or she is already attempting to do" (p. 200). Of necessity, this involves assisting clients to develop new resources as they repeatedly experience exposure and reprocessing of their terror and trauma.

Regardless of what theoretical framework one may use to understand and work with the child, adult, and family, cultural competency is always important. Abney (2002) promoted the use of a "culturally diverse" model that combines the subjective worldview of a particular culture with that of a broader cross-cultural base. Because of many destructive cultural practices that leave children at risk for serious and long-term harm, she rejected the concept of cultural relativism that holds behavior is acceptable if it is based on one's culture. With the diverse model, one recognizes that cultures vary and there is no single ideal culture. Cultural competency refers to making the best effort to try to understand the worldview of another person from a different culture and then adapting one's practice to meet the person's needs within his or her culture. Professionals need to adopt the cultural-competency approach because of increasing diversity in the United States, the underrepresentation of health-care professionals from diverse cultures, and the lack of access to quality and cost-effective health care. Abney maintains that if we do not, we will not be able to meet the needs of abused children and their families.

CHARACTERISTICS OF FAMILY MEMBERS

The incestuous family is viewed most typically as endogamous or enmeshed. These families are characterized by relatively closed boundaries to the outside world and a lack of boundaries within the family. Because they are physically, socially, and psychologically isolated from outsiders, they become excessively dependent on each other for satisfaction of physical, social, and psychological needs. Courtois (1988) noted that despite the fact that these family members are excessively dependent on each other, emotional and physical deprivation prevails. Thus, the only source of love and affection for the children in these families may be through sexual contact.

Many researchers have claimed that incestuous behaviors become repetitive generational patterns. Young girls who are abused may grow up to become adults who fail to protect their own children. Summit (1989) reported that 90% of mothers who seek help for child abuse have a history of being sexually abused as children. Other researchers have reported that these women often choose cruel and neglecting husbands because they view themselves as immoral and undeserving.

Because of their lack of self-esteem, unresolved anger, and sense of powerlessness, such women have difficulty maintaining healthy interpersonal relationships and are unable to protect themselves or their children. But it is vitally important to understand that although a person has been victimized as a child, she or he will not necessarily fail to protect or become a victimizer as an adult. Statistics of mothers who fail to protect their children and of fathers who abuse their children are drawn from sexual-abuse treatment programs and do not represent all men and women who have been sexually abused as children. The majority of people who have been abused do not grow up to be abusers. It is critical that adults with childhood incest experiences understand that they are not doomed to revictimize others.

CHARACTERISTICS OF OFFENDERS

Research on child sexual offenders is still in its infancy, evidenced by the fact that the majority of studies recruit subjects (adult males) from the criminal-justice system. These subjects involve a small percentage of the total number of child sexual abusers. In Russell's study (1986), only 2% of the incest offenders were reported to the police. Among the offenders that are reported, only a few are apprehended and go to trial. The even smaller number convicted probably represents the most flagrant and repetitive sexual offenders (Chaffin, Letourneau, & Silovsky, 2002; Finkelhor, 1986). In addition to samples culled from the criminal-justice system, the studies usually only look at male offenders in father–daughter relationships. Therefore, it is clear that samples from the criminal-justice system are not representative of all offenders. More research is needed to develop primary-prevention sexual-abuse programs, to identify people at risk for offending, and to predict the likelihood of identified offenders repeating their sexual abuse.

Glasser and colleagues (2001) examined the link between being a victim of childhood sexual abuse and becoming a perpetrator. They based their study on a retrospective clinical review of 843 predominantly male subjects ($n = 747$) attending an outpatient forensic psychotherapy center in London, England. Most of this sample were antisocial and sexually deviant. In the male component of the sample, 18% were victims and 30% were perpetrators. For males, the greatest predictor for becoming a perpetrator was being abused by a sister or mother. Of the females in the sample, although 43% of them had been sexually abused, only one female became a perpetrator. Of the total sample, 82% were not victims and 72% were not perpetrators. Thus, only a third of men who were sexually victimized in childhood became perpetrators and only 2% of women became perpetrators. The number of women perpetrators was so low that the researchers claimed "being a woman" may actually protect the victim from becoming a victimizer. They concluded that although their data did not provide strong support for a "cycle of sexual abuse," prior victimization may have some effect on male abusers, particularly those with a history of pedophilic abuse and even more so those with both an incestuous and pedophilic abuse history. Although the sample for the study was not a representative sample of abusers, other studies support their conclusions (Murphy & Smith, 1996). Chaffin and others (2002) reported that self-reported histories of childhood sexual abuse stabilized between 20% to 30% for both juvenile and adult offenders once polygraph tests were used for verification.

Some researchers have claimed that the percentage of female abusers is higher than research indicates because it is more difficult to identify them, as they perpetrate the abuse under the guise of child-care activities (Barnett, Miller-Perrin, & Perrin, 1997). Others have reported that female perpetrators operate as accomplices to male perpetrators in families with multiple-partner sexual abuse (Elliott, 1993; Urbancic, 1992).

In recent years, researchers have begun directing more reporting attention to juvenile sexual offenders, who are significantly underreported (Barnett et al.,

1997). In the NIS-3, 22% of children had been sexually abused by a perpetrator that was less than 26 years old. Ryan and Lane (1991) reported that, based on self-report surveys, approximately one-third of sexual-abuse offenders are less than 18 years old. Sexual-abuse treatment centers are also seeing greater numbers of adolescent referrals, and most of the victims are other children. Besides the growing concern about the number of juvenile sex offenders, professionals are reporting increasing numbers of children with sexual behavior problems (Chaffin et al., 2002). Adler and Schultz (1995) claimed that although sibling incest is probably the most common form of incest, it is the least researched. In their Caucasian, middle-income sample of sibling-incest offenders from intact families, 92% had a history of childhood physical abuse, whereas only 8% were sexually victimized. Ryan and Lane reported that the adolescent offender is similar to the adult in that both are primarily male from all ethnic, racial, and socio-economic levels.

In the 1970s and 1980s, Groth's description of offenders as either fixated or regressed was commonly accepted (1978). Today, this typology is no longer accepted. Conte (1990) reported that most offenders are a mixture of both types. As an example, Conte described a sample of 159 incest offenders who abused their daughters but also abused nonrelated male children (12%) and nonrelated female children (49%) and raped adult females (19%).

The American Psychiatric Association Task Force (1999) on sex offenders uses the FBI typology for sexual abusers. Offenders include:

- The regressed, immature male who interacts with children on a peer level
- The morally indiscriminate (antisocial) abuser who abusers anyone who is vulnerable and who provides him with the opportunity
- The sexually indiscriminant, polymorphous perverse who will experiment with any type of sexual behavior
- The inadequate abuser (social misfit) who may be developmentally disabled, psychotic, or senile and who takes advantage of a child's vulnerability, to satisfy his own curiosity.

Herman (2000) and Chaffin and colleagues (2002), in summarizing the literature on incest offenders, reported that there is no scientific psychological profile for them because they are so varied and appear so normal. Therefore, the majority of offenders do not qualify for any psychiatric diagnosis. Most are successful in all aspects of their lives with the sexual abuse being a hidden component that they have great difficulty controlling. Herman describes incest offenders as being addicted to sexual fantasy that they feed with pornography. They are also typified by their denial, rationalizations, and lack of remorse. In Urbancic's therapy groups with offenders who were mandated by the courts to participate, few expressed guilt, shame, or remorse. Instead, they presented a variety of scenarios, including accusing the child of lying about the abuse, admitting to the abuse because of a need to "get even" with the mother, accusing the child of initiating and seeking the sexual activity, and frank denial of their actions.

Offenders offer a variety of reasons for their abusive behavior, and it is clear that the reasons are complex and multifactorial. Many theories about offenders have never been tested empirically and others, only minimally. Therefore, more research is needed before any can be accepted. Regardless of the cause, the offender makes a conscious decision to abuse the child, and the responsibility for the abuse is always his (or hers), despite circumstances. According to Finkelhor

(1986), certain preconditions must be met for child sexual abuse to occur: the offender must be motivated to sexually abuse the child, must overcome internal inhibitions and external barriers to the abuse, and must overcome the child's resistance to the abuse.

Although the research on offenders is very limited and weak methodologically, recent studies are consistent in reporting success with reducing recidivism (Chaffin et al., 2002). Across studies, recidivism rates for sexual offenders who receive treatment range from 3% to 39%; untreated offenders ranged from 12.5% to 57%. Offenders who complete their treatment tend to have lower recidivism rates, and incest offenders have lower recidivism rates than extrafamilial offenders (Proulx, Tardif, Lamoureux, & Lussier, 2000). The biomedical treatments such as surgical castration, antiandrogens, and antidepressants have been successful in reducing recidivism rates, as has cognitive-behavioral therapies (American Psychiatric Association, 1999). These successes fly in the face of traditional beliefs that the sex offender is always a treatment failure. Hudson, Ward, and Laws (2000) reported that the public is educated about offenders by the media that focuses on 1% of all sex crimes; therefore, people are unaware that successful interventions exist for sex offenders. For interventions to be effective, they must be matched with offender risk level, use cognitive-behavioral modalities, focus on criminogenic need, and promote prosocial skills. Hudson and colleagues maintained that high-risk offenders who need treatment the most are often the ones least likely to receive it. Currently, all states have registries for sex offenders, and some states even make the information public by placing it on the Internet.

FEMALE SEX OFFENDERS

There are few reports specifically on female offenders; however, there is consensus that males are the perpetrators in the majority of sexual-abuse cases and the victims are most typically female. Finkelhor (1986) claimed that 95% of female child abuse and 80% of male child abuse involve male offenders. Even when female offenders are identified, abuse is often at the instigation of male partners. In Russell's (1986) probability sample of 930 women in the community, only 10 cases of incestuous abuse by females were identified. These 10 cases comprised 5% of the incest offenders in Russell's study and provided strong support for the argument that female child abuse by adult females represents only a small portion of the total abuse cases. The data from NIS-3 (Sedlak & Broadhurst, 1996) supported these statistics, with 89% of all the sexual abuse perpetrated by males and 12% by females. In addition to the infrequency of female offenders, abuse that was perpetrated by females was less severe (Finkelhor, 1986; Russell, 1986). However, when females do abuse, they are more likely to target male rather than female children (Berliner & Elliott, 2002).

In Urbancic's (1993) convenience sample of 147 female incest survivors, 6.6% ($n = 16$) of the total offenders ($n = 243$) were women. All 16 of the female offenders were part of a multiple family-abuse system, and none acted in isolation. Of the cases with female offenders, 13 involved an abusing father or stepfather. Research suggests that when women sexually abuse children, it is usually at the instigation of male family members (Elliott, 1993; Finkelhor, 1984; Urbancic, 1993).

Some writers claim that adult females abuse male children more frequently than females, and because these activities are hidden they are seriously underreported. Since Russell's study (1986) involved abused females only, no inferences can be made about male child abuse from her work. However, if females do abuse males more frequently, it should be reported in self-reported surveys such as Finkelhor (1994) conducted with college students; this has not occurred. Both Finkelhor and Russell assert that no evidence exists to support the claim that adult females more commonly abuse male children than female children.

THE CHILD VICTIM
IN THE INCESTUOUS FAMILY

The child victim in the incestuous family is usually the oldest daughter, with the average age of approximately 9 years (Berliner & Elliott, 2002) and with a range of infancy to 17 years. In Russell's study (1986), 11% of the abuse occurred before age 5, 19% from 6 to 9 years, 41% from 10 to 13 years, and 29% 14 years of age and later. Early sexual abuse rarely involves attempts at vaginal intercourse but oral penetration is not unusual.

The incestuous relationship may extend over a period of many years; the average length of time is approximately three years. It is common for the severity of incest to increase as the incestuous activity continues over the years. Most typically, it begins with fondling and gradually evolves into oral sex and vaginal intercourse. Few incestuous relationships involve violence or force, although coercion is usually present.

It is normal and healthy for a young female to practice her female wiles on her father, and regardless of her behavior, she needs controls and limits set by the adults in her family. Parents have the roles of teachers and protectors, not exploiters, and although all parents may experience some sexual feelings toward their children at times, it is the incestuous parent who acts on those feelings.

The majority of child incest victims never disclose, but some are able to extricate themselves from the situation in a variety of ways. If the child is able to escape the abuse, often the next daughter is forced to assume the servicing of the offender's needs. Sometimes it is the victimization of a younger sibling that motivates the oldest daughter to disclose the incestuous activity.

Cessation from the sexual abuse may occur when the daughter becomes older and more able to assert herself in a way that protects her from further abuse. If she begins dating, it often leads to serious conflict with the father because it may engender jealousy. The escalating tension and anger may result in acting-out behavior in terms of drug use and sexual promiscuity. It is not unusual for the victim to accuse the offender of sexual abuse during a heated family argument over her delinquent behavior. The mother may join the father in accusing the daughter of lying to seek revenge on the father for setting limits on the daughter's behavior.

The daughter may choose to disclose the incest to a friend or teacher, who then would report the abuse to protective services. Running away from home is another frequent way of coping with the sexual abuse; therefore, anyone working with runaway teenagers should carefully assess them for a history of sexual abuse.

MOTHERS AS NONOFFENDING PARENTS

Many investigators insist that the key to the incestuous family is the mother. She has been described as rejecting and dominating of both husband and daughter. Although the mother sometimes may be physically or mentally incapacitated, in the past researchers (Henderson, 1972; Justice & Justice, 1979) reported that she imposed the mother–wife role on her daughter and expected the daughter to provide nurturance for her also.

These earlier writers also maintained that the role reversal of mother and daughter is instrumental in keeping the dysfunctional family together because the father's needs are satisfied, the mother is relieved of her responsibilities, and the daughter assumes a position of power with many payoffs. Some even suggested that the father and daughter unite to gain revenge on the rejecting mother.

Today, researchers and clinicians contest the assertions that place all the responsibility and blame on the mother (Elliott & Carnes, 2001; Herman, 2000). They maintain that the mother is often depressed or physically incapacitated and therefore unable to care for herself or her family. Although the mother-blaming theory may be correct in some instances, it is unreasonable to assume that the mother consciously or unconsciously arranges and encourages the father–daughter relationship. It is argued that some mothers often tolerate physical abuse, humiliation, and poverty because of their social and economic status. Deblinger, Hathaway, Lippman, and Steer (1993) reported that mothers of sexually abused children are more likely to be battered by the abusive partner than are mothers of children abused by other relatives or nonrelatives. In Herman and Hirschman's study (1977), the daughters viewed their mothers as weak and downtrodden and unable to provide protection for anyone. Thus mothers are accused of being dependent or dominating, frigid or promiscuous, rejecting or domineering. Whatever language was used, blaming the mother for the incest was common, instead of blaming the offender.

In families where the mother possesses power, incest is less likely to occur. This phenomenon can be explained by Finkelhor's (1986) disinhibition factor; that is, if the father believes that the child will disclose to the mother and that the mother will take steps against the offender, then internal inhibitions against the incest will be strengthened rather than weakened, and incest is less likely to occur.

Because the literature on incest focuses on the victim and the offender, little research or clinical literature was available about nonoffending mothers until recently. Traditionally, child-protective-service, social-service, and law-enforcement personnel maintained that the majority of mothers did not believe or protect their children in sexual-abuse cases. In my experience with nonoffending mothers, many initially do not know whom to believe, especially when they trust and love the offender and he vehemently denies the incest charges. If the woman believes that her partner loves her and that the relationship has been successful, the revelation of an incestuous relationship can be overwhelming and profoundly distressing. No one can be trusted. Nothing makes sense. Her partner has betrayed her for a younger woman, and this younger woman is her own daughter. Therefore, it is much less devastating to believe that it did not happen.

In my clinical practice, many mothers come to therapy groups feeling angry, confused, and ambivalent, but most gradually believe their daughters, understand the dynamics of the situation, place the blame and responsibility on the offender, and accept that they must learn how to protect their children to prevent future abuse. This clinical scenario has been supported by other clinicians (Cammaert, 1988; Deblinger et al., 1993) For many mothers, belief of her victimized daughter usually involves a crisis, followed by a grief process or working through feelings of shock, disbelief, ambivalence, acceptance, and eventually strong support for the daughter. However, as the mother grapples with her own pain and guilt, she also must address her daughter's pain. The daughter will be experiencing the trauma of abuse and rage and blame toward the mother for not believing and protecting her. It is not unusual for the daughter to place more blame and anger on the mother than on the offender.

If social-service agencies do not follow the mother closely for a long enough period, they may only remember her as being in denial and shock and not appreciate acceptance as a gradual process. Certainly, some mothers consistently deny their daughters' claims of sexual abuse and choose to join their partners in accusing the daughter of lying. To relatives and friends, both parents may appear to be conscientious caretakers who are being victimized by their own daughter. Mothers reinforce this victimization role by trying to convince others that the daughter is a "bad seed." They make statements such as "she began to lie as soon as she started to speak."

One explanation for the mother's denial may relate to the fact that many mothers are themselves victims of childhood incest. It is well established that women who were child victims of sexual abuse frequently fail to protect their own daughters from abuse. Some clinicians have suggested that the mother's denial and failure to protect may be the result of the unconscious coping mechanism of dissociation. Each time any cue in the environment threatens to trigger memories of her own abuse, the mother psychologically (unconsciously) separates herself from the threat (Dolan, 1991; Fredrickson, 1991). These researchers maintain that offenders, nonoffending parents, and child victims all use dissociation to some degree to cope with abuse.

Pintello and Zuravin (2001) described four factors that predicted whether or not the mother believed the child's allegations about sexual abuse: the mother was not the current partner of the abuser; the mother was an adult, not a teenager; the mother did not have knowledge of the sexual abuse before the child disclosed; and the child did not display sexualized behaviors prior to disclosure.

Contrary to traditional beliefs about nonoffending parents, current research supports the belief that most mothers believe their children when they disclose sexual abuse (Elliott & Carnes, 2001; Strand, 2000). No research exists that examines the belief patterns of nonoffending fathers. In a review of the literature, Elliott and Carnes reported that although a substantial number of parents do not believe their children's allegations, the majority do believe regardless of whether it is extrafamilial or intrafamilial abuse. In their review of nine studies, mothers believed their children 69% to 78% of the time. In a summary of another four studies, Elliot and Carnes reported even higher numbers of mothers who believed at least some portion of their children's allegations (83% to 84%). They also claimed that given the shock of the disclosure, it should not be surprising that some parents may initially disbelieve their children or express ambivalence, as reported by Urbancic (1993). Elliot and Carnes emphasized that belief does not guarantee that the nonoffending mother will protect the child.

EFFECTS OF INCEST

Abuse Effects on the Child's Developing Brain

In recent years, because of advanced, noninvasive technology, we have seen an explosion in the research on early brain development and the effects of abuse and neglect in infancy and early childhood. Today, we know that by the time normal children are three years old, their brains have achieved 90% of their size. The development of the brain is dependent on the child receiving ongoing stimulation. Stimulation results in the process of learning or in neurobiological terms, the development of brain connections called synapses. These first three years of life are critical, as during this time trillions of neuronal pathways are established because very few are present at birth (Shore, 1997). Researchers believe that this time of rapid neurobiological development is a critical period for establishing the foundation for future human functioning (National Clearinghouse on Child Abuse & Neglect, 2001).

Perry (2001) maintained that childhood memories are the organizing framework for brain development, and it is with repeated stimulation of neuronal pathways that memories are established. Through these memories, a child's lasting impression of the world is created. Therefore, if the child experiences trauma such as sexual or physical abuse or neglect, neuronal pathways that create memories of this trauma are established; they have the potential for impacting the child's perception of the world forever. The child who experiences chronic stress and abuse will also have oversensitized regions of the brain, whereas other regions will be undersensitized or undeveloped. For example, a child who is a victim of ongoing sexual or physical abuse may need to concentrate on using her brain's resources to survive the abuse by adapting to a negative environment. Other pathways of the brain, in which a child may learn to respond to a loving caregiver, will not be stimulated, and therefore, neuronal pathways for learning healthy human functioning may not develop.

Chronic abuse is also involved in a variety of neurochemical changes in the brain. Perry (2001) explained that chronic fear can cause an overstimulation of the hypothalamic-pituitary-adrenal (HPA) axis, which will then impair the development of the subcortical and limbic systems. This overstimulation of the HPA axis may also result in a state of hyperarousal or hypervigilance so that the child tends to interpret the world as a threatening and harmful place in which one must always be on guard. The impairment can be expressed as hyperactivity, aggressiveness, anxiety, sleep problems, and depression. Although some children become overly aggressive as a way to survive, others learn to withdraw through dissociation. Thus, many of these children are unable to realize their own feelings or empathize with others, and consequently they fail to develop healthy attachments to others. Perry claims that children do not just "get over it." As they strive to survive in their harsh worlds, their brains adapt to this negative environment, and their potential for emotional, behavioral, cognitive, and social growth is significantly lessened.

Short-Term Effects of Incest

Despite the influence of Freudian theory, the last 25 years have seen a wealth of clinical and research articles and books that have supported the belief that the occurrence of childhood incest has both short- and long-term traumatic effects. These studies were initially stimulated by the feminist movement and most recently by the research on neurophysiology of psychological trauma. Clinicians and researchers have identified a variety of short-term effects of incest in children as well as long-term effects in adults. The degree of damage depends on many variables. Still, studies over the past 20 years have consistently indicated that children who have been sexually abused have more psychological and behavioral problems than children who have not.

One disadvantage with the research on child victims of sexual abuse is the sampling bias; most of the children are clinically accessed through child-protection agencies or the criminal-justice system. Research studies of childhood incest are becoming more rigorous in that many have begun to use standardized measures, adequate sample size, and comparison groups. Because most studies on sexual abuse are retrospective, one cannot claim a causal relationship between the abuse and subsequent life functioning. Significantly, one prospective study that followed sexually abused children to adulthood reported a strong relationship between childhood sexual abuse and adult PTSD and depression (Boney-McCoy & Finkelhor, 1996).

Most researchers appear to agree that serious effects are not inevitable, particularly if the child and family are given support and treatment. In a review of literature, Kendall-Tackett, Williams, and Finkelhor (1993) found that approximately 40% of children who were sexually abused did not demonstrate any of the expected abuse-related problems. However, one must be cautious about interpreting the absence of symptoms as meaning that the sexual abuse was not harmful.

Some believe that the effects of discovery and consequent stressful legal involvement are more traumatic than the actual incest experience, particularly if the child is removed from the home or the father is incarcerated. The child may feel guilty and may interpret removal from the home as her punishment. She also may blame herself for the destruction of the family if the father is removed. Berliner and Elliott (2002) pointed out that dysfunctional families not only are at greater risk for intrafamilial sexual abuse, but also once the abuse occurs the family chaos may increase the sexual-abuse trauma.

Some researchers have concentrated on documenting the short-term effects of incest on young children. Berliner and Elliott (2002), in synthesizing the literature, reported that sexually abused children demonstrate higher rates of depression, anxiety, and low self-esteem than nonabused comparison children do. The abused girls from disturbed families have more internalized aggression, lower self-esteem, and poorer relationships with their mothers than nonabused girls from the same type of families do. Briere (1992) pointed out that children who are abused develop an internal framework for viewing the world as hostile and dangerous. Because of the helplessness and powerlessness they were forced to experience, they tend to overestimate danger and adversity and become fearful and anxious, thereby predisposing themselves to depression and other emotional distress. Sexually abused children are also more likely to experience symptoms of PTSD, with about one-third qualifying for the diagnosis.

Sexually abused children also have a consistent pattern of increased sexual-behavior problems. Researchers have documented premature sexual behavior such as open masturbation, frequent exposure of genitalia, and a tendency to become involved sexually with other children. Berliner and Elliott (2002) cited several studies that found more of these problem behaviors among the sexually abused children than among their counterparts who were neglected, physically abused, or psychiatrically disturbed. However, nonabused children who are exposed to family nudity, sexual activities among family members or on TV, and serious family stress may also express problem sexual behaviors. These erotic behaviors present a problem in placement and maintenance in foster-care facilities. Nightmares, encopresis, enuresis, anorexia, school phobias, learning problems, genitourinary problems, and depression also are commonly seen. Infants and very young children may have reddened and swollen genitalia, sleep and eating disturbances, as well as changes in activity levels (Browne & Finkelhor, 1986; Berliner & Elliott, 2002).

Many of the sexually abused children have interpersonal difficulties because of their shame, guilt, and perception of being different. In addition, these children tend to have more cognitive deficits in school achievement than do nonabused counterparts.

Adolescent incest victims tend to have many of the same problems and additional ones, such as teenage pregnancy, promiscuity, truancy, running away from home, drug and alcohol abuse, eating disorders, self-mutilation, panic attacks, suicide attempts, and depression. Older girls may exhibit hypersexuality, whereas older boys are more likely to engage in sexual exposure or coercion (Kendall-Tackett, Williams, & Finkelhor, 1993). Berliner and Elliott (2002) claimed that 10% to 24% of the sexually abused children do not improve over time and some even decline further.

The conflicting role of child and lover is extremely difficult to fulfill. Sometimes it also entails the role of being a physical caretaker. Such demands on the child create confusion and interfere with the normal developmental tasks of childhood and adolescence. It typically causes rage and resentment toward authority figures as well. As previously noted, the daughter may feel deep anger and resentment toward the father figure, but she may harbor even deeper anger toward her mother for not protecting her. In addition to feeling betrayed by her father (or other surrogate male) and mother, she also may feel betrayed when she seeks professional assistance because of the blame, disbelief, or unconcern she may encounter.

Long-Term Effects of Childhood Incest

Survivors may experience a broad range of long-term effects, from an overwhelming variety of symptoms to a total absence of them. Male and female survivors both suffer from long-term effects. Briere (1996) placed the long-term effects of childhood sexual abuse into four categories: posttraumatic stress, cognitive effects, emotional effects, and interpersonal effects. These categories approximate those identified by Kendall-Tackett. However, like Wilson and colleagues, (2001) Briere placed more emphasis on the PTSD, whereas Kendall-Tackett subsumes PTSD under emotional pathway.

Posttraumatic Stress

Berliner and Elliott (2002) reported that approximately 36% of adult survivors of childhood sexual abuse suffer from PTSD as adults. Other survivors may not have all the symptoms to qualify for the PTSD diagnosis, but approximately 80% (Briere, 1996) do experience some of its disabling symptoms, including nightmares, flashbacks, intrusive thoughts, intense fear, numbing, hypervigilance, and hyperarousal. In particular, survivors tend to reexperience the abuse through flashbacks and intrusive thoughts. Survivors also frequently experience dissociation as a protective response for coping with their childhood trauma. This defense mechanism protects the survivor from reliving the trauma by splitting off painful thoughts, feelings, and memories. Dissociation may take the form of amnesia as a way of defending from the traumatic memories (Foa, Keane, & Friedman, 2000; Wilson et al., 2001). Many survivors exhibit this amnesia through partial or fragmentary memories of abuse. Whereas survival techniques such as dissociation and amnesia are productive during childhood, they are counterproductive in adulthood.

Cognitive Effects

Because of their traumatic and violent childhood, survivors develop many cognitive distortions about themselves, others, and the safety of the environment. These cognitive distortions are reflected in the survivors' beliefs about themselves as being unworthy, bad, shameful, helpless, and ineffectual. They believe other people are rejecting and scornful of them and that the world is a hostile and unsafe place.

Emotional Effects

Emotional effects of childhood sexual abuse include anxiety disorders, depression, suicidal behaviors, and problems with anger regulation. Zlotnick, Mattia, and Zimmerman (2001) reported that survivors of childhood sexual abuse are a subgroup of depressed patients who are at especially high risk for psychiatric disorders and prolonged depression. They often have difficulty regulating their anger, which can explode into rage and result in injury to themselves or others. Survivors often express the trauma of their sexual abuse through somatic symptoms that are an extension of sympathetic-nervous-system hyperarousal; these symptoms include headaches, gastrointestinal disturbances, pelvic and back pain, and muscle tension (Berliner & Elliott, 2002; Kendall-Tackett, 2002). In primary-care settings, health-care providers who inquire about sexual abuse histories of their patients note that women survivors report more physical and psychosocial symptoms (including chronic pain) and incur more primary-care costs than do their nonabused counterparts (Finestone et al., 2000). Survivors may externalize their emotional distress through alcohol and substance abuse, obesity and other eating disorders, and self-mutilating activities.

Interpersonal Effects

Because of their challenges with trust and their poor self-esteem, survivors have difficulties becoming intimate with men and women. They often choose abusive partners, which continues their childhood patterns of abuse. Researchers have begun to document the repeated victimization patterns of survivors, particularly women. Banyard, Arnold, and Smith (2000) reported that childhood sexual abuse among female college students was significantly related to having experienced increased physical and psychological dating aggression. Research (Arata, 2000; Briere, 1996; Herman, 2000; Kendall-Tackett, 2002) also has supported the probability that incest victims are more likely to experience sexual and physical revictimization as adults by strangers, husbands, and boyfriends. Russell (1986) found that from 33% to 68% (depending on definition of abuse) of the childhood sexually abused women in her probability sample were subsequently raped, as compared to 17% of women without histories of childhood sexual abuse. In addition to being physically and sexually revictimized in an adult relationship, these women were more likely to have attempted suicide in the past.

Survivors also report difficulties across the sexual domain from sexual dysfunction to sexual promiscuity. Recently, some researchers have begun documenting the relationship between early sexual abuse and adult HIV-risky sexual behaviors (Parillo, Freeman, Collier, & Young, 2001). Kendall-Tackett reported that childhood physical and sexual abuse was a strong predictor of homelessness in women. In a review of the literature on interpersonal functioning in women with histories of childhood sexual abuse, DiLillo (2001) indicated that these women often have significant difficulties parenting their children, particularly in maintaining boundaries and meeting emotional needs of their children.

Concluding Thoughts on Effects of Incest

The growing body of research indicates that childhood incest experiences can have serious effects on both child and adult functioning and health. However, it is important to emphasize that not all of the effects can be classified as serious and long term and that many people who have had childhood sexual experiences have recovered without formal psychotherapy and professional assistance. There is no profile for the sexually abused child or the adult survivor. Instead there are myriad symptoms that abuse survivors may demonstrate across a wide range of psychiatric problems, particularly those relating to posttraumatic stress.

NURSING INTERVENTIONS

Primary Prevention

Primary-prevention interventions for childhood sexual abuse began to proliferate in the 1980s. Because most victims do not disclose or have treatment, the potential for short- and long-term effects is significant. Sexual-abuse educational programs for children, parents, and professionals are the first step in eliminating the trauma of sexual abuse. Although nurses are not always in a position to present such programs, it is essential that they value the critical importance of the programs and support them in their schools and communities. Nurses, as health-promotion advocates, must insist that these programs balance themes of violence and abuse with those of healthy touch and intimacy.

Many agencies and institutions provide sexual-abuse primary-prevention programs for children, parents, and mental-health professionals. Storybooks, coloring books, videos, and films are available for children on the topic, as are workshops that incorporate art and role-plays into primary-prevention education. The developmental level and cultural background of the children are important to consider when developing or selecting materials. Past educational programs focused on the "stranger" as the abuser, but today the message contains the possibility that someone whom the child knows and trusts may try to involve them in sexually inappropriate behavior. If they are involved in such an activity, children are taught to tell someone they trust and also to try to resist the offender in whatever manner they are able.

The programs can help not only nonabused children but also those who have experienced sexual abuse. Improving self-esteem and the sense of mastery over their lives may prevent revictimization for many children. In a review of the literature on primary prevention of childhood sexual abuse, Daro and Connelly (2002) reported that such programs are effective in not only increasing children's knowledge about how to protect themselves but also creating an environment that facilitates disclosures. Daro and Connelly emphasized that although results from these primary education programs are inconsistent, results can be maximized by individualizing the materials to the child's developmental level;

providing practice and feedback for the children; developing more intensive programs, especially for at-risk children; teaching children basic assertive and communication skills; repeatedly emphasizing the need to tell someone; and involving parents.

Programs of primary prevention for children are not enough to stem the tide of childhood sexual abuse. Parents also must be involved in the primary prevention of childhood sexual abuse. However, studies indicate that parents are not involved. In a study by Finkelhor (1984), only 29% of parents claimed to have discussions about sexual abuse with their children, although almost all warned their children about the possibility of kidnapping. Even when discussions about sexual abuse did occur, they began when the child was too old (older than nine years), and crucial facts about sexual abuse were omitted. Parental difficulty in addressing sexual issues with their children is common across all socioeconomic, religious, and educational levels. It is crucial that parents become aware of the high incidence of abuse among all socioeconomic, ethnic, and religious groups and are assisted in discussing the sensitive issue of sexual abuse with their children. Lowering the anxiety of parents about sexual-abuse issues may be more important than the materials presented.

Families with high risk for abuse, such as those that have stepfathers, parents with a childhood history of physical or sexual abuse, or children with developmental or emotional problems, need special and concentrated attention. Nurses who teach parenting classes should emphasize the role of both parents in the caretaking of their children. In addition to the involvement of fathers, it also may be appropriate for older siblings and other caretakers to participate. Research strongly suggests that fathers who are involved in the early care of their children are more likely to bond with their children and are less likely to sexually abuse them. Unfortunately, too often only the mothers attend parenting classes or sexual-abuse workshops. Nurses who conduct parenting classes must creatively devise methods for involving both parents.

Professionals also need special training and education about childhood sexual abuse to educate the public formally and informally and to become child advocates in the prevention of abuse. Nurses must demand that content on sexual abuse be incorporated into the curricula of their nursing schools and that in-service training on the topic be conducted periodically at their places of employment.

Daro and Connelly (2002) pointed out that prevention efforts must involve the community because stress and isolation are strong predictors for all child abuse and neglect. Therefore, communities need to support the strengthening of at-risk parents and at-risk communities.

Secondary Prevention: Interventions for the Sexually Abused Child and Her Family

All professionals must be prepared to quickly and effectively intervene whenever necessary in cases of sexual abuse. Nurses are in a special position to intervene because they have intimate and frequent interactions in a variety of settings with children and adolescents, as well as adults who have been sexually molested as children. But nurses cannot be effective in primary- and secondary-prevention efforts unless they examine their own feelings and educate themselves.

Many nurses and other professionals are uncomfortable dealing with the issues of incest, as shown by an evasive, punitive manner and the failure to respond to child sexual-abuse statutes that mandate reporting if suspicion exists. If nurses and other professionals do not identify and report victims of sexual abuse, they support its proliferation. In addition, failure to invite the victim to disclose and discuss the abuse will probably make them think that their secret is too terrible to discuss, and their shame, guilt, and sense of helplessness may increase. Every state requires both physicians and nurses to report suspected cases of child sexual abuse. The American Academy of Pediatrics (1999) has published guidelines for assisting professionals in reporting cases of sexual abuse. Jenny (2002) also developed guidelines for interviewing caretakers of the sexually abused child.

Identifying children who have already been abused has not been an easy task because many do not disclose their abuse and do not fit the typical textbook picture of the abused child. Their response depends on their cognitive, behavioral, and emotional development. Sometimes a child may be able to spontaneously give a clear and detailed report of the abuse. Jenny (2002) recommended first establishing rapport with the child, asking open-ended, nonleading questions, and also inquiring about pain, bleeding, dysuria, or other problems. Children need to be able to ask questions and have them answered at the level they will understand. A majority of sexually abused children will not demonstrate physical signs of sexual abuse. Even when the abuse is quite severe, tissue may heal without significant physical signs of the abuse. In cases where vaginal or rectal penetration had occurred, physicians reported abnormal medical findings in only 5.5% of the children. Therefore, the child's history is by far the most critical component in establishing the presence of sexual abuse (Giardino, Datner, Asher, Faugno, & Spencer, 2002).

Physical Indications of Sexual Abuse

Anytime child sexual abuse is suspected, a complete physical examination should be performed. Before a child is examined for the possibility of sexual abuse, the nurse and doctor must establish trust and gain the child's cooperation to prevent further victimization through the exam. In addition, a child who is frightened and tense will most likely tighten pubococcygeal muscles so that it is difficult to evaluate the vaginal canal or hymen. It is critical to document in her exact words the history the child relates. The first priority in dealing with a sexually abused child is to determine if it is safe for the child to return to her home.

Even though the majority of children will have normal physical findings, they still should be examined for bruises on the entire body as well as evidence of trauma to the external genitalia, vagina, and rectum. Cultures of the pharynx, urethra, vagina, penis, and rectum for sexually transmitted diseases (STDs) need to be obtained. Children can acquire all of the STDs that adults have. Gonorrhea can be misdiagnosed as vulvovaginitis, which is merely the result of poor hygiene. Adams (2001) reported that it is possible that *Condyloma accuminata* and human papilloma virus may be transmitted nonsexually.

The physical position for a child to assume during a genital examination depends on the age of the child. Children younger than three years may be most comfortable sitting on the mother's lap. Children older than three will usually cooperate and lie on an examining table if rapport has been established. Dolls can be used to demonstrate desired positions to the child. Jenny (2002) recommended either a supine (frog-leg) or prone (knee-chest) position. Sometimes exam findings may appear abnormal in the supine position but normalize in the prone position. The use of colposcopy for magnification is more common today. Jenny reported that in most cases, the typical examination is noninvasive and without pain to the child. If instruments are needed, the child may need sedation.

More recent research indicates that notches or clefts in the posterior rim of the hymen are not necessarily positive for sexual abuse in female children. Berenson and others (2000) reported that both abused and nonabused female children may have shallow posterior notches but only abused females have deep notches that penetrate through more than 50% of the posterior rim of the hymen. Some physical conditions may present as sexual abuse in a child. These include anal and vaginal streptococcal infections, lichen schlerosis, and straddle injuries. Sexual abuse of boys most typically involves trauma to the anus rather than the genitals (Frasier, 2002; Jenny, 2002).

Additional Interventions for Secondary Prevention

Even when all the data strongly indicates that the child has been abused, she may deny it and may do so because of her relationship to the offender. Disclosure by the child is easier if the offender is not a close, trusted person to whom the child feels a sense of commitment or loyalty.

Another reason for the child's ambivalence may be threats the offender has made regarding disclosure. They may provoke a variety of anxious fantasies about physical harm to herself or other family members. In addition, she may fear the breakup of the family, with the offender going to prison and the rest of the family blaming her for the breakup. The victim also may fear removal from the family and placement in foster care. These fears can provide powerful motivation for not disclosing or even for later retraction. Some children might choose to sacrifice themselves rather than have their dysfunctional family destroyed, whereas others feel that the positives of their relationship with the offender outweigh the negatives of the abuse. Therefore to make sense of the child's denials, retractions, and vacillations, it is essential to consider and process all possible concerns, fears, and perceptions of the child.

Initial interventions focus on stabilizing the crisis that results from the disclosure. For nurses who are in a position to work with incestuous families, the focus of care is on the individual needs of the child, but all family members need support. Organizations that offer groups for offenders, nonoffending parents, victims, and siblings are urgently needed for effectively treating these families. These groups are beginning to develop across the country.

Because the nonoffending parent is a critical element in the child's recovery from the abuse, it is important to support her as well. Recent literature indicates that the nonoffending parent, usually the mother, may suffer from PTSD symptoms and depression. Because symptoms may take time to emerge, the parent will need to be assessed at different points in time. The assessment of the parent needs to be followed with treatment, if indicated (Cohen & Mannarino, 1998; Elliott & Carnes, 2001).

Many more resources are becoming available for the nonoffending parent and professionals working with them (Levenson & Morin, 2001a, 2001b; Strand, 2000). Initially, the mother may be so overwhelmed by the disclosure and threatened loss of her children, spouse, and economic security that without support she may side with the offender against the daughter. Therefore, the mother needs immediate support to process the meaning and implications of the abuse and often to address her own denial. The workbook by Levenson and Morin is an excellent resource for nonoffending parents. It addresses these issues and assists the parent to process her own grief and loss as well as to understand the child and prepare a safety plan for reunification of the family if this is feasible and therapeutic.

Using cognitive-behavioral therapy (CBT) in both individual and group modalities, a number of researchers have reported a significant difference in outcomes with nonoffending parents, as compared to using supportive therapy. These researchers reported that a variety of CBTs are effective in assisting the nonoffending parent to address and process the sexual abuse of her child. Exposure techniques and artwork can facilitate the parent's ability to gradually discuss the abuse without becoming overwhelmed. Eventually, joint session with the child and parent can be conducted using cognitive restructuring to correct some of the distorted beliefs about the abuse. Often, the parent can benefit from stress management and child management as well as psychoeducation about childhood sexual abuse (Berliner & Cohen, 2000; Deblinger, Stauffer, & Steer, 2001; Wilson et al., 2001).

Crisis intervention with the incestuous family requires a direct, swift, and active approach to ensure that the abuse will end and the child will be protected. It also requires coordination with protective services, law-enforcement agencies, and counselors. Usually, the court mandates that the offender leave the home. If the offender may continue to abuse and the mother cannot or will not protect the child, then she may be removed from the home. Because this approach is usually traumatic for the child, it is avoided if possible.

When addressing the needs of the sexually abused child, the nurse must realize that not all destructive effects from the abuse will be obvious immediately. Therefore, a physical and psychological assessment and intervention are always necessary regardless of whether the child appears traumatized. The child's age and developmental level are determining factors in choosing the type of therapy. In reviewing the research on treatment for sexually abused children, most studies have indicated that the best outcomes involve extending and modifying existing clinical child-psychology treatment models for the sexually abused child. Recently, several metanalytic studies have examined well-controlled research on effective treatments with children and adolescents who have been sexually abused (Fonagy, 1998; Kasdin & Weisz, 1998; Saywitz, Mannarino, Berliner, & Cohen, 2000). CBT and behavioral therapies are the most researched modalities

In general, studies have indicated that those therapies are more effective than nonbehavioral interventions, especially for children with depression, anxiety symptoms, or behavior problems. The CBT is combined with gradual-exposure sessions, psychoeducation, stress management and safety skills, and parent-management training. These modalities can be used individually, with parent and child, or with groups.

Saywitz and colleagues (2000) claimed that sexually abused children fall into four groups, and these groups need to be considered when deciding on interventions. The first group is those children with no discernible symptoms from their abuse. This group accounts for 30% of sexually abused children. Approximately 70% of these children will remain asymptomatic, probably because the event was not traumatic even if it was exploitative and illegal. But 30% of them will develop symptoms later (i.e., have a sleeper effect). Because there is not a reliable method to predict who will experience later symptoms, all children who have been abused should have basic treatment that includes psychoeducational interventions to prevent future abuse and sleeper effects. A second group of children will present with mild symptoms that do not exceed the symptoms seen in a general clinical population. The third group presents with serious psychiatric problems, including depression, anxiety, sexualized behaviors, aggression, and components of PTSD. The fourth group meets the full criteria for PTSD and comorbidity for depression, anxiety disorders, and sleep disorders. Treatment needs to be individualized and targeted to specific symptoms. For some children, pharmacotherapy may be indicated.

Group therapy for sexually abused children can be a powerful modality for assisting all children older than three years. Using CBT, the group can be effective in correcting many of the traumatic sexualization behaviors that abused children exhibit, as well as in improving their sense of power and esteem, in decreasing feelings of being stigmatized, and in reestablishing a sense of trust and assertiveness with people in their world. In addition, the group can address the child's understanding of the abuse so that misconceptions about her role and the roles others played can be examined and corrected. Often, the child has overwhelming guilt about the pleasurable aspects of the abuse and the fact that she sometimes initiated the interactions. A major component of therapy is directed toward decreasing anxiety and fear related to the abuse. As the child repeatedly addresses different aspects of the abuse and learns to express her anger, sadness, and grief about them, the memories of the event gradually lose their power for negative arousal. In addition, age-appropriate sex education should be provided, along with discussions of cues that indicate a situation is becoming sexually threatening.

Even though the offender completes treatment, develops new coping skills, and admits full responsibility for the abuse, the mother and children must always be on guard for a loss of the offender's inner control and resumption of the sexual abuse. Family therapy is never appropriate until the family has reached some level of stability. It is important for nurses to be aware of community resources so that referral of the family to the appropriate agency can be made.

Tertiary Prevention with the Adult Sexually Abused as a Child

The word "victim" has generally been replaced by the word "survivor" in describing the adult who was abused in childhood. The shift in terminology places the focus on the process of recovery rather than on being helpless, injured, or destroyed.

As with the child who has been sexually abused, nurses in a variety of settings have opportunities to assist the adult survivor of abuse. Because the survivor requires support on many different levels, nurses need not be expert therapists to be helpful. Briere (1996) emphasized that the most important aspect of psychotherapy with survivors is a caring, reliable, nonexploitative therapist who creates a therapeutic environment by facilitating self-awareness, self-acceptance, and the careful processing of traumatic experiences. Thus, nursing interventions with adult survivors can encompass a variety of helping techniques that can mitigate the guilt and shame of the survivor's long-kept secret, as well as the denial, minimization, and blame that she has experienced from family, friends, and other professionals.

Agreement exists that trauma-based treatment for adult survivors involves three stages (Chu, 1998; Courtois, 1999; Draucker, 2000; Herman, 1997). The first stage consists of establishing safety by stabilizing, containing, and reducing symptoms and learning self-care skills; the second stage involves the processing and resolution of traumatic memories; and the third stage focuses on personality integration and relational development.

Because incest is based on abuse of power, a demand for secrecy, betrayal of trust, and disregard for the child's needs, the potential for developing profound feelings of helplessness, shame, guilt, and confusion is significant. Therefore, interventions for resolving incest trauma must focus on support to empower the victim to develop a sense of self-worth, mastery, competence, and control. For nursing interventions to be effective and empowering, they must involve collaborative effort rather than the traditional patriarchical relationship of the all-knowing professional and the unknowing client. Instead, the relationship becomes a partnership in which both nurse and client collaborate in establishing and achieving objectives to resolve the incest trauma. The nurse must support the survivor to believe that she is the ultimate expert on herself and therefore has the ability to make appropriate decisions for her health and well-being. In addition, the nurse and client should identify and develop strategies that will build on client's strengths and increase her sense of control while supporting her to take action to change her life. The following discussion covers empowerment-support interventions for nurses to use with adult survivors of incest. A basic level of intervention will be discussed, followed by an advanced level.

The first step for the survivor is to disclose the incest to someone she trusts. The nurse must support the survivor in discussing the incest whenever and however she chooses. Too often, the nurse may be uncomfortable with the disclosure, and this discomfort is communicated nonverbally to the client and interpreted as a sign that she is not to discuss her incest experiences. It is crucial that the survivor feels she has permission to disclose and that the nurse will be a therapeutic listener.

In addition to supporting the survivor to control the discussion and details of the disclosure, the nurse must refrain from expressing horror, shock, or dismay, as these reactions may add to the survivor's existing feelings of being alienated and unworthy. Rather than asking repeated intrusive questions, basic therapeutic communication techniques are highly effective when supporting the survivor to disclose. This includes simply "being with" the survivor in silence if she chooses, reflecting on her comments, encouraging a discussion of her perception and expression of feelings, following her cues, offering to strategize with her, and considering behavioral options that might help her. In addition, the nurse can assist the survivor in recognizing that self-disclosure is a strength that requires great courage.

The survivor needs reassurance of her power to decrease any painful flashback episodes she may be having. Reassurance about the reality of her world in the present is helpful as well. Survivors also need assistance in learning to constructively express feelings of anger without fear of losing control, to express needs without feeling frightened or guilty, and to come to terms with the failure of her mother or other family members to protect her. In addition, she needs encouragement to try new experiences and relationships and to set time aside for herself.

Many of the empowerment support strategies that the nurse uses with the survivor involve teaching. New behaviors and corrections of myths and distortions about incest are taught. Because the myths and distortions have shaped the survivor from childhood, corrective learning is a lengthy, ongoing process for the survivor. Before the nurse can be helpful, she must learn the difference between myth and fact.

The nurse will be called on repeatedly to reinforce that the adult is always the responsible party in childhood sexual abuse, but women who have derived pleasure and even sought the childhood sexual activity may become especially ashamed and guilt-ridden. Thus basic principles of normal physiology and child development are taught, and it is emphasized that children normally seek that which is rewarding, feels good, and is adaptive. Understanding the traumatic sexualization (Finkelhor, 1986) can be helpful to the survivor who is having difficulty forgiving herself. If the survivor has young children, she must learn how to protect her children from abuse and become more sensitive to their needs.

Weaknesses are realistically discussed and analyzed, and the survivor is recognized for her courage to address these areas. Many troublesome behaviors and habits that the survivor currently identifies are explained as being linked to the incest; although these behaviors may have been necessary and adaptive in earlier years, they no longer are helpful to the survivor and may even be destructive. Nevertheless, it is reinforced that these behaviors, which could include hyperventilation, self-abuse, somatization, dissociation, denial, repression, and substance abuse, were creative self-care behaviors.

Advanced-practice nurses who work with adults sexually abused as children often have opportunities to use more developed interventions. Research on outcomes for these interventions with adult survivors is beginning to appear in the literature. Price, Hilsenroth, Petretic-Jackson, and Bonge (2001) conducted a review of eight study outcomes for individual therapy for these adults. The studies involved four different therapeutic methods: cognitive-behavioral, experiential, psychodynamic/interpersonal, and psychoeducational/supportive. The results indicated that all the individual psychotherapy methods were successful in reducing symptoms of adult survivors. Although the results were significant across the eight studies, Price and associates recognized that the studies each had multiple weaknesses that needed to be addressed in future studies. DeJong and Gorey (1996) conducted a review of seven studies on group-therapy effectiveness. As with individual-therapy outcomes, the group modalities were also effective in reducing symptoms and improving self-esteem and overall functioning. For many survivors of childhood sexual abuse, both individual and group psychotherapy are concurrently recommended.

Of all the treatment modalities, cognitive-behavioral therapy (CBT) has been the most researched. It is based on the premise that a person's beliefs about oneself influence the person's affect and behavior in profound ways. Therefore, a critical and early task of therapy is to work with the client to assist her to understand that how and what she thinks is an important part of therapeutic change. CBT includes a wide variety of interventions that have been reviewed extensively in the literature. Treatment guidelines using CBT for patients with partial, full, or complex PTSD are described in many books and publications (Chu, 1998; Courtois, 1999; Foa, Keane, & Friedman, 2000; Wilson et al., 2001).

Foa and others (2000) reviewed the effectiveness of eight different CBT techniques in relieving PTSD symptoms of intrusion, numbing/avoidance, and hyperarousal. The techniques consisted of exposure therapy, systematic desensitization, stress inoculation training, cognitive processing therapy, cognitive therapy, assertiveness training, biofeedback, relaxation training, and various combinations of these. Most of these interventions require special training for the therapist. Foa and colleagues rated the studies according to the "gold" standard for evaluating clinical studies. They found that exposure therapy was the most effective of the eight techniques, and, therefore, they recommend some form of its use with PTSD populations. Exposure therapy involves PTSD education, breathing retraining, in vivo exposure, and imaging exposure. Although exposure therapy has various forms, the common theme is confronting dangerous stimuli in the belief that with repeated exposure, anxiety will gradually diminish. Therefore, the individual will eventually not have to result to escape or avoidance behaviors. The other seven modalities were more difficult to evaluate because of mixed results or poor research methodology, and the combination of therapies was not more effective than individual ones alone. Nevertheless, significant results have been reported for all of the CBT interventions.

Researchers (Foa et al., 2000; Friedman, 2001) have also evaluated across multiple randomized clinical trials the effectiveness of pharmacotherapy in relieving symptoms of PTSD. Although results again were mixed, some patients experienced significant improvement in symptoms. The selective serotonin reuptake inhibitors (SSRI) antidepressants were seen as the best drug and recommended as first-line treatment. Across studies, the SSRIs diminished PTSD and comorbid disorders as well as associated symptoms that were barriers to daily functioning. The SSRIs also produced less distressing side effects than other medications that were prescribed for PTSD.

Another intervention that has received much attention is eye movement desensitization and reprocessing (EMDR). It is viewed as a unique application of imaging exposure because it involves having the client imagine the trauma while using saccadic eye movements. Researchers (Foa et al., 2000; Zoellner, Fitzgibbons, & Foa, 2001) have reported that the studies examining the efficacy of EMDR are weak methodologically, so no conclusions could be made about its effectiveness. Several studies reported by the researchers did not have significant results between EMDR and traditional exposure.

Foy and others (2001) reviewed the research outcomes on group psychotherapy with clients suffering from PTSD; the types of groups were supportive, psychodynamic, and cognitive-behavioral. The supportive approach is considered more of a covering approach in that the focus is on current life issues, whereas the other two modalities generally use an uncovering approach. With the uncovering, the focus is on the actual trauma. Group psychotherapy promotes a sense of trust, commonality, community, and validity for its members, as well as a safe, respectful and therapeutic place to process their pain as well as their successes and growth. Although research methodology on the effectiveness of group therapy has been weak, results have been consistently significant for positive outcomes across the three types of group modalities. Foy reported that these outcomes were effective against a broad range of symptoms, including PTSD.

Many other therapeutic modalities are used in the treatment of the adult survivor of childhood sexual abuse. Psychodynamic psychotherapy is commonly used to explore the unconscious meanings of the trauma and other significant events in the survivor's life. Marital or family therapy may also be helpful. A wide variety of creative therapies have been found to be helpful, including art, dance/movement, drama, music, poetry, and bibliotherapy, as have a variety of body therapies, including relaxation and exercise. Survivors report positive results from learning assertiveness skills and anger control techniques. Research on these modalities is limited at this time.

No treatment can be successful without the consideration and integration of the client's culture. Because a person's culture may define what is normal and abnormal, when it is appropriate to seek help from an outsider, and what is appropriate to share with an outsider, respect and acceptance of the client's world view is critical. Therefore, nurses and other health-care professionals need to be patient and flexible with people from cultures different from their own, appreciate the strengths of the culture, and honestly and candidly negotiate common goals.

SUMMARY

Child sexual abuse can be a profoundly disturbing experience for many children and adults. Some carry their burden for their entire life. It is believed that most children and adults who have been abused do not disclose their experiences. Failure to disclose may have serious short- and long-term effects on the victim. Because nurses work in a variety of settings and practice on many different levels, they have many opportunities to assist victims and their families. However, nurses cannot help these families unless they first understand their own experiences and feelings about sexual abuse. Nurses also must become knowledgeable about the dynamics of incestuous behavior and the appropriate evidenced-based interventions for all levels of prevention.

Kendall-Tackett (2002) reminded us that "health" is dependent on complex and multiple interacting factors as identified under the long-term effects of incest. However, mental health cannot be separated from physical health. Each of many problems and symptoms discussed has the potential to influence health. Nurses and other health-care professionals must make a concerted effort to address all these factors if health outcomes for survivors of childhood abuse are to improve.

The ultimate nursing goal is the rehabilitation of all members of the incestuous family and reconstitution of the family, if feasible and therapeutic. The concerned, caring, and knowledgeable nurse who is willing to listen and learn from family members and to establish collaborative goals with them, but take firm action to protect its weaker members when necessary, is a valuable resource for survivors and their families, as well as for society and the nursing profession.

References

Abney, V. D. (2002). Cultural competency in the field of child maltreatment. In J. B. Myers, L. Berliner, J. Briere, C. T. Hendrix, C. Jenny & T. A. Reid (Eds.), *The APSAC handbook on child maltreatment* (2nd ed., pp. 477–486). Thousand Oaks, CA: Sage.

Adams, J. A. (2001). Evolution of a classification scale: Medical evaluation of suspected child abuse. *Child Maltreatment, 6,* 31–36.

Adler, N. A., & Schultz, J. (1995). Sibling incest offenders. *Child Abuse and Neglect, 19*(7), 811–819.

American Academy of Pediatrics, Committee on Child Abuse and Neglect. (1999). Guidelines for the evaluation of sexual abuse of children: Subject review. *Pediatrics, 103,* 854–857.

American Psychiatric Association. (1999). *Dangerous sex offenders. A task force report of the American Psychiatric Association.* Washington, DC: Author.

Arata, C. M. (2000). From child to adult victim: A model for predicting revictimization. *Child Maltreatment, 5,* 28–38.

Banyard, V. L., Arnold, S., & Smith, J. (2000). Childhood sexual abuse and dating experiences of undergraduate women. *Child Maltreatment, 5,* 39–48.

Barnett, O. W., Miller-Perrin, C. L., & Perrin, R. D. (1997). *Family violence across the lifespan.* Thousand Oaks, CA: Sage.

Bender, L., & Blau, A. (1937). The reaction of children to sexual relations with adults. *American Journal of Orthopsychiatry, 7,* 500–518.

Berenson, A. B., Chacko, M. R., Woemann, C. M., Mishaw, C. O., Friedrich, W. N., & Grady, J. J. (2000). A case-control study of anatomic changes resulting from sexual abuse. *American Journal of Obstetrics and Gynecology, 182,* 820–834.

Berliner, L., & Cohen, J. (2000, July). *Guidelines for the treatment of trauma in child victims.* Paper presented at the Eighth Annual Colloquium of the American Professional Society on the Abuse of Children, Chicago, IL.

Berliner, L., & Elliott, D. M. (2002). Sexual abuse of children. In J. B. Myers, L. Berliner, J. Briere, C. T. Hendrix, C. Jenny & T. A. Reid (Eds.), *The APSAC handbook on child maltreatment* (2nd ed., pp. 55–78). Thousand Oaks, CA: Sage.

Boney-McCoy, C. & Finkelhor, D. (1996). *Is youth victimization related to PTSD and depression after controlling for prior symptoms and family relationships? A longitudinal, prospective study.* Unpublished manuscript, University of New Hampshire.

Briere, J. (1992). *Child abuse trauma.* Newbury Park, CA: Sage.

Briere, J. (1996). *Therapy for adults molested as children: Beyond survival.* New York: Springer.

Briere, J. (2002). Treating adult survivors of severe childhood abuse and neglect: Further development of an integrative model. In J. B. Myers, L. Berliner, J. Briere, C. T. Hendrix, C. Jenny & T. A. Reid (Eds.), *The APSAC handbook on child maltreatment* (2d ed., pp. 175–203). Thousand Oaks, CA: Sage.

Briere, J., & Zaidi, L.Y. (1989). Sexual abuse histories and sequelae in female psychiatric emergency room patients. *American Journal of Psychiatry, 146,* 1602–1606.

Browne, A., & Finkelhor, D. (1986). Impact of child sexual abuse: A review of the literature. *Psychological Bulletin, 99,* 66–77.

Burgess, A., Hartman, C. R., Wolbert, W. W., & Grant, C. (1987). Child molestation: Assessing impact in multiple victims (part 1). *Archives of Psychiatric Nursing, 1,* 33–39.

Cammaert, L. P. (1988). Nonoffending mothers: A new conceptualization. In L. E. Walker (Ed.), *Handbook on sexual abuse of children* (pp. 309–325). New York: Springer.

Carmen, E., & Rieker, P. P. (1989). A psychosocial model of the victim-to-patient process. *Psychiatric Clinics of North America, 12,* 431–443.

Chaffin, M., Letourneau, W., & Silovsky, J. (2002). Adults, adolescents and children who sexually abuse children. In J. B. Myers, L. Berliner, J. Briere, C. T. Hendrix, C. Jenny & T. A. Reid (Eds.), *The APSAC handbook on child maltreatment* (2nd ed., pp. 205–232). Thousand Oaks, CA: Sage.

Chu, J. A. (1998). Rebuilding shattered lives: The responsible treatment of complex-post-traumatic and dissociative disorders. New York: Wiley.

Chu, J. A., Frey, L. M., Ganzel, B. L., & Matthews, J. A. (1999). Memories of childhood abuse: Dissociation, amnesia and corroboration. *American Journal of Psychiatry, 156,* 749–755.

Cohen, J. A., & Mannarino, A. P. (1998). Interventions for sexually abused children: Initial treatment outcome findings. *Child Maltreatment, 3,* 17–26.

Conte, J. R. (1990). The incest offender: An overview and introduction. In A. L. Horton, B. L. Johnson, L.

M. Roundy & D. Williams (Eds.), The incest perpetrator: A family member no one wants to treat (pp. 19–28). Newbury Park, CA: Sage.

Courtois, C. (1988). *Healing the incest wound.* New York: W. W. Norton.

Courtois, C. (1999). *Recollections of sexual abuse: Treatment principles and guidelines.* New York: Norton.

Daro, D., & Connelly, A. C. (2002). Child abuse prevention: Accomplishments and challenges. In J. B. Myers, L. Berliner, J. Briere, C. T. Hendrix, C. Jenny & T. A. Reid (Eds.), *The APSAC handbook on child maltreatment* (2nd ed., pp. 431–448). Thousand Oaks, CA: Sage.

Deblinger, E., Hathaway, C., Lippman, J., & Steer, R. (1993). Psychosocial characteristics and correlates of symptom distress in nonoffending mothers of sexually abused children. *Journal of Interpersonal Violence 8*(2), 155–168.

Deblinger, E., Stauffer, L. B., & Steer, R. A. (2001). Comparative efficacies of supportive and cognitive behavioral group therapies for young children who have been sexually abused and their nonoffending mothers. *Child Maltreatment 6,*(4), 332–343.

de Jong, T., & Gorey, K. (1996). Short-term versus long-term work with female survivors of childhood sexual abuse: A brief meta-analytic review. *Social Work with Groups, 19,* 19–27.

DiLillo, D. (2001). Interpersonal functioning among women reporting a history of childhood sexual abuse: Empirical findings and methodological issues. *Clinical Psychology Review, 21,* 553–576.

Dolan, Y. M. (1991). *Resolving sexual abuse: Solution focused therapy and Eriksonian hypnosis.* New York: W. W. Norton.

Draucker, C. (2000). *Counseling survivors of childhood sexual abuse.* Thousand Oaks, CA: Sage.

Eilenberg, J. (1996). Quality and use of trauma histories obtained from psychiatric outpatients through managed inquiries. *Psychiatric Services, 47,* 165.

Elliott, D. M. (1993). *Female sexual abuse of children.* New York: Guilford.

Elliot, D. M., & Briere, J. (1995). Posttraumatic stress associated with delayed recall of sexual abuse: A general population study. *Journal of Traumatic Stress, 8,* 629–647.

Elliott, D. M., & Carnes, C. N. (2001). Reactions of nonoffending parents to the sexual abuse of their child. A review of the literature. *Child Maltreatment, 6,* 314–331.

Epstein, M. A., & Bottoms, B. L. (2002). Explaining the forgetting and recovery of abuse and trauma memories: Possible mechanisms. *Child Maltreatment, 7,* 210–225.

Faller, K. C. (2002). Disclosure in cases of child sexual abuse. *Newsletter of the Michigan Professional Society on the Abuse of Children, Inc., 7,* 3–6.

Finestone, H. M., Stenn, P., Davies, F., Stalker, C., Fry, R., & Koumanis, J. (2000). Chronic pain and health care utilization in women with a history of childhood sexual abuse. *Child Abuse and Neglect, 24*(4), 547–556.

Finkelhor, D. (1984). *Child sexual abuse: New theory and research.* New York: Free Press.

Finkelhor, D. (1986). A sourcebook on child sexual abuse. Beverly Hills, CA: Sage.

Finkelhor, D. (1994). Current information on the scope and nature of childhood sexual abuse. *The Future of Children, 4*(2), 21–53.

Finkelhor, D., & Browne, A. (1986). The traumatic impact of child sexual abuse: A conceptualization. *American Journal of Orthopsychiatry, 55*, 530–541.

Foa, E. B., Keane, T. M., & Friedman, M. J. (2000). *Effective treatments for PTSD: Practice guidelines from the International Society for Traumatic Stress Studies.* NewYork: Guilford Press.

Fonagy, P. (1998). Prevention, the appropriate target of infant psychotherapy. *Infant Mental Health, 19*, 124–150.

Foy, D. W., Schnurr, P., Weiss, D., Wattenberg, M. S., Glynn, S. M., Marmar, C. R., & Gusman, F. (2001). Group psychotherapy for PTSD. In J. P. Wilson, M. J. Friedman & J. D. Lindy (Eds.), *Treating psychological trauma and PTSD.* New York: Guilford Press.

Frasier, L. (2002). Child abuse or mimic? *Consultant,* 769–771.

Freidman, M. J. (2001). Allostatic versus empirical perspectives on pharmacotherapy for PTSD. In J. P.Wilson, M. J. Friedman, & J. D. Lindy (Eds.), *Treating psychological trauma & PTSD* (pp. 94–124). New York: Guilford Press

Fredrickson, R. M. (1991, October). *Advanced clinical skills in the treatment of sexual abuse.* Paper presented at a workshop held at Wayne State University, Detroit, MI.

Freud, S. (1954). *The origins of psychoanalysis: Letters to Wilhelm Fliess, drafts and notes. 1887–1902.* New York: Basic Books.

Giardino, A., Datner, E., Asher, J., Faugno, D., & Spencer, M. (2002). *Sexual assault: Victimization across the life-span.* Maryland Heights, MO: G. W. Medical Publishing

Glasser, M., Kolvin, I., Campbell, D., Glasser, A., Leitch, I., & Farrelly, S. (2001). Cycle of child sexual abuse: Links between being a victim and becoming a perpetrator. *British Journal of Psychiatry, 179*, 482–494.

Greenfield, S. F., Strakowski, S. M., Tohen, M., Batson, S. C., & Kolbrener, M. L. (1994). Childhood abuse in first-episode psychosis. *British Journal of Psychiatry, 164*, 831–834.

Groth, N. A. (1978). Guidelines for assessment and management of the offender. In A. Burgess, N. A. Groth, L. Holstrom, & S. Sgroi (Eds.), *Sexual assault of children and adolescents* (pp. 25–42). Lexington, MA: Lexington Books.

Heger, A., Ticson, L., Valasquez, O., & Bernier, R. (2002). Children referred for possible sexual abuse: Medical findings in 2,384 children. *Child Abuse & Neglect, 26*, 545–659.

Henderson, D. J. (1972). Incest: A synthesis of data. *Psychiatric Association Journal, 17*, 299–313.

Henley, J., & Kristiansen, C. (1997). An analysis of the impact of prison on women survivors of child sexual abuse. In J. Harden & M. Hill (Eds.), *Breaking the rules: Women in prison and feminist therapy. Women and Therapy: A Feminist Quarterly, 20*, 29–44.

Herman, J. (1997). *Trauma and recovery.* New York: Basic Books.

Herman, J. (2000). *Father-daughter incest.* Cambridge, MA: Harvard University Press.

Herman, M., & Hirschman, L. (1977). Father-daughter incest: Signs. *Journal of Women in Culture and Society, 2*, 735–756.

Hudson, S. M., Ward, T., & Laws, D. R. (2000). Whither relapse prevention? In D. R. Laws, S. M. Hudson & T. Ward (Eds.), *Remaking relapse prevention with sex offenders* (pp. 503–522). Thousand Oaks, CA: Sage.

Jacobson, A., & Herald, C. (1990). The relevance of childhood sexual abuse to adult psychiatric inpatient care. *Hospital and Community Psychiatry, 41*, 154–158.

Jenny, C. (2002). Medical issues in child sexual abuse. In J. B. Myers, L. Berliner, J. Briere, C. T. Hendrix, C. Jenny & T. A. Reid (Eds.), *The APSAC handbook on child maltreatment* (2nd ed., pp. 235–237). Thousand Oaks, CA: Sage.

Jones, L., & Finkelhor, D. (2001). *The decline in child sexual abuse cases.* Washington, DC: U.S. Department of Justice.

Justice, B., & Justice. R. (1979). *The broken taboo: Sex in the family.* New York: Human Sciences Press.

Kasdin, A. E., & Weisz, J. R. (1998). Identifying and developing empirically supported child and adolescent treatments. *Journal of Consulting and Clinical Psychology, 66*, 19–36.

Kendall-Tackett, K. (2002). The health effects of childhood abuse: Four pathways by which abuse can influence health. *Child Abuse & Neglect, 26*, 715–729.

Kendall-Tackett, K., Williams, L. M., & Finkelhor, D. (1993). Impact of sexual abuse on children: A review and synthesis of recent empirical studies. *Psychological Bulletin, 113*, 164–180.

Legal Information Institute (1995). *The Child Abuse Prevention and Treatment Act (CAPTA)* [Online]. (US Code Colleection, Title 42, Chapter 67-subchapter I, Sec. 510g.) Available: http://www.4law.cornell.edu/uscode/42/5106g/html.

Levenson, J., & Morin, J. W. (2001a). *Connections workbook.* Thousand Oaks, CA: Sage.

Levenson, J., & Morin, J. W. (2001b). *Treating nonoffending parents in child sexual abuse cases.* Thousand Oaks, CA: Sage.

McEwen, B. S. (1998). Protective and damaging effects of stress mediators. *Seminars in medicine of the Beth Israel Deaconess Medical Center, 338*(3), 171–179.

Mueser, K. T., Goodman, L. B., Trumbetta, S. L., Rosenberg, S. D., Osher, F. C., Vidaver, R., Auciello, P., & Foy, D. W. (1998). Trauma and posttraumatic stress disorder in severe mental illness. *Journal of Consulting and Clinical Psychology, 66*, 493–499.

Murphy, W. D., & Smith, T. A. (1996). Sex offenders against children. Empirical and clinical issues. In J. Briere, L. Berliner & A. Bulkley (Eds.), *The APSAC handbook on child maltreatment* (pp. 175–192). Thousand Oaks, CA : Sage.

National Clearinghouse on Child Abuse and Neglect. (2001). Understanding the effects of maltreatment on early brain development [Online]. Available:

http://www.calib.com/nccanch/pubs/focus/earlybrain.cfm.

Parillo, K. M., Freeman, R. C., Collier, K., & Young, P. (2001). Association between early sexual abuse and adult HIV-risky sexual behaviors among community-recruited women. *Child Abuse & Neglect, 25,* 335–346.

Perry, B. D. (2001). The neurodevelopmental impact of violence in childhood. In D. Schetky & E. Benedek (Eds.), *Textbook of child and adolescent forensic psychiatry.* Washington, DC: American Psychiatric Press.

Pintello, D., & Zuravin, S. (2001). Intrafamilial child sexual abuse: Predictors of postdisclosure maternal belief and protective action. *Child Maltreatment, 6*(4), 344–352.

Polusny, M. A., & Follette, V. M. (1996). Remembering childhood sexual abuse: A national survey of psychologists' clinical practices, beliefs, and personal experiences. *Professional Psychology: Research and Practice, 27,* 41–52.

Price, J. L., Hilsenroth, M. J., Petretic-Jackson, P. A., & Bonge, D. (2001). A review of individual psychotherapy outcomes for adult survivors of childhood sexual abuse. *Clinical Psychology Review, 21,* 1095–1121.

Proulx, J., Tardif, M., Lamoureux, B., & Lussier, P. (2000). How does recidivism risk assessment predict survival? In J. R. Laws, S. M. Hudson & T. Ward (Eds.), *Remaking relapse prevention with sex offenders: A sourcebook.* Thousand Oaks, CA: Sage.

Rush, P. (1980). *The best kept secret: Sexual abuse of children.* Englewood Cliffs, NJ: Prentice Hall.

Russell, D. (1986). *The secret trauma.* New York: Basic Books.

Ryan, G., & Lane, S. (1991). *Juvenile sexual offenders.* Lexington, MA: Lexington Books.

Saywitz, K. J., Mannarino, A. P., Berliner, L., & Cohen, J. A. (2000). Treatment of sexually abused children and adolescents. *American Psychologist, 55,* 1040–1049.

Sedlak, A. J., & Broadhurst, D. D. (1996). The third national incidence study of child abuse and neglect. [Online]. Available: http://www.calib.com/nccanch/pubs/statinfo/nis3cfm.

Sedney, M. A., & Brooks, B. (1984). Factors associated with history of childhood sexual experience in a nonclinical female population. *Journal of the American Academy of Child Psychiatry, 23,* 215–218.

Shore, R. (1997). *Rethinking the brain.* New York: Families and Work Institute.

Smith, D. W., Letourneau, E. J., Saunders, B. E., Kilpatrick, D. G., Resnick, H. S., & Best, C. L. (2000). Delay in disclosure of childhood rape: Results from a national survey. *Child Abuse and Neglect, 24,* 273–287.

Strand, V. C. (2000). *Treating secondary victims: Intervention with the nonoffending mother in the incest family.* Thousand Oaks, CA: Sage.

Summit, R. C. (1989). The centrality of victimization: Regaining the focal point of recovery for survivors of child sexual abuse. *Psychiatric Clinics of North America, 12,* 413–430.

Urbancic, J. C. (1992). *The relationship between empowerment support, mental health self-care, incest trauma resolution, and subjective well-being.* Unpublished doctoral dissertation, Wayne State University, Detroit.

Urbancic, J. (1993). Intrafamilial sexual abuse. In J. Campbell & J. Humphries (Eds.), Nursing care of survivors of family violence. St. Louis, MO: Mosby.

Weiss, J., Roger, E., Darwin, M., & Dutton, C. (1955). A study of girl sex victims. *Psychiatric Quarterly, 29,* 1–27.

Williams, L. M. (1994). Recall of child trauma: A prospective study of women's memories of childhood sexual abuse. *Journal of Counseling and Clinical Psychology, 62,* 1167–1176.

Wilsnack, S. C., Wonderlich, S. A., Kristhanson, A. J., Vogeltanz-Holm, N. D., & Wilsnack, R. W. (2002). Self reports of forgetting and remembering childhood sexual abuse in a nationally representative sample of U.S. women. *Child Abuse and Neglect, 26,* 139–147.

Wilson, J. P., Friedman, M. J., & Lindy, J. D. (2001). Treating psychological trauma & PTSD. New York: Guilford Press.

Wyatt, G. E. (1985). The sexual abuse of Afro-American and White-American women in childhood. *Child Abuse and Neglect, 9,* 507–519.

Wyatt, G. E., & Powell, G. J. (1988). Lasting effects of child sexual abuse. Beverly Hills, CA: Sage.

Zlotnick, C., Mattia, J., & Zimmerman, M. (2001). Clinical features of survivors of sexual abuse with major depression. *Child Abuse and Neglect, 25,* 357–367.

Zoellner, L. A., Fitzgibbons, L. A., & Foa, E. B. (2001). Cognitive-behavioral approaches to PTSD. In J. P. Wilson, M. J. Friedman, & J. D. Lindy (Eds.), Treating psychological trauma and PTSD (pp. 159–182). New York: Guilford Press.

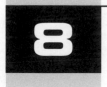

Nursing Care of Families Using Violence

- Kären Landenburger, Doris W. Campbell, and Rachel Rodriguez

Breaking Away

I have to escape from beneath this dark cloud cold,
ominous easy to hide in
Need to let sunshine into my life
I'll be blinded by the sudden burst of light
Like a child taking first steps
Falling down sometimes
Get up and try again
Raising my children not to hide beneath the cloud
Laughing and free, we'll grow together
getting our strength
from warmth
of the light

Reprinted from *Every Twelve Seconds*, compiled by Susan Venters
(Hillsboro, Oregon: Shelter, 1981) by permission of the author.

A violent family is in pain. Without understanding the underlying dynamics or necessarily labeling the violent behavior as a problem, violent family members are hurting each other emotionally and physically. Even those members who are not victims or perpetrators are learning that violence is acceptable and are highly at risk to use violence themselves, either in the family or outside it. They are also hurt by the destructive family dynamics. Their homes are schools in which the children learn to become violent adults. Nurses see such families in hospitals, clinics, homes, and mental-health settings. Effective nursing care is crucial in preventing further violence and in helping these families to end the pain.

A violent family is considered to be one in which at least one family member is using physical or sexual force against another, resulting in physical and emotional destructive injury or both. The issue of when physical discipline of children becomes destructive is important; it is discussed in Chapter 3. In most cases, there is also intent to injure on the part of the violent family member, although this is frequently difficult to determine. A violent family can be one in which there is child abuse, wife abuse, abuse of elderly members, severe physical aggression between siblings, violence by adolescents against parents, or any combination thereof. A family in which there is incest is also considered to be violent, because even if physical force is not used it is implied, and destructive injury is a consequence.

This chapter describes the nursing care of violent or potentially violent families in which the family as a whole is considered the focus of intervention. This chapter also suggests nursing measures for decreasing violence in society in general, which will have the effect of decreasing the legitimacy of violence within families.

Four areas of theoretical background are important in setting the stage for nursing care of violent families. It is necessary to understand:

- Family theoretical perspectives and approaches
- Why the family seems especially prone to use violence as a conflict-resolution strategy
- The evidence suggesting the intergenerational transmission of violence
- The connections between wife abuse and child abuse

FAMILY THEORY AND FAMILY-THERAPY PERSPECTIVES

A theoretical framework is useful in guiding clinical efforts in any area of nursing. Theories from nursing, family social sciences, and family therapy may all be useful in assessing problems, defining goals, and planning appropriate interventions with families experiencing violence. Relevant discussions of nursing theories and family nursing process are found in Oermann (1991), and Friedman (1998). Goldenberg and Goldenberg (2000) provided an overview of basic models of family therapy. McGoldrick (1998) expanded traditional views of family and family therapy and offered a more inclusive cultural perspective than one usually finds in conventional family-therapy literature. Empirical studies based on many of these theories and models provide important information on their utility for guiding the involvement of professionals with violent families. With more research, it is likely that the formulation of more effective family intervention and prevention strategies will become possible.

The following frameworks from the family social sciences and family therapy are some prominent family theoretical perspectives.

Systems Approach

Based on a systems-theory framework, the family is viewed as an open social system with boundaries, self-regulatory mechanisms, interacting and superordinate systems, and subcomponents. The family system is composed of a set of logically related, interacting subsystems (e.g., a spouse subsystem, a parent–child subsystem, and a sibling subsystem). Important assumptions of a systems perspective are the following: a change in one member of the system ultimately results in changes in the entire system; the system is greater than the sum of its parts; and the system is capable of self-regulation and can adapt and change (Friedman, 1998).

A nurse whose practice is guided by a systems perspective assesses the individual members of the family as well as the family as a whole. Intervention strategies should be directed toward the family as an interacting system as well as toward the larger systems with which the family must relate.

Structural-Functional Approach

This perspective also views the family as a social system, but with more of an outcome orientation than a process orientation. The structural-functional approach is grounded in Gestalt psychology, which emphasizes that one must view the whole and its parts and explore the interrelationships between them. The general assumptions of the structural-functional perspective are that the family is a social system with functional requirements, a small group possessing certain generic features common to all small groups, and a social system that accomplishes functions that serve the individual in addition to the society (Friedman, 1998).

The concept of structure refers to how the family is organized, the manner in which units are arranged, and how these units relate to each other. Important dimensions of family structure include role structure, value systems, communication processes, and power structure. These elements are intimately interrelated and interacting. Family structure is ultimately evaluated by how well the family is able to fulfill its functions—the goals important to its members and society.

Family functions are defined as outcomes or consequences of the family structure (e.g., what the family does). Examples of family functions to be assessed from this theoretical perspective are the family's affective function, socialization and social-placement function, reproduction function, economic function, and health-care function. Relationships between the family and other social systems (e.g., the health-care system) are also examined (Friedman, 1998; Oermann, 1991).

The nurse whose practice is grounded in structural-functional theory finds it a useful framework for examining the family as a holistic unit and assessing how the family interacts with other institutions. This approach is compatible with general systems theory and interfaces well with a developmental perspective of the family.

Developmental Approach

Theories of family development attempt to account for changes in the family over time, based on the idea that families are long-lived groups with a natural history or life cycle. Family development theory describes family life over time by dividing the family life cycle into a series of discrete stages (such as changes in the family when new members are added or subtracted, changes in the developmental stages of the oldest child, and changes in child-rearing and discipline practices). The most widely used formulation of family developmental stages is the eight-stage family life cycle devised adapted by Duvall and Miller (1985).

Family developmental theory does not address situational or nonnormative stressors, and this is its major weakness. The assumption of homogeneity of families and stability within each stage presents a middle-class bias that fails to consider the diversity in American families. Despite these limitations, family developmental theory does increase understanding of families at different points in their life cycles and generates "typical" descriptions of family life during the various stages. Variations from the traditional family are accounted for in examining the family life cycle from different perspectives, such as those of divorced families, domestic-partner relationships, and families with disabilities or long-term illness (Friedman, 1998; Oermann, 1991).

The nurse can use a developmental perspective to guide the assessment of the family's developmental stage and its performance of the tasks appropriate to that stage. The nurse can then develop guidelines for analyzing family growth and health promotion needs and should be able to better provide the support needed for smooth progression from one stage to another.

Interactional/Communication Approach

The interactional/communication approach focuses on how family members relate to one another; family dynamics or family processes are the core of the framework. Processes considered important to investigate include roles, status relations, communication patterns, decision-making patterns, and socialization. The interactional/communication perspective does not examine the family within its external environment nor how the external social system interfaces with the family. The interactional approach is therefore limited because the family is viewed as self-contained (Friedman, 1998; Oermann, 1991). However, it is a valid approach to use when exploring the meaning or perception various acts or symbols have for people in an interaction.

Family Ecological Perspective

The family ecological perspective incorporates the family environment into any examination of the family. It is sometimes referred to as the ecosystem approach because it explores relationships between a changing environment and a changing family. The major concepts of the theory are the environed unit (family), the environment, and the patterning of interactions and transactions between them (Oermann, 1991). The family ecomap can be used to perform an ecological assessment of the family.

The family ecological framework proposed by Bronfenbrenner (1979) is an example of a systems approach in which the family is pictured as part of three nested structures: the microsystem, mesosystem, and macrosystem. The individual family members are nested within the immediate setting that includes the family (the microsystem). The microsystem is situated within and affected by a mesosystem, which includes not only the individual family members but also the immediate larger social environment. The mesosystem is nested within a macrosystem, an even larger environment and social setting that includes a community's ideology, values, and social institutions (Friedman, 1998).

Family Paradigm Theory

Family paradigm theory assumes that the family's basic beliefs guide its interpretation of and responses to a variety of social situations. This model of the family, developed by Reiss (1981), explains variations in families that are based on their shared beliefs about the social world and their family's place within it.

Four family paradigms based on distinct approaches used by families to problem-solve are consensus-sensitive (closed) families, achievement-sensitive (random) families, environment-sensitive (open) families, and distance-sensitive (synchronous) families. Reiss (1981) and a team of researchers have presented some evidence in support of the major concepts of this theory.

Family rituals are mechanisms used by families to stabilize identity, clarify roles, delineate boundaries, and thus conserve the family's paradigm or worldview. Examples of family rituals are family traditions, family celebrations, and patterned family interactions (Campbell, 1991). Ritual use in families can be explored to provide clues to difficulties families face in maintaining the family's paradigm and its shared identity, during challenging periods of change or conflict (Campbell, 1991).

The nurse can use ritual assessment to evaluate the extent to which the family has had to give up certain rituals and routines because of a severe clinical problem such as family violence. The nurse can also help the family consider ways to adapt cherished rituals or develop new and meaningful ones.

Family Stress Perspective

Hill (1949) conceptualized the family stress model (ABCX) to describe variations in how families cope with stress. Hill postulated that A (the stressor event) interacting with B (the family's crisis-meeting resources) and with C (the definition the family makes of the event) produces X (the crisis). In this model, Hill defined a stressor as a situation for which the family has had little or no prior preparation. A crisis is defined as any sharp or decisive change from which old patterns are inadequate (McCubbin & Patterson, 1982).

Hill's original conceptualization has been expanded by McCubbin and Patterson (1982), who added postcrisis variables to the model to describe the additional life stressors and changes that may influence the family's ability to achieve adaptation. The model is referred to as the Double ABCX model of family stress and coping. In this framework, the aA factor represents family demands or pileup, which include event-related stressors and family hardships as well as prior strains that continue to affect family life. The double-B (bB) factor refers to the family's existing resources as well as those strengthened or developed in response to the demands of the crisis. The double-C (cC) factor is the meaning the family gives to the total crisis situation, which includes the stressor believed to have caused the crisis as well as stressors and strains that have accumulated since the onset of the event. The double X (xX) factor refers to the outcome of family efforts or family adaptation (Oermann, 1991).

A more recent version of the Double ABCX Model is the T-Double ABCX Model of Family Adjustment and Adaptation proposed by McCubbin and McCubbin (1987). This variation adds the T-factor, which addresses those family types, strengths, and capabilities that explain why some families are better suited than others are to adjust and adapt to changes. Four family types identified by McCubbin and McCubbin (1987) are regenerative, resilient, rhythmic, and ritualistic. The typologies are based on dimensions of family strength, such as family hardiness, family coherence, family bonding, family flexibility, family time and routines, valuing of that time, family celebrations, and family traditions (Artinian & Conger, 1997; Oermann, 1991).

Family stress models have relevance for nursing because they provide a framework for assessment and intervention with the family in a variety of areas. For example, the aA factor can guide the nurse to view family violence in terms of the stressors and hardships it has placed on the family. The cC factor can guide the nurse to try to understand the meaning the family gives to the violence and to the total crisis situation surrounding it.

Feminist Perspectives

Feminist theory focuses on women and attempts to understand patterning of the human experience from a paradigm that incorporates assumptions and beliefs about the origins and consequences of gendered social organization, as well as strategic directions and actions for social change. Issues of gender, inequality, power and privilege, patriarchy, and the subordination of women can all be examined from a feminist perspective. Yllö (1993) and Bograd (1999) proposed that current family theories and the therapies based on them are inadequate explanatory and treatment models, and they described how feminist theory can foster knowledge and understanding of both generational and gender issues. Research based on perspectives from feminist theory is needed to help answer such questions as why the family takes the form it does at the present time. Could families be constituted differently? Feminist theory could also provide a framework for studying the social genesis of such problems as wife-battering, incest, and other problems that occur frequently among women but have been largely neglected by family therapists (Bograd, 1999; Yllö, 1993). This approach guides nurses to be aware of the gender-related power imbalances within families that maintain many forms of family violence.

Object Relations Theory

Although feminist theory has broadened the scope of traditional theories, Kozol (1995) and McGoldrick, (1998) critiqued the strengths and limitations of feminist theories and domestic violence, stating that individuals may experience multiple forms of oppression. A focus on gender oppression alone does not fully explain experiences or attack the issue from a broad perspective within contexts of racism, heterosexism, or classism.

Zosky (1999) claimed that no one theory is adequate in examining family violence. Whereas feminist theory is helpful in understanding violence on a macro or social level and systems theory assists in explaining the dynamics within the family, object relations theory directs analysis on the intrapsychic level. Cultural perspectives are emphasized in the work of Yick (2001) and Hamby (2000). Yick, focusing on the Asian-American population and Chinese Americans in particular, and Hamby, focusing on American Indians, suggested that it is essential that we understand how cultural beliefs and norms influence responses to family violence. Both writers emphasized how it is common to assume similarities across different ethnic or tribal groups and how these assumptions can hinder our ability to work effectively with violence in these communities. Bograd (1999) emphasized that by not explicitly examining domestic violence from multiple perspectives we may in a sense make invisible the experiences of those who are not members of the dominant culture.

Collectively, the various family theories and family therapy approaches provide partial perspectives for understanding the individual, family, societal, cultural, and contextual factors that contribute to family violence. Future directions of practice must be more inclusive of issues of race, sexual orientation, and the multiple stereotypes that prejudice the care of various groups of people. Increased understandings in these areas can lead to more effective intervention with families experiencing violence.

No unifying family theory ties together the various types of family violence under one conceptual umbrella, and it is unlikely that such a model can be constructed, given the qualitatively unique developmental and life-span issues associated with violence directed toward children, adults, and the elderly (Ammerman & Hersen, 1991). Because numerous factors mediate the extent, severity, and impact of family violence, the level of intervention required for treatment (primary, secondary, or tertiary) varies.

The essence of family-centered nursing involves understanding the dynamics of the family and all the forces, both internal and external, that affect it. Nurses may be required to gain insights into concepts from a variety of highly complex theoretical and intervention models to deliver effective care to families experiencing violence.

THE FAMILY AS A VIOLENCE-PRODUCING INSTITUTION

Through work with a nationally representative sample, Gelles and his associates (1997) estimated that 28% of conjugal pairs report some form of physical violence during marriage. This research is supported by the National Violence against Women Survey (Tjaden & Thoennes, 2000) that reports 25% of women and 7.6% of men report having experienced, in their lifetime, some form of physical violence while in an intimate partner relationship. A national survey conducted by the National Committee to Prevent Child Abuse (Weise & Daro, 1995) found that 33% of children were victims of child abuse or neglect. Female parents were more likely to neglect or physically abuse their children, whereas male parents were more likely to sexually abuse their children (National Institute of Justice, 2001). Margolin (1992) asserted that if research were to control for the time spent caring for children, males would be more likely to physically abuse their children than females. Children experiencing child abuse and neglect were 29 percent more likely to be involved in criminal activity as a juvenile or an adult (National Institute of Justice, 2001).

Most of the literature on intimate partner violence focuses on heterosexual violence among young-to-midlife couples. Populations that have been overlooked in surveys on domestic violence are siblings and the elderly. There is a dearth of literature on violence in gay and lesbian relationships, and further research needs to be conducted to corroborate what results there are and to determine the extent of violence in these types of relationships. The latest National Violence against Women Survey (Tjaden & Thoennes, 2000) found that women in lesbian relationships experience less violence than do women in heterosexual relationships. There is also a need to better understand family violence among ethnic minorities. If nurses are to assist individuals from various cultures, it is important to acknowledge differences and similarities across the types of violence as well as among different groups of people experiencing family violence.

Gelles (1997) stated that sibling violence is the most common form of violence in intimate relationships. Social norms that support aggression, particularly in boys, hinder obtaining a clear picture of the extent and nature of the abuse that takes place. Limited data has shown that boys are more violent than girls are and that sibling violence decreases as children grow older. In addition, there is growing evidence that elderly family members are abused. Elder abuse takes many forms and can include physical and emotional abuse, neglect of the elderly person's physical and emotional needs, and financial abuse in the form of fraud and money mismanagement (Kleinschmidt, 1997; Wilber & Reynolds, 1996). In some cases, the roles of victim and perpetrator of abuse are reversed. The elderly person who once was the perpetrator of abuse may become the victim of abuse and neglect (Baron & Welty, 1996).

There appears to be substantial reductions in the rates of child abuse between 1993 and 1999 (National Clearinghouse on Child Abuse and Neglect,

1999). It is difficult to determine if there have been changes in the incidence of intimate partner violence because of variability in how data has been collected over the last 25 years (Tjaden & Thoennes, 2000).

Such family-violence data explodes the myth that the American family is a nonviolent institution. Gelles (1997) identified several factors that he believes contribute in general to violence in the family. He asserted that some of the very characteristics that make families prone to domestic violence also contribute to the supportive atmosphere of the family group.

One characteristic is that there is a great deal of "time at risk" for violence between family members. They spend many hours of every day interacting with each other, which could provide the occasion for violence. Closely related is the idea that the wide range of family activities and interests affords many possible areas of conflict.

The intensity of involvement in families is another potentiating factor. What may be a minor irritation in a relationship with a friend or coworker may be seriously upsetting between family members. The activities of family members may also impinge on each other's privacy, usage of family equipment, and ability to engage in activities of their own. The many different ages and the difference in gender among family members are also conflict-generating factors (Gelles, 1997; Straus & Gelles, 1990).

Some family members may believe that they have the right to try to influence the behavior and values of each other, which sets the stage for disagreements. Children have no choice about belonging to the family; thus, solving problems by leaving the group is usually impossible for them. Major life stressors, inherent in the development of the family, also contribute to the possibility of physical aggression, yet the nuclear family of today is frequently isolated from the support systems of relatives. Finally, the American culture sanctions a certain amount of violence within families both overtly, as in approval of physical punishment for children, and covertly, as in the widespread tolerance if not approval of men hitting their female partners (Gelles, 1997; Straus & Gelles, 1990).

Because of these characteristics, the family can become very stressful and produce conflict. Ascribed roles, conflicting agendas among family members, and the intensity of interaction all are factors that contribute to family violence (Gelles, 1997). Adults also may have been taught in their childhood that violence is an acceptable way to solve problems and therefore be more apt to use physical aggression in response to stresses.

THE INTERGENERATIONAL TRANSMISSION OF VIOLENCE

Social learning theory (see Chapter 1) provides the background for understanding the possibility of intergenerational transmission of violence within families. When children are hit by their parents, even as a disciplinary measure, they learn a powerful message. First, the parents are demonstrating that violence is an acceptable way to deal with conflict and, second, that love and violence are intertwined. Through the family, children may learn not only modes of violence but justification to support it in the family (Gelles, 1997).

The family functions within the context of a larger society. Social norms of masculinity, the socialization of both female and male children, and societal views of women all contribute to the transmission of violence (Miedzian, 1995).

Neither childhood victimization nor the witnessing of violence mandates later adult perpetration of abuse. Nor does the absence of childhood victimization insulate the family against violence perpetration, especially if the learning of social skills or controls against violence was inadequate during childhood (Gelles, 1997). Therefore, one must be careful when attributing family violence to childhood learning. Although some children who have grown up in abusive households may become abusive parents, most children will not transmit violence from one generation to the next (Harrington & Dubowtiz, 1993).

THE CONNECTIONS BETWEEN WIFE ABUSE AND CHILD ABUSE

Child abuse and intimate partner violence often co-occur in the family. Estimates vary regarding the amount of overlap. Most research, though, has indicated a higher rate of child abuse for violent couples, as compared to families without intimate partner violence, and a higher rate of wife abuse in husbands documented as child abusers, as compared to families without child abuse (O'Leary, Smith-Slep, & O'Leary, 2000; Rumm, Cummings, Krauss, Bell, & Rivara, 2000). This evidence provides support for the view that certain families tend to use violence as their principal conflict-resolution strategy.

In homes with intimate partner violence, children may suffer both directly and indirectly. Children may be the direct recipients of abuse by either parent figure. Although a child may not be physically abused directly, emotional abuse may be experienced through witnessing abusive incidents. In addition, a child may also experience emotional trauma indirectly if his or her primary caretaker suffers from depression and anxiety (Hughes & Luke, 1998; Salzinger et al., 2002). In families experiencing co-occurrence of violence, children have greater difficulties handling stress and experience more behavioral problems than their peers do (Shipman, Rossman, & West, 1999).

The studies of abused women and children have also emphasized the interrelationship between spouse and child abuse. The factors associated with the family as a violence-prone institution—the intergenerational transmission of violence and the connections between wife abuse and child abuse—suggest that families that are violent or prone to being violent need interventions as a total unit. Nursing interventions with these families are based on the nursing process and begin with assessment of the family. Nursing care should take place within the context of the family's social and cultural background.

CULTURALLY SENSITIVE CARE

Culturally sensitive family nursing care is based on understanding and respect for the diversity of backgrounds and perspectives found in American families. The United States is a multicultural society with many ethnic and cultural groups. Practitioners, researchers, and policy makers are becoming increasingly aware of the need for cultural understanding in the area of domestic violence. Although current literature addresses specific populations, such as African Americans, Latinos, Native Americans, and Arab Americans to name a few, much work remains to be done to avoid the trap of stereotyping or creating a "recipe" approach to caring for battered women of diverse cultures. In many areas of the United States, particularly in small rural areas, communities are experiencing for the first time an influx of people of diverse ethnic backgrounds, skin color, and religious beliefs. Nurses and other health-care providers may feel overwhelmed by the increasing numbers of diverse clients requesting services. Because of this, they may be looking for quick answers regarding how to care for this diverse clientele. It is often frustrating to realize that there are no quick and easy "recipes" to follow when caring for clients from a different cultural group.

Warrior and colleagues (2002) provided a critical definition of culture as "shared experiences and commonalities that evolve under changing social and political landscapes" (p. 662). They further stated that previous definitions that included the idea that culture is something passed on from generation to generation are outdated because culture is not static. Warrior and colleagues also explained that we "must look at how race, class, gender, sexual orientation, and other axes come together for different communities in different locations during different times" (p. 662). Finally, and probably the most important, these researchers stressed that "culture is part of all of us. It does not exist outside of us" (p. 663).

Assessment of the family's cultural orientation is critical to understanding and working effectively with families from cultures different from the nurse's own background. It is important to realize that discussions of how to assess and intervene with various cultural groups run the "risk of promoting stereotypes that misrepresent and oversimplify the cultures involved" (Gary & Kavanagh, 1991, p. 149). Nonetheless, the nurse must be willing to try to understand the complexities and life conditions under which different groups have developed their worldviews and under which they function.

It is equally important for nurses to understand that regardless of whether they have participated in cultural-competency or cultural-awareness training, they must first and foremost become aware of their own cultural lens through which they interpret the world. Thus, the key to creating a positive interaction between nurse and client(s) is to realize that the meeting of the two (or more) cultures is what is important.

Friedman (1998) recommended that the following factors be used when assessing a family's cultural orientation:

- Ethnic/racial identity
- Languages spoken
- Place of birth
- Geographical mobility
- Family's religion
- Ethnic-group affiliation
- Neighborhood affiliation
- Dietary habits, dress
- Household appearance
- Use of folk systems
- Acceptance by community

Cultural-assessment questions that cover these basic areas should be integrated throughout the entire family assessment. The results will provide the nurse with comprehensive data about cultural influences related to family organization (role, power, values, and communication patterns), child-rearing practices, affective responses, health-care practices and beliefs, and coping strategies (Friedman, 1998). This information is invaluable in developing an effective database from which to plan care for the family experiencing family violence.

ASSESSMENT

Before nurses can make effective assessments for violence in families, they must examine their feelings and thoughts about the subject and be committed to the idea that violence is an important health problem and within the scope of nursing. Violence is not an easy area to explore with families, and it is usually easier to just avoid it. Strong feelings of anger and despair may be aroused in family members, and of justifiable fear in nurses. Nursing educational programs now routinely discuss violence in families as part of their basic curricula. For nurses who still feel ill at ease, attendance at workshops on the issue and arrangement for group discussions with colleagues may go far to alleviate anxiety around the routine exploration of violence in families. In both settings, role-playing can help nurses anticipate dealing with confrontations within families.

Once a family member has been identified as violent or potentially violent, that information affects the nurse's interactions with him or her. Nurses need to be able to share their fear with peers and explore ways of handling it through discussion. Established protocols are often available in primary-care and emergency-practice settings. Consensus guidelines have been developed by several professional organizations dealing with specific types of family violence (e.g., child abuse and neglect, intimate partner violence, and elder abuse). In addition, several states mandate regular continuing-education requirements in specific areas such as domestic violence.

The incidence of physical injury and death from violence outside and especially within the home indicates the seriousness of the problem. Nurses are in people's homes probably more than any other professionals are. If nursing care of families does not include assessing for and intervening against violence, it will probably not be identified until someone has been seriously injured or killed. Rather than waiting for that to occur and letting the police, courts, or social worker intervene at that point, with demonstrably poor results, nurses can work for early identification and prevention, as with any other serious health problem. After self-examination of feelings and acquisition of knowledge, the nurse is in a prime position to make a significant impact in the prevention of morbidity and mortality from violence.

The nurse should examine whether she or he thinks that family conflict resolution is a private, family matter. This belief can be discussed in workshops or nursing conferences in the institution of employment. The families may also share this view and perceive their privacy as being invaded by questioning. If the nurse handles questions in this realm as if they were routine, with a matter-of-fact demeanor, the inquiry will seem more comfortable. If the family questions the need for such exploration, the nurse can share the facts about the prevalence of abuse and injuries from violence. This is valuable not only in making the family feel more at ease but also in educating the public about the problem. The first few times that assessment about violence is discussed may be uncomfortable, but just as nurses have learned to include sexual-functioning assessment without discomfort, assessment of violence in the family can also be learned, with practice, to be handled easily.

An equally important area to consider in any family assessment is family strengths. The healthy areas of family functioning need to be explored with the family, both to see the total picture and to identify areas that can be built on in nursing interventions. McCown and Artinian (1997) used an intersystem approach to look at the family as a dynamic unit within a sociocultural environment. Using this model, the nurse assesses the family using the framework of three interactive subsystems: biological, psychological, and spiritual subsystems. Each subsystem identifies specific areas for assessment.

The biological subsystem assesses areas of family development, role functioning, and ability of the family to meet basic needs. The psychological subsystem assesses coping strategies, decision-making patterns, communication, and family rituals and traditions. Religious socialization or spiritual beliefs are explored in the spiritual subsystem.

Through this assessment, past and present areas of family functioning in which individual members' needs are met by the family and in which the family has adequate physical and affective resources can be identified. An inventory of social supports both within and outside the family can be developed. Such an inventory can be used to identify those who are providing direct aid, emotional support, or affirmation to members or the total family unit. Relationships that can be strengthened and further enhanced become evident. Healthy coping mechanisms used to deal with normative life changes and developmental issues are identified. Areas in which the family feels a sense of accomplishment and in which past problems were effectively solved need as thorough an exploration as areas of difficulty. Family actions that foster appropriate help-seeking and utilization behavior can be identified as actions to be encouraged for future referrals. As a general indication of family well-being, each individual member can be asked about his or her life as a whole and his or her perception of the family. Family functions that have enhanced individual and total unit perceptions of well-being are identified as important family mechanisms and should be commended.

Assessment of a total family is usually done in primary health-care, community, and mental-health settings when an entire family has been referred. Whenever a family history is being taken, it is important that patterns of family conflict-resolution are explored. Questions about this should also be included in the social/personal section of the history of individuals. Physical assessment of family members includes looking for signs of trauma. Observations of intrafamilial interactions are also important in family assessment. The history, physical examination, and nursing observations, if conducted with awareness, reveal potential and actual family-violence problems.

History

Several areas of family history can indicate the potentiality or actuality of violence problems. These areas, along with at-risk findings, have been outlined in Table 8-1. In addition, as part of the data collection, the nurse should directly ask about physical aggression. Questions about methods of disciplining children, including physical punishment, are usually routinely asked in the nursing history of families, but in the past direct inquiry about other forms of violence has often been neglected. The nurse needs to ask about the existence of hitting or other unwanted physical contact between any family members.

Nursing judgment is required in assessing how many of the at-risk findings indicate a real problem with physical aggression. Physical punishment of children is considered by many to be normal and to require little follow-up questioning. On initial assessment, the nurse needs to inquire more about such child-rearing practices, how often physical punishment is used, whether or not

Table 8-1 • **Nursing-History Indicators of Potential or Actual Violence in a Family**

AREA OF ASSESSMENT	AT-RISK RESPONSES
Information from genogram	Severe physical punishment or husband-wife violence in parental families of origin Violent death or serious injury from violence Family members in parental families of origin using violence outside the home Wife abuse in husband's previous marital relationship
Family structure	Single-parent home Dependent grandparent in home Blended family (involving stepparents and/or stepchildren)
Family resources	Unemployment; poverty Inadequate housing Elderly member with controlled resources Financial problems Total control of monetary resources by male head of household Perception of inadequate "fit" of family resources to family demands
Family roles	Rigid traditional sex roles Individual or family dissatisfaction with roles family expects individuals to fulfill Incompatible roles Rigid, unchangeable roles
Family boundaries	Rigid boundaries; mistrust of all outsiders
Family communication patterns	Nonnurturing family communications, destructive to some members Communications ambiguous Lack of communication among family members
Family conflict-resolution patterns	Extensive use of verbal aggression; many threats of violence Evidence of physical aggression used in husband-wife, parent-child, sibling-sibling, or parent-grandparent conflict resolution
Family power distribution	Autocratic decision-making by father Children have no power Grandparent in home who is powerless Frequent power struggles
Family values	Violence considered acceptable or valued Great incongruence of values among family members or between family and society Intolerance of differing values among family members
Emotional climate	High tension in home Lack of visible affection Scapegoating High anxiety in family members(s) Lack of support between family members Frequent disparagement between family members
Division of labor	Rigid division of labor according to gender Member highly dissatisfied with division of labor
Support systems	Family isolation Family inhibitions to help seeking Children not forming close, supportive peer relationships (especially same-sex peer relationships) Lack of support systems considered useful for direct aid, emotional support, and/or affirmation Relatives are highly critical; tension among extended family

(continued)

Table 8-1 • Nursing-History Indicators of Potential or Actual Violence in a Family (Continued)

AREA OF ASSESSMENT	AT-RISK RESPONSES
Developmental stages	More than one family member facing difficult developmental crisis Lack of knowledge in parents of what to expect at various developmental stages of children, selves, and grandparents
Stressors	At-risk scores on stress scale Lack of past successful coping mechanisms to deal with stress Situational crises Stress-related physical symptoms in family members
Socialization of children	Physical punishment used Only one parent disciplines children Lack of nurturance of children Children displaying aggressive behavior, at home or outside of home Juvenile delinquency or sexual promiscuity in children
Health history	Frequent trauma injuries to family members Adolescent suicide attempts Serious illness in a family member History of treatment for mental illness or vaginal trauma History of venereal disease or genital trauma in children Substance abuse by any family member

such implements as belts are ever used, and whether the form of such punishment is spanking, slapping, or hitting with fists. After a relationship with the family is established, this area can be readdressed, and the nurse can discuss the implications of even the mildest forms of physical punishment.

Nurses and other practitioners are increasingly recognizing the prevalence and damaging effects of psychological maltreatment or emotional abuse in families. There is emerging evidence, although the literature is still small, that psychological maltreatment occurs on a continuum of hurtful behaviors, from speaking in angry, verbally aggressive tones on one end to pervasive, one-sided, severe psychological torture paralleling intentional brainwashing and mistreatment of prisoners of war (Tolman, 1992). The nurse must assess for psychological maltreatment of individuals in families, especially women and children. Categories of assessment include discussing threats that create fear; verbal put-downs and degrading behaviors that make the individual feel less competent, less adequate, or even less human; isolation; economic abuse (limited or no access to financial resources); rigid sex-role expectations; and emotional or interpersonal withholding. Besides physical abuse, it is equally important to assess for emotional abuse or psychological maltreatment because they often occur in combination. Further, emotional or psychological maltreatment may continue even if the physical violence stops during treatment. Psychological maltreatment of children threatens their psychological integrity and may lead to a significant pervasive psychological dysfunction (Vondra, Kolar, & Radigan, 1992).

Sibling fighting is typically not fully explored. Gelles (1997) stated that if "normal" interactions among siblings are considered, sibling violence is the most common form of family violence. Hitting between siblings is so common that it is rarely considered violence. Children often learn how to handle anger in their relationships with brothers and sisters and from their parents' guidance in such interactions. When brothers and sisters are allowed to use unrestricted physical aggression against each other, they also learn that violence is endorsed as a way to solve problems. The potential for severe violence in such conflicts is also frequently overlooked. Extrapolating from their findings in the large national survey of family violence, Straus, Gelles, and Steinmetz (1980) estimated that "2.3 million children in the United States have at some time used a knife or gun on a brother or sister" (p. 117). Sibling physical aggression no longer can be considered either normal or as something to be overlooked.

Sexual abuse within the family is difficult to assess and may only be revealed after intense involvement with the family. Nurses must be aware of the possibility of incest and try to elicit information about its occurrence when there are indications that it may be a possibility. Incest involves secrecy, fear, guilt, shame, and coercion. Child victims in incestuous families frequently fear bodily harm and withdrawal of affection. These may be powerful in eliciting compliance with the perpetrator's demands (Damon, Card, & Todd, 1992). Taking an individual history on each family member before, during, or after conducting the physical examination in private may be an avenue for uncovering sexual abuse.

Victims of incest may experience problems with trust. Sexual abuse often destroys a child's sense of trust because the very person who should offer protection exploits the child (Faller, 1993). Therefore, the development of trust is the first step in the assessment.

Changes in the behavior of the child or indications of vaginal irritation or trauma are important suggestions that incestuous activities have occurred. It is also important to assess the relationship, by observation and history, of female children to adult males who are in and around the home frequently. It must be remembered that sexual abuse is frequently carried out by uncles, cousins, and close family friends as well as by fathers and stepfathers. The mother of the child may have suspicions of the incest, and as the relationship with the nurse develops she may ask oblique questions concerning "normal" sexual activity or make general references to problems in the sexual relationship between herself and her spouse. It is important that these questions are followed up; if there is any indication of possible sexual abuse, direct queries should be made about it. For a young child the question might be "has anyone ever touched your private parts or other parts of your body with their private parts or hands or body in a way that hurt you or made you feel bad?" The nurse should substitute the term the child uses for vagina or penis for "private parts." For an adolescent, the question could be "has anyone ever forced or pressured you into sexual activities you did not wish to participate in?"

The incestuous family is often very closed and tends to isolate itself from helping professionals. A tone of secrecy in the family and a closed attitude toward the nurse's questions during the history-taking phase may be an indicator of incest. It is important to keep the lines of communication open with these families and delay closing the case until further assessment can be made. It may take a long time before trust can be engendered in these families, and the nurse must be patient. Another way to obtain the needed information is to elicit the help of another adult who the child trusts; often a teacher or school nurse can be helpful in this regard. The nurse can share concerns and uneasiness about possible sexual abuse in the family and ask the other professional to conduct a similar assessment. If the suspicions of incest are strong, protective services must be informed as with any other case of child abuse. There is no such thing as consensual sex between an adult family member and a child. A child is powerless in relation to an adult and is not free to refuse a sexual advance. The child's trust of caretakers and desire to comply with adults leave a child open to manipulation and violation of boundaries. As a result, the child is overwhelmed and feels betrayed, powerless, and traumatized (Faller, 1993).

Assessment Tools

The genogram or kinship diagram is an important tool of family assessment. The genogram can include questions on violence as well as other health problems and concerns. Violence must be asked about specifically or it will not be revealed. Because of intergenerational transmission of violence, the genogram should include inquiries about wife and child abuse, violent injury and death, histories of incarceration for violent crime, and family members' use of violence in interpersonal relationships outside the home. Cultural sensitivity and an awareness of differential treatment by the law according to race and class is necessary when assessing this information, however. Specific questions like "have you ever been hit?" with follow-up questions as to how often the hitting occurred and its severity are more useful than using the word abuse. Many people do not recognize a history of significant violence as abuse when it has happened to them or a family member.

Nursing assessment of families may include more formal assessment tools that tap areas of concern, especially for determining potential for violence. The Feetham Family Functioning Survey (FFFS) has been shown to be a reliable and concurrently valid nursing measure that can quickly indicate perceptions of dissatisfaction with family functioning (Roberts & Feetham, 1982). The instrument is designed to be self-administered and can be completed in 10 minutes. When scores on this instrument indicate perception of problems in family functioning, it provides a useful starting point for discussion about the areas indicated as problematic (for example, the FFFS indicator "Disagreement with Spouse"). McCubbin, Thompson, and McCubbin (1996) developed a series of inventories useful for family assessment in the areas of resiliency, coping, and adaptation. Blau, Dall, and Anderson (1993) suggested other individual and parenting scales that are helpful in the assessment of family violence.

Physical Assessment

In addition to physical examination of individual family members, an important part of the objective portion of assessment is observations of family interactions. Physical at-risk findings of child abuse can be found in Chapter 11 (Box 11-5). Table 8-2 lists other observational indicators of possible family violence. Family interactions sometimes show discrepancies between what actually happens and what has been described. Home visits with as many family members present as possible are invaluable in this regard. Community-health nursing-home visits often take place when only the mother, preschool children, and possibly a grandparent are at home, and the nurse may miss important elements. Creativity is needed to ensure a total assessment of the family, and interventions for family violence are almost impossible if the nurse only has a relationship with the mother. The nurse should attempt to have fairly lengthy visits of initial assessment. Children may be able to maintain their "best behavior" for a short time, but a longer visit often allows interactions to become nearly what they normally are.

AREA OF ASSESSMENT	AT-RISK RESPONSES
	Table 8-2 • **Nursing Observations Indicating Potential or Actual Violence in a Family**
General considerations	Observations differ significantly from information gathered on history
Family resources	Family members inadequately clothed and groomed One family member inadequately clothed and/or groomed, but the rest are not Household totally disorganized, and family members indicate displeasure with the lack of organization
Family roles	One parent looks at the other to have major interaction with children One parent answers all questions One parent looks at other for approval before answering questions
Family communication patterns	Members continually interrupt each other Members answer questions for each other; one member never talks for him or herself Negative nonverbal behavior in other members when one family member speaks Members frequently misunderstand each other Members do not listen to each other
Family conflict resolution	Verbal aggression used in front of nurse
Family power distribution	Members act afraid of another member One person makes all decisions Power struggles
Emotional climate	Members who don't speak or who are unhappy, anxious, or fearful Excessive physical distance maintained between members Members never touch each other Tense atmosphere Secretive atmosphere Voice tones sharp, nonaffectionate, or disparaging

(Also include observations from Table 9-1 and Boxes 11-4 and 11-5.)

The nurse also often finds that complete assessment regarding possible violence comes over time. The family may reveal more about the nature of their relationships as the helping relationship is formed. Later, the nurse can return to areas of the family history that previously appeared to be sensitive. It is often useful for the nurse to show empathy, knowledge, and helpfulness in other more concrete or traditionally nursing areas of family concern before attempting to fully assess the possibility of violence or to intervene.

NURSING DIAGNOSIS

The first priority of the final stage of assessment, that of synthesizing assessment data into a family diagnosis, is a listing of family strengths as both the nurse and the family perceive them. This starts diagnosis in a positive note and identifies areas of competence that can be further developed. Even the family badly disintegrated by violence has strengths that need to be recognized by all as a basis for confidence that problems can be resolved.

Problems with violence may not be the primary concern of the family at first. If, in the nurse's judgment, no serious danger to family members or suspicion of abuse of a child or other dependent person exists (any such observation must be immediately reported), observations concerning potential violence can be offered but action deferred until the family is ready or has had its more immediate health problems dealt with. It is often useful to state the concern about violence in terms of ways of solving disagreements or methods of disciplining children rather than using the words "violence" or "abuse," which can appear judgmental and threatening to the family.

The sample nursing process in Box 8-1 indicate several possible nursing diagnoses used for a family experiencing potential or actual violence. These are only hypothetical, but they may be helpful in providing a base for modification according to each particular family.

PLANNING

The first step of the planning process is to ensure the safety of the woman, her children, and other dependent persons. It may be difficult to work with an entire family, as participation in a family conference can place individuals in further danger from the abuser because of comments during the session. It may be necessary for the nurse to meet individually with different family members at different times. The perpetrator may or may not be living in the household, depending on what, if any, legal action has been enforced. The perpetrator may be attending batterer-intervention or other group-counseling sessions as mandated by a court proceeding. In some cases, the perpetrator may attend these sessions voluntarily. One drawback of such intervention programs is that currently very few of them offer culturally and linguistically appropriate services.

The nurse may need to help an elder or the woman and her children secure a safe place to live. The nurse may also need to help secure important documents and decide on how the elder or woman can gain financial support. Although emergency shelters are only a short-term solution, they may afford safety and time to rest and plan for the future. If a shelter is not an option, the nurse must help to set realistic goals for the future. If the woman or elder decide to leave the abuser, the nurse must help the individual find the appropriate legal, health, and social services to meet the family's needs.

NURSING INTERVENTIONS

Nursing interventions can occur at the societal and family levels. At both levels, the nurse must remember to consider the cultural implications of designing specific interventions. Nursing care is directed toward the prevention of violence in families and the identification and treatment of families that are already affected. From incidence statistics and the aspects of family life that make violence a possibility, it is readily apparent that much is to be accomplished. The first task is to prevent the seeds of violence from being planted in the family.

Primary Prevention

Primary prevention of violent families is to be undertaken by many segments of our society, including nurses. To prevent families from becoming violent, nursing must promote nonviolence in family interactions and in society in general, take specific measures to try to eliminate physical aggression from the family arena, and identify and intervene with families who are at risk to become violent. Primary prevention of family violence involves strengthening individuals and families in ways that enable them to better cope with multiple life stressors.

BOX **8-1**   **SAMPLE NURSING PROCESS**

ASSESSMENT

BRIEF BACKGROUND

The Smith family is a white middle-class family consisting of the mother, Dora; her second husband, Bill; Patty, a 14-year-old daughter from Dora's first marriage; Billy, a 10-year-old son from this marriage; and Eileen, Dora's mother.

SIGNIFICANT HISTORY

Dora states that she and Bill have a satisfactory sexual life. Bill is under a great deal of stress because of a new boss and being "behind" with the bills. He is extremely irritable toward Dora, and she does not feel as close to him as she would like. Bill makes all the decisions in the family and believes in "taking a belt to the kids" when they don't behave. She expresses horror at the news that Bill has tried to have a sexual relationship with Patty. Eileen is totally quiet during the interview, and Dora talks for her, even when a question is directly asked of Eileen. Dora says that Eileen is becoming very difficult to care for as her arthritis worsens. Billy has been in trouble in school because of frequent fights with other children and cursing at teachers. Dora expresses a high degree of commitment to "making this marriage work."

SIGNIFICANT OBSERVATIONS

Nonverbal communications are highly anxious, and Eileen looks afraid of Dora. Patty sits very close to Dora and they occasionally touch. Affectionate tones of voice and glances are used between them. Both Eileen and Billy sit apart from the other two. Billy has a sullen expression and answers questions abruptly and without elaboration. Dora's tone of voice is disparaging when she talks about Eileen.

NURSING DIAGNOSES, OUTCOMES, AND INTERVENTIONS

Three of the family nursing diagnoses identified are described in order of priority.

POTENTIAL FOR VIOLENCE (INCEST)

The potential for violence (incest) is related to spousal marital problems, family stress, inadequate family and individual (father) coping mechanisms, unequal power relationships, and dysfunctional communication patterns.

OVERALL FAMILY GOAL

No further sexual advances toward Patty as evidenced by:

- Patty reporting no further advances
- Protective-services investigation showing no further advances
- Patty's fear of stepfather diminishing

NURSING INTERVENTIONS

- Report incident to protective services after discussion of such with family during first home visit.
- nitiate and maintain contact with protective services to coordinate care.
- Refer family for family therapy with a family nurse practitioner working in a community mental-health center.
- Initiate and maintain contact with family nurse practitioner to reinforce and support therapy.
- See Patty regularly in school to discuss the progress being made in the family, monitor events in the home according to her perception, and help her express feelings about what has been happening.
- Make regular home visits when all family members are present to obtain the perceptions of other family members and to make continued assessments.

BOX **8-1** **SAMPLE NURSING PROCESS** (*Continued*)

- Build on observed strength of closeness between Patty and Dora by encouraging mother–daughter interactions.

LONG-TERM FAMILY GOAL

Increased satisfaction with marital relationship at the end of three months, as evidenced by:

- Signs of decreased tension in the home
- Dora reporting feeling closer to husband

NURSING INTERVENTIONS

- Form therapeutic relationships with family by doing below listed activities.
- Discuss fully with Dora and Bill the marital relationship.
- Help Dora and Bill see the relationship of the stress in home with their relationship.
- Build on Dora's commitment to marriage as a motivator to improve relationship.
- Support expression of feelings to nurse and of partners to each other.
- Help partners develop more effective coping mechanisms to deal with stress and to help each other cope.
- Suggest regular times for partners to be together alone, including weekends away. Help to arrange for baby-sitting and suggest Patty learn to care for grandmother at times.
- Teach family how to listen effectively to each other and communicate with respect for the other person.
- Teach Dora and Bill how to encourage each other to express feelings, as a coping mechanism for dealing with stress and as a relationship-enhancing strategy.

POTENTIAL FOR VIOLENCE (ELDERLY)

The potential for violence (elderly) is related to family stress, dysfunctional communication patterns, chronic illness in grandmother, increased role responsibilities (mother), and inadequate family and individual (mother) coping mechanisms.

SHORT-TERM FAMILY GOAL

Increased family sharing of responsibilities of physical care of Eileen at the end of two weeks as evidenced by:

- Dora feeling less tied down
- Signs of decreased anxiety in Eileen
- Less disparaging communication

NURSING INETERVENTIONS

- Refer Eileen to physician for complete medical work-up and suggestions of arthritis treatment.
- Encourage contact of Dora's siblings for help in caring for Eileen on selected weekends.
- Help family work out a schedule of care for grandmother that all can participate in.
- Point out the communication patterns that Dora has been using in relationship to Eileen and teach more effective communication skills.
- Help Eileen express feelings about situation.
- Help Eileen and Dora really communicate with each other, by role-modeling and pointing out blocks as they occur.
- Praise Dora's care of Eileen and encourage other family members to express appreciation for it.

(*continued*)

BOX 8-1 SAMPLE NURSING PROCESS (*Continued*)

LONG-TERM FAMILY GOAL

Demonstration of improved individual and family coping mechanisms at the end of three months as evidenced by:

- Dora feeling less tension
- Family showing less conflict in communications
- Family holding regular discussions to solve problems

NURSING INTERVENTIONS

- Support coping mechanisms being developed in family therapy.
- Encourage family to problem-solve with health concerns together during regular home visits; praise their efforts.
- Teach supportive communication techniques.
- Help mother develop individual coping mechanisms, such as relaxation techniques, spending time with friends while other family members take care of Eileen, and expressing feelings openly.

AGGRESSIVE BEHAVIOR PATTERNS (FATHER AND SON)

The aggressive behavior patterns (father and son) is related to corporal punishment, observations of aggressive behavior, family stress, and destructive conflict resolution patterns.

SHORT-TERM FAMILY GOAL

Recognition within family of the connections between aggressive behavior in Billy and aggressive behavior in Bill at the end of two weeks as evidenced by:

- A decision by Bill to refrain from physical punishment
- Reports from family therapist of constructive conflict resolution
- Reports from Patty of same

NURSING INTERVENTIONS

- Discuss the intergenerational transmission of violence with family.
- Identify with father how he learned violence in family of origin.
- Encourage and praise efforts made.
- Suggest family members keep a log of conflicts, how they were solved, and how effective the solutions were perceived to be. Discuss these logs with the family.

LONG-TERM FAMILY GOAL

Less aggressive behavior in Billy at the end of three months as evidenced by:

- Less nonverbal negativity in Billy
- Fewer reports of aggressive behavior in school

NURSING INTERVENTIONS

- Support interventions being given to Billy through his school; maintain coordination with professionals there; and provide communication between Billy's school and family.
- Encourage father to spend at least half an hour every day with Billy in some type of one-to-one activity.
- Encourage feeling expression between Billy and father.
- Praise Billy for nonaggressive behavior and efforts to change. Encourage family to use a great deal of praise with Billy also.

EVALUATION

- Evaluation is based on achievement of goals as perceived by family and as indicated by criteria met.

Promotion of Nonviolence

Elimination of violence from our society is an awesome undertaking. However, there are some specific measures that nurses can advocate for on a societal level that can make a difference. The first is to decrease the amount of violence in the media. Based on social-learning theory, less violence on television, in children's books, and in movies will decrease the amount of modeling for violence.

Measures have been instituted to rate movies for violence (and sex) so that young children may be prevented from seeing films that are problematic for them. These ratings are unclear guidelines for parents concerned about violence. The PG (Parental Guidance) rating is the most troublesome in terms of violence. Diligent reading of movie reviews and inquiries of other parents are needed to determine if a movie rated PG contains a great deal of violence. The raters seem to be more concerned with graphic sex than with the murder and mayhem depicted in some PG films. When the hero of the film uses force to achieve laudable aims or violent characters are not punished for their acts, a message of the legitimacy of using violence is conveyed. Nurses need to advocate a rating system that differentiates PG films on the basis of violence.

Violence on television continues to be a problem for parents. Despite the laudable efforts of the Parent Teachers Association and American Medical Association, children's television programming continues to be violent, and evening programs, even in the so-called family hour, are filled with physical aggression. Parental supervision of children's TV viewing is only part of the solution. Whenever public outcries lose momentum, the networks seem to return to violence. Nurses need to help in maintaining pressure on the programmers to decrease the violence being shown.

Nurses can also lend support for gun-control legislation. Guns in the home play a significant role in family injuries and deaths (Kellerman & Heron, 1999). The Violence Against Women Act includes provisions that prohibit gun ownership of person's convicted of domestic violence. Research has shown that enforcing gun-control laws can reduce homicide rates (Sherman, 2000). Advocating gun control is not the only answer to violence, but it is a start. Gun control would not only prevent some arguments from becoming lethal but also would create a climate of sanction against violence. The nurse should assess for the presence of a handgun in the home and strongly advocate gun-free households.

Historically, nurses have not been involved in political advocacy. However, the American Nurses' Association (ANA) and state nurses' associations are beginning to lead the profession in using their political power. Individual nurses can write their legislators, but this impact can be magnified many times by working through the local and state units of the ANA. Linkages can be formed with other organizations concerned about these issues, and nurses can spearhead national campaigns that could have considerable power. There is considerable support for gun control legislation and decreasing media violence. What remains is mobilization and effective political action.

Nurses can also have considerable impact on child-rearing. Whole cultures are totally nonviolent, and their way of living can be largely traced to the way their children are raised and the strong sanctions against aggression in their cultures. High school parenting classes and childbirth-education classes are places to start with strong messages about raising children without using physical punishment. Both laboratory studies of aggression and anthropological research on nonviolent cultures suggest that cooperation, empathy, nurturance, tenderness, sensitivity to feelings, and an abhorrence of violence need to be taught as primary values to young children of both sexes. Nurses can also be useful in supporting the teaching of nonaggressive problem-solving to children in preschools. The use of physical punishment in schools must be abolished wherever it is found. When schools allow physical aggression to discipline students, they are only teaching that our society sanctions the use of violence. They teach it not only to the children being punished but also to the rest of the students. Wherever nurses have contact with parents, the message of nonviolence can be spread.

Another important societal and community intervention is for nurses to advocate and teach special classes on sex and violence to schoolchildren. Important gains can be made in the prevention and early detection of incest if children know what is inappropriate sexual contact and whom they should tell if any occurs. A full discussion of incest with children, covering the threats to not tell and protestations of normalcy and affection by the offender, arms children with the knowledge necessary to get help immediately before serious physical and emotional damage has been done. Such discussions are best held within the context of a general health curriculum, which includes general sex education, health promotion, and emotional health content, with information on how to deal with violence and the promotion of nonviolent values and problem-solving methods incorporated. The curriculum would be taught at every grade level, with age-appropriate teaching methodologies. Nurses can advocate the establishment of such a curriculum both as health professionals and as concerned citizens and parents.

Another way in which nurses can make broad intervention is in the promotion of healthy attitudes toward the elderly and advocacy of programs that allow older Americans independence and useful functioning as long as possible. Nurses can be in the forefront in helping the young respect the aging process, rather than dread and fear it. Learning institutions and social-service agencies need to take advantage of the participation of older adults. Programs that provide home health care or daycare to the elderly must be advocated. It is unrealistic to expect that all dependent elderly can be totally cared for in their children's homes. Nurses are ideal to begin and administer such programs. Promotion of third-party payments for nurse-administered day-care centers is also needed.

Families at Risk

Identifying families at risk to become violent includes both performing assessment in one's own professional practice and advocating its inclusion by other health professionals. Any family that uses physical punishment or any form of physical aggression can be considered at risk to become violent, because violence tends to escalate under stress. Families under a great deal of stress, from poverty, unemployment, recent divorce, death in the family, severe illness in a family member, developmental crises in family members, remarriage, or changes in location or job can be considered to be at risk also. This is especially true if their methods of conflict resolution are problematic to any of the family members. In addition, families in which communications are unclear, discordant or lacking can be identified as at risk to become violent. Psychological abuse or an absence of emotional nurturance can be considered at-risk indicators. Families with a dependent elderly person in the home are at risk, especially if there is a history of verbal or physical aggression or if the elderly family member is adding considerable financial or emotional stress to the home (see Chapter 5). An overall framework to identify families at risk is to evaluate the "fit" of family resources to demand.

Interventions with such families consist primarily of helping them to develop democratic ways of solving problems. Nurses need to help families develop more constructive ways to deal with the inevitable disagreements that characterize family life. It is useful to meet with the entire family and help members work through a relatively minor conflict. Once the family has seen how this type of disagreement can be solved without creating a power struggle or aggressive argument, they can start to practice the same methods with more difficult problems.

Effective means of disciplining children without the use of physical punishment need to be discussed and modeled by the nurse. This idea may seem foreign to some parents, and careful groundwork is necessary before any suggested alternatives will be considered. It is frequently useful to explore with the parents how they were punished as children and how they perceived hitting by their parents. The perceptions of the physical aggression can also be explored with the children. Demonstration of the effectiveness of positive reinforcement with the family's children is a powerful teaching method. Getting the parents to at least try other methods of correction and carefully evaluating their results is also useful. If children are becoming aggressive, the nurse can associate their behaviors with the use of physical punishment in the home. The development of a firm, trusting relationship is necessary before parents will listen to the nurse on the subject of discipline.

The nurse can help the family develop and more fully use various support systems. Today's nuclear family has become more isolated from relatives, neighbors, and community resources. Families are more likely to move frequently than families of the past were. Community agencies and groups may be able to take the place of some of the more traditional support systems, but the family may need help in finding groups that are suitable and of interest to them. They also may want someone to attend such a group with them for the first time. The nurse may be that person, or she may be able to suggest another individual. The nurse can positively intervene as well with those who are part of the growing population of immigrants. With an eye toward the stressors that immigrants encounter, the nurse can assist immigrant families in obtaining services such as health care, housing, and child care.

When working with at-risk families, it is helpful to alleviate stressors. The nurse may be able to work with social services in helping family members obtain jobs, further education, or find work training. Guidance for anticipated developmental crises, such as adolescence, birth of the first child, and retirement, can be helpful. Part of the intervention is to help the family assess how much stress they are experiencing and the normal level of tension in the home. How the family members can help each other with stress, including helping to arrange for times and places of privacy for individuals, can be useful.

Problems with family communications and a lack of nurturance of family members can best be addressed through sessions conducted with the whole family to improve communications. The professional nurse can easily conduct such family intervention with the extensive background in therapeutic communications that is provided in most nursing education. The principles are the same; the family is helped to see blocks that the members are presently using in communication with each other, and members are taught to use active listening and therapeutic techniques of exploration of feelings. The most widely used block in family interactions is giving advice; the nurse can model the solving of shared problems as an alternative. Family members can be taught to present clear, unambiguous messages. They need to be helped to respond to each other in ways that are nurturing rather than destructive. Almost all families at risk can benefit from at least a few sessions of this type of family intervention.

Finally, nurses can make referrals to agencies directed toward the prevention of child abuse or offering classes in parenting or other such services. Some of these programs offer respite care of children for families under a great deal of stress, along with a variety of groups for parents to help them deal with stress. These types of alternatives are useful as an adjunct to nursing care. Day-care programs for the elderly or home-health agencies that offer help with household management and health care for dependent elderly persons can offer the same type of assistance.

Secondary Prevention

Secondary-prevention interventions include identification of families that are beginning to use violence beyond the physical punishment of children. Such families may be referred because of possibilities of abuse or because a child is becoming violent in school. Nurses may identify incestuous families secondary to the diagnosis of venereal disease in young children. The diagnosis may be considered a definite sign of sexual abuse and most likely incest, as the child is far more likely to have reported sexual contact with a stranger rather than a relative or close family friend. Male and female runaways may be fleeing violence in the home. Adolescents in trouble with the criminal justice system often reflect the violence in their families, and sexually promiscuous teenage girls are frequently the victims of incest and other forms of violence. When a child (or adolescent) is identified as a problem because of aggression toward his or her parents, it must be remembered that the child may be retaliating for abuse received, or he or she may be intervening to protect the mother from wife abuse. These families need intervention as quickly as possible to prevent further physical and emotional damage.

Immediate intervention frequently takes the form of crisis intervention. If a particularly violent episode resulting in serious physical injury has occurred, a son or daughter has run away or been arrested, or incest has just been discovered, the family may have no previously learned coping mechanisms to deal with the situation. The family may thus be open to assistance offered by the nurse, but high anxiety may prevent family members from fully participating in mutual assessment and planning. The nurse may need to make a quick assessment, based primarily on the crisis situation, and offer concrete assistance that will decrease the anxiety.

Crisis intervention also includes helping the family members define the situation for each of them in terms of their feelings about it and their intellectual understanding of what has happened. The nurse may be able to clarify for family members exactly what is likely to happen next, because much of the anxiety generated in a crisis is fear of the unknown. Supportive networks need to be established; for instance, relatives, friends, or clergy should be called, so that the family will have continued support after the nurse has gone. It is important that family members indicate whom they perceive as supportive; the sources may be nontraditional.

The healthy coping mechanisms that the nurse observes should be encouraged and family members helped to understand that strong feelings are normal and may not always be handled well. The family may experience much denial regarding the crisis, especially at first. The denial must be allowed (although not encouraged), and insight must be supported as it begins to appear. Family members are often adept at helping each other begin to see the ramifications of the crisis and should be encouraged to interact as much as possible.

The entire family is affected by violence and thus needs to be considered the focus of intervention. Younger children may misunderstand or be frightened by what has happened, and the first impulse of parents is often to send them away to a friend or relative. This may be useful for infants and toddlers, and the nurse can help to arrange it, but older children are better served if they are allowed to stay and participate in discussion. The nurse can make sure that the children understand what is happening, reassure them that they are not to blame, and help them determine whether they would rather stay or go.

The final part of crisis intervention is to ensure that concerned professionals will follow up with the family. The primary nurse, depending on professional role, may ensure that situation, or another nurse or professional to whom the family is referred may do so. During the four to six weeks immediately following the crisis-precipitating event, the family is particularly open to learning new coping mechanisms and working on eliminating violence from the home. It is imperative that this time of crisis be used to the fullest extent to promote growth. The crisis period may be the only time when violent family members are willing to accept help; referral must be swift and appropriate. Thus, the nurse must be sure that the referral agency or person is acceptable to the family and that they will be seen immediately.

Nursing intervention at the secondary-prevention level frequently involves working with protective services. If violence or sexual abuse is directed toward children, a report to protective services is mandatory. Protective services can be helpful by providing counseling and a variety of social services. The same is true of adult branches of protective services that operate in most cities. Reporting elder abuse is mandated by law, although spouse abuse is not. Currently, only 13 states have laws for reporting domestic violence, gunshots, and life-threatening injuries: California, Colorado, Florida, Kansas, Kentucky, Maine, Minnesota, Missouri, New Hampshire, Rhode Island, Texas, Vermont, and Washington (Family Violence Prevention Fund, 2001). It is important for nurses to be informed of the domestic-violence reporting laws for their state.

An investigation by the protective service agency will ensue; it will impress on the family the seriousness of the problem. Family members may be prompted to seek help through protective services or other agencies. The nurse may have the advantage of being able to work with the family during and after adult or child protective service investigation. Even when evidence does not warrant abuse or assault charges, the nurse can continue to work with the family in preventing further violence. In advance of referral, nurses need to be aware of exactly how protective services operates in the particular community. They need to be able to explain to families precisely what will ensue and how much time will be involved. It is helpful if the nurse is on personal terms with the professionals at the local protective services so that coordination and continuity efforts are successful and the nurse is informed of current agency protocol and policy.

The nurse may use other agencies as referrals. Community mental-health clinics and private psychiatrists, psychologists, and social workers knowledgeable about violence in families may be helpful. Nurse-to-nurse referrals are often preferable, when the identifying nurse's professional role does not include the type of long-term home visitation or therapy sessions required by some families. Psychiatric mental-health clinical nurse specialists, nurse family therapists, and family nurse practitioners are often available as consultants in community health agencies or as part of community mental-health centers or primary-care clinics. Nurses practicing in other settings need to contact these nurse specialists and make sure they are knowledgeable about violence. Then linkages can be formed so that the nurse-to-nurse referrals are conducted with a minimum of red tape.

The identifying nurse may continue to work with the family in resolving some of their other health concerns and in reinforcing and supporting the therapy being conducted by other professionals. It is beyond the scope of this book to teach the basics of family therapy with a seriously dysfunctional family. However, some basic descriptions of family therapy specific to family violence follow.

Family therapy with violent families requires the nurse to have a firm, support system of colleagues with whom she can discuss the progression of therapy. Violent families, including those who are incestuous, engender strong feelings in the nurse and can be extremely draining. In addition, the intrafamily dynamics are powerful, and the nurse can easily become caught up in them. Frequent discussions with a supervisor or colleague can help the nurse remain objective. It also must be kept in mind that these families have usually taken several years to reach such a destructive stage, and the roots of the violence may have preceded the present situation by several generations. Therefore, progress in eliminating the violence requires much time and hard work on the part of all participants.

A behavioral family-therapy model is frequently suggested for working with violent families. This is helpful in assisting the family with understanding how violent interaction patterns are learned and in keeping the interactions focused on the present situation, thereby escaping a pattern of blaming individual members. At the same time, it is imperative for individual members to take responsibility for their own violent behavior. Regardless of the model of family therapy used, it may be necessary for the nurse to use considerable confrontation in making sure that this occurs. The therapy then focuses on the extinction of violent behavior on the part of all family members by establishing enforceable, definite, and undesirable consequences of further violence, coupled with reinforcement of nonviolent behaviors and the teaching of new ways to deal with stress and arguments. Contracts with the nurse and among family members may be helpful in specifically delineating the consequences of physically aggressive behavior. The family members must monitor each other's behavior between therapy sessions, and it is imperative that everyone understands exactly what will happen. It is not sufficient that the violent relationship of primary concern (such as wife abuse) is the subject of behavior elimination or reinforcing; all the physical aggression in the household must be stopped, and the dynamics of power and control must be understood by all.

In addition to using behavioral techniques, it is important that the communication patterns between family members be analyzed and improved. Family members should also have a chance to express their feelings and learn how to accept both positive and negative feelings from their kin. The power distribution among family members also should be analyzed and equalized in most violent families. These interventions are difficult and demanding.

If possible and especially if the family is large and includes several adolescents, a cotherapist arrangement is ideal. There is so much happening in a violent family that two therapists are more likely to be able to detect all the underlying dynamics. They can also support each other during confrontation and prevent triangulation attempts that frequently occur with just one therapist in a violent family. Because many family problems stem from sex-role difficulties, it is helpful if the therapists are male and female.

Secondary prevention measures may also include working with the criminal justice system. The nurse may be called on to testify in court or to create liaisons between the enforcement agencies or lawyers and the family and other professionals involved. She may also help by being a supportive, knowledgeable person for the family in the courtroom and during the court proceedings. All these activities necessitate a working knowledge of the law as it applies to family violence and of the criminal justice system. Background information on these subjects can be found in Chapter 13. In addition, the nurse needs to advocate education and sensitization of judges, district attorneys, police, and defense lawyers regarding the issues surrounding family violence and the plight of the victims.

Furthermore, the nurse can participate in community coalitions, sometimes known as Community Coordinated Response Teams in her or his county. These groups are made up of providers working on issues of family violence in communities, such as representatives of the court system, domestic-violence advocates, law-enforcement representatives, and others working in social-service agencies. These groups will welcome participation by the nurse to add the important dimension of health care.

Secondary prevention of violence in families can thus be seen as an area for nursing to make considerable impact. Identification of families using violence in conflict resolution may take place in many nursing settings, including inpatient areas, where this is routinely assessed. Nurses in community-health settings, mental-health agencies, and primary-care facilities may be in prime positions to provide effective interventions, case coordination, and important referrals. Nurse specialists in family therapy and family functioning may continue the interventions in the form of family therapy and long-term case management and follow-up.

Tertiary Prevention

Tertiary-level nursing interventions for violence are usually carried out with families that have broken up because of violence. Nurses may work with parents who have had a child or children placed in foster homes because of abuse; families that have a member incarcerated because of sexual, elderly, wife, sibling, or child assault or intrafamilial homicide; and families that have gone through a divorce or have a child who has run away permanently because of violence. Some significant emotional and perhaps physical damage will have been done, and the nurse should be mainly concerned with helping the family to return to as healthy a level of functioning as possible and to grieve for its losses.

Part of intervention on the tertiary level is to work with the children. They need to have the emotional effects of the violence assessed and handled and to be involved with learning different ways to cope with anger to counteract the learning of violence. More detailed means of working with the children are outlined in Chapter 9.

The adolescents of violent families may act out their disturbances in school, run away, or engage in sexual or delinquent activities. Nurses need to coordinate with the professionals who work directly with these teenagers. Nurses can significantly contribute to runaway programs for adolescents. Teenagers who are runaways are frequently housed at these agencies temporarily. It would be helpful for a nurse to be part of the paid staff of such agencies. Adolescents staying there may have a variety of health problems, including sexual abuse, other sexual concerns, drug abuse, and alcohol misuse; a nurse can effectively manage these problems. Group sessions on health matters are a useful mode of intervention with these young people. If a full-time or part-time nurse cannot be hired for the program, community-health nurses or volunteer nurses can involve themselves with such agencies on the planning level as well as in direct services.

The family needs to grieve for a lost family member and the loss of the family as a total unit. The nurse can support family members through their stages of mourning and encourage expression of feelings. The family should also examine the impact of violence on their lives and work to eliminate any remaining physical aggression between members. Identification of serious psychological or physical aftereffects is also needed, and appropriate referrals should be made. When an abused child is hospitalized, the nurse can intervene with the mother and other siblings during hospital visits by helping to devise a safety plan for her and the children.

Because of the increase in immigration to the United States in recent years, there are a number of battered women whose immigration status influences their decisions about whether or not to leave the batterer. Nurses must not assume that all women from a certain ethnic group are immigrants but instead must work with each individual to see if this is an issue for her. For immigrant women, particularly undocumented women (i.e., those who entered the country without the proper documentation), it is important for the nurse to know the community resources for obtaining proper and safe legal assistance. A number of agencies can assist the nurse in identifying the safest alternatives for battered immigrant women. The National Organization for Women, Battered Immigrant Women's program in Washington, DC and the Family Violence Prevention Fund, Immigrant Women's Program in San Francisco are two national agencies that can be of assistance.

When working with populations that are not primarily English speaking, language accommodation is critical. Offer services in the language of choice for the family. Having providers or volunteers who speak the language is the best approach, leaving telephone interpreters as the last alternative. *Never* use children as interpreters! This is very stressful for the adult as well as the child, and can be potentially dangerous if children are also being abused. The Department of Health and Human Services as well as the Department of Justice mandate any agency receiving federal funds (including Medicare) to provide language-appropriate services for clients.

EVALUATION

The evaluation of nursing care of violent families is based on achievement of the goals set with the family during the planning stage of intervention. It is an ongoing process that begins with the short-term goals, with revisions of the plans and long-term goals as needed. As part of evaluation, it is important to reassess the family periodically. When dealing with issues of family functioning it is vital to conduct evaluation with the entire family so that praise can be given for progress achieved. It may be important to deal with individuals privately to identify conflict areas that need to be brought to attention. When talking about specific cases of violence, assess individuals alone so that an individual feels safe and has the privacy to discuss experiences fully. Ongoing evaluation also includes frequent contacts with other professionals and agencies involved.

The nurse can evaluate herself based on the goals set. When working with violent or potentially violent families, the nurse should continually reevaluate her perceptions and feelings. The problems may be more extensive than was originally assessed. The full extent of the violence often does not become evident until after the nurse has worked with the family for some time. Long-term interventions can thus be draining, and the nurse may decide that her effectiveness as primary therapist or case manager has eroded. In such cases, it is best to discuss these feelings with the family and a supervisor. If the nurse transfers the family to another professional without a full airing of the dilemma, the family may feel abandoned or fear that its case is hopeless.

Final evaluation is the time when the family is encouraged to make realistic plans for the future. If nursing intervention is ending before the problems with violence have been completely resolved, the family needs referrals for future interventions. The family can make these contacts during times of particular stress when the physical aggression is apt to erupt. If the family can anticipate problems and seek help early, another round of violent interaction may be prevented.

SAMPLE NURSING PROCESS

A sample nursing process for a hypothetical case is included here. (See Box 8-1.) The case illustrates how nursing care can be provided to victims of family violence. It is not meant to be all-inclusive, of course; it merely provides a basic understanding. The background given is brief, and the history and observations only indicate findings related to the violence. In actual nursing care, a much more detailed and holistic history and physical assessment would be conducted.

SUMMARY

The theoretical framework of family violence suggests that violence can occur because of the nature of family interaction, that physical aggression is taught through family socialization from one generation to the next, and that families abusive in one form may also be abusive in another. Thus, nursing care based on the total family unit is frequently indicated. The nature of the nursing practice is necessarily based on clinical experience and family nursing principles because of the paucity of nursing research specific to family violence. Assessment of families for possible violence includes direct questioning about forms of conflict resolution. Other indications that the family may experience or be at risk for violence were summarized in Tables 8-1 and 8-2. The assessment for violence ends with nursing diagnoses being formulated with the family, which should include identification of family strengths. On the basis of the problems listed, the family works together with the nurse to formulate short-term and long-term goals and interventions. This process of planning together can itself be a form of intervention.

Interventions are based on the three levels of prevention and are made at the societal and family levels. The nurse is in an excellent position to work with the entire family, as well as to be a liaison between the family and other professionals and agencies. Nursing care is finally evaluated with the family on the basis of the goals set. The nursing care of violent families is both challenging and rewarding and allows nurses to make a significant impact on decreasing the violent nature of American society.

References

Ammerman, R. T., & Hersen, M. (1991). Family violence: A clinical overview. In R. T. Ammerman & M. Hersen (Eds.), *Case studies in family violence* (pp. 3–12). New York: Plenum.

Artinian, B. M., & Conger, M. M. (Eds.). (1997). *The Intersystem model: Integrating theory and practice.* Thousand Oaks, CA: Sage.

Baron S., & Welty, A. (1996). Elder abuse. *Journal of Gerontological Social Work, 25*(1/2), 33.

Blau, G. M., Dall, M. D., & Anderson, L. M. (1993). The assessment and treatment of violent families. In R. L. Hampton, T. P. Gullotta, F. R. Adams, E. H. Potter & R. P Weissberg (Eds.), *Issues in children's lives: Family violence: prevention and treatment* (pp. 198–227). Newbury Park, CA: Sage.

Bograd, M. (1999). Strengthening domestic violence theories: Intersections of race, class, sexual orientation, and gender. *Journal of Marital and Family Therapy, 25*(3), 275–289.

Bronfenbrenner, U. (1979). *The ecology of human development: Experiments by nature and design.* Cambridge, MA: Harvard University Press.

Campbell, D. W. (1991). Family paradigm theory and family rituals: Implications for child and family health. *The Nurse Practitioner: The American Journal of Primary Health Care, 16,* 22, 25, 26, 31.

Damon, L. L., Card, J. A., & Todd, J. (1992). Incest in young children. In R. T. Ammerman & M. Hersen (Eds.), *Assessment of family violence: A clinical and legal sourcebook* (pp. 148–172). New York: Wiley.

Duvall, E. M., & Miller, B. L. (1985). *Marriage and family development* (6th ed.). New York: Harper & Row.

Faller, K. C. (1993). *Child sexual abuse: Intervention and treatment issues.* Washington, DC: U.S. Department of Health and Human Services Administration for Children and Families.

Family Violence Prevention Fund. (2001). *Health care report card* [Online]. Available: http://www. endabuse.org.

Friedman, M. M. (1998). *Family nursing: Research, theory, & practice* (4th ed.). Stamford, CT: Appleton & Lange.

Gary, F., & Kavanagh, C. K. (1991). *Psychiatric mental health nursing.* Philadelphia: Lippincott.

Gelles, R. J. (1997). *Intimate violence in families.* Thousand Oaks, CA: Sage.

Goldenberg, I. & Goldenberg, H. (2000). *Family therapy: An overview* (5th ed.). Belmont, CA: Wadsworth.

Hamby, S. L. (2000). The importance of community in a feminist analysis of domestic violence among American Indians. *American Journal of Community Psychology, 28*(5), 649–669.

Harrington, D., & Dubowitz, H. (1993). What can be done to prevent child maltreatment? In R. L. Hampton, T. P. Gullotta, G. R. Adams, E. H. Potter & R. P. Welsberg (Eds.), *Family violence: Prevention and treatment* (pp. 258–280). Newbury Park, CA: Sage.

Hill, R. (1949). *Families under stress.* New York: Harper & Row.

Hughes, H. M., & Luke, D. A. (1998). Heterogeneity in adjustment among children of battered women. In G. W. Holden, R. Geffner & E. N. Jouriles (Eds.), *Children exposed to marital violence* (pp. 185–221). Washington, DC: American Psychological Association.

Kellerman, A. L., & Heron, S. (1999). Firearms and family violence. *Emergency Medicine Clinics of North America, 17*(3), 699–716.

Kleinschmidt, K. C. (1997). Elder abuse: A review. *Annals of Emergency Medicine, 30,* 463–472.

Kozol, W. (1995) Fracturing domesticity: Media, nationalism, and the question of feminist influence. *Signs, 20*(3), 646–667.

Margolin, L. (1992). Beyond maternal blame: Physical child abuse as a phenomenon of gender. *Journal of Family Issues, 13,* 410–423.

McCown, D. E., & Artinian, B. M. (1997). The family as client: An interactive interpersonal system. In B. M. Artinian & M. M. Conger (Eds.), *The intersystem model: Integrating theory and practice* (pp. 130–154). Thousand Oaks, CA: Sage.

McCubbin, H. I., Thompson, A. I., & McCubbin, M. A. (1996). *Family assessment: resiliency, coping, and adaptation-inventories for research and practice.* Madison, WI: University of Wisconsin.

McCubbin, M. A., & McCubbin, H. I. (1987). Family stress theory and assessment: The T-Double ABCX model of family adjustment and adaptation. In H. I. McCubbin & A. L. Thompson (Eds.), *Family assessment inventories for research and practice* (pp. 14–32). Madison, WI: University of Wisconsin.

McCubbin, M. A., & Patterson, J. M. (1982). Family adaptation to crises. In H. I. McCubbin, A. E. Cauble, & J. M. Patterson (Eds.), *Family stress, coping and social support* (pp. 26–47). Springfield, IL: Charles C. Thomas.

McGoldrick, M. (Ed.). (1998). *Re-visioning family therapy: Race, culture, and gender in clinical practice.* New York: Guilford.

Miedzian, M. (1995). Learning to be violent. In E. Peled, P. G. Jaffe, & J. L. Edleson (Eds.), *Ending the cycle of violence: Community responses to children of battered women* (pp. 10–24). Thousand Oaks, CA: Sage.

National Clearinghouse on Child Abuse and Neglect. (1999). *10 years of reporting child maltreatment.* Washington, DC: U.S. Department of Health and Human Services, Administration on Children, Youth and Families.

National Institute of Justice. (2001). *Research in brief: An update on the "cycle of violence."* Washington, DC: U.S. Department of Justice, Office of Justice Programs.

Oermann, M. H. (1991). *Professional nursing practice: A conceptual approach.* Philadelphia: Lippincott.

O'Leary, K. D., Smith-Slep, A. M., & O'Leary, S. G. (2000). Co-occurrence of partner and parent aggression: Research and treatment implications. *Behavior Therapy, 31*(4), 631–648.

Reiss, D. (1981). *The family's construction of reality.* Cambridge, MA: Harvard University Press.

Roberts, C. S., & Feetham, S. L. (1982). Assessing family functioning across three areas of relationships. *Nursing Research, 31*(4), 231–235.

Rumm, P. D., Cummings, P., Krauss, M. R., Bell, M. A., & Rivara, F. P. (2000). Identified spouse abuse as a risk factor for child abuse. *Child Abuse & Neglect, 24*(11), 1375–1381.

Salzinger, S., Feldman, R. S., Ng-Mak, D. S., Mojica, E., Stockhammer, T., & Rosario, M. (2002). Effects of partner violence and physical child abuse on child behavior: A study of abused and comparison children. *Journal of Family Violence, 17*(1), 23–52.

Sherman, L. (2000). Gun carrying and homicide prevention. *Journal of the American Medical Association, 283*(9), 1193–1195.

Shipman, K. L., Rossman, B. B. R., & West, J. (1999). Co-occurance of spousal violence and child abuse: Conceptual implications. *Child Maltreatment, 4*(2), 93–102.

Straus, M. A., & Gelles, R. A. (1990). *Physical violence in American families.* New Brunswick, NJ: Transaction.

Straus, M. A., Gelles, R. J., & Steinmetz, S. K. (1980). *Behind closed doors.* Garden City, NY: Doubleday.

Tjaden, P., & Thoennes, N. (2000). *Extent, nature, and consequences of intimate partner violence.* Washington, DC: National Institutes of Justice.

Tolman, R. M. (1992). Psychological abuse of women. In R. T. Ammerman & M. Hersen (Eds.), *Assessment of family violence: A clinical and legal sourcebook* (pp. 291–310). New York: Wiley.

Vondra, J. L., Kolar, A. B, & Radigan, B. L. (1992). Psychological maltreatment of children. In R. T. Ammerman, and M. Hersen (Eds.), *Assessment of family violence: A clinical and legal sourcebook* (pp. 253–290). New York: Wiley.

Warrior, S., Williams-Wilkins, B., Pitt, E., Reece, R., Groves, B., Lieberman, A., & McNamara, M. (2002). Culturally competent responses and children: Hidden victims. *Violence Against Women, 8*(6), 661–686.

Weise, D., & Daro, D. (1995). *Current trends on child abuse reporting and fatalities: The results of the 1994 fifty-state survey.* Chicago: National Committee to Prevent Child Abuse.

Wilber, K. H., & Reynolds, S. L. (1996). Introducing a framework for defining financial abuse of the elderly. *Journal of Elder Abuse and Neglect, 8*(2), 61–80.

Yick, A. G. (2001). Feminist theory and status inconsistency theory: Application to domestic violence in Chinese immigrant families. *Violence Against Women 7*(5), 545–562.

Yllö, K. A. (1993). Through a feminist lens: Gender, power, and violence. In R. J. Gelles & D. R. Loseke (Eds.), *Current controversies on family violence* (pp. 47–62). Thousand Oaks, CA: Sage.

Zosky, D. L. (1999). The application of object relations theory to domestic violence. *Clinical Social Work Journal, 27*(1), 55–69.

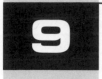

Nursing Care of Abused Children

• Faye A. Gary and Janice Humphreys

Nursing care of abused and neglected children requires current, theory-based knowledge and individualized application. The nurse may become aware of child abuse and neglect at almost any point during practice with families. The maltreated child may be obvious or may have less apparent indications of abuse and neglect. Nursing care of families is based on prevention, however, and therefore does not require evidence of a problem for the nurse to intervene. Assessment for potential and actual child abuse is thus an integral part of the nursing care of every child and parent. This chapter assists in the application of the theory and research presented in previous chapters. It also discusses suicide prevention and highlights the need for the nurse to be alert and diligent in prevention and early intervention.

Early theories of child abuse and neglect tended to suggest that only one or a few factors contributed to the occurrence of child maltreatment. More recent theoretical developments recognize the importance of multiple factors. (See Chapter 3 for a discussion of theories of child abuse and neglect.) Child abuse and neglect are complex, serious health problems requiring the best efforts of professionals from a variety of disciplines. The need for a multidisciplinary approach to interventions with abusive and neglectful families is generally recognized. Although some discussion of the benefits and difficulties of multidisciplinary interventions is presented, the primary purpose of this chapter is to discuss the nurse's role with abused and neglected children and their families.

SELF-AWARENESS

Self-awareness begins when the nurse is able to recognize any conflicting thoughts and feelings she or he may have; although getting in touch with feelings is helpful, it can also be frightening for the nurse.

When thoughts and feelings are incongruent with desired behavior, discomfort typically occurs. Denying a certain feeling or being caught off guard by others' responses produce discomfort and thus are clues that indicate inner conflict. Dissatisfaction with the result of the outcome of an interaction is another typical example (Cox, Kershaw, & Trotter, 2000; Lapham-Alcorn, 1991). The nurse should strive to identify her true feelings and thoughts, even though they may not be pleasing to others. Getting in touch with feelings is one characteristic of maturity; it is good for oneself and others (Cox et al., 2000; Lapham-Alcorn, 1991). The following example illustrates the concept of incongruence between feelings and desired behavior:

A pediatric nurse is working in the emergency department of a large hospital when a mother and a young child who had been burned rush in for service. The mother states, "Here, you take her, she has burns on her stomach and legs and I can't stand to look at her." The pediatric nurse looks at the young child and comments to the mother, "You tell me how this happened right now!" Without waiting for the mother to respond, the nurse takes the child and asks the mother to wait in the hall while she begins assessment. Child abuse is immediately suspected. During the assessment, the pediatric nurse is anxious, angry, and accusatory toward the mother. As she begins to incorporate her perceptions into the documentation about the event, the nurse manager intervenes after determining that the pediatric nurse, who has had a fine nursing reputation, was upset and not able to be objective. After the assessment and treatment plan is complete, the nurse manager requests a conference with the pediatric nurse, and they review her reactions. At this time, the pediatric nurse shares with the nurse manager that she had been maltreated when she was a child but had never shared that information with anyone. She also comments, "I was not aware that I had such strong memories about those horrible years in my life."

The nurse must be empathic, respectful, kind, and genuine in her approach to children and families. These key elements are necessary for the development of a therapeutic alliance between the nurse and the family (Webster-Stratton, 1998). Some experts suggest that the nurse or other professionals working with the family display genuineness and concern by sharing personal experiences, feelings, and selected problems of their own. This approach is sound only if the professional strategically thinks through the information to be shared; the purpose is to demonstrate more effective methods of problem-solving and crisis management (Webster-Stratton, 1998). The nurse will also find humor, reframing, positive feedback, and reinforcement to be useful. Here is an example of positive reinforcement; it is effective in reinforcing desirable parental behaviors (Webster-Stratton, 1998; Wolfe & Yuan, 2001):

Mother: When we were getting dressed for school this morning, Ken could not find his schoolwork, and instead of looking for it he was watching television. I became so very angry, walked over to him and hit him on his backside while shouting, "You can do some stupid things. You had better not make any bad grades or I will fix you good." I caught myself, stopped the yelling, and folded my arms. After we were in the car, I calmed down and reflected. I had no doubt lost control and made the situation worse for Ken, the rest of my family, and me. I was upset all day while working on my job.

Nurse: I commend you for recognizing your own actions and amending them. Also, you were able to reflect on your own behaviors and conclude, correctly, that you were not handling the situation in the best manner. In addition, you became aware that your behavior was upsetting to Ken and other members of your household. I praise you for having the courage to confront how you impacted the situation. Since that incident, have you thought about other more useful ways to handle your anger? If you could recreate this same morning, how would it unfold now? Can we role-play the situation? I will act as if I am Ken. During the role-play, try to include the new thoughts and behaviors that you have learned since the two of us began our discussions about Ken and the other children in your family.

ASSESSMENT

Nurses need to be aware that the standards for assessment of family competence measure minimal adequacy. The standards reflect the notion that state intervention should be the final option. Families are treated as autonomous units. The nurse should remember that final judgment about the adequacy of parenting is social, and clinical judgments are bound in culture. Nevertheless, these standards help determine the safety and well-being of the child and help the nurse to fulfill professional responsibilities in a more objective manner. The five standards, income; physical care; affection; education; and guidance, are shown in Table 9-1.

The nurse who works with small children should be knowledgeable about human growth and development. Psychosexual and psychoanalytic theories reflect the thinking of theorists like Freud and Erikson whereas cognitive developmental theories are grounded in the works of Jean Piaget. Anna Freud (1967) introduced the concept of developmental lines, which is still quite useful for nurses who work in pediatric settings. (See Table 9-2.) Her conceptualization traces child development from complete dependence through mastery over the internal and external environment. However, it is not uncommon for children to show some irregularities in their development; the nurse should then make a determination about underlying causes. The nurse should ask if a physiological or environmental factor is impacting the child's normal development. The following example illustrates the application of Anna Freud's theory of developmental lines.

William is a smart, independent child who is considered to be well-adjusted. When he came into the pediatric clinic for his annual check-up, the nurse examined him, took a history, and determined that William still wets the bed at night and falls asleep in his grandmother's bed each evening. Otherwise, he cries and has temper tantrums until the parents and grandmother give in to him. He confided in the nurse, "I wish I did not wet the bed—I am a big boy now, and I want to stay over with my cousin, Bobby. But I might wet the bed, and then my mama will not let me go to his house." The nurse can incorporate the lines of development into her assessment to aid her in determining the irregularities that William experiences. It can also help in planning the nursing care.

Assessment is always one of the key elements in treatment and should be done with care, based on practical and theoretical knowledge. The following "quick methods" should be helpful to the nurse, regardless of settings. The mnemonic ARM PAIN is useful for remembering (Robinson, 1998):

Altered state of consciousness (delirium, intoxication, sleep deprivation)
Repeated attacks (violence in the family)
Male gender (men abuse women more often than women abuse men)
Paranoia (rule out schizophrenia, mood disorders, mania, and delusional disorders; narcissism; and jealousy)
Age (younger people are more likely to be violent than older people)
Incompetence (brain injury, cognitive deficits, psychosis)
Neurologic diseases (Huntington's chorea, dementia)

Psychiatric disturbances may increase the risk of violence, and the nurse should be aware that abuse against the child might be related to one or more of such disorders. Here is a quick way to remember the psychiatric disorders that

STANDARD	INDICATORS

Income and Money Management

Income

The family has sufficient income to meet the family's basic needs for food, shelter, clothing, education and health care

Employability of parents
Employment history
Income earned from employment
Income from other sources (disability, etc.)
In-kind value of rent subsidies, food stamps, other
Parental ability to access community resources as needed

Money Management

Parents demonstrate skills necessary to meet the basic needs of the family

Budgeting skills
Shopping skills
Menu-planning skills
Expenditure history
Nonessential expenditures (alcohol, tobacco, etc.)
Banking skills
Knowledge of resources for low-cost essential items (clothing, food, health care)

Physical Care

Food

Parents are able to obtain the quality and quantity of food necessary to assure adequate health and development for family members

Presence of sufficient quantities of nutritional food
Number of meals prepared each day
Nutritional balance of daily menu
Shopping patterns
Menu-preparation skills
Cooking equipment usable in home
Food-storage hygiene
Kitchen-area hygiene

Shelter

Parents provide a safe and protective living environment

Electrical safety throughout the home environment
Properly operating, safe heating and cooling sources
Roof, walls, doors, windows, floors, ceilings adequate
Residence can be locked
Adequate plumbing
Adequate water sources; safe, clean wells as water source
Overall sanitary conditions in and outside the home
Garbage is disposed
Child-safe storage of medicines, cleaning materials, and other potentially dangerous substances

Clothing

Parents provide and maintain clothing that is of sufficient quality and quantity

Presence and use of clothing as determined by season
State of repair of clothing
Cleanliness of clothing
Shopping skills to obtain clothing

Personal Hygiene

Parents assure personal hygiene of child

Bathing and washing frequency
Dental-care patterns
Hair-care patterns (washing, combing, brushing)
Utilization of personal-hygiene supplies

Medical Care

Parents provide medical care to children

Examination frequency
Immunization history
Utilization of home health-care supplies (bandages and such)
Regular appointments and treatment when needed
Parental knowledge about children's medical needs
Ablity to obtain care in case of emergencies

(continued)

255

Table 9-1 • **Parental Standards for Determining Safety and Well-Being of a Child (Continued)**	

STANDARD	INDICATORS
Affection	
Spouse-to-Spouse	
Parents display high regard for each other	Behaviors related to positive physical interactions
	Behaviors related to positive verbal interactions
	Behaviors related to negative physical interactions
	Behaviors related to negative verbal interactions
Parent-to-Child	
Parents show positive affection	Behaviors related to positive physical interactions
	Behaviors related to positive verbal interactions
	Behaviors related to negative physical interactions
	Behaviors related to negative verbal interactions
Sibling-to-Sibling	
Interaction between siblings displays positive, age-appropriate affection	Behaviors related to positive physical interactions
	Behaviors related to positive verbal interactions
	Behaviors related to negative physical interactions
	Behaviors related to negative verbal interactions
Education	
Social Education	
Parent displays the competency to educate the child in social skills, within the context of age and culture	Health-care and hygiene skills
	Clothing-procurement and -care skills
	Personal interaction and problem-solving skills
	Nutrition and eating skills
	Transportation skills
	Child care skills
	Safety and security skills
Academic Education	
The parent fosters the child's age-appropriate academic achievement	Preschool, day-care participation
	Reading, writing, and math skills
	School enrollment
	Homework patterns and parent interaction
	Presence of educational toys
	Parental visits, communication with school personnel
	School-attendance pattern
	Special diagnostic testing when indicated
Guidance	
The parent displays positive methods of providing age-appropriate guidance to the child	Behaviors related to providing advice and feedback to child
	Level of understanding regarding child development
	Philosophy and methods of providing child supervision
	Philosophy and methods of providing discipline and limit-setting for the child
	Attitude and ability to access community resources to secure professional guidance and counseling for the child and parent as needed

Sources: Adapted from Illinois Department of Children and Family Services. (1985). *Child welfare services practice handbook*; and Greene, B., & Kilili, S. (1998). How good does a parent have to be? Issues and examples associated with empirical assessments of parenting adequacy in cases of child abuse and neglect. In J. Lutzker (Ed.), *Handbook of child abuse research and treatment*. New York: Plenum.

could be associated with violence and abuse. The mnemonic MADS BADS is helpful (Robinson, 1998):

Manic (impulsivity, grandiosity, and psychotic behaviors)
Alcohol (intoxication and withdrawal)
Dementia (diminished judgment and compromised inhibition)
Schizophrenia (command hallucinations and delusions)
Borderline personality disorder (anger, uneven emotions, impulsivity)
Antisocial personality disorder (indifferent about the safety of others)
Delirium (hallucinations, delusions)
Substance abuse

NURSING INTERVENTIONS

Primary Prevention

Bonding between the child and mother is essential in the relationship, and it should be preserved and nurtured. Bonding is considered to be the base for all other human relationships; if it does not take place, the child will be compromised and will experience difficulties in the future. Bowlby wrote that children who experience loss and separation at an early age, and who therefore have normal attachment interfered with, are predisposed to various types of mental disorders and maladjustments (Barthel & Herman, 1991; Gage, 1990). Yet other researchers have reminded us that abuse can be present and affect the child even before birth. Low birth weight babies could be the result of the pregnant women having been battered. The nurse should, therefore, become suspicious of intimate partner abuse in these instances (Bullock & McFarlane, 1989). Moreover, if there is a history of substance abuse in the family, the assessment could include information about alcohol and drug abuse in the current household. An astute nurse would also want to know if others who abuse substances would have the responsibility of caring for the child, and ask questions to determine risk (Cappell & Heiner, 1990; Justice & Justice, 1976).

The hospital-based nurse can facilitate the parent–child bond by encouraging parents to participate in the care of their children as soon as they are ready. Having a newborn in a nursery separate from the postpartum mother may inhibit the mother's ability to develop a healthy relationship with her child. Keeping the newborn with his or her mother during hospitalization has been shown to correlate with fewer subsequent cases of parenting inadequacy; therefore it is encouraged. During the daily, extended contact among mother, father, and newborn, the nurse can praise and reassure the parents. Criticism of parental behavior can be replaced with identification of strengths.

In addition to the traditional class on bathing the baby, the nurse on a postpartum unit can guide the parents in terms of what they can expect when they go home. Topics to be covered include infant crying, feeding patterns, and developmental milestones. The nurse should emphasize that parenting is hard work and that it is okay to ask for help. Parents can be encouraged to identify and call on others who can help them adjust to the changes and stress they experience.

Nursing intervention may be even more important in the case of the birth of a handicapped or a premature infant. These infants are frequently whisked away from parents to initiate life-sustaining measures. The parents are unable to expe-

Table 9-2 • Anna Freud's Developmental Lines

	INFANT	TODDLER	PRESCHOOL	SCHOOLAGE	ADOLESCENT
Body to toy	Own body source of play and orientation	Transitional objects to symbolic objects	Utilizes play material	Pleasure in finished products and self accomplishments	
Play to work	Autoerotic play	Parallel play	Constructive play	Task completion, decision-making, and problem-solving	Capacity to love and work
Egocentricity to companionship	Others are intruders in mother-child relationship	Other children are communicated with as if objects	Other children are perceived as helpers	Other children are perceived as separate individuals and partners	
Wetting and soiling to bowel and bladder mastery	Complete freedom	Ambivalence about body products, and external control imposed by mother or caregiver	Identification with others; autonomous, and internal controls		

Source: Freud, A. (1967). Normality and pathology in childhood. New York: International Universities Press; and Barthel, R., & Herrman, C. (1996). Psychiatric mental health nursing with children. In F. Gary, & C. Kavanaugh, Psychiatric nursing. Philadelphia: Lippincott.

rience early contact with their children. In addition, they are grieving the loss of the anticipated perfect child and must adjust to their "imperfect" baby. Nursing interventions include providing emotional support to the family of the infant, encouraging parents to have contact whenever possible with the child, and educating parents in the care of their child. Parents are encouraged to be as involved as possible in the daily child care. Many neonatal intensive care units (NICUs) now routinely encourage active parent participation. Nurses can advocate such policies in hospitals where they do not already exist.

The handicapped child or the child who is hospitalized for long periods, particularly during infancy, is a special concern to the nurse who practices on a pediatric unit. In a study of 51 abused children, Stern (1973) observed that "one-third of these children had either been seriously ill in the newborn period or had a persistent congenital defect" (p. 119). The separation of the parent and child or the existence of some anomaly is associated with child maltreatment. It may be simplistic to think that prematurity or birth defect alone predisposes a child to abuse or neglect. Chronic health problems, particularly in offspring, are a source of stress. In addition, financial strain, absence from work, and the need to identify alternative sources of other child care may occur. Primary prevention of child abuse and neglect in the case of the premature or handicapped child includes attention to more than just the child. Professional nurses include among their interventions contact with community social agencies, contact with child-care services, visits (by community-health nurses), and parent groups whenever appropriate.

Community

Professional nurses who can make primary-prevention interventions include community-health nurses, public-health nurses, school nurses, and clinic nurses because each is in a position to assess families for risk factors before maltreatment occurs and to refer them to appropriate resources.

The community-health nurse (CHN) provides skilled nursing care to the child with an identified health problem. The CHN can use frequent home visits to assess family functioning and to provide parents with guidance as to what to expect. The frequent family contact in the home environment allows the CHN to assess the family in a natural setting. Generally, behavior in the home is free from influences associated with the hospital (i.e., acute illness, foreign environment). In addition, the CHN maintains contact with the family over time, which allows for assessment of parental behavior changes toward the child. "Red flags"—behaviors that may signal a potential for maltreatment—include keeping the child dirty or unkempt visit after visit and continuous negative references to the child. A major component of the CHN visit is a history and physical assessment. Factors that may indicate a potential for maltreatment include weight gain inappropriate for age; a parental report of the child being very fussy, inconsolable or irritable; and lack of follow-up with the pediatrician or absence of immunizations for the child. The CHN should also assess support systems—those people the mother can rely on in times of need. The parent who is isolated and reports poor or nonexistent support systems is also at risk for maltreatment.

Another component of the CHN visit is teaching. Although a majority of teaching revolves around disease, routine teaching should include guidance as to what to expect for growth and development, nutrition, and preventive health care. Finally, the CHN should be familiar with community-support services and refer families when risk factors are identified.

The public-health nurse's scope of practice tends to be broader than the CHN. The public-health nurse (PHN) is funded through a county or city health, department. The goal of public-health nursing is promotion of health through prevention. The PHN makes home visits to clients referred from a variety of sources, including schools, clinics, child-protection agencies, hospitals, and home-health agencies after skilled care is no longer needed. Because of the goal of public-health nursing, the PHN is in an optimal position to prevent maltreatment. Several demonstration programs funded and operated through public-health departments have shown great promise in prevention. The most noteworthy programs are the maternal–child support programs that provide home visitation by professionals or paraprofessionals to pregnant and new mothers. Examples include the Child Parent Enrichment program (Barth, Hacking, and Ash, 1988) and several demonstration projects sponsored by the National Center on Child Abuse and Neglect (Gray, 1982).

Both the CHN and the PHN are in an excellent position to connect parents to appropriate resources in the community to meet their needs. Parents of children with special health-care needs who are overwhelmed or experiencing isolation or financial burdens can be referred to community-based support programs. For parent-to-parent support, parents can be referred to local support groups. The groups may be diagnosis-based (e.g., a seizure-disorder support group), or they may be response-based (e.g., a support group for parents of children with special health-care needs). If the nurse is unfamiliar with locating such groups, she may contact the local hospital pediatric ward or the regional children's hospital. The clinical nurse specialist in the area of interest should be able to provide contacts for such groups. The local United Way is another source of information because it provides funding to many community-based groups. For families that need financial help, the nurse should contact the local health department to determine whether the state offers a program of services to crippled children. (In some states, this program has been changed to one of services to children with special health-care needs.) Although the program may vary from state to state, a majority of them offer a low-cost or no-cost insurance, family assessment, case management, ombudsman services, and, in some states, a parent-support network.

Preventive services, sponsored by the state department of social services, aims at assisting families encountering myriad stressors. It is a voluntary help program directed at prevention of maltreatment through coordination of appropriate community-based services. Anyone can make a referral to preventive services; the family can even "refer" themselves. When a referral has been accepted, the family is assigned a caseworker. The caseworker visits the home to make a family/environmental assessment. The prevention worker then puts the family in contact with appropriate agencies geared toward meeting the family's needs. Preventive services can assist families in meeting a variety of needs, from adequate housing and furniture to daycare and job training. Because the program is voluntary, families must be motivated to work with the agency to accomplish their goals. Preventive services continues to work with a family until all the goals are met, even if the process takes a year or longer.

Nurses who practice in schools can intervene with adolescents who are just entering the childbearing years. Nursing interventions include sex-education programs that allow adolescents to be knowledgeable about sexuality and contraception. The decision of when and if to have children can be made more intelligently if adolescents and young adults are well informed about the prevention of pregnancy. Child-development courses that expose the adolescent to the realities of being a parent can also assist the potential parent's decision-making. If the adolescent becomes a parent, she or he is more likely to understand the child's behavior after exposure to information about child growth and development.

The nurse can intervene with the pregnant adolescent to prevent child abuse and neglect. The school or clinic nurse can present available options. If the adolescent chooses to keep and raise the child, the nurse can work closely with the mother-to-be. The primary-care nurse working with the pregnant adolescent should refer the client to available community-based maternal–child support programs.

It is important that the nurse approach the pregnant adolescent with the same respect given to any other client. The pregnant adolescent does not need recriminations from the nurse. The nurse who seeks to punish or lecture the adolescent on past behaviors ceases to be therapeutic. When the adolescent father is also involved in prenatal planning, the same nonjudgmental, supportive approach is appropriate. Group programs for pregnant mothers that allow them to complete their education by assisting with child care, parent education, and peer contacts are useful.

Clinic-based nurses who provide primary care to children and their parents routinely include guidance as to what to expect as part of their health-promotion teaching. Parents can be prepared for the various behaviors and changes in their children as they grow and develop. For example, if parents have been forewarned about stages of development, they may not find the negativism of a two-year-old as aggravating as it would be if they weren't prepared. In addition, parents need to be prepared for situations that can prompt anger or make them want to hit their child. The nurse can problem-solve with the parents to identify alternative methods of dealing with their frustration and anger and to learn effective, nonviolent methods of discipline.

Parents should routinely be praised for evidence of good child care. Even if there are 99 problems with child care identified by the nurse, the parent can be praised for the one aspect of positive parenting. Doing so cannot be overemphasized. Parents rarely hear from health-care providers about what they did right. Praise from the nurse can be easily included during the history examination or physical examination. For example, the nurse can say, "You've really done an excellent job at seeing that your child has a nutritious diet" or, "Her skin is so beautiful. I can see that she's really getting the kind of care she needs." Parents are usually pleased and surprised to have their hard work noticed. The praise increases the likelihood of it continuing, helps parents to see strengths, and increases parental self-esteem. Parents should also be encouraged to spend some time away from the child; they can be supported and reassured that time for themselves is not selfish.

An excellent way to give both parents and preschool children time apart is to enroll the child in Head Start or another stimulating preschool program. Clinical experience has revealed that Head Start is a blessing to many parents and a delight to the children. Head Start has also been shown to assist children in their personal development; that is, self-esteem and advanced reading, arithmetic, and language scores are registered at all grade levels, even 15 years after Head Start experience. In a long-term follow-up of individuals 19 to 22 years of age, those who had attended Head Start had a higher high school completion rate, a greater likelihood of attending college, less tendency to use welfare, a higher rate of employment, and lower arrest rates than those who had attended no preschool (Weikart, 1980). Programs like Head Start were developed to help break the cycle of poverty. Considering the major contribution that poverty makes to family violence, the nurse who is truly a client advocate will work for the continuation of programs that assist the poor.

Social Interventions

Several authors and reports (Child Welfare League of America, 1989) have recommended changes in social policy and services that could significantly enhance the lives of children and their families. Vondra and Toth (1989) concluded that interventions that fail to address the multiple problems confronting families are unlikely to provide the full range of services necessary to help them recover and gain control of their lives. In 1971, Gil clearly identified several changes that must occur if maltreatment of children is to be eliminated in the United States. Gil's suggestions are still the most basic and potentially the most pervasive form of primary prevention. The nurse who is more than just a "responder" can be actively intervening at the social-policy level.

Gil (1971) recommended that efforts be made in all areas to change the cultural sanction of the use of physical force against children. He said that "changing this aspect of the prevailing child-rearing philosophy and developing clear-cut cultural prohibitions and legal sanctions against such use of physical force are likely to produce over time the strongest possible reduction of the incidence and prevalence of physical abuse of children" (p. 646). Gil did not suggest that children be treated with such permissiveness that they are never punished. He recommended that constructive, educational, nonviolent discipline be used. As he pointed out, "rarely, if ever, is corporal punishment administered for the benefit of an attacked child, for usually it serves the immediate needs of the attacking adult who is seeking relief from his uncontrollable anger and stress" (p. 647).

Gil also suggested the active pursuit of the elimination of poverty and racism. Social inequalities that prevent individuals of every race from experiencing the same opportunities result in the overrepresentation of minorities in the lowest socioeconomic strata. In addition, current social policies allow for levels of poverty that were heretofore unacceptable. Racial discrimination and poverty contribute in a complex fashion to child maltreatment. The nurse cannot expect to eliminate the maltreatment of children by family education or support alone. The culture and social environment in which the harming of children occurs and is at times condoned requires nursing intervention.

Social support and social interaction repeatedly have been identified as significant factors in child maltreatment. Although in a literature review Seagull (1987) concluded that there is little evidence that social support plays a significant role in the cause of child abuse, she suggested that a relationship between child neglect and lack of social support exists. Others (Hamilton, 1989; Hoffman-Plotkin & Twentyman, 1984) have identified the social isolation that is frequently associated with child neglect. Cowen and Work (1988) proposed that availability of support in early childhood and continuing support in later childhood strengthen resilience in children. Social interventions that support families and enhance their interactions with members in their communities are primary preventions of child maltreatment. "It is not the quantity but the quality of social support [and its timing] that is vital" (Hamilton, 1989, p. 32). Community-based (municipal, church, volunteer) and employer-supported child care assists families by providing child services and family resources. If families need additional services, existing relationships can support families through life events. Some authors have argued that home visitors reduce both felt and actual isolation and should be supported (Cohn, 1981).

Child-care services that provide help in case of minor illness can be invaluable. Even a minor childhood illness can seriously affect families who rely on all adult members for employment income and benefits. Clearly, nurses can be involved in establishing and, if necessary, initiating community- or employer-supported child-care services. They can reasonably be developed in association with health-care institutions and other providers. As direct client providers, nurses are an obvious choice for such programs. Given the finding in at least one study (Sherrod, O'Connor, Vietze, & Altemeier, 1984) that maltreated infants tend to be ill more often than other infants, nursing involvement with minor illness and care services can provide an additional opportunity for early diagnosis and treatment of child abuse and neglect.

Finally, Gil recommended that comprehensive programming be undertaken in every community to reduce abuse and neglect of children. Included in each community program should be the following (Gil, 1971, p. 647):

- Comprehensive family-planning programs, including repeal of all legislation concerning medical abortions
- Family-life and education counseling programs for adolescents and adults in preparation for, and after, marriage
- A comprehensive, high-quality neighborhood-based, national health service, financed through general tax revenue and geared not only to the treatment of acute and chronic illness but also to the promotion and maintenance of maximum feasible physical and mental health for everyone
- A range of high-quality, neighborhood-based social services geared to the reduction of environmental stresses on family life and especially on mothers who carry major responsibility for child-rearing
- A system of social services and child-care facilities geared to assisting families whose members cannot live together because of severe relationship or reality problems

Nurses can include Gil's or similar recommendations as part of primary prevention of child abuse and neglect at the community level. The community provides the framework for the child abuse and neglect seen in the family.

In 1982, Michigan income-tax forms had a new option for taxpayers: people receiving a refund could elect to allot two dollars (or four dollars for a joint return) for child-abuse prevention. Funds collected were placed in the Children's Trust Fund of the Michigan Department of Treasury. Half of the money collected each year since then has been invested, and half has been spent for local child-abuse prevention programs. Funds have been distributed by a citizen's board, appointed by the governor, for local child-abuse councils and local prevention services through hospitals, churches, schools, and other community organizations.

Every year since its implementation, the Children's Trust Fund has received increased funds from the tax check-off (Children's Trust Fund, 1988/1989-1989/1990). As of the fifth funding cycle, 133 child-abuse and -neglect prevention grants had been awarded. However, only 6 to 7% of the people eligible for tax returns contribute to the fund. Even after a legislative appropriation of $500,000 for increasing public awareness of the fund, fewer than 6% of all eligible people contributed.

Secondary Prevention

At the moment a child experiences harm at the hands of parents or some other responsible adult, professional nursing interventions are termed "secondary prevention." The goals of secondary prevention are early diagnosis and intervention to prevent recurrence and to limit impact of the abuse and neglect.

Secondary prevention of child abuse and neglect needs to target several areas. Clearly, the health and safety of the children must be a first priority. Within families, however, interventions must be directed at the individual needs of members, interactions among members, and the larger family environment. Each family must be assessed, and a specific program of care should be established. Nurses will be required to contribute their expertise to a multidisciplinary effort on behalf of the maltreating family. Within this general framework, the nature of nursing practice with abusive and neglectful families varies depending on the nurse's role and practice setting.

Hospital

The most important type of secondary prevention of child abuse and neglect is the early identification of the maltreated child. In the case of the nurse who practices in an acute-care setting, abused and neglected children may or may not be medically diagnosed at her first contact. Some forms of child abuse and neglect are not readily obvious. (See Tables 8-1 and 8-2 for a complete listing of pertinent assessment findings.) Some children are admitted directly to pediatric or intensive care units with the diagnosis of child abuse or neglect. Other children with reported "accidental" injuries seen in emergency rooms are more correctly identified as abused or neglected.

The less obviously maltreated child is medically diagnosed as other than abused or neglected. The child with a fractured femur who "fell out of bed" certainly needs health care to aid in the healing process. However, treating the fracture alone is profoundly inadequate.

The first step in early identification of child abuse and neglect is a thorough nursing assessment. Other professional nursing interventions may involve consultation with other health professionals. Diagnostic tests to definitely determine child abuse and neglect usually require a physician's order. The nurse, with extended, intensive contact with hospitalized children and their parents, coupled with thorough assessment and theory-based knowledge, often has the greatest insight into family health needs. The nurse should accurately record an assessment and alert other professionals involved in the care of the child and family.

Child abuse and neglect should be handled via collaboration by a group of health professionals. Ideally, a child-abuse-and-neglect team should exist in every hospital. The team is composed of interested representatives from several different professions—nursing, social work, and medicine, for example—and meets on a regular basis and as needed to review suspected cases, develop plans of care, and educate other members of the hospital community. These teams can be invaluable resources in early detection and treatment of child maltreatment. An important nursing intervention is the development of such teams in hospitals in which they do not already exist.

Multidisciplinary efforts are extremely important. Cupoli and Newberger (1977) noted that neither health nor social interventions alone will allay the impact of child maltreatment. However, interdisciplinary management of child abuse can be difficult. In an article showing the physician's perspective on inter-disciplinary management of child abuse, Newberger (1976) identified several fac-tors that prevent professionals from various disciplines from working most effectively. Professionals from one discipline are often ignorant of the concep-tual basis of practice for another discipline. Thus, communication among mem-bers of different disciplines is often poor and compounded by institutional isolation. Professionals may have a general distrust or lack of confidence in col-leagues in different fields. Newberger suggested that, in general, all profession-als suffer from too much work, a sense of hopelessness, punitive public policies, and cultural isolation from clients. The result is often multiple professionals functioning independently in a fashion that can hurt, not help, violent and ne-glectful families. For the benefit of the family, the nurse can therefore ensure that a coordinated approach to child abuse and neglect among professionals is used. The nurse is in a prime position to coordinate such multidisciplinary func-tioning. At the minimum, the nurse can be systematic and thorough in his or her assessments and assertive in interventions.

Schmitt and Mauro (1989) described an outpatient approach to the medical treatment of children diagnosed with nonorganic failure to thrive. Nursing in-volvement in such an approach is obvious. They categorized types of nonorganic failure to thrive as accidental, neglectful, and deliberate. Accidental failure to thrive is the result of errors in formula preparation, diet selection, or feeding technique. A mother who switches from concentrated formula to ready-to-feed formula and still continues to dilute it is an example of a mother who acciden-tally contributes to the failure of her child to thrive. Deliberate failure to thrive is the direct result of the intentional undernourishing of a child. Schmitt and Mauro suggested that this type of failure to thrive is rare and that such children usually require placement in foster care. Neglectful failure to thrive occurs be-cause the parent is overwhelmed or psychologically distressed.

In neglectful cases, the parent caretaker does not spend enough time with the baby and neglects feeding. This neglect may occur because the parent is busy with external problems, perhaps overwhelmed with work or overburdened by more children than the caretaker can handle. In other cases, the parent is preoc-cupied with psychological stresses—for example depression, very poor self-esteem, marital strife, or even psychosis.

Schmitt and Mauro (1989) recommended that the care of children and fami-lies experiencing any type of failure to thrive begin with a detailed history with par-ticular attention to nutrition. A detailed 24-hour recall of the child's diet provides essential information. Every effort must be made to avoid leading the parent as he or she recounts the process of feeding preparation. Schmitt and Mauro concluded that in families with good mother–child interaction, normal child development, and no deprivational behaviors or inflicted injuries, management of the failure to thrive can be maintained on a monthly outpatient basis. "If the infant is over 12 months of age, the parents have a support system, or the parents have sought med-ical care for some previous sickness or immunizations, an outpatient approach is even safe" (pp. 243–244). The authors recommend a multidisciplinary outpatient management of mild neglectful failure to thrive according to the following steps: clearly written dietary and stimulation instructions, twice-weekly visits by the pub-lic-health nurse, and referral to child protective services. Even with the prospect of successful outpatient management, the providers cannot forget that every case of even suspected child abuse and neglect must be reported.

Community

Lutzker and Newman (1986) defined child abuse and neglect as a community-health problem and suggested a community-based treatment approach. Hence community-health nurses and public-health nurses play an integral role in intervention at the secondary prevention level, namely case-finding and treatment.

Risk factors were discussed in the section on primary prevention. Once the nurse identifies the family at risk, the assessment must be carried one step further and the nurse must assess if child maltreatment is occurring. Behavioral assessment data that leads the nurse to strongly suspect abuse includes the following (Heindl, Krall, Salus, & Broadhurst, 1979):

- The child is wary of physical contact with adults and may even shrink away from such contact.
- When an adult hand is raised, the child winces or flinches.
- The child responds to the nurse's questions with one-word answers and often glances toward the parent or caregiver before answering, as if to seek approval.
- The child demonstrates extremes of behavior, ranging from overt aggression to profound withdrawal.

When behavioral cues suggest abuse, a physical examination must follow. Physical assessment data suggestive of abuse includes bruises or welts in unusual places and in various stages of healing. It is unlikely that a child would incur numerous bruises on the expanse of the back from a fall. A fall would be expected to injure a bony prominence. Abuse injuries are often to the trunk area of the body, since this area is easy to cover to prevent discovery of the injury. Other signs include unexplained burns, fractures, and dislocations. When questioned regarding injuries, parents often appear nervous and have a "hard time remembering" what happened. Frequently, the parent blames the child for being "clumsy" and may even state that the child did not inform him or her about the injury when it occurred. The caregiver should also be asked why the child was not brought for medical treatment after the injury.

Assessment data for neglect is distinctly different than those for abuse. Behavioral "red flags" for neglect include frequent truancy from school; when he or she does attend school, the child may often arrive late and leave early. School nurses are in key positions to identify and follow up on such behaviors. Physical indicators of neglect include poor physical growth of the child, who may also fail to meet appropriate developmental milestones. The infant who is not stimulated and left in the crib all day may have a bald spot in the back of the head. Neglected children often are dirty, and their clothes may be old, dirty, or inappropriate for environmental conditions. The children often do not receive proper preventive health care (such as well-child visits or immunizations) and treatment of health problems (injuries or colds).

Once child maltreatment has been identified, the professional nurse's next intervention is to report the fact to the appropriate child-protective agency. Each state has mandatory child abuse and neglect reporting laws; the nurse is legally responsible to report all cases. (See Chapter 13 for a detailed discussion.) Often, the quickest way to report is a referral to the local Child Protective Services Agency (CPSA) followed shortly thereafter by the written report. It is important to have definite, objective data to support the claim when reporting child mal-treatment. Physical findings are important, as are environmental findings, school-attendance records, and verbatim parental accounts. Reports of findings such as "the mother constantly yells at the child and he seems afraid" will proba-bly not meet CPSA standards for maltreatment. Reporting of child abuse can be made anonymously; however, CPSA may appreciate knowing who reports the abuse because this helps determine the credibility of the report. Once the nurse has given the intake person the data, it is the responsibility of the CPSA to assign the case and begin action. Many states have a mandatory time frame in which the CPSA must take action. In addition, many states also have a time frame within which the written report must be sent to the CPSA. The state's child-protection law outlines the guidelines in these areas.

Next, the CPSA worker makes a home visit to the family and informs the members of the referral. Ideally, the parent should be informed that the referral is being made; however, most families react with anger and hostility to such accu-sations. The professional nurse must consider the impact of such a revelation on the therapeutic relationship with the family. It is important that the nurse not mistakenly assume that abusive and neglectful parents do not want help and that they are content with their maltreatment. It is possible that some parents do not wish to change their behavior, yet clinical experience more often reveals anxious, frightened people who do not want to lose custody of their children and who fear what harm they may do in the future. Once the CPSA worker has met with the family, the nurse can assist the family members in using a variety of services available from the protective service agency. Parents often suffer under the mis-conception that the sole function of protective service agencies is to remove chil-dren from their families. Child protective agencies often offer a wide range of services from crisis-telephone lines to emergency respite child-care services.

The primary focus of secondary prevention is to assure safety of the child vic-tim. In some cases, the child will be placed in temporary foster care until the par-ent has completed treatment; in other cases the family will be closely monitored by CPSA while the family is in treatment. This intervention is very important; Cohn and Daro (1987) reported, after an analysis of the research findings on child abuse and neglect treatment programs, that approximately one-third of parents in treat-ment programs continue to maltreat their child(ren) during the course of therapy. The CHN or PHN may also be following such families and should be attuned to the possibility of continued maltreatment despite treatment interventions.

Secondary-prevention treatment programs are focused on the family as a unit, rather than on select individuals. Scharer (1979) used six subroles to de-scribe the role of the nurse who intervenes with abusive and neglectful families: mother surrogate, manager, technical advisor, teacher, nurse-psychotherapist, and socializing agent. Essentially, nursing interventions are focused on gaining trust, role-modeling, teaching problem-solving and limit setting, attending to the parent, and facilitating the development of extrafamilial resources. Carter, Reed, and Reh (1975) saw the role of the professional nurse as service coordinator. In-tervention techniques used by the nurse included relationship building, model-ing appropriate methods of child care, supporting the mother psychologically, collaborating with the mother in planning health care, and coordinating of other agency services. Modeling and reinforcement of desirable behaviors were also used. In suggested interventions with abusive and neglectful families, derived from both studies, nurses are called on to use the full range of their skills.

In the few instances in which child abuse and neglect is committed by a mentally ill parent, intensive treatment by the appropriate professional should be aimed at alleviating the illness. However, since 95% of the adults who abuse and neglect children are not psychotic, psychiatric treatment is not a frequently used treatment option (Justice & Justice, 1976).

Treatment modalities and interventions are custom-tailored to meet the family's needs. When intervening with maltreating families, the nurse must use assessment data to set long- and short-term goals. Short-term goals must be directed to alleviate immediate stressors, as abusive and neglectful parents most often experience tremendous stress combined with inappropriate methods of child-rearing. Quick action by the professional nurse to alleviate some of the family stress can not only prevent recurrence of child abuse and neglect but also demonstrate to the family the nurses' commitment and ability to "deliver." The power of definitive interventions like emergency housing, supplemental food, and short-term child care should never be underestimated. Horowitz and Wintermute (1978) described an emergency fund established in New Jersey precisely for the purpose of providing direct services to child abusive and neglectful families that were not covered by any other resource. One result of the pilot study was the realization that small, immediate stress-reducing interventions could successfully eliminate the need for more extensive agency action later.

More long-term stress-reducing interventions call for the nurse to involve the family in available community social and economic-assistance programs. Even limited social and economic assistance may be enough to reduce the strain on the family and allow the members to attend to alternative methods of coping and child-rearing. Ideally, the cause of their poverty would be addressed as well. For example, if a father is laid off from his job as a manual laborer, he would be provided with assistance in retraining, thereby increasing his ability to get a satisfactory job, to raise his status of living, and to allow his family to be self-sufficient. Although the financially independent, nonpoor families may still commit child abuse and neglect, the chances are significantly less.

The ultimate long-term goal for abusive families is to achieve a change in behavior. Many modalities exist to accomplish this. One approach is parental education, commonly referred to as "parenting classes." Classes are usually structured around a learning theory or approach. Four common approaches used in parenting classes are (Gaudin & Kurtz, 1985):

- Supportive, unstructured discussion (a parent-driven approach)
- The teaching of child development, with the hope that doing so will provide insight into the child's behavior and a framework for discipline (a developmental approach)
- Improvement of the communication pattern between parent and child (a child-centered approach)
- The teaching of the principles of social-learning theory as a basis for parenting (a social learning theory approach)

The effectiveness of parenting classes, particularly of individual approaches, is difficult to assess because different outcome measures have been used to determine "success." The most frequently used outcome measure was the absence of recurrent abuse. This has inherent faults because abuse may still occur though not be reported. Hence, the effectiveness of parenting classes at this time is at best inconclusive.

Another intervention modality is the parent support group. Such groups exist to provide social support and a format for discussion and friendship for maltreating parents. Parents Anonymous is based on the theoretical approach to child abuse that states that abuse results from unresolved conflict from the parent's childhood, current unmet parental needs, and stressful events that are presently occurring. The group focuses on parental factors that contribute to the occurrence of such situations. These factors include social isolation, low self-esteem, impulsiveness, passivity, negative attitude toward the child, inadequate knowledge of child development, inadequate problem-solving skills, inability to cope with stress, and inappropriate child-management techniques.

Hunka, O'Toole, and O'Toole (1985) empirically evaluated the effectiveness of a Midwest Parents Anonymous group by use of interviews and a Likert questionnaire to assess the 18 subjects' progress in the aforementioned factors. Overall, the majority of the parents reported positive change in each one of the factors. Self-esteem was reported to be the most problematic area for the subjects and also demonstrated the greatest degree of improvement after treatment. Hence it appears that this particular program was effective for these participants. It should be noted that the longer the subjects attended the sessions and the more frequently the subjects attended, the greater the differences in pretreatment and posttreatment scores (Hunka et al., 1985).

Another treatment option is parenting classes that also function as support groups. Soditus and Mock (1988) discuss one such program developed and implemented by public-health nurses in Sacramento. The goals of the eight-week program were to increase parents' skills as nurturers, to facilitate positive parent–child interactions, and to encourage parents to see their children as individuals. Although the classes were structured, parents were encouraged to participate and share. Soditus and Mock reported that participation in the classes increased the parents' self-esteem, shown by more relaxed posture by participants over time, more smiling, and increased interaction between parents. No other empirical measures of program effectiveness were reported and there was no follow-up of families after completion of the program to assess for any recurrent abusive behavior.

The federal government has funded four major studies aimed at evaluating interventions aimed at treating child abuse and neglect (Cohn et al., 1981). The evaluation concluded that lay services (such as Parents Anonymous) were most effective within a treatment program that included parenting classes and individual therapy. In addition, the findings identified an optimal length of treatment to be between 7 and 18 months. Clients involved in treatment less than 6 months or longer than 19 months scored lower on success indicators than those who stayed in treatment for the optimal time did. Success rates, however, for all the demonstration projects evaluated were disappointing—only fair to poor. Physical abuse continued to occur during the course of treatment in 30% to 47% of the cases evaluated. The authors concluded that overall current treatment efforts are not very effective.

Kempe and Kempe (1978) estimated that 20% of maltreating families experience no change in behavior, regardless of intervention; 40% of parents experience a long-term behavior change; and 40% cease to physically maltreat their children but continue to emotionally and mentally maltreat. The findings of the government studies suggest the percentages for continued maltreatment are much higher than Kempe and Kempe estimated. Kempe and Kempe used their findings to advocate increased funding for primary prevention because secondary prevention does not appear to be effective.

Family

When a father is absent from the home, the male child is deprived of his emotional support, guidance, and direction. Girls are adversely affected too. As the female child approaches puberty, the father often withdraws from the child, in part because of his feelings about sexuality, the inability to separate paternal caring emotions and thoughts from his own sexuality, and the inability to acknowledge clear boundaries in the father–daughter relationship (Fiese, Wilder, & Bickham, 2000; Saunders, 1991). Conversely, when mothers behave in a seductive manner toward their sons, they, as a rule, are more hostile toward their daughters. This behavior is also a violation of mother–child boundaries (Fiese et al., 2000).

Research has documented that mothers tend to be more abusive toward daughters than the father is, perhaps because mothers spend much more time with their children than fathers. But the probability of a mother abusing her child is linked with the father's proviolence attitude and behaviors. Husbands who direct aggression toward their wives indirectly places the child at risk because the mother is more likely to scapegoat and abuse the child to channel her own sense of victimization (Fiese et al., 2000; Mierendorf & Sarandon, 2000; Saunders, 1991). See Box 9-1 for factors that tend to increase violence between intimate partners.

Men in this society value self-reliance, autonomy, and freedom. These values sometime make it extremely difficult for men to seek help for physical health conditions and even more difficult, as a rule, for them to seek psychiatric care. Nurses can implement some basic psychodynamic techniques that will aid men in having more positive attitudes about seeking psychiatric help (Cicchetti, Toth, & Maughan, 2000; Swanson & Woolson, 1973):

- Involve the patient in developing goals and timelines for his own treatment.
- Focus on the patient's pleasant memories and here-and-now thoughts and feelings.
- Set realistic and straightforward goals and timelines for treatment.
- Discuss the potential positive outcomes of treatment.
- Introduce realistic and practical change in a positive, step-by-step manner.
- Provide regular feedback, with many positive statements and incentives.

Issues related to maltreatment in families also have a societal component that must be considered. Issues of ethnicity and race contribute to parental violence toward children. Racism, unfair treatment, and other types of oppression create stressors and interrupt dreams, resulting in destabilization of families and making it almost impossible for the father and mother to provide a stable, enduring, and safe home for their children (Cicchetti et al., 2000). The frequent display of violence on television and film suggests that this society condones violence (Cicchetti et al., 2000; Strauss, Gelles, & Steinmetz, 1980).

The nurse who provides services to children and families should always be alert to the potential for child abuse and know how to appropriately respond. Crisis intervention is useful in helping the nurse when developing interventions for these families. The strategies listed in Box 9-2 will be helpful to the nurse who is involved in child-abuse interventions.

BOX	9-1	**FACTORS THAT INCREASE THE POTENTIAL FOR VIOLENCE BETWEEN INTIMATE PARTNERS**

Dating Violence: Intimate courtship in which violence has occurred.

Youth: Marriage or steady intimate partnerships at a young age after a brief courtship.

Premarital Pregnancy: Dependency—a possibly lethal combination of youth and premarital pregnancy.

Stepchildren: The provocation of a child by another male partner.

Isolation: Severed or limited relationships with others and little social support from family, friends, or health and social agencies.

Unknown History: Insufficient information about the male partner's former intimate relationships or about the partner in general, including parents, coworkers, and friends.

Dependence: Inability to function as an independent person because of health, language limitations, education, occupation, geography, or caregiver responsibilities.

Adapted from Pagelow, M. (1984). *Family violence.* New York: Praeger Special Studies (Louie, 1991; Lutzker, 1998).

Parents with intellectual disabilities require special consideration and skills. Over the past several decades, individuals with intellectual disabilities have lived in communities and not in institutions, as they did earlier. Laws regulating their human and civil rights have provided them with many "normative" opportunities, among which are marriage and parenting.

Many of the parents were victims of child abuse and neglect. Too often, they live in poverty, are stigmatized and unemployed, and live in substandard housing. Many of them live in unsafe neighborhoods and do not enjoy the support of other families and friends. Numerous such families receive a variety of social services and may be monitored by Child Protective Services (Feldman, 1998a; Feldman & Walton-Allen, 1997). These parents may manifest some deficits in feeding, washing hair, sleep safety, cleaning baby bottles, and nutrition. They can, however, be trained and assisted to provide adequate care for their children (Feldman, 1998b).

Research has documented that these parents function not only with limited resources but also under a tremendous amount of stress, including the threat of having their children removed from the home. The stress is greater when these parents have children who also have intellectual disabilities or chronic physical or mental illnesses. These circumstances will require that the nurse assess the family situation, the parental capacity to care for the child, and the resources available to the parents. In some, but not all, instances, the mother may be the only parent in the home and have the sole responsibility of providing for the child (Feldman, 1998; Feldman & Walton-Allen, 1997; Fiese et al., 2000).

About 80% of mentally retarded parents have had their children removed from their homes, and their parental rights terminated because of potential, perceived, or actual child maltreatment and neglect, including sexual abuse. These statistics suggest that there might be professional biases that mitigate against these parents and children. On the other hand, there could also be a real or potential threat to the child that requires intervention and monitoring (Feldman, Sparks, & Case, 1993). Nurses need to approach these families with an open mind, focus on a thorough and unbiased assessment, and then be guided by the

BOX 9-2 STRATEGIES FOR CHILD-ABUSE INTERVENTIONS

Maintain a neutral, mater-of-fact attitude about the alleged maltreatment. Avoid using words or body language that conveys shock, disappointment, or disapproval. The nurse should monitor his or her behavior.

Be supportive. Use responses such as "Young children can be stubborn" or "I know it's difficult for you to talk about this." These types of statements should be made with affect and verbal responses matching the context of the discussion.

Provide validating statements and recognize positive interventions. For example, a statement such as "You did an excellent job in treating the child's burn immediately after the incident" conveys positive reinforcement to the parent for the actions taken to assist the child.

Keep the focus on the best interest of the child and the parents or caregivers. Make statements such as "Now we will make plans for getting the child the treatment needed, and we will need your help in scheduling an appointment for you [parents] to talk with a social worker about stress management and time management."

Keep attention on what the parents and caregivers reveal and what is known and observable. Avoid innuendoes, accusations, and interpretations of the information available from other sources, especially informal information.

Reassurance is essential. Parents and caretakers need to be reassured that the worker is viewing the incident with an open mind and is working to provide the necessary care for the child, based on authentic and confirmed evidence. The nurse can provide information about policies and procedures likely to be followed in relation to the incident and then help the parents or caregivers with their fears and anxieties. The nurse should make the legal implications for child abuse clear to the parents and caregivers, but in the context of support and respect. Information about services and resources, public and private, can be shared with the parents and other family members. Efforts should be made to help the adults work through the crisis and learn alternative behaviors to the abuse.

Always be aware of nonverbal communication and look for signs of hostility, fear, and affection among family members. Nonverbal communications are highly significant for the assessment process. Be alert to nods, eye contact, seating arrangements, spatial clues, and other nonverbal methods of communicating.

Talk with family members individually. Individual family members can have different perceptions about the incident. A thorough assessment involves their individual input and then a validated description of the situation.

Open-ended questions provide more clinical data. For example, instead of asking who burned the child, ask how the child got burned. Or ask, "How do you think the child got burned?"

Recognize and label feelings. Statements such as "That must have been frightening and upsetting to you" or " You must have been angry when you hit your child" helps to facilitate the discussion and conveys to the parents that you are sensitive to the complexities of the situation.

Restate the parents' answers to make sure that they understand and give them the opportunity to provide information, ask questions, and clarify your statements. The nurse might say, "Now let me review what you have said. You became angry when Joe wet his pants and pulled the boiling pot off the stove—is that correct?"

Avoid agreeing with or seeming to condone everything that the parents share, while making sure that you understand the facts, the emotions, and the context. Statements such as "That was upsetting to you" or "That made you fearful" will help to convey your concern without passing judgment. Avoid statements like "I would have done the same thing" or "No wonder you hit him."

Do not make verbal abuse a personal experience. Frequently, the person being interviewed who is in a stressful situation will be defensive and fearful. He or she could become hostile, angry, and even disrespectful to the interviewer. This behavior should not be taken personally but should be understood as a reaction to being interviewed.

(continued)

BOX	9-2	**STRATEGIES FOR CHILD-ABUSE INTERVENTIONS** *(Continued)*

Convey a goal of alleviating the stress and assisting with changing the situation in the service of the child's best interest. Saying "I have confidence that you can manage the morning meals and the children" tells the parents that you think they can change. However, the parents need to be clear about your willingness and capacity to take charge of the situation if needed. That is, the highest priority is the child's safety and well-being.

Source: Adapted from Borgman, R., Edmunds, M., & MacDicken, R. (1979). *Crisis intervention: A manual for child protective workers* (DHEW Publication No. OHDS 79-30196). Washington, D.C.: Department of Health, Education, and Welfare; Cicchetti, D., Toth, S., & Maughan, A. (2000). An ecological-transactional model of child maltreatment. In A. Sameroff, M. Lewis, and S. Miller (Eds.), *Handbook of developmental psychopathology* (2nd ed., pp. 689–722). New York: Kluwer Academic/Plenum Publishers.

data that is available. Again, the best interest of the child should be the framework that guides and directs any intervention plan. Good nursing care is based on an informed assessment, an understanding of the cultural and political context within which the child or adolescent lives, and the assets and limitations of the parents.

Social Interventions

The nurse concerned about the status and treatment of children is likely alarmed at dramatic cutbacks of social services to children and their families. The nature of child abuse and neglect requires the involvement of many disciplines; yet, the exact agencies that are needed the most by families with the fewest resources are the agencies that experience the most severe funding cuts. The individuals who preach the sanctity of the American family are often the advocates of the elimination of the few services that might help a family stay nonviolent and together. The American Bar Association's Juvenile Justice Standards Project (1977) cited the prevailing low quality of protective child welfare services in the United States and therefore recommended a sharp restriction of access to those services. A technique suggested for decreasing the number of referred cases of child abuse and neglect is to change mandatory reporting to discretionary reporting. Social policies and beliefs that promote such a backward movement of child-welfare services are of great concern and a focus of intervention for nursing.

Over the past 30 years, the problem of child abuse and neglect has become more familiar to both the professional and general public. Of the cases of child abuse and neglect reported to child protective services in 1988, 26% came from sources other than institutions and community agencies (National Center on Child Abuse and Neglect, 1988). Approximately 68% of the reports were from professionals (in education, health care, law enforcement, and social agencies). Hospitals and public-health agencies accounted for 10%. Unfortunately, as many cases and possibly even more went unreported.

Friedrich (1977) reported that after a two-week media campaign in Houston, Texas, aimed at educating the public and professionals about their role in child abuse, a significant increase in reported cases of child abuse occurred. The greatest apparent effect of the campaign was on the professionals, and the increase in reports came under the category of the "less severe" type of abuse (such as soft-tissue abuse or abuse with neglect). "Possibly the campaign had the effect of increasing potential reporters' awareness of the many types of abuse rather than just the severe types like burns, fractures, and gunshot" (pp. 161–162). Because cases go unreported, nurses have a responsibility to see that media campaigns like the one described by Friedrich take place in their communities. Until abusive families are identified and given assistance, the child/victim will likely continue to suffer.

The increasing literature reports on resilience in children offer hope to professionals and families alike. The work of Cowen and Work (1988) has been cited for its insight into the role of support in the ability of children to develop resilience as they experience adversity. Mrazek and Mrazek (1987) concluded that generic life circumstances (good health, educational, and social-welfare services) and abuse-specific protective factors (quick and full offender acknowledgment of abuse and timeliness and permanence of legal actions affecting the child's custody) can help children to be less vulnerable. Generic life circumstances that can support children include good health, education, and social-welfare services. According to Mrazek and Mrazek (1987), these circumstances can foster resilience in children regardless of the stressors. Although abuse-specific protective factors alone cannot ensure that detrimental effects are minimized, they are recognized as significant factors that should be considered in the development of any plan of care for abused and neglected children.

Tertiary Prevention

Ideally, child abuse and neglect is never allowed to progress to the tertiary level of intervention; however, as social resources are eliminated, more children are likely to need this intervention. Tertiary prevention is required when the damage of child abuse and neglect is done and the disability is irreversible. The goal of tertiary prevention is rehabilitation to the maximum level of functioning possible within the limitations of the disability.

Tertiary prevention is also required when, after thorough assessment and interdisciplinary consultation, it becomes clear that the abusive and neglectful family cannot safely function together. Out of necessity, the child is removed from the home, either voluntarily or by court action. At the time of the removal, the child is placed in an alternative-living arrangement, usually a foster home. The nurses in such emergency-custody programs are in an excellent position to provide services from crisis intervention to health promotion.

The Standards for Service for Abused or Neglected Children and their Families (1989) were developed by the Child Welfare League of America, through a multidisciplinary committee that sought to address both the generic components of child welfare practice and specific information on children and families experiencing abuse and neglect. These standards provide guidelines for multidisciplinary practice with maltreated children and their families and for community responsibilities for the protection of children. They are valuable for the nurse who seeks to restore these individuals to their highest level of functioning.

Separating children from their families is often necessary to ensure the safety of the children, but it does not solve the family's problems. If prior separation from children is thought to be at least partly responsible for the lack of positive parent–child relationship, subsequent separations can only be expected to exacerbate the problem (Watters, Parry, Caplan & Bates, 1986).

Foster-home placement for an abused and neglected child is often described as a "temporary" action designed to provide care to the child when the family cannot. However, in Massachusetts, Derdeyn (1977) reported that in a cross-sectional study 60% of the children in foster care had been there for four to eight years. Interestingly, one of the factors impeding return of children to their families, cited by the Jenkins and Norman (1975) study of children in foster care in New York City, was the extreme poverty of their mothers.

Derdeyn also explained that foster-home placement often is not temporary and that many children live in multiple homes during their placement. Adoption is often impossible. Even when a family wishes to adopt a child, the biological parents usually refuse to give up custody. It appears that foster children, in the eyes of the court, have even fewer rights than children in general. Derdeyn recommended permanent foster placement for children who cannot be returned home or placed by adoption.

Generally, institutions—foster homes, group homes, and large child-welfare institutions—are unacceptable and do not benefit the abused and neglected children in them (Bush, 1980). The 370 children surveyed by Bush lived in a variety of settings at the time of the study. The majority living in institutions "felt less comfortable, loved, looked after, trusted, cared about, and wanted than children [did] in any other form of surrogate care (foster home) or than children who had been returned to their families [did]. In general, institutions were reported to be run on the basis that the children in them had 'problems' and were in need of 'treatment'" (p. 249). Another frequent comment of the children interviewed by Bush was that environment and activities were organized primarily to facilitate the running of the institution.

When the child is in poor physical condition as the result of parent maltreatment, the nurse can intervene based on the child's symptoms. Obviously, the malnourished infant requires nursing interventions that alleviate the child's alteration in nutrition. The burned child experiences the same alterations in skin integrity as any other burn victim. In addition to physical needs, though, the abused and neglected child is likely to have difficulties relating to adults, to be limited in communication, and to otherwise be developmentally delayed.

The appropriate nursing interventions directed at the child's psychological, social, and developmental needs, at the level of tertiary prevention, are rehabilitative. The harm inflicted on the child is irreversible, and nursing care must seek to limit the extent of the disability as much as possible.

The most important intervention for the abused and neglected child is the securing of a positive, loving home. If the home of the biological parents cannot be made safe, then the nurse should support the other professionals involved in the welfare of the child in foster-home placement. Though safe, such an alternative living arrangement is questionably healthy. It is doubtful that an abused and neglected child would learn to be a successful parent in either setting. Ideally, the biological parents' home should be made safe and the child returned as soon as possible.

The plan of care with the abusive and neglectful parents should aim to reduce stress on the parent and increase parent self-esteem, problem-solving skills, and knowledge of child development. Family counseling and therapy are most likely necessary to terminate the maladaptive family members' interactions. See Chapter 8 for a detailed discussion of overall family nursing care.

While in foster care, the abused and neglected child needs ongoing nursing intervention. Indeed, it is possible that the nurse is the only consistent person in the life of the child in the transition from abusive and neglectful home to foster home. The nurse seeks to ensure that the foster home provides the child with an environment that is supportive, understanding, consistent, and nonviolent. Often, the move to a foster home involves relocation to another part of town. Nursing intervention can ensure that schooling and health-care services continue in the new location where past services ended. A child need not restart his or her immunizations just because no one kept track of the shot records.

To help the child overcome past trauma, the nurse may refer the child to psychological therapy, special education, or both. The child who does not require special assistance in school still needs the support of his or her school nurse, who received a referral from the public-health nurse.

Preschool children can be involved in an educational program appropriate to their needs. Many abused and neglected children have received either no developmental stimulation or the wrong kind. As soon as possible, they need to experience developmentally appropriate, positive stimulation.

Many severely abused and neglected children experience permanent physical disabilities as a result of their maltreatment. These children are entitled to many of the same state, federal, and charitable health and financial benefits available to other disabled children. The nurse can see that such children use all available services as soon as possible in an effort to reduce the impact of physical disability.

In a qualitative study, Korbin (1989) proposed a framework for understanding the most severe form of child abuse and neglect, fatal maltreatment. Korbin, whose study was limited to mothers, concluded that although extreme in outcome, fatal maltreatment was not a homogeneous entity. She further noted that although the specifics of each case varied, each was characterized by a recurrent pattern of abuse culminating in fatality. The women in Korbin's study reported life histories rampant with adverse conditions and risk factors, such as past or current family violence, difficulties (real or perceived) in child management, and financial stressors. Korbin reported that within a pattern of recurrent abuse, the women give signals to others that problems existed. "Like suicide victims, abusive parents may give signs or clues that they consciously or unconsciously hope will be interpreted as pleas for help and alert others to the problems that they are experiencing. Such signals may be provided to professionals and public-service agencies or to individuals such as kin, neighbors, or friends in their personal networks" (p. 484).

Especially noteworthy was Korbin's finding that the presence of visible injuries was a significant point in the evolution toward child fatality. When the mothers were faced with visible evidence of their maltreatment, they were often shocked into seeking help or telling others of their behavior. For the women in Korbin's study, however, these warnings and pleas for help went unrecognized and therefore untreated. This was a pivotal stage in the progression toward the fatality. The women could exit the cycle into intervention (that might or might not be successful), or they could deny the seriousness of their actions. Two of the women in Korbin's study had been reported to child protective services and either the child who subsequently died or another had been removed from the home.

Fontana and Alfaro (1987) found that a previous court-ordered placement was among the few factors that differentiated fatal from nonfatal abuse. Korbin concluded that regardless of the reason for removing a child, the reuniting period may be particularly dangerous. Korbin's research supported the need for early identification and intervention with families at risk or experiencing child abuse and neglect. Her findings further suggested that removal of the child from the home ensures the safety of the child often only in the short term.

It would seem that leaving an abused and neglected child in an unsafe home is unacceptable. However, placing a child in a foster home, group home, or state institution is also no solution. The energies of the nurse are best directed toward an earlier level of prevention, ideally primary. The nurse needs to see social policies in the United States as intolerable until children are given the same rights and opportunities granted by the Constitution to adults.

All three levels of prevention of child abuse and neglect may be necessary in the nursing interventions with an individual family. For example, the professional nurse may intervene to safely return an abused child to his or her home from foster care (tertiary prevention), secure supplemental-food-program benefits for underfed siblings (secondary prevention), and provide health education to parents of a healthy newborn (primary prevention). The demands on the nurse are great and require skillful, creative nursing care.

SPECIAL EMPHASIS ON SUICIDE AMONG CHILDREN AND ADOLESCENTS

Child and adolescent suicide has reached an alarming level over the past decades. Special emphasis is given to suicide prevention here because it may be one of the most devastating outcomes related to the battering of women and child abuse. Children who have been abused frequently experience feelings of hopelessness and helplessness, basic antecedents for suicidal ideation and behaviors.

Suicide is now the third leading cause of death in children aged 10 to 14 years (303 deaths among 19,097,000 children) and among 15- to 24-year-olds (1.4 of every 100,000 persons). Among adolescents aged 15 to 19 years (1,802 suicide deaths among 19,146,000), the numbers continue to increase. More males (4:1 ratio) than females commit suicide, though more females express suicidal ideation and make attempts (National Clearing House on Child Abuse and Neglect Information, 2000; National Institute of Mental Health, 2001; Children's Bureau Administration on Children, Youth & Families, 2002).

Models for Understanding Suicide

It is necessary for the nurse to understand suicide from a theoretical perspective. We briefly describe psychoanalytic, behavioral, sociological, and biological models here.

The psychoanalytic model suggests that the intrapsychiatric (inside the mind) phenomenon is an unconscious hostility directed toward an introjected love object for which the person has feelings of both love and hate. Rage, hatred, guilt, anxiety, depression, dependency, hopelessness and helplessness are some of the psychiatric correlates associated with suicide (Louie, 1991).

Shneidman, in his classic writings about suicide, delineated three basic characteristics that are present, and the nurse who works with abused children or adults should be aware of all of them. First, the intense period of suicide is a lethal time where self-destruction is deemed to be the best solution to a situation; its duration is about 24 hours or even less. Second, the person might make detailed plans for self-destruction and simultaneously construct plans for a rescue mission. This state exists because of the depth of ambivalence that the individual is experiencing regarding the suicide. Third, suicide is a dyadic event. The suicidal person's significant other could be a mother, a child, or a lover (in adolescence) who is involved in some intense dynamic with the child. If the child or adolescent completes the suicidal act, then the emotional needs of the survivors emerge as being of paramount importance to the nurse and other health-care professionals (Shneidman, 1976).

Behavioral models are distinguished from other models by the underlying premise that behavior is learned and reinforced by events in the environment (Bandura, 1977a, 1977b). Hence, by inference, suicide is a learned behavior that is added to the child's range of possibilities transmitted through the environment within which he or she lives. Suicide can also function as a reward and punishment system for the child, and this fact makes it even more essential that the nurse not reinforce the suicidal thoughts and behaviors. The therapeutic goal is to extinguish the suicidal behaviors and help the child to test out other alternatives (Kaplan, Pelcovitz, Salzinger, et al., 1997).

Sociological models are grounded in understanding the child's relationships to society. Durkheim, about 50 years ago, discussed three types of suicide. Altruistic suicide exists when the individual (adolescent) accepts rigid and unrealistic rules and customs generated by a particular society (Durkheim, 1951; Shneidman, 1976). Egoistic suicide is related to the person's lack of connectedness to family and society. Typically, the person feels lonely, isolated, depressed, anxious, and fearful (Shneidman, 1976; Swenson & Hanson, 1998). Anomic suicide happens when the individual perceives that the relationship between self and society are broken with little possibilities of them being set right. The loss is considered a permanent one (Durkeim, 1951; Louie, 1991).

Finally, the biological model suggests that norepinephrine metabolism, adrenal-cortical function, and electrolyte metabolism play a role in suicide. These systems are integrated and are not easily separated. It has been hypothesized that depressed individuals have elevated sodium levels in the nerve cells, which helps to support the use of lithium for patients who are manic-depressive. At the cellular level, lithium interrupts the exchange of sodium and helps with symptom relief.

In recent years, researchers have concluded that neurotransmitter components play an important role in human behavior, and certain classifications of drugs can aid in altering those behaviors. The components include dopamine, serotonin, acetylcholine, norepinephrine, glutamate, and aminobutyric acid. Monoamine oxidase (MOA) enzyme breaks down norepinephrine, inhibits the enzyme for metabolizing biogenic amines that accumulate, and increases the concentration of neurotransmitters that are released when the nerves are stimulated. Researchers have also found that thyrotropin-releasing hormone (TRH) helps to lower the levels of thyroid-stimulating hormone (TSH). These hypotheses have helped to advance the understanding of biological underpinnings of mood disturbances and depression, antecedents to suicide (Louie, 1991; Wilcox, Gonzales, & Miller, 1998). (For more details about biological psychiatry and suicide, see Wilcox, Gonzales, & Miller, 1998.)

Assessment of Adolescent Suicide

Adolescents often engage in suicidal-type behaviors without the intent to die. They are frequently expressing a desire for help. The nurse should be aware of several clues (Bureau of Emergency Medical Services, 2000; Louie, 1991; Reducing Suicide: A National Imperative, 2002):

- Withdrawal from family, peers, and friends
- The giving away of highly personal and valued possessions
- Substance abuse (alcohol, marijuana, cocaine)
- Eating disorders (anorexia, bulimia)
- Changes in personality, mood, and interests
- Change in school performance (usually school failure) or dropping out of school
- Numerous physical complaints (headaches, stomach aches)
- Highly personal thoughts about death, letters to friends about morbid topics
- Irritability and ambivalence regarding relationships and their outcomes
- Familial conflict at home
- High risk behaviors, such as driving recklessly and under the influence of substances
- Involvement in aggressive behaviors and provocative acts
- Numerous crises and losses

The child or adolescent who has attempted or is thinking about suicide should never be left alone. Instead, the nurse or a responsible adult should remain with the individual until the acute phase has passed. Nurses can educate parents and caregivers about the importance of limiting the suicidal person's access to large amounts of medications. All lethal weapons such as guns and large, sharp knives should be removed from the environment.

The following sources can provide more information about suicide:

The National Institute of Mental Health (NIMH)
301-443-4513
www.nimh.nih.gov

American Association of Suicidology
202-237-2280
www.suicidology.org

American Foundation for Suicide Prevention
212-363-3500
www.afsp.org

Suicide Prevention Advocacy Network
770-998-8819
www.spanusa.org

A FOCUS ON SAFETY WHEN THE PATIENT IS VIOLENT

A major consideration in nursing care is safety, and the degree to which it exists should also be assessed. When nurses and other health professionals anticipate violence from parents, practical approaches for safety should be considered:

- The nurse should always be alert to the potential for violence and be prepared to prevent harm to themselves and others.

- When the nurse is interviewing the patient, the door to the room should never be closed, and other staff ought to be aware of the whereabouts of the nurse.
- Interview rooms can be engineered for safety: desks can be bolted to the floor, emergency alarms can be installed, cameras can be mounted on the walls and linked to a system with monitoring screens strategically placed for continuous view and assessment.
- Breakable glass and heavy objects should be removed from the environment.

The nurse who works in emergency and crises situations ought to be well informed about crisis-management theory and practice methods.

CHILDREN'S RESPONSES TO FAMILY VIOLENCE AND IMPLICATIONS FOR TREATMENT

One of the most devastating life events that a child can experience is the death of one parent at the hands of the other. The child has to deal with the loss of a parent, usually the mother; changes in residence; possible placement in a foster home; shame; fear; and anxiety. The child may be stigmatized as "a child of a murderer" and may become depressed and at risk for developing other childhood psychiatric disorders (Fantuzzo & Mohr, 1999; Kilpatrick & Williams, 1997a; Osofsky, 1999; Plass, 1993).

Few scientifically based estimates of the prevalence of children who witness violence in intimate relationships currently exist, but the data that are available suggest that children are negatively affected. Even though violence in intimate relationships has been a public health problem for years, its impact on children did not attract the attention of researchers until the 1980s (Fantuzzo & Mohr, 1999). Hence, it is not yet known how children's exposure to violence in intimate relationships affects them developmentally in the short or long term; neither are their specific experiences known. The protective factors and at-risk factors are not well understood (Fantuzzo & Mohr, 1999; Kilpatrick & Williams, 1997a,b; Osofsky, 1999).

Kilpatrick & Williams examined 20 child witnesses to intimate-partner violence, along with 15 matched controls. They determined that, relative to posttraumatic stress syndrome, the effect of the violence is not mediated by maternal emotional well-being, age and gender of the child witness, and the child's method of coping with parental conflict. The study suggests that intimate-partner violence has a long-term devastating effect on children (Kilpatrick and Williams, 1997a).

Researchers interviewed 228 children between 8 and 14 years of age residing in a shelter for battered women and identified specific patterns of behaviors that existed among them, including multiple problems associated with externalizing (acting out) and internalizing (depression, suicide), mild distress, and no manifest problems. Children with high levels of depression and anxiety tended to display anger and acting-out behaviors. Research findings raise issues regarding the variability of child responses to family violence (Grych, Jouriles, Swank, McDonald, & Norwood, 1999). Further studies are needed to help determine which factors or variables influence which patterns of responses over the child's lifespan.

Little is known about the influence of the mother's aggression relative to the father's level of aggression. This is a fertile area for nurse researchers.

A group of researchers in London examined the responses of 95 children who had witnessed one of their parents kill the other. They reported a significant number of these children developed posttraumatic stress syndrome, but the children who did not witness the killing showed less PTSD. A correlation between witnessing a killing between parents and the development of PTSD is also in need of scientific exploration (Harris, Black, Kaplan, 1993; Kaplan, Black, Hyman, and Knox, 2001).

INTERVENTION PROGRAMS

In the case of suicide prevention, specific intervention programs must be evaluated for short-term and long-term effects. One important research finding suggests that school-based, information-only programs are not effective in the prevention of suicide among children and adolescents and could possibly increase the children's vulnerability (Vieland, Whittle, Garland, Hicks, & Shaffer, 1991). Intervention programs, including those that highlight suicide prevention, should have a broad-based approach, encompassing mental health, coping skills, stress management, control of substance use and abuse, anger and aggressive-behavior management, and positive relationships with adults (Mierendorf & Sarandon, 2000; National Institute of Mental Health, 2001; Vieland, Whittle, Garland, Hicks, & Shaffer, 1991; Wolfe & Yuan, 2001).

EVALUATION

The final step of the nursing process is evaluation, when the professional nurse reviews the changes that have occurred based on the identified goals. Again, the nurse must be realistic in her evaluation of child abuse and neglect. She can praise even small evidence of progress. Praise to a parent who is having difficulty in child-rearing can be a new experience and a strong reinforcer.

SAMPLE NURSING PROCESS

A sample nursing process in a hypothetical case of child abuse and neglect is included in this chapter to demonstrate how each of the four steps can be applied. An in-depth assessment composed of both historical and physical findings would naturally have preceded its development; the total assessment is not completely presented. The nurse should remember that a child and his or her family are unique and require individualized plans of care. The sample nursing process (see Box 9-3) can be used as a starting point.

SUMMARY

Nursing care of the abused and neglected child is based on a family framework and on the limited available nursing research. It involves four steps: assessment, goals, planning, and evaluation. Assessment for child abuse and neglect can be included in the practice of every nurse who provides care to children and their families. Particular attention should be paid in assessment to certain warning signs that can indicate potential or actual abuse. Although three levels of prevention of child abuse and neglect are discussed, nursing practice should be mainly directed toward primary prevention, as no level of maltreatment of children can be acceptable to the nurse whose philosophy is to promote the life, health, and well-being of her clients.

BOX 9-3 SAMPLE NURSING PROCESS

ASSESSMENT

BRIEF BACKGROUND

Kent is a 15-month-old white boy admitted to the general pediatric unit of the hospital with a medical diagnosis of child abuse and neglect. Kent lives with his 22-year-old mother and two siblings. The family's sole source of income is Aid to Dependent Children. Kent's mother describes him as a "difficult" child who willfully disobeys her and refuses to be toilet trained. She reports that he holds his bowel movements "just to make me angry." In addition, Kent's mother reports that he "won't eat" and drinks only Kool-Aid in his bottle. Kent's mother is the primary caretaker and knows no one in the neighborhood; she moved to the area to be with Kent's father, who has since deserted the family.

PHYSICAL EXAMINATION

The nurse's physical examination of Kent includes, but is not limited to, the following:

- General appearance: Thin, 15-month-old white boy who appears to watch all activities in the room but remains quiet and passive through all procedures, including blood drawing
- Vital statistics: Height and weight below third percentile
- Skin: Multiple discrete, circumscribed, 1cm in diameter second-degree burns in various stages of resolution about the distal arms and legs. Scant purulent drainage noted at lesions. Generalized decreased subcutaneous tissue
- Neurological: Abnormal score on DDST (Failed language and personal/social)

NURSING DIAGNOSES, OUTCOMES, INTERVENTIONS, AND EVALUATIONS

Three of the nursing diagnoses identified are described in order of priority.

ALTERED FAMILY PROCESS

This is a family-focused nursing diagnosis. The altered family process results in a potential for subsequent violence (child) related to lack of parent support systems, inadequate financial resources, mother's knowledge deficit regarding growth and development, and ineffective parent behavior.

SHORT-TERM CLIENT GOAL: Family will not experience additional violence before discharge from the hospital as evidenced by:

- No additional child injuries during hospitalization
- Demonstration of nurturing behavior by parent toward child
- Mother's discussion of factors contributing to past episodes of violence toward child
- Mother's identification of alternative methods of expressing anger
- Mother's identification of key aspects of child behavior and development during the toddler stage
- Mother's agreement to participate with child-protective and other agencies

NURSING INTERVENTIONS:

- Provide continuous but discrete supervision of mother–child interaction.
- Provide mother with age-appropriate child-safety precautions for hospitalization.
- Model nurturing child-care behaviors for mother, especially during bath, play, and feeding
- Encourage mother to actively participate in daily child care.

(continued)

BOX 9-3 SAMPLE NURSING PROCESS (*Continued*)

- Praise mother's attempts at nurturing behaviors, expecting close approximations of goal.
- Spend at least 20 minutes in discussion with mother, encouraging her to talk about herself.
- Use therapeutic-communication techniques to elicit factors that contribute to the violence toward child.
- Use therapeutic-communication and problem-solving techniques to assist mother in identification of nonviolent expressions of anger.
- Provide mother with information about child development.
- Demonstrate to mother how information about child development can be used in daily life (e.g., in discipline, play, feeding, and toileting).
- Provide mother with information about child-protective and other agencies.
- Contact appropriate agencies and initiate client contact before discharge.
- Reassure mother that all agencies are concerned with child safety and helping her to care for her child.

EVALUATION: Because the nursing process is still in the development phase, no evaluation is possible. When appropriate, evaluation should be ongoing and based on the achievement of identified family goals measured against the stated criteria.

LONG-TERM CLIENT GOAL: Remain free of violence six months after discharge as evidenced by:

- No additional child injuries after hospitalization
- Improved DDST age-appropriate score
- Demonstration of consistent nurturing parental behaviors
- Documented demonstration of mother using nonviolent methods of dealing with anger
- Demonstration by mother of age-appropriate techniques of child discipline
- Documented active participation with other agencies
- Documented use (as appropriate) of alternative child-care services
- Mother's participation in social or other organizations (e.g., church or school) that increase circle of acquaintances

NURSING INTERVENTIONS:

Refer to public-health nursing for continued, intermittent monitoring of child, home, and family. The public-health nurse will:

- Have contact with mother and child before discharge.
- Secure and coordinate child-protective and other agency services to family.
- Enroll child in an educational preschool program. School will educate, encourage, and support mother in parenting skills.
- Administer DDST six months postdischarge. (Alternatively, the school nurse could do so.)
- Praise all attempts by the mother to use nonviolent discipline.
- Provide information to mother regarding day-care centers and emergency child-care services.
- Use problem-solving techniques to assist mother in identifying friends and relatives who might assist or exchange child care.
- Assess mother for areas of social, educational, recreational, religious, or community interest.
- Provide information about appropriate organizations in community and arrange for personal contact as desired.
- Praise all evidence of the mother decreasing her social isolation

EVALUATION: Long-term evaluation will be carried out by the public-health nurse, be ongoing, and be based on the achievement of identified family goals as measured against the stated criteria.

(continued)

BOX **9-3** **SAMPLE NURSING PROCESS (*Continued*)**

IMPAIRMENT OF SKIN INTEGRITY

Impairment of skin integrity is related to partial-thickness burns and poor hygiene.

OVERALL CLIENT GOAL: Client will experience improved skin integrity during hospitalization (two weeks) as evidenced by:
- Healing of skin lesions and no additional child injuries during hospitalization
- Decreased signs of infection (redness, tenderness, swelling)
- Evidence of good personal hygiene

NURSING INTERVENTIONS:

- Note size, shape, location, and condition of lesions. Exact diagram of lesions will be recorded and included in initial nursing assessment.
- Clean and gently débride skin lesions after 15 minutes of soaking during morning bath.
- Leave lesions open to air.
- Monitor progress of lesions.
- Provide adequate diet (see next nursing diagnosis).
- Monitor vital signs.
- Monitor skin lesions for increased redness.
- Monitor laboratory data (e.g., CBC).
- Keep client's fingernails clean and short.
- Inform mother of all signs of improvement.
- Monitor client's skin.
- Provide supervision of mother–child interaction.
- Serve as role model to mother.
- Provide information to mother.
- Praise mother's efforts to assist in attainment of goal and identify strengths.

EVALUATION: Because the nursing process is still in the development phase, no evaluation is possible. When appropriate, evaluation should be ongoing and based on the achievement of identified client goals measured against the stated criteria.

INADEQUATE NUTRITION

There is an alteration in nutrition. It is less than body requirements and is probably related to parent knowledge deficit and inadequate financial resources.

CLIENT GOAL: Client will experience adequate nutrition during hospitalization (two weeks) as evidenced by:

- No loss in weight
- Good skin turgor and moist mucous membranes
- Laboratory findings that show no worsening of physical condition
- Mother's identification of key aspects of nutrition, child behavior, and development during the toddler stage and identification of appropriate available resources

NURSING INTERVENTIONS:

- Provide client with age-appropriate diet: Protein, 1.8 (g/kg); Energy, 100 (kcal/kg); Fat, > 30%, < 50%; Carbohydrate, 50 to 100 g
- Record all food and fluid intake.
- Provide a varied (in color, taste, and texture) selection of food.
- Prepare food so that it is mild and of comfortable temperature.
- Provide three nutritious finger-food snacks (at 10:00 A.M., 3:00 P.M., and 7:30 P.M.).

(*continued*)

BOX 9-3   SAMPLE NURSING PROCESS (*Continued*)

- Encourage mother's involvement in feeding.
  - Serve as role model to mother.
  - Provide information to mother.
  - Praise mother's efforts to assist in attainment of goal and identify strengths.
- Weight
- Provide client with adequate fluid intake: 120 to 125 ml/kg.
- Record all fluid intake.
- Offer 4 oz of fluid (vary type) every waking hour.
- Encourage drinking from cup.
  - Assist as necessary.
  - Praise mother's and child's efforts.
- Measure urine-specific gravity each shift.
- Monitor laboratory tests and alter diet as necessary.
- Inform the mother about nutrition, growth, and development.
- Arrange consultation with nutritionist.
- Inform the mother about available supplemental food programs.
- Recommend parent–child educational day-care center to the mother.
- Contact social-service agency to arrange for enrollment before discharge.

EVALUATION: Because the nursing process is still in the developmental phase, no evaluation is possible. When appropriate, evaluation should be ongoing and based on the achievement of identified client goals measured against the stated criteria.

References

American Bar Association Juvenile Justice Standards Project. (1977). *Students relating to abuse and neglect.* Cambridge, MA: Harper & Row.

Bandura, A. (1977a). Self efficacy: Toward a unifying theory of behavioral change. *Psychological Review, 84,* 191–215.

Bandura, A. (1977b). *Social learning theory.* Englewood Cliffs, NJ: Prentice Hall.

Barth, R. P., Hacking, S., & Ash, J. R. (1988). Preventing child abuse: An experimental evaluation of the child–parent enrichment project. *Journal of Primary Prevention, 8,* 201–217.

Barthel, R., & Herrman, C. (Eds.). (1991). *Psychiatric mental health nursing with children.* Philadelphia: Lippincott.

Borgman, R., Edmunds, M., & MacDicken, R. (1979). *Crisis intervention: A manual for child protective workers.* National Center on Child Abuse and Neglect Children's Bureau, Administration for Children, Youth and Families Office of Human Development Services. U. S. Department of Health, Education and Welfare. DHEW Publication No. (OHDS) 79-30196.

Bullock, L. F., & McFarlane, J. (1989). The birth weight/battering connection. *American Journal of Nursing, 89,* 1153–1155.

Bureau of Emergency Medical Services (2000). *Adolescent suicide prevention plan task force report to the Florida Department of Health* [Online]. Available: http://www.ac.wwu.edu/~hayden.spsp/states/fla.

Bush, M. (1980). Institutions for dependent and neglected children: Therapeutic option of choice or last resort? *American Journal of Orthopsychiatry, 50,* 239–255.

Cappell, C., & Heiner, R. B. (1990). The intergenerational transmission of family aggression. *Journal of Family Violence, 5,* 135–152.

Carter, B. D., Reed, R., & Reh, C. J. (1975). Mental health nursing intervention with child abusing and neglectful mothers. *Journal of Psychiatric Nursing and Mental Health Services, 13,* 132–140.

Cersonsky, J. (1988). Cocaine abusers as mothers. *Pediatrics, 82,* 136.

Children's Trust Fund, (1988/89-1989/90). *State plan for years 1988/89 and 1989/90.* Lansing, MI: Author.

Child Welfare League of America (1989). *Standards for service for abused or neglected children and their families.* Washington, DC: Author.

Cicchetti, D., Toth, S., & Maughan, A. (Eds.). (2000). An ecological-transactional model of child maltreatment. In A. Sameroff, M. Lewis, and S. Miller (Eds.), *Handbook of developmental psychopathology* (2nd ed., pp. 689–722). New York: Kluwer Academic Plenum Publishers.

Cohn, A. H. (1981). *An approach to preventing child abuse.* Chicago: National Committee for Prevention of Child Abuse.

Cohn, A. H., & Daro, D. (1987). Is treatment too late: What ten years of evaluative research tells us. *Child Abuse and Neglect, 11,* 433–442.

Cowen, E. L., & Work, W. C. (1988). Resilient children, psychological wellness, and primary prevention. *American Journal of Community Psychology, 16,* 591–607.

Cox, P., Kershaw, S., & Trotter, J. (2000). *Child sexual assault: Feminist perspectives.* New York: Palgrave.

Cupoli, J. M., & Newberger, E. H. (1977). Optimism or pessimism for the victim of child abuse? *Pediatrics, 59,* 1356–1360.

Derdeyn, A. P. (1977). A case for permanent foster placement of dependent, neglected, and abused children. *American Journal of Orthopsychiatry, 47,* 604–614.

Durhkeim, E. (1951). Suicide. (J. A. Spaulding & G. Simpson, Trans.). New York: Free Press.

Fantuzzo, J., & Mohr, W. (1999). Prevalence and effects of child exposure to domestic violence. *The Future of Domestic Violence and Children, 9*(3), 21–32.

Feldman, M. (Ed.). (1998). *Parents with intellectual disabilities: Implications and interventions.* New York: Plenum Press.

Feldman, M., Sparks, B., & Case, L. (1993). Effectiveness of home-based early intervention on the language development of children of mothers with mental retardation. *Research in Developmental Disabilities, 14,* 387–408.

Feldman, M., & Walton-Allen, N. (1997). Effects of maternal mental retardation and poverty on intellectual, academic, and behavioral status of school-age children. *American Journal on Mental Retardation, 101,* 352–364.

Fiese, B., Wilder, J., & Bickham, N. (Eds.). (2000). *Family context in developmental psychopathy.* New York: Kluwer Academic Plenum Publishers.

Fontana, V., & Alfaro, J. (1987). *High risk factors associated with child maltreatment fatalities.* New York: New York Mayor's Task Force on Child Abuse and Neglect.

Freud, A. (1967). *Normality and pathology in childhood.* New York: International Universities Press.

Friedrich, W. N. (1977). Evaluation of media campaign's effect on reporting patterns of child abuse. *Perceptual and Motor Skills, 45,* 161–162.

Gage, R. B. (1990). Consequences of children's exposure to spouse abuse. *Pediatric Nursing, 16,* 258–260.

Gaudin, J. M., & Kurtz, D. P. (1985). Parenting skills training for child abusers. *Journal of Group Psychotherapy, Psychodrama and Sociometry, 38,* 35–54.

Gil, D. G. (1971). Violence against children. *Journal of Marriage and the Family, 32,* 637–648.

Gough, D., & Taylor, J. (1988). Child abuse prevention: Studies of ante-natal and post-natal services. *Journal of Reproductive and Infant Psychology, 6,* 217–228.

Gray, E. B. (1982). Perinatal support programs: A strategy for primary prevention of child abuse. *Journal of Primary Prevention, 2,* 138–152.

Grych, J., Jouriles, E., Swank, P., McDonald, R., & Norwood, W. (1999). Patterns of adjustment among children of battered women. *Journal of Counseling and Clinical Psychology, 68*(1), 84.

Hamilton, L. R. (1989). Variables associated with child maltreatment and implications for prevention and treatment. *Early Child Development and Care, 42,* 31–36.

Harris, H. J., Black, D., & Kaplan, T. (1993). *When father kills mother: Guiding children through trauma and grief.* London: Routledge.

Heindl, C., Krall, C. A., Salus, M. K., & Broadhurst, D. D. (1979). The nurse's role in the prevention and treatment of child abuse and neglect (DHEW No. 79-30202). Washington, DC: U.S. Government Printing Office.

Herzberger, S. D., & Tennen, H. (1988). Snips and snails and puppy dog tails: Gender of agent, recipient, and observer as determinants of perceptions of discipline. *Sex Roles, 12,* 853–865.

Hoffman-Plotkin, D., & Twentyman, C. T. (1984). A multimodal assessment of behavioral and cognitive deficits in abused and neglected preschoolers. *Child Development, 55,* 794–802.

Horowitz, B., & Wintermute, W. (1978). Use of an emergency fund in protective services casework. *Child Welfare, 57,* 432–437.

Hunka, C. D., O'Toole, A. W., & O'Toole, R. (1985). Self-help therapy in parents anonymous. *Journal of Psychosocial Nursing, 23,* 24–31.

Jenkins, S., & Norman, M. (1975). *Beyond placement: Mothers view foster care.* New York: Columbia University Press.

Justice, B., & Justice, R. (1976). *The abusing family.* New York: Human Sciences Press.

Kaplan, S., Pelcovitz, D., Salzinger, S., et al. (1997). Adolescent physical abuse and suicide attempts. *Journal of the American Academy of Child and Adolescent Psychiatry, 36*(6), 799–808.

Kaplan, T., Black, D., Hyman, P., & Knox, J. (2001). Outcome of children seen after one parent killed the other. *Clinical Child Psychiatry, 6*(1), 9–22.

Kempe, R. S., & Kempe, C. H. (1978). *Child abuse.* Cambridge, MA: Harvard University Press.

Kilpatrick K., & Williams, L. (1997a). Potential mediator of post-traumatic stress disorder in child witnesses to domestic violence. *Child Abuse and Neglect, 22*(4), 319–330.

Kilpatrick, K., & Williams, L. (1997b). Post traumatic stress disorder in child witnesses to domestic violence. *American Journal of Orthopsychiatry, 67*(4), 639–644.

Korbin, J. E. (1989). Fatal maltreatment by mothers: A proposed framework. *Child Abuse and Neglect, 13,* 481–489.

Lapham-Alcorn, G. (Ed.). (1991). *Communication theory.* Philadelphia: Lippincott.

Louie, K. (Ed.). (1991). *Psychological crises.* Philadelphia: Lippincott.

Lutzker, J. (Ed.). (1998). *Handbook of child abuse research and treatment.* New York: Plenum Press.

Lutzker, J. R., & Newman, M. R. (1986). Child abuse and neglect: Community problem, community solutions. *Education and Treatment of Children, 9,* 344–354.

Mierendorf, M. (Producer, Director, Writer), & Sarandon, S. (Narrator). (2000). *Broken child* [Film]. (Available from Films for the Humanities & Sciences, P.O. Box 2053, Princeton, NJ 08543-2053.)

Milner, J. S., & Chilamkurti, C. (1991). Physical child abuse perpetrator characteristics. *Journal of Interpersonal Violence, 6,* 345–366.

Mrazek, P. J., & Mrazek, D. P. (1987). Resilience in child maltreatment victims: A conceptual exploration. *Child Abuse and Neglect, 11,* 357–366.

National Center for Injury Prevention and Control. (2000). *Fact book for the year 2000: Suicide and suicide behavior.* [Online]. Available: www.cdc.gov/ncipc/pub-res/FactBook/suicide.htm.

National Center on Child Abuse & Neglect (1988). *Study of national incidence and prevalence of child abuse and neglect: 1988* (Contract No. 105-85-1702). Washington, DC: U.S. Department of Health and Human Services.

National Institute of Mental Health. (2001). *In harm's way: Suicide in America* [Online]. Available: www.nimh.nih.gov.publicat/harmaway.cfm.

Newberger, E. H. (1976). A physician's perspective on the interdisciplinary management of child abuse. *Psychiatric Opinion, 2,* 13–18.

Osofsky, J. (1999). The impact of violence on children. *The Future of Children: Domestic Violence and Children, 9*(3), 33–49.

Pagelow, M. (1984). *Family violence.* New York: Praeger Special Studies.

Plass, P. (1993). African American family homicide. *Journal of Black Studies, 23*(4), 1–15.

Robinson, D. (1998). *Psychiatric mnemonics and clinical guides.* Fort Gratiot, Michigan: Rapid Psychler Press.

Saunders, D. (Ed.). (1991). *Psychiatric mental health nursing in men.* Philadelphia: Lippincott.

Scharer, K. (1979). Nursing therapy with abusive and neglectful families. *Journal of Psychiatric Nursing and Mental Health Services, 17,* 12–21.

Schmitt, B. D., & Mauro, R. D. (1989). Nonorganic failure to thrive: An outpatient approach. *Child Abuse and Neglect, 13,* 235–248.

Seagull, E. A. (1987). Social support and child maltreatment: A review of the evidence. *Child Abuse and Neglect, 11,* 41–52.

Sherrod, K. B., O'Connor, S., Vietze, P. M., & Altemeier, W. A. (1984). Child health and maltreatment. *Child Development, 55,* 1174–1183.

Shneidman, E. (Ed.). (1976). *Suicide among the gifted.* New York: Grune and Stratton.

Soditus, C., & Mock, D. (1988). Interrupting the cycle of child abuse, *MCN: The American Journal of Maternal Child Nursing*, 13, 196–199.

Steele, B. F. (1987). Psychodynamic factors in child abuse. In R. E. Helfer & C. H. Kempe (Eds.), *The battered child* (4th ed., pp. 81–114). Chicago: University of Chicago Press.

Steele, B. F., & Pollock, C. B. (1974). A psychiatric study of parents who abuse infants and small children. In R. E. Helfer & C. H. Kempe (Eds.), *The battered child* (2nd ed., pp. 92–139). Chicago: University of Chicago Press.

Stern, L. (1973). Prematurity as a factor in child abuse. *Hospital Practice, 8,* 1–19.

Strauss, M., Gelles, R., & Steinmetz, S. (1980). *Behind closed doors: Violence in the American family.* New York: Anchor Publishers.

Swanson, M., & Woolson, A. (1973). Psychotherapy with the unmotivated patient. *Psychotherapy: Theory, Research, and Practice, 10*(2), 175–183.

Swenson, C., & Hanson, R. (Eds.). (1998). Handbook of child abuse research and treatment. New York: Plenum Press.

Twentyman, C. T., & Plotkin, R. C. (1982). Unrealistic expectations of parents who maltreat their children: An educational deficit pertaining to child development. *Journal of Clinical Psychology, 38,* 497–503.

Vieland, V., Whittle, B., Garland, A., Hicks, R., & Shaffer, D. (1991). The impact of curriculum-based suicide prevention programs for teenagers: An 18-month follow-up. *Journal of the American Academy of Child and Adolescent Psychiatry, 30*(5), 811–815.

Vondra, J. I., & Toth, S. L. (1989). Ecological perspectives on child maltreatment: Research and intervention. *Early Child Development and Care, 42,* 11–29.

Watters, J., Parry, R., Caplan, P. J., & Bates, R. (1986). A comparison of child abuse and child neglect. *Canadian Journal of Behavioural Science, 18,* 449–459.

Webster-Stratton, C. (1998). Parent training with low-income families: Promoting parental engagement through a collaborative approach. In J. Lutzker (Ed.), *Handbook of child abuse research and treatment.* New York: Plenum Press.

Weikart, D. P. (1980). *Research report.* Ypsilanti, MI: High/Scope Education Research Foundation.

Wilcox, R., Gonzales, R., & Miller, J. (Eds.). (1998). *Introduction to neurotransmitters, receptors, signal transduction, and second messengers* (2nd ed). Washington, DC: American Psychiatric Press.

Wolfe, D., & Yuan, L. (2001). *Health Canada: A conceptual and epidemiological framework for child maltreatment surveillance.* Ottawa: Minister of Public Works and Government Services Canada.

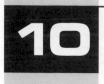

Nursing Care and Adolescent Dating Violence

• M. Christine King and Josephine M. Ryan

Research has clearly demonstrated that adolescent women experience abuse in dating relationships. Although the rates of violent crimes have declined for all age groups since 1994, adolescents between the ages of 12 and 19 remain at highest risk for both perpetration and victimization of violent crimes (Office of Justice Programs, 1998). Approximately one in five female high school students reports being physically and/or sexually abused by a dating partner (Silverman, Raj, Mucci, & Hathaway, 2001). A review of dating-violence research found that prevalence rates of nonsexual, courtship violence range from 9% to 65%, depending on whether threats and emotional abuse or verbal aggression were included in the definition (Sugarman & Hotaling, 1989). Forty percent of girls aged 14 to 17 report knowing someone their age who has been hit or beaten by a boyfriend (Commonwealth Fund, 1997).

Teen dating violence is a serious crime that includes sexual assault, physical violence, and emotional abuse committed by someone whom an adolescent is dating. Teen dating violence can occur in the context of casual dating relationships or in more serious, long-term relationships. Although dating violence has been documented as occurring in gay and lesbian relationships and as initiated or engaged in by adolescent girls in relationships with boyfriends, the focus of this chapter will be on interventions to use with adolescent girls who experience abuse in the context of heterosexual dating relationships.

Why do young women today, who appear confident, sassy, and assertive, continue to become involved in physically and emotionally unhealthy dating relationships? The underlying reasons are quite similar to the reasons adult women find themselves involved in abusive relationships. An interplay of sociocultural, intrapersonal, and interpersonal factors predispose young women to abuse in dating relationships. Contributing social and cultural influences include the historical legacy of patriarchy, the media portrayal of gender inequality and violence, the sexualization of women and girls, the general acceptance of violence in our culture, and societal denial of the problem of interpersonal violence. This is augmented by the lack of education girls receive about intimate relationships in general and the silence on the issues of dating violence in particular. In fact, young women often do not even realize they are being abused until it is too late.

The desire for involvement in a dating relationship is ever present in the lives of young women. Cultural norms for adolescence dictate that to be considered "normal," one must be popular. Popularity is coupled with physical attractiveness, which is then coupled with having a boyfriend. Sometimes, young women know little more than that they have a "crush on a cute guy," leaving them ready to drop everything in order to have a boyfriend. Adolescent girls are eager to get involved with guys they think everyone likes, often failing to examine the dynamics of the relationship until it is too late.

THE ADOLESCENCE CONTEXT

Adolescence is a time of transition and change. It is a period of intense physical growth and development coupled with major transformations in cognitive and emotional development. During this time, adolescents are engaged in a variety of developmental tasks, such as gaining mastery, pursuing intimacy, and separating from parents. The most striking aspect of adolescence is change. Puberty marks the adolescent's most profound change and has an effect on the adolescent's biology and psychosocial functioning. It is gradual, however. Selected hormone levels increase in all adolescents but vary in timing, depending on the gender and on the individual. Increasing hormone levels lead to physiological and behavioral changes. Boys normally enter puberty at age 12 and girls at age 11. Changes include increases in body hair, in the activity of sweat glands, and in the activity of oil glands (leading to acne). There are also increases in height and weight, usually involving a growth spurt followed by a period of more gradual growth. Body-fat distribution changes and is different for boys and girls. These are typical changes for adolescents but vary in the individual.

These physical changes, and the timing of them, affect psychological and social development in the adolescent. Society sets social norms for what is attractive. As the body changes, so does self-evaluation. Self-evaluation is strongly related to viewing one's self as meeting society's norms. This association is thought to be stronger for girls than for boys. The timing of biological changes also affects self-evaluation, with early or late maturation having different effects. In girls, weight changes and breast development have a profound influence on self-evaluation. The image of a long-limbed and lithe body is a culturally idealized image that the girl who has gone through puberty typically does not approximate. All these changes are further mediated by contextual factors of family, school, community, media, ethnicity, class, and gender.

During adolescence, there are also major cognitive changes that exert an influence on the adolescent's personal and social spheres. How adolescents organize and structure knowledge is marked by a change from concrete to abstract thinking. Changes in self-understanding include self-definition, personal agency, and consciousness of self in public and in private.

During adolescence, boys and girls begin the process of searching for intimate relationships outside the family. While the term "dating" may not appear relevant to today's teenagers, they clearly display a pattern of engaging in intimate relationships, with 89% of adolescents aged 13 to 18 years reporting some type of intimate relationship with another teen (Cohall et al., 1999; Wolfe & Feiring, 2000). What is even more significant is that the majority of adolescents are "dating" teenagers who are not in their age-related peer group. One study documented that 75% of 8th and 9th grade girls were dating boys in higher grades, with a similar 75% of boys in these same grades dating girls in lower grades (Foshee et al., 1996). Given the enormous changes that occur in physical, emotional, social, and cognitive development over the course of one adolescent year, this dating pattern has major import for the nature and dynamics of teen dating relationships.

Adolescence is often described as a time of turmoil: a period of personal angst and interpersonal conflict between the adolescent and the family. Differentiating between normal "turmoil" and transient or deeper disturbances is difficult during adolescence. Whereas most teenagers are well-adjusted and cope effectively with the physiological, cognitive, emotional, and social changes experienced in this time of transition, those who experience violence and abuse are at great risk for depression and engagement in risky and unhealthy behaviors.

DEFINITION OF DATING VIOLENCE

Dating violence can be defined as a cycle of emotional, physical, or sexual abuse performed by one person to control or dominate another, within a dating relationship. The Centers for Disease Control and Prevention (CDC) IPV surveillance and uniform definitions document divides dating violence into four categories: physical violence, sexual violence, threats of physical or sexual violence, and psychological/emotional abuse (Saltzman, Fanslow, McMahon, & Shelley, 1999). All forms of dating abuse are designed to make the boyfriend feel "in control" and to "keep the girlfriend in line." Dating violence serves to violate, humiliate, degrade, or otherwise threaten or compromise the safety, health, and wellness of young women. Key dynamics found in abusive relationships include the violation of trust, the threat to repeat the abuse, and an overwhelming feeling of blame.

Abusers often excuse their own behavior by placing blame on the victim: "She made me do it" or "She knew I would hit her if she did that." Young women may also internalize these beliefs and blame themselves in an effort to make sense of their situation or to hold on to that which is considered essential, a boyfriend.

TYPES OF DATING ABUSE

Emotional abuse consists of words or actions designed to harm a young woman's self-image and to isolate her from her life outside the dating relationship. Emotional abuse can have a profound effect on the young woman's self confidence, emotional state, and opinions about herself. Emotional abuse is manifested in the following ways: insults, name-calling, swearing, remarks designed to make the young women feel helpless and childlike, jealousy, and guilty accusations. A major component of emotional abuse is control. Abusers repeatedly tell lies, spread rumors, and fail to keep promises. These behaviors center around controlling friendships and behaviors: what friends she may have, where and when she can go out with friends, what she can wear or eat, how well she can do in school, and whether she can have a job and what type of job. Besides damage to emotional development, emotional abuse may also jeopardize physical safety.

Physical abuse consists of actions designed to cause pain and physical injury, such as hitting, pushing, slapping, kicking, shaking, grabbing parts of the girl's body, biting, hair-pulling, attacking or threatening with a weapon, destroying the girl's personal property, and engaging in physical acts that are unwelcome, such as tickling, holding/hugging, and wrestling.

Sexual abuse consists of unwanted sexual advances and contacts, comments, and innuendo. These behaviors are used to obtain sex and to make the young woman feel intimidated, used, dirty, ashamed, and trapped. Young women are especially vulnerable to sexual abuse as they are just beginning to develop a personal sexual identity. They often feel that they must engage in sexual acts, despite not always wanting to, to keep their boyfriend. They may feel pressured to have oral, rectal, or vaginal sex. Sexually abusive behaviors include unwanted touching, sexual name calling, use of pornography in sexual encounter, forced sex, hurtful sex, and unfaithfulness and promiscuity on the part of the abuser. Many young women feel unable to demand the use of condoms, putting themselves at great risk for pregnancy and sexually transmitted disease. The most extreme act of sexual abuse is rape, the act of forcing sexual intercourse on an unwilling person. In many cases of adolescent rape, the consumption of drugs and alcohol, by both the perpetrator and the victim, is present. The use of "date-rape drugs" such as Rohypnol has become a widespread social problem. These drugs immobilize the victim and impair memory, making it easy for an abuser to force sex, leaving her feeling guilty, with vague or no memories of the sexual assault. In most cases of adolescent date rape, not only does the young woman remember the rape for the rest of her life, but also it often affects every sexual decision and encounter she makes in the future.

The behaviors demonstrated by abusive adolescent males in abusive dating relationships are similar to those seen in adult relationships. In general, abusers usually feel that they are entitled to behave in a controlling manner, often minimizing and denying their abusive behaviors. They often blame others for their actions, refusing to take personal responsibility. Jealousy and possessiveness are common, with the harm increasing when drugs and alcohol are involved. Young men do not receive adequate education about intimate relationships and have been raised in a society that does not foster adequate communication skills in boys and men. (See Box 10-1.)

The feelings and behaviors demonstrated by young women are likewise similar to those seen in abused adult women; however, the intensity of adolescent feelings and emotions is often markedly increased. Abused young women display denial, disbelief, embarrassment, blame and guilt, humiliation, violation, fear, powerlessness, anxiety, stress, sadness, and anger. The emotional reactions experienced by teens also include indecisiveness, mood swings, depression, and suicidal thoughts. Behaviors include use of drugs and alcohol, eating and sleep disturbances, nightmares, self-mutilation, poor grades, truancy, phobias, and increased social isolation. (See Box 10-2.)

Teen dating violence most certainly affects the healthy growth and development of young women. Most teens lack experience with intimate relationships

---

BOX 10-1   ADOLESCENT MALE INNER VOICES

- Guys are supposed to be in charge.
- Girls are supposed to act like "girls" and cater to guys.
- She led me on; she made me do it.
- She really meant yes, of course she wants to have sex.
- I lost control; I couldn't stop.
- I'm only teasing or playing with her.
- She makes me so angry and causes me to act this way.
- It's the liquor or drugs that make me act this way.
- But she hits, too; everyone gets hit.
- She deserves it; she's my "wifey."

BOX	10-2	ADOLESCENT FEMALE INNER VOICES

- I don't want to be unpopular.
- Having a boyfriend will make me fit in.
- Dating someone is better than dating no one.
- He loves me; he needs me.
- If he's jealous, it means he really loves me.
- No one else will want me or love me.
- I can change him with love.
- He won't do it again.
- If we have sex, things will get better.
- Everyone gets put down or hit sometimes.
- You always hurt the one you love.
- Having a baby will improve things.

and are reluctant to voluntarily discuss relationship issues with adults. Isolation and control, hallmarks of abusive dating relationships, interfere with emotional and social development of teens. Academic progress and life plans are often hindered. It is therefore imperative that interventions be designed and implemented to assist adolescent girls in their developmental tasks of creating a positive self-image as a woman and in forming healthy, supportive, intimate relationships.

INCIDENCE AND PREVALENCE OF VIOLENCE IN ADOLESCENT DATING RELATIONSHIPS

Although the literature on teen dating violence is relatively recent, a number of studies have investigated the prevalence of physical and sexual violence in dating relationships during adolescence. Prevalence data have varied significantly across studies, with ranges reported from 9% to 46% of adolescent females and males involved as victims or perpetrators (Avery-Leaf, Cascardi, O'Leary, & Cano, 1997; Coker et al., 2000; Foshee et al., 1996; Halpern, Oslak, Young, Martin, & Kupper, 2001; Malik, Sorenson, & Aneshensel, 1997; Molidor, Tolman, & Kober, 2000; O'Keefe & Treister, 1998; Rhynard, Krebs, & Glover, 1997; Reuterman & Burcky, 1989; Silverman et al., 2001; Spencer & Bryant, 2000; Watson, Cascardi, Avery-Leaf, & O'Leary, 2001; Wingood, DiClemente, McGree, Harrington, & Davies, 2001). Several issues can explain this wide variation, including lack of uniform definitions of dating violence, variations in the instruments used to assess dating violence, variations in ages considered to comprise adolescence, and the length of time for which results are reported (current versus past few months, versus lifetime).

Various studies seem to indicate that teen dating violence is mutual and reciprocal (Foshee et al., 1996; Molidor et al., 2000; Watson et al., 2001; Wingood et al., 2001). In a study of rural primarily European-American eighth- and ninth-grade adolescents (*n*=1,405), Foshee and colleagues (1996) reported victimization in a dating relationship at least once by 36.5% of girls and 39.4% of boys. Adolescent dating violence was examined by Watson and colleagues (2001) in a sample of ethnically and economically diverse urban youth (*n*=476). They reported that physical dating violence (current or past relationship) affected 45.5% (*n*=217) of participating girls and boys, with a much smaller percentage (9%) of girls and boys reporting exclusive victimization. African-American boys and girls reported the highest rates of victimization, and Latina girls reported significantly higher rates of physical-violence victimization than Latino boys did (Watson et al., 2001). In a dating violence study of 522 single, African-American girls aged 14 to 18 who were seeking care in a family medicine clinic, Wingood and colleagues (2001) found that 18.4% reported a history of dating violence, with 30.2% having been assaulted in the past six months (Wingood et al., 2001).

Data reported by Moskowitz and colleagues (2001) indicate that since 1994 adolescent girls are responsible for a higher proportion of assaults involving a penetrating weapon than boys are. Although these data may indicate that adolescent girls are becoming increasing violent, it might also indicate an increase in the severity of dating violence and abuse (Moskowitz et al., 2001).

The percentages of adolescent boys and girls who report being the recipient or perpetrator of abuse in dating relationships are quite close to equal, but severe physical and sexual victimization in dating relationships has been shown to be more prevalent among adolescent girls (Coker et al., 2000; Foshee et al., 1996; Molidor et al., 2000; Moskowitz et al., 2001). Foshee and colleagues (1996) found that girls reported more injuries from physical violence and that girls (14.5%) were significantly more likely to report sexual violence than boys (6.9%). Coker and colleagues (2000) reported that in their survey of students from small, medium, and large public high schools in South Carolina, severe dating-violence victimization rates were higher among females (14.4%) compared to male students (9.1%). Among girls in the study who were sexually active, 16.2% reported forced sex victimization and 5.3% reported forced sex perpetration.

In studies that look at context of interpersonal violence in teen dating relationships, considerable gender differences appear. In their study of an ethnically diverse group of 635 high school students, Molidor and Tolman (1998) reported significant gender differences in the experience of interpersonal violence for boys and girls. For students who had ever dated, 36.4% of females and 37.1% of males reported that they had experienced physical violence while in a dating relationship. However, they report that boys and girls react to incidents of violence in completely different ways: boys did not find the incidents of violence as threatening as the girls did, and girls indicated that they found the incidents frightening and had damaging physical and emotional effects. Another reported significant finding was that much of the girls' perpetrated violence was, in fact, reported as self-defense (37%) versus self-defense reported by only 6% of the boys in this study. There were also significant differences in the severity of the violence. Using subscales of severe and moderate violence, the data reveal girls reporting more severe violence (27.1%) with boys reporting significantly less severe forms of violence (16.4%). Drugs and alcohol were involved in many violent encounters, but the use of the substances was deemed too complex for the authors to draw any conclusions.

In a study of 939 multiracial and mixed-class high school students in a large urban area, O'Keefe and Trieste (1998) found that although dating violence may look mutual, a careful examination of their study indicated that the quality of violence inflicted on males and females was different. The rate of dating violence in their study was greater than the rate of some previous studies (males, 45.5%; females, 43.2%). Males reported being slapped or hit with a fist more frequently than females (males, 17.3%; females, 14.7%), but females reported considerably more sexual violence (females, 17.0% versus males, 9.6%). The authors concluded that the violence that males received may have resulted from the forced sexual activities perpetrated against their partners. Males were also more frequently found to initiate violence. Males thought their experiences of violence "was funny" and girls reported that their responses to the violence were "fear" and "emotional hurt." Neither racial nor socioeconomic factors were found to predict receiving or perpetrating violence in dating relationships.

Few studies have examined the contextual factors of teen dating violence. One study indicated a number of factors that increase the probability of dating violence, including exposure to family and community violence, poor parenting practices and family functioning, access to firearms, and neighborhoods characterized by high rates of poverty, transiency, family disruption, and social isolation (Dahlberg, 1998).

ANTECEDENTS OF ADOLESCENT DATING VIOLENCE

A popular belief concerning dating violence is that it is directly related to intergenerational transmission of interpersonal violence. Interpersonal violence is seen as a learned behavior that occurs as a result of witnessing aggression between parents. In an extensive review of the literature, Widom (1989) concluded that little empirical evidence demonstrates that witnessing spousal abuse in the home leads to either being the abuser or abused in dating relationships or in intimate-partner relationships. She cites flawed studies and poor research design in the persistent misinformation of intergenerational transmission of violence as a prevailing causative factor in interpersonal violence. This conclusion is supported by a prospective study by Simons (1998), who found that data failed to support the common notion that abusive behavior between parents increases the chances that children will grow up to be either abused or abusive. He argues that violence between parents is not seen by children as an effective way of reaching solutions and therefore will be equally ineffective in influencing a dating partner.

Yet other studies indicate that exposure to multiple forms of family violence, including child maltreatment, spousal/partner violence, and a climate of fighting and hostility, has a strong effect on future victimization or perpetration of violence (Dahlberg, 1998). In a study of 250 ethnically diverse urban high school students, O'Keefe (1997) reported that more than half (51%) of the students who reported having experienced dating violence witnessed parental spouse abuse. Similarly, Thornberry's (1994) longitudinal study demonstrated that 60% of adolescents exposed to one form of family violence, and 78% of adolescents exposed to three forms of family violence, reported involvement in violent behavior. This was in contrast to Thornberry's finding that 38% of adolescents from nonviolent families reported involvement in violent behavior.

Although this research is inconclusive in regard to exposure to family violence increasing the risks of subsequent dating violence, some studies indicate that parental neglect might increase the risks for dating violence. Widom (1989) concluded that neglect, not abuse of children by their parents, may lead to increased levels of violence. Abused and neglected children show more aggressive behaviors than those who are not abused and neglected. Aggression seems to be a fairly stable personality trait and may be predictive of later antisocial behavior.

She was reluctant to make further conclusions because she inferred from the literature that abuse and neglect are conceptually different and the research to discriminate between these two is scanty and methodologically difficult. From his study, Simons (1998) concluded that although frequent exposure to corporal punishment may increase the risk of dating violence, low support or low involvement of the parents (i.e., neglect) is associated with delinquency and substance abuse, which, he felt, predicts dating violence. He acknowledged that much more research needs to be conducted to delineate intergenerational transmission of violence.

Jessor took a more epidemiological approach to the study of risk behaviors and risk factors. Based on his work, he suggested that adolescent problem behaviors, such as abusive dating relationships, are only one part of a whole constellation of problem behaviors. He believed that these behaviors stem from a host of risk factors rather than one causal factor. He warned, as other epidemiologists have, not to look for the immediate cause of risk behaviors but to the interplay of risk factors. The factors influencing behavior may be biology and genetics, the social environment, the perceived social environment, and personality. Within each of these domains, risk factors and protective factors exist. Reducing risk factors or increasing protective factors can decrease risky behavior (Jessor, 1991). Thus, it is perhaps more efficient to focus on lifestyle as a whole rather than on one risky behavior.

In a study looking at the interrelationships among health-enhancing behaviors (such as seat-belt use, sleep, and tooth brushing), Donovan, Jessor, and Costa (1993) noted that a single underlying factor (unknown) may account for the correlation among health-enhancing behaviors. This single factor appeared to hold true across gender and cultural boundaries and across age (middle school and high school). They posited that it is worth pursing a research track that investigates whether multidimensional modes for health-related behavior, which encompass both health-enhancing and risk behaviors, exist.

Some studies have sought to examine the relationship between alcohol and substance use and current adolescent dating violence. Dahlberg (1998) found that this correlation was unclear, and O'Malley, Johnston, & Bachman (1993) reported that whereas males were more likely to use substances than females were, the difference was relatively small. However, in a small sample of Canadian high school students, alcohol was associated with dating violence, with 31% of girls and 53% of boys reporting the use of alcohol before or during the date where violence occurred (Rhynard, Krebs, & Glover, 1997).

The media is considered a significant contextual factor for violence in society. Adolescents are especially vulnerable to the powerful influence of the media, particularly music, music videos, movies and television, and teen magazines. Popular media may have different effects not only on how adolescents define themselves but also on their views of interpersonal relationships, including dating violence. Critics of contemporary media argue that exposure to negative depictions and treatment of women may affect attitudes and behavior regarding violence against women. One study reported that exposure to violent music led to a normalization of the use of violence among listeners (Johnson, Adams, Ashburn, & Reed, 1995).

Little research allows us to say with any assurance what array of variables may contribute to dating violence. We are unsure of the interplay among peer influence, family, community, media, increasing urban violence, substance abuse, and commercialized, sexualized, and violent popular culture that influence protective or risk-producing behaviors (Schubiner, Scott, & Tzelepis, 1993; Schwab-Stone et al., 1999; Singer et al., 1995). However, interpersonal risk factors probably include attitudes of peers about violent and abusive behaviors, a family history of violent and abusive behavior, level of parental and other adult acceptance of abuse in intimate violence, and the level of family and adult interaction.

Intrapersonal risk factors for dating violence and abuse may then include the adolescent and peer attitudes toward violence and gender roles, the extent of rebelliousness and perceived entitlement, the extent of alienation and depression, the adolescent's sexual activity and possible pregnancy, the extent to which the adolescent engages in problem behaviors, and physiological factors such as the adolescent's response to alcohol or drugs (Ellickson & McGurgan, 2000; O'Keefe, 1997).

HEALTH EFFECTS OF DATING VIOLENCE

Although few studies report the health effects of teen dating violence on mental or physical health, dating violence has been shown to result in serious negative health outcomes for adolescent victims and perpetrators, including depression, unhealthy weight control, sexual-risk behaviors, and substance use (Coker et al., 2000; Plichta, 1996; Sells & Blum, 1996; Silverman et al., 2001; Wingood et al., 2001). The U.S. Department of Justice reported in national survey data that girls receive more severe violence in dating relationships than do boys and 10% of intentional injuries to girls are from male dating partners (Tjaden & Thoennes, 2000). Plichta (1996) found rates of depression, eating disorders, and substance use to be twice as high among girls who reported physical or sexual dating violence than among girls who did not. Wingood and colleagues (2001) reported that girls who indicated a history of dating violence were three times more likely to have had a sexually transmitted disease than girls who had not experienced dating violence. Their study data also indicated that girls reporting dating violence were two times more likely to have ever been pregnant and half as likely to have used condoms consistently during the previous six months (Wingood et al., 2001).

For these reasons, researchers in Massachusetts decided to focus their attention on the effects of dating violence on girls in Massachusetts (Silverman et al., 2001). Massachusetts, in 1997, became the first state to include a question assessing the prevalence of lifetime physical and sexual abuse in the Youth Risk Behavior Study conducted biannually by the CDC in schools in all states. Using data collected in 1997 and 1999, the authors reported that adolescent girls who experienced interpersonal violence from their dating partners were more likely to partake in serious health-risk behaviors such as substance abuse, unhealthy weight control, sexual-risk behavior, pregnancy, and suicide. Unhealthy weight control was more associated with physical abuse than with sexual abuse.

IMPLICATIONS FOR CLINICAL PRACTICE

To effectively assist adolescent girls through the unfolding process of maturity, nurse clinicians must be cognizant of the impact of dating violence. Specifically, nurses need to develop an awareness of the problem of dating violence and gain informed knowledge concerning the dynamics and effects of abuse on the lives of adolescent girls. Quality intervention includes changing personal attitudes, becoming comfortable with routine inquiry, and improving developmentally appropriate supportive counseling skills. These areas of knowledge and skill are then most effectual if coupled with an awareness of community resources and the ability to collaborate with others in the school and community. Nurse clinicians must be especially sensitive to the need to rescue teenagers, to make everything better for them. Rescue fantasies only distance adolescents and result in adult caregivers and helpers feeling overwhelmed by teen issues. It is pivotal to remember that the adult role is to listen and to help teens discover what they are feeling, not to work miracles or to make feelings go away. The nurse's role is to help teens decide what they want to do and to help them discover their own strength, assisting them in their transformation to adulthood.

Nurses need to set intervention goals for teen dating violence at both the individual and community levels. Reaching out to adolescent girls is essential. A nurse's mandate is to assist young women to live safe and productive lives while raising consciousness of the risks they face in intimate relationships.

Interventions at the individual level include:

- Identifying teens who are at risk or who are currently experiencing abuse in dating relationships (see Box 10-3 and Box 10-4).
- Creating an environment in which they will feel comfortable discussing their relationship and the situation they find themselves in.
- Assisting teens to strategize for the future and to enlarge their personal support system.
- Providing information on community resources and services to aid in accessing support for emotional growth and development.

ADVOCACY AIMED AT ELIMINATING DATING VIOLENCE

Advocacy for teens in regard to dating violence is essential. Dating violence is often hidden because teenagers typically are inexperienced with dating relationships, have "romantic" views of love, and do not seek out adults to help them with their problems. Advocacy efforts must focus on the critical areas of assessment, intervention, and prevention. Protocols for assessment and identification must be incorporated in all settings in which nurses encounter adolescents. Rou-

---

BOX	10-3	**DATING-VIOLENCE WARNING SIGNS FOR CLINICIANS**

- Physical bruises or other signs of injury
- Sudden or increased social isolation
- Sudden changes in mood or personality
- Use of alcohol or drugs
- Difficulty in making decisions
- Truancy, failing, or dropping out of school
- Withdrawing from activities
- Sexually transmitted diseases/pregnancy

| BOX | 10-4 | **DATING-ABUSE INDICATORS FOR ADOLESCENT GIRLS** |

Jealousy and Possessiveness: He won't let you have other friends or see your friends; checks up on you constantly; thinks everyone else *wants* you; thinks you are flirting with, spending time with, or sleeping with someone else; expects you to spend every minute with him; won't accept breaking up; and possibly threatens to commit suicide if you leave him.

Controlling Behaviors: He tries to control you by being bossy, making all the decisions, keeping track of whom you're with and where you are, picking your friends, picking your clothes, keeping you from getting good grades or getting a job, and spreading gossip or rumors about you if you don't act like he wants or if he is jealous.

Minimization: Your boyfriend doesn't take your ideas, future dreams, school accomplishments, or choice of friends seriously. He treats you as a little girl.

Economic Abuse: He takes your money or lavishes gifts on you and then makes you feel obligated to him.

tine assessment should be conducted in school health and guidance offices, in community primary-care clinics and offices, and in family-planning centers. School and youth-group presentations on dating issues, focused on teaching relationship rights and skills, assertiveness skills, and communication and negotiation skills, are essential prevention strategies. Targeted interventions for adolescents experiencing dating abuse as well as for those at risk can be implemented at the individual level and coupled with psychoeducational support and learning groups. The hallmark of individual intervention is providing a sustained and readily available presence in the lives of adolescents.

ASSESSMENT

Adolescence may be the last best chance to effect changes leading to healthy behaviors and positive developmental pathways (Scales & Gibbons, 1996). Adolescents involved in teen dating violence rarely report to parents, teachers, and law enforcement about their experiences (Molidor & Tolman, 1998). So adolescents need to be frequently asked about what is occurring in their dating relationships (Campbell, 2002; Williams & Martinez, 1999).

Because episodes of interpersonal violence in teen dating relationships often occur in the school or on school grounds (Molidor & Tolman, 1998), school is an excellent place to intervene. Most public schools and many nonpublic schools in the United States employ a school nurse; he or she is the obvious agent for universal screening of adolescents. Nursing has a long history in the research of and practice related to interpersonal violence. Nurses are perceived as helpful and caring. Nurses are also skilled interviewers. A clinical instrument for screening adult women for violence and abuse appears elsewhere in this volume; a slightly different screening is useful for teenagers. As with adult women, all girls should be screened regardless of whether physical injuries or mental-health symptomatology is present. At every health encounter, the nurse should determine if the teenager is or has been dating. A neutral statement that adolescence is sometimes stressful and that dating is not always idyllic can precede this question. The nurse can then go on to generalize about the prevalence of abuse during adolescent dating.

Ideally, routine assessment for dating violence should be included in every health encounter with adolescent girls. Many barriers to authentic communication between adolescents and caring adults exist in our society. The encounters nurses have with teenage girls are windows of opportunity for addressing this significant health concern. Routine screening need only take a few minutes and not only identifies at-risk youth but also raises consciousness about dating violence. When talking with a young woman suspected of being in an abusive relationship, a nonconfrontational and indirect manner may work. The nurse could perhaps remark that she doesn't seem as happy as usual or ask if something is bothering her in life. Box 10-5 lists some possible screening questions, which can be tailored according to the nurse's interviewing style.

Though the usefulness of these screening questions has not been tested, they make intuitive sense. It is important, as it is with adult women, to be direct. Asking how their relationship is in general may not be sufficient to elicit complete responses. If responses to any of these questions indicate an abusive dating relationship, then empathize and generalize: "I'm sorry this is happening to you, it is not your fault." Then the nurse should schedule follow-up counseling appointments with any teen who indicates abuse. Because abuse in dating relationships has a positive correlation with suicide ideation for girls (Silverman et al., 2001), girls who indicate abuse should be screened for suicide risk before she leaves the nurse's office.

NURSING INTERVENTIONS

Once an adolescent girl has disclosed an abusive relationship, the next step is to respond effectively. It is important to validate what she has said, letting her know that you have heard what she has said. Adolescents are quite vulnerable to

---

BOX 10-5	SCREENING QUESTIONS FOR TEEN DATING VIOLENCE

- What do you like about your relationship with your partner?
- What things don't you like?
- Have you had fights with your partner? Have you been injured in any of these fights?
- Have you developed a method to avoid having a fight?
- Has your partner ever hit, kicked, punched, or otherwise physically hurt or threatened you?
- Does your partner make fun of you or put you down?
- Is your partner jealous of other people you talk to or spend time with?
- Does your partner try to keep you from hanging out or talking with others?
- Does your partner try to make you think a certain way or dress a certain way?
- Are you afraid of your partner or afraid of your partner's behavior or anger?
- Does your partner make or ask you to do things you don't want to do?
- Does your partner try to make you perform sex acts that you do not want to do?
- Does your partner refuse to let you use condoms?
- Can you say "no" to sex? Can you say "no" to performing sexual acts?
- Can you be in charge of making decisions?
- Can you say "no" to anything?
- Are your friends or parents worried about you in this relationship?

feeling like an outcast; therefore, it is important to empathize while also generalizing. Letting them know that other teenage girls have found themselves in similar abusive relationships will help to reduce the stigma they feel. To help empower these young women, it is also essential at the point of disclosure to let them know how courageous they are and how strong they can become. "Girl power" is one of the most significant interventions that can be employed with teenage girls as they struggle with personal problems and life changes.

When intervening, nurses should emphasize respect, concern, perpetrator responsibility, advocacy, resources, and support. More specifically, nurses should make sure to:

- Respect the adolescent's independence and decision-making ability.
- Address issues of safety and concern.
- Constantly focus on not alienating or distancing the teen.
- Teach personal safety and assertiveness skills.
- Link teens to peer-support networks and community resources.
- Maintain a sustained, caring presence regardless of the choices made.

Patience is crucial. Allow teens to connect with you, to tell their stories, and to express their feelings. It is important to listen without judging, condemning, or giving unwanted advice. Teenagers are particularly sensitive to adult criticism and may be unwilling to hear any negative comments about their boyfriend. Understand that the value teens place on relationships may be different that the value adult women place on relationships, and this may vary from culture to culture. However, it is important to remember that these individual values will affect how teens behave and the choices they see. Teens will be highly ambivalent about ending their relationship; making changes is a process. Continued support is essential, coupled with allowing her to decide what is best for her. (See Box 10-6.)

Change is a gradual process for everyone. Because adolescent girls are already in a period of major physical, emotional, and cognitive change, making changes in intimate relationships may seem overwhelming and frightening. Nurses must re-

---

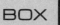 **GUIDE TO INDIVIDUAL INTERVENTION WITH ADOLESCENT GIRLS IN ABUSIVE RELATIONSHIPS**

Discuss and chronicle the relationship and the abuse. When did she start going out with her boyfriend? For how long? What types of sexual activities has she engaged in? What is it like for her? What are the good things about the relationship? What are the bad things? Has it gotten worse? Focus on helping her to talk about the different types of abuse she may be experiencing.

Discuss where has she gone for help. Who has she talked to about this? What do other people say to her? What do her parents say or think? What is she most afraid of when she thinks of ending the relationship?

Assess her level of danger and personal risks to self and others: Assess violence perpetrated by boyfriend against her or others, self-mutilation, suicide, anorexia and bulimia, overeating, unprotected or hurtful sex, and substance use.

Strengthen her social support system: Tell her who will listen to her, who has been in a similar situation, who can she confide in, and who will support her.

Help her to develop and strengthen her effective coping mechanisms.

Reaffirm her decision-making power and understand her ambivalence.

main cognizant of how difficult this process may be. Initially, teens often do not recognize their relationship as being abusive. They have a dream of what they desire in a boyfriend, and the warning signs are often overlooked. They focus on the good parts of the relationship and consider the abusive behaviors as minor or something that will go away over time or disappear once their boyfriend feels more secure. Concerted efforts are made to please their boyfriend. They tolerate the negative aspects of the relationship because they are committed to having it. This is particularly true when they are sexually active. Unfortunately, the good feelings they have of themselves are gradually being replaced by self-doubt, self-blame, and overwhelming feelings of inadequacy. Disengaging has everything to do with recognizing the danger involved, the unhappiness they feel, and the limits to the relationship. Disengaging has everything to do with their ability to heal, to lead a life without a boyfriend, and the ability to find another relationship in the future. The important first step is to begin to see their abusive boyfriend as part of the past, to grieve the loss of the relationship, and to believe that the abuse was not their fault. Assisting adolescent girls through this process of disengagement will result in helping her to regain self-importance and develop goals and dreams for the future. (See Box 10-7.)

Safety must be a fundamental concern when working with adolescents who are involved in abusive dating relationships. (See Box 10-8.) The reality of the risk of danger is significant, particularly when teens decide to break off a relationship. It is not easy to leave a relationship at any age. This is often even more difficult for teens because of fewer resources, more peer pressure, and uninformed adults who do not realize the seriousness of dating violence. It is important to remember that adolescents are able to obtain civil orders of protection and can be assisted with this by abused-women's organizations and offices of the district attorney.

It is essential to assure the adolescent of continued support and a sympathetic ear. It is necessary to remember that health behaviors covary. If the adolescent is involved in one type of risk behavior, then that teen is probably involved in others. A relationship with at least one interested, caring adult may be the single most important element in protecting youth who have multiple risk factors and the possibility of participating in risky behaviors (Scales & Gibbons, 1996). If parental, caring adults are not available to the adolescent, then

---

BOX 10-7   CHECKLIST FOR INTERVENTION

- Provide a safe, confidential place for talking, particularly while in a crisis.
- Focus on the issue, help clarify, and be honest.
- Affirm the injustice.
- Listen, respect, and support.
- Respect and safeguard her confidentiality.
- Provide resources and peer support specifically on this issue.
- Help the teen to create a new enlarged friendship circle (support system).
- Foster involvement in activities targeted to young women.
- Respect the teen's choices and limits.
- Highlight inner strength and point it out to the teen; help her draw on that strength.
- Compliment the teen on her hard work.

BOX 10-8	**SAFETY PLAN FOR ADOLESCENTS: IF YOU THINK IT'S TIME TO CALL IT OFF**

- Get out safely and get help. If you think a situation is dangerous, get out of it.
- Talk with someone you trust—a nurse, teacher, counselor, parent, or adult friend.
- Don't abruptly break it off. Don't threaten to break it off. Plan ahead, and talk to someone you trust.
- When you are dating, make sure that a responsible friend, sympathetic adult, or parent knows where you are.
- Always have some reserve money for transportation.
- Remember that you can obtain civil orders of protection.
- Call the Domestic Violence Hotline (800-838-8238) or the Youth in Crisis Hotline (800-442-4673).

---

another caring adult can be helpful. In some communities, these individuals may be difficult for the adolescent to find. Health-care providers and teachers may then be a substitute.

PREVENTION AND EDUCATION: WORKING TO EDUCATE OTHERS ABOUT DATING VIOLENCE

In most abusive dating relationships, adults are usually not informed. The adolescent will sometimes tell a friend, and many will tell no one (Molidor & Tolman 1998). This finding not only underscores the need for screening but also indicates the need for education of peers and adults in the school and community. The mission of the school is to provide an atmosphere where learning can take place so that adolescents may achieve academically and be productive adults. Therefore, not only do adolescents need to be healthy and free from stress, but also the atmosphere of the school must be one of caring and respect and one in which bullying and violence is not tolerated. Though violence in schools has been well-discussed since Columbine, dating violence is still largely hidden. The nurse can be instrumental in ensuring that when setting up plans and policies to ensure safer schools that dating violence is on the agenda. This may mean educating teachers, parents and administration about the pervasive problem and the adverse effects it can have on the students' ability to be healthy and succeed in school. In providing education to faculty, staff, and administration, local shelters for abused women can be of enormous help. All states have grass-roots organizations dedicated to educating and providing shelter for abused women. The educative arm of these organizations can provide tested interventions and educational and training sessions for faculty, staff, and administration on the prevalence and incidence of teen dating violence. Although more severe violence is often perpetrated when pairs are alone, acts of violence do occur when others are around. This underscores the need for education in the classrooms and through peer groups (Molidor & Tolman, 1998).

As with other risky behaviors, adolescents may believe that "everyone is doing it." Caught up in their peer group, adolescents may see abuse and violence in their relationships as normal and not see it leading to injury, arrest, and incarceration. Classroom discussions may make these erroneous beliefs transparent. For this type of intervention to work, a culture of openness in the school, requiring the education of teachers, administration, and school health personnel, is necessary. Setting policies and developing school-wide plans of intervention need to occur with input from students through classroom discussion. During this process, a strong link with community organizations should be forged.

Adolescent partners frequently confuse jealousy and controlling behaviors with love. There is a belief that violence and abuse in the relationship will end once the partners marry or live together. Classroom discussion is an ideal way to prevent dating violence and promote healthy dating. Currently, no dating-violence programs or curricula for prevention or intervention have sufficient research evidence to support utility (Wekerle & Wolfe, 1999). Because research is ongoing, it is hoped that a powerful prevention program based on research may emerge. Wekerle and Wolfe (1999) have isolated some characteristics of programs that show promise:

- When putting together peer discussion groups on dating violence, try to include a wide age group. If only one grade at a time is used, girls in the class may be dating older boys and boys in the class may be dating younger girls, making discussion difficult.
- Do not rely on one method. Interventions are more powerful when the preponderance of methods are interactive rather than didactic.
- Skill-building is important. Have students do behavioral rehearsing when learning skills such as refusal.
- Always include a section on where to go for help inside and outside of school. If possible, distribute a list of inside resources and community resources.
- Students learn from each other. Do not set up a group composed of adolescents who are behaving antisocially. Instead, include in the group some students who behave ordinarily and some that display antisocial behaviors.
- Try to design into the group some type of social action. This can be as simple as allowing students to prepare a poster or a flier relative to dating violence or as complex as developing an antiviolence school-action plan.

The focus of dating-violence prevention efforts should be on raising consciousness and changing behaviors. The key elements of prevention programs include exploring actual rather than perceived social norms concerning gender roles and dating relationships, providing information about the social consequences of abuse in dating relationships, utilizing peer leaders and peer educators, and involving parents, teachers, and community members in the prevention effort. Peer leaders are trained to emphasize the social rather than the personal, to acknowledge perpetrator responsibility, and to lend peer support in changing attitudes and behaviors.

Prevention programs should help adolescents to recognize healthy and unhealthy behaviors and norms that exist in the community and to understand their susceptibility to violence and abuse in intimate relationships. Dating-violence education should begin with an examination of attitudes held about women and women's roles in society. This underpinning is an essential component of consciousness-raising. Prevention education proceeds to include content on incidence and prevalence of dating violence, myths and biases about dating violence, the dynamics of abuse in intimate relationships, and the characteristics of healthy relationships. This should be coupled with activities that help adolescents recognize the pressures that put them at risk and help them see the protective factors in their lives that minimize the effect of these risks. Effective prevention programs not only raise consciousness and impart knowledge but also include opportunities for adolescents to practice ways to engage in better communication. Dating-violence prevention education develops relationship skills, assertiveness skills, and negotiation and conflict-resolution skills that are based on an awareness of gender issues. Skill-based intervention includes observation, modeling, coaching, rehearsal, feedback, and self-evaluation. Behavioral rehearsals or role-playing scripts can be used to aid in developing sound decision-making skills, goal-setting, assertiveness, and conflict-resolution skills.

It is important to remember that adolescents must become engaged in their own learning. Interventions based solely on information, as well as single-shot interventions, have not been demonstrated to change attitudes and behaviors. Interventions that do not address normative values, do not reflect reality, and do not go beyond the individual are also ineffective. Qualified youth educators must present prevention interventions, as interventions delivered by poorly trained or nonenthusiastic individuals will not impress an adolescent audience.

SUMMARY

Abuse not only threatens the immediate health and safety of teenagers but also influences the developmental progress of adolescents as they grow from childhood into adulthood. The effects of physical, emotional, and sexual violence pose significant obstacles to adolescents in their search for meaningful intimate partnerships. Dating violence may also be a risk factor for a host of interrelated health problems that are only beginning to be understood.

The tasks facing professional nursing regarding dating violence are multiple. Of paramount concern is that we establish a sustained focus on the issue, educating adults about the seriousness of dating violence. We must develop policies and protocols that mandate routine screening for dating violence, advocacy-based interventions for youth experiencing dating violence, and developmentally appropriate, skill-based prevention education. The establishment of coordinated efforts in the clinical-practice arena, coupled with coalition building within the community, is essential.

Fortunately, adolescents are amazingly resilient and resourceful. They are eager to learn, experience, grow, and change. With adult support and connection, all teenagers can examine the effect of violence and abuse not only in their own lives but also in the cultural messages they receive on a daily basis. Only by recognizing the deleterious effect of dating violence will nurses be capable of assisting adolescents on their safe passage to adulthood.

References

Avery-Leaf, S., Cascardi, M., O'Leary, K. D, & Cano, A. (1997). Efficacy of a dating violence prevention program on attitudes justifying aggression. *Journal of Adolescent Health, 21,* 11–17.

Campbell, J. C. (2002). Health consequences of intimate partner violence. *Lancet, 359,* 1331–1336.

Campbell, J. C., Rose, L., Kub, J., & Nedd, D. (1998). Voices of strength and resistance: A contextual and longitudinal analysis of women's responses to battering. *Journal of Interpersonal Violence, 13,* 743–761.

Cohall, A., Cohall, R., Bannister, H., & Northridge, M. (1999). Love shouldn't hurt: Strategies for health care providers to address adolescent dating violence. *Journal of the American Medical Women's Association, 54,* 144–148.

Coker, A. L., McKeown, R. E., Sanderson, M., Davis, K. E., Valois, R. F., & Huebner, E. S. (2000). Severe dating violence and quality of life among South Carolina high school students. *American Journal of Preventive Medicine, 19,* 220–227.

Commonwealth Fund, Survey of Adolescent Girls, November, 1997.

Dahlberg, L. L. (1998). Youth violence in the United States: Major trends, risk factors, and prevention approaches. *American Journal of Preventive Medicine, 14,* 259–272.

Donovan, J. E, Jessor, R., & Costa, F.M. (1993). The structure of enhancing—enhancing behavior in adolescence: A latent variable approach. *Journal of Health and Social Behavior, 34,* 346–362.

Ellickson P. L, & McGuigan, K. A. (2000). Early predictors of adolescent violence. *American Journal of Public Health, 90,* 566–572.

Family Violence Prevention Fund. (1999). *Preventing domestic violence: Clinical guidelines on routine screening.* San Francisco: Author.

Foshee, V., Linder, G. F., Bauman, K. E., Langwick, S. A., Arriaga, X. B., et al. (1996). The Safe Dates Project: Theoretical basis, evaluation design, and selected baseline findings. *American Journal of Preventive Medicine, 12,* 39–47.

Halpern, C. T., Oslak, S. G., Young, M. L., Martin, S. L., & Kupper, L. L. (2001). Partner violence among adolescents in opposite-sex romantic relationships: Findings from the National Longitudinal Study of Adolescent Health. *American Journal of Public Health, 91,*1679–1685.

Jessor, R. (1991). Risk behavior in adolescence: A psychosocial framework for understanding and action. *Journal of Adolescent Health, 12,* 597–605.

Johnson, J. D, Adams, M. S., Ashburn, L., & Reed, W. (1995). Differential gender effects of exposure to rap music on African American adolescents' acceptance of teen dating violence. *Sex Roles, 33*(7/8), 597–605.

Malik, S., Sorenson, S. B., & Aneshensel, C. S. (1997). Community and dating violence among adolescents: Perpetration and victimization. *Journal of Adolescent Health, 21,* 291–302.

Molidor, C., & Tolman, R. (1998). Gender and contextual factors in adolescent dating violence. *Violence Against Women, 4*(2), 180–194.

Molidor, C., Tolman, R. M., & Kober, J. (2000). Gender and contextual factors in adolescent dating violence. *The Prevention Researcher, 7,* 1–4.

Moskowitz, H., Griffith, J. L., DiScala, C., & Sege R. D. (2001). Serious injuries and deaths of adolescent girls resulting from interpersonal violence: Characteristics and trends from the United States, 1989–1998. *Archives of Pediatric Adolescent Medicine, 155,* 903–908.

Office of Justice Programs. (1998). Bureau of Justice statistics factbook: Violence by intimate —analysis of data on crimes by current or former spouses, boyfriends, and girlfriends. Washington, DC: Department of Justice.

O'Keefe, M. (1997). Predictors of dating violence among high school students. *Journal of Interpersonal Violence, 12*(4): 546–568.

O'Keefe, M., & Treister, L. (1998). Victims of dating violence among high school students: Are the predictors different for males and females? *Violence Against Women, 4*(2), 195–223.

O'Malley, P. M., Johnston, L. D., & Bachman, J. G. (1993). Adolescent substance use and addictions: Epidemiology, current trends, and public policy. *Adolescent Medicine, 4,* 227–248.

Plichta, S. B. (1996). Violence and abuse: Implications for women's health. In M. M. Falik & K. S. Collins (Eds.), *Women's Health: The Commonwealth Survey* (pp. 237–272). Baltimore, MD: Johns Hopkins University Press.

Reuterman, N. A., & Burcky, W. D. (1989). Dating violence in high school: A profile of the victims. *Psychology, 26,* 1–9.

Rhynard, J., Krebs, M., & Glover, J. (1997). Sexual assault in dating relationships. *Journal of School Health, 67*(3), 89–93.

Roscoe, B., & Callahan, J. E. (1983). Adolescent's self-report of violence in families and dating relationships. *Adolescence, 10,* 545–563.

Roscoe, B., & Kelsey, T. (1986). Dating violence among high school students. *Psychology, 23,* 198–202.

Saltzman, L. E., Fanslow, J. L., McMahon, P. M., & Shelley, G. A. (1999). *Intimate partner violence surveillance uniform definitions and recommended data elements.* Atlanta, GA: Centers for Disease Control and Prevention.

Scales, P. C., & Gibbons, J. D. (1996). Extended family members and unrelated adults in the lives of young adolescents. *Journal of Early Adolescence, 16*(4), 365–389.

Schubiner, H., Scott, R., & Tzelepis, A. (1993). Exposure to violence among inner-city youth. *Journal of Adolescent Health, 14,* 214–219.

Schwab-Stone, M., Chen, C., Greenberger, E., Silver, D., Lichtman, J., & Voyce, C. (1999). No safe haven II: The effects of violence exposure on urban youth. *Journal of the American Academy of Child and Adolescent Psychiatry, 38*(4), 359–367.

Sells, C. W., & Blum, R. W. (1996). Morbidity and mortality among U.S. adolescents: An overview of data and trends. *American Journal of Public Health, 86*(4), 513–519.

Silverman, J. G., Raj, A., Mucci, L. A., & Hathaway, J. E. (2001). Dating violence against adolescent girls and associated substance use, unhealthy weight control, sexual risk behavior, pregnancy, and suicidality. *Journal of the American Medical Association, 286,* 572–579.

Simons, R. (1998). Socialization in the family of origin and male dating violence: A prospective study. *Journal of Marriage and the Family, 60,* 467–478.

Singer, M. I., Anglin, T. M., Song, L. Y., & Lunghofer, L. (1995). Adolescents' exposure to violence and associated symptoms of psychological trauma. *Journal of the American Medical Association, 273,* 477–482.

Spencer, G. A., & Bryant, S. A. (2000). Dating violence: A comparison of rural, suburban, and urban teens. *Journal of Adolescent Health, 27,* 302–305.

Sugarman, D. B., & Hotaling, G. T. (1989). Dating violence: A review of contextual and risk factors. In B. Levy (Ed.), *Dating Violence: Young Women in Danger* (pp. 100–118). Seattle, WA: Seal Press.

Thornberry, T. P. (1994). *Violent families and youth violence* (Fact sheet No. 21). Washington, DC: U.S. Department of Justice, Office of Juvenile Justice and Delinquency Prevention.

Tjaden, P., & Thoennes, N. (2000). *Extent, nature and consequences of intimate partner violence: Findings from the national violence against women survey* (Publication No. NCJ 181867). Washington, DC: U.S. Department of Justice, Office of Justice Programs.

Watson, J. M., Cascardi, M., Avery-Leaf, S., & O'Leary, K. D. (2001). High school students' responses to dating aggression. *Violence and Victoms, 16*, 339–348.

Wekerle, C., & Wolfe, D. A. (1999). Dating violence in mid-adolescence: Theory, significance, and emerging prevention initiatives. *Clinical Psychological Review, 19*, 435–456.

Widom, C. S. (1989). Does violence beget violence? A critical examination of the literature. *Psychological Bulletin, 106*(1), 3–28.

Williams, S. E., & Martinez, E. (1999). Psychiatric assessment of victims of adolescent dating violence in a primary care clinic. *Clinical Child Psychology and Psychiatry, 4*(3), 427–439.

Wingood, G. M., DiClemente, R. J., McGree, D. H., Harrington, K., & Davies, S. L. (2001). Dating violence and the sexual health of black adolescent females. *Pediatrics, 107*, E72.

Wolfe, D. A., & Feiring, C. (2000). Dating violence through the lens of adolescent romantic relationships. *Child Maltreatment 5*, 360–363.

Wolfe, L. R. (1994). "Girl stabs boy at school": Girls and the cycle of violence. *WHI, 4*(2), 109–116.

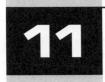

Nursing Care of Survivors of Intimate Partner Violence

- Jacquelyn C. Campbell, Sara Torres, Laura Smith McKenna, Daniel J. Sheridan, and Kären Landenburger

scared frightened and all alone
cant go back to my home left with only the clothes on my back
wondering if I'll make it on the right track
all i have is my daughter and me made it to the shelter we are free
now all i have to do is make a life for katie and me
you gave me hope, courage and most of all love
and so now i can spread my wings take off again and go on

N.L.

I am writing a poem
and it is one of thanks
to the women who've come seeking shelter to those who have given me strength it's
     easy to share all your laughter
its harder to share your own tears so thank you my sisters, my neighbors for helping
     me deal with my fears
its you who have given me courage to face my own life as it is
and its you who have taken the 1st step so your children can grow up and live
there are some who can't work in a shelter
and you're right it's not all peaches and cream But it's worth all the petty displeasures
just to watch someone learning to dream
(we grow from each other's growing)

Kathy Clair

Both poems reprinted from *Every Twelve Seconds*, compiled by Susan Venters (Hillsboro, Oregon: Shelter, 1981) by permission of the authors.

This chapter focuses on the planning of nursing care with and for survivors of intimate partner violence (IPV) in a variety of health care settings. Professional nursing care of battered partners (primarily women) is based on theoretical foundations (see Chapter 2) and is individualized to the needs and goals of battered women dealing with various types and levels of abuse. In any health care setting, routine assessment for battering of all women seeking care, especially in situations identified as high risk for battering, must be a priority for nursing. Nursing interventions are needed at all three levels of prevention. An awareness of the scope of the problem, combined with a knowledge base that directs nursing assessment and interventions, is basic to developing and retaining sensitivity to the significance of cues of abuse presented by clients. Research on nurse identification and intervention in cases of domestic violence has suggested that the nurse's responsibilities begin before the initial client interaction.

ESTABLISHING THE NURSE-CLIENT RELATIONSHIP

Although nurses already have the necessary skills to plan client care in a variety of clinical settings, and the majority of nurses accept addressing IPV as part of the nursing role, experience and research has demonstrated that nursing interventions with victims and survivors of domestic violence continue to be inadequate. King and Ryan (1989) found that the identification of such clients in health care settings is impeded when nurses continue to believe in societal myths about domestic violence, and that inappropriate interventions result from nurses' misperceptions of the cues presented by women. The nurses consistently deferred direct questioning that might lead to the woman's disclosure of the violence. Barriers to effective intervention also involved the nurse's fears of the client's response and fears of inability to respond to the client's needs. The majority of nurses (90%) in this study reported lack of basic content in educational programs about abuse of women.

More-current research has suggested that a majority of nursing curricula, at least in baccalaureate programs, contain content on domestic violence, but that nurses continue to fail to routinely screen and intervene for IPV (American Association of College Nursing, 1999; Institute of Medicine, 2001; Glass, Campbell, & Dearwater, 2001). For example, in a recent multisite survey of emergency services, emergency staff were aware of only 13% of the women who had experienced domestic violence from a male partner (Abbott, Johnson, Koziol-McLain, & Lowenstein, 1995).

Nurses must examine their beliefs and values related to violence against women and create learning situations that allow survivors to explore the dynamics of and alternate solutions to the problem. Desensitization to women's stories, exploration of one's own exposure to violence in the family, and information about available community resources will lead to appropriate interventions with such clients. It is necessary to take into account the stereotypes nurses may have about battered women and the effect of the client on the nurse. For example, frustration can occur when the nurse suspects abuse, sees the woman only once, and battering is denied. Such frustration may be easily transmitted into anger at the abused woman. It is helpful for the nurse to know that denial is a normal response to battering and an important step in grieving the losses experienced by the woman abused in an intimate relationship. It also is a part of the avoidance cluster that is part of the trauma response to any violent experience (Woods, 1999; Woods & Campbell, 1993). The nurse should facilitate disclosure but not aggressively confront; the abused woman would thus be allowed this defense until she can confront the situation. However, for some nurses, allowing denial means condoning it, and nurses fear they will be responsible for the woman remaining in the abusive situation.

Nurses are better prepared to intervene effectively if they have thoroughly examined their own attitudes about wife abuse and have anticipated their possible responses to such clients. They must carefully sort their own reactions to the myths

BOX 11-1	PRINCIPLES OF EMPOWERMENT

- Mutuality and reciprocity
- Sharing information
- Giving choices
- Brainstorming solutions
- Making sense of it

about battering and examine their general responses to victims of violence. It is helpful for the nurse to imagine being the victim of abuse at the hands of an intimate partner who is deeply loved, as impossible as that may seem, and to place that scene at a time when her or his own self-esteem was at its lowest ebb. Once nurses realize that abuse could have happened or could happen to them in the future, they can better empathize with the woman, accept her reactions, and anticipate their own responses. Clinical discussion groups and role-plays with other nurses also help develop the sensitivity and provide the support necessary to continue working with this vulnerable population.

The general model of nursing care in this chapter is an empowerment model derived from several nursing frameworks (e.g., Orem, 1991; Parse, 1987) and the advocacy of the battered-woman's movement (e.g., Gondolf, 1990). The general principles of empowerment are outlined in Box 11-1. They are referred to throughout the chapter. In this spirit, we refer to abused women as survivors rather than victims, in recognition of their strengths and survival skills. We also recognize that men and women in same-sex relationships can and often are survivors of IPV (Greenwood et al., 2000; Relf, 2001; Renzetti, 1992; Tjaden, Thoennes, & Allison, 1999; Turell, 2000) and that women are sometimes more violent than their male partners. Even so, by far the largest numbers of persons physically or sexually assaulted by current and former intimate partners are females (Tjaden, Thoennes, & Alison, 1999), and we will therefore assume in this chapter that the recipients of abuse are women. The chapter also is based on the premise that the nurse needs to be sensitive to the cultural background of the abused woman.

WORKING WITH BATTERED WOMEN FROM DIFFERENT CULTURES

The nurse must be aware of cultural issues important to the battered woman that may affect her response to treatment. Unless culture is considered, interventions with battered women will fail (Bohn, 1998; Campbell & Campbell, 1996; Torres, 1987, 1998; Rodriguez, 1998).

"Culture" refers to the cumulative deposit of knowledge, experience, meanings, beliefs, values, attitudes, religion, concepts of self and the universe, self-to-universe relationships, and time concepts acquired by a large group of people in the course of generations. Culture manifests itself both in patterns of language and thought and forms of activity and behavior.

Culture is central to how a battered woman organizes her experience. For instance, Torres (1991) found that although there were more similarities than differences between the two groups, Anglo-American battered women perceived more types of behavior as abusive and exhibited a less tolerant attitude toward abuse than did a group of Mexican-American abused women. Thus, culture shapes how a battered woman views violence, whether or not she sees herself as abused, the degree of hopefulness or pessimism she has about the violence ending, how she seeks assistance, what she understands as the causes of psychological difficulties, and the unique, subjective experience of being a battered woman. Certain cultural beliefs, values, and practices are likely to increase the number of stressors to which the battered woman is exposed. Culture also determines the battered woman's attitudes about sharing troublesome emotional problems with nurses, attitudes toward her emotional pain, expectations of the treatment, and what she believes is the best method of addressing the difficulties presented by the abuse.

Most cultural behaviors make sense within the culture even if they do not outside the culture. The nurse must view the woman's behavior from inside the culture, taking into account the woman's family structure, gender roles, marriage patterns, sexual behavior, contraceptive patterns, pregnancy and childbirth practices, child-rearing practices, diet, dress, personal hygiene, housing arrangements, sanitation arrangements, religion, migrant status, occupation(s), use of chemical comforters, leisure pursuits, self-treatment strategies, and lay therapies. Rural women have their own culture and set of circumstances that makes their experience of abuse particularly isolating and needing a particular set of interventions (Fishwick, 1998). Women and men in same-sex relationships who experience intimate partner violence can also have particular needs for sensitive nursing care (Hall, 1994; Relf, 2001).

Socioeconomic class and the degree of assimilation are important factors. The degree of acculturation or assimilation into the dominant culture determines the degree to which women identified as ethnic minorities have assumed the values and customs of the dominant culture. In a study of abuse during pregnancy, Torres and colleagues (2000) found that Latina women who were less acculturated also were less severely and frequently abused than Latina women who were more acculturated, perhaps indicating that they challenged the traditional male dominant roles of their culture less. Acculturation may also determine how likely it is that a woman perceives herself as abused and is willing to seek help through the American system. Any ethnic minority may particularly mistrust the criminal-justice system. African Americans and immigrants from many countries have experienced or heard about violence and unfair treatment from the police and the courts here as well as in other lands (Campbell & Gary, 1998; Moss, Pitula, Campbell, and Halstead, 1997).

An immigrant woman may be particularly concerned about citizenship issues; an abusive husband could tell her that he can prevent her from getting citizenship if he does not sponsor her. According to the provisions of the 2001 Violence Against Women Act, a battered immigrant can self-petition for citizenship, and documentation of her abuse from a health care setting can be instrumental in her success. (See Box 11-2.) It is also important to remember that even the most acculturated middle-class person has a tendency to revert to his or her cultural past when organizing coping strategies after a stressful event.

There are instruments that measure the degree of acculturation. However, in the clinical setting, the nurse can assess acculturation by determining:

BOX	11-2	RESOURCES FOR IMMIGRANT BATTERED WOMEN

- Violence Against Women Act—self petition for citizenship if abused
- English-language classes
- Citizenship classes
- National Organization of Women Legal Defense Fund 202-326-0040
- AYUDA 202-387-0434
- Family Violence Prevention Fund (http://www.FVPF.org)

- Command of English
- Language spoken at home and language preference with friends, television, and radio programs
- Length of time in the United States
- Religion, influence of religion, and degree of religious faith
- Stresses of migration
- Community of residence and opportunities for linking with fellow countrymen/women

The nurse can determine this information through regular contacts with battered women and by asking specific questions in a culturally sensitive manner. The nurse must realize that the stresses of migration can make women more vulnerable to abuse and limit their social networks and resources for coping with the abuse. An abusive husband may be reluctant for his wife to learn English, knowing her lack of English skills may further isolate her. One of the most important and empowering first interventions for such a woman may be to help her enroll in an English-speaking class. The nurse or physician can tell her husband that in order for her to better negotiate the health care system for herself and the children, English-language skills are necessary.

Nurses must prepare for cross-cultural work. First, it is important for the nurse to explore her own attitudes to minimize biases. What are her racial, cultural, and class biases? Does she tend to be culture blind, a "bleeding-heart" liberal, culturally sensitive, or culturally competent? Cultural competence suggests attitudes beyond cultural sensitivity, with in-depth knowledge of the language and patterns and advocacy for the cultural group (Orlandi, 1986). The nurse's attitude is critical. It is important to respect the cultural traditions of the woman and not assume that complete acculturation is the most healthy state. Cultural insensitivity or inappropriate treatment procedures can inadvertently retraumatize clients.

The battered woman from a different culture or ethnic group feels different from the nurse and may therefore feel that the nurse cannot help or understand her. The nurse must work to overcome this feeling by becoming familiar with the woman's culture. She can read about the culture, become a participant in that culture, and talk to informants and experts from that culture. However, familiarity with the woman's culture is not enough. Nurses must develop skills for cross-cultural care (Barcelona de Mendoza, 2002).

Credibility and being perceived as giving can overcome the client's feeling of "difference." There are two types of credibility: acquired and ascribed. Acquired credibility is gained by status (position) and education. Ascribed credibility is gained not only by being empathic and having knowledge but also by communicating an awareness of the woman's worldview. Thus, the woman ascribes to the nurse the ability to help her. Giving is important because the culturally different battered woman must feel that she is benefiting from the helping relationship with the nurse. Giving can occur in many forms; for instance, the nurse can teach stress reduction or assist with obtaining or negotiating social services.

The nurse can use several strategies to increase communication effectiveness when working with a battered woman who has difficulty with English. The nurse can learn some words of greeting and basic sentences in the woman's language. Even better is to learn the language of at least one other cultural group that the nurse is likely to practice with. Recognizing that persons of Hispanic descent are the largest minority in the United States and that Spanish speakers are the majority in many health care settings, many schools of nursing are requiring knowledge of Spanish medical terminology and health assessment. Especially in sensitive areas, like family violence, a working knowledge of the woman's language is enormously helpful (Barcelona de Mendoza, 2002). This makes the woman feel that the nurse cares and respects her culture.

If the nurse does not know the woman's language, speaking slowly and clearly in English, without using slang, idioms, or difficult medical terminology, and allowing time for the woman to respond aids communication. Women whose first language is not English go through a process that includes hearing in English, translating mentally to the native tongue, thinking of a response in the native language, then translating mentally, and finally responding in English.

A three-way relationship is required when an interpreter is used. To build rapport between the interpreter and woman, it is helpful to introduce the two. It is important to have the interpreter translate exactly what the woman says. The nurse should look directly at the woman, not the interpreter, when she speaks, watching her facial expressions and body language. It is better to use a trained interpreter than a family member, because it would often be impossible for the woman to discuss issues like abuse in front of family members.

Considering a woman's culture in nursing intervention is a difficult task. If possible, nurses should be supervised by experts when they begin to work with battered women from other cultural groups. Ideally, the expert would be a woman from the cultural group who is familiar with both the minority and dominant culture, to assist the nurse in translating cultural behaviors into nursing care. The expert should also be sensitive to the issues battered women face.

ASSESSMENT

The nurse's initial approach to the battered woman is important in establishing a nurse–client relationship that allows the woman to disclose her abusive situation. Nurses may encounter battered women in any health care setting. However, nurses are more likely to encounter abused women in emergency and urgent-care departments, perinatal and women's health care settings, gynecological and family-planning centers, community-health centers, primary-care settings, occupational-health settings, and inpatient and outpatient mental health locations. In addition to assessing women for abuse, if there are overt injuries or signs of conflict in a marital or cohabiting relationship routine questions related to intimate partner violence should be asked. Tilden and Shepherd (1987) suggested that the question be framed to normalize the event: "Many families have difficulty expressing anger. What is that like in your family?" (p. 30). Another way to frame the assessment within the context of inquiring about the person's most important relationship is to ask, "How do you and your partner (husband) resolve disagreements?" The nurse should then listen for indications that one partner is invested in power and control or for mention of frequent fighting. If fighting is mentioned, the nurse can ask, "Does the fighting ever get physical?" The question about solving disagreements can be followed by "What happens when he (or she) gets really angry? Does it ever involve pushing or shoving?" Pushing or shoving is the least violent of aggressive conflict-resolution methods and often is the start of abuse. It is also the easiest for a survivor to acknowledge. If a woman admits to pushing and shoving or more violent tactics, then a more thorough assessment of the nature of the violence can begin.

It is important that the nurse develop a personal repertoire of abuse-related questions that are comfortable, natural, and culturally sensitive. For instance, Torres and her colleagues (2000) found that white pregnant women were more likely to disclose abuse on a written history form, whereas women of color were more likely to disclose when asked face-to-face by an empathetic nurse. McFarlane, Christoffel, Bateman, Miller, and Bullock (1991) found face-to-face questioning most effective in a family-planning setting, but some providers are successfully using computerized questions. Rachel Rodriguez, a nurse researcher and advocate, has found that an icon is most useful in assessing IPV with migrant farm-working women (Short & Rodriguez, 2002).

The Nursing Research Consortium on Violence and Abuse (Parker & McFarlane, 1991) developed a four-question assessment tool (the Abuse Assessment Screen, or AAS) that directly asks about the characteristics of abuse in a relationship and can be incorporated into the nurse–client interview or a written history. (See Appendix A.) These questions can be prefaced or followed by giving the client information about the incidence of battering in the United States, acknowledging the sensitivity of the issue and the woman's possible emotional response, and assuring the client of the routine nature of assessment of abuse in intimate relationships, given its prevalence. Indication of the nurse's familiarity with and the widespread nature of the problem is usually helpful in reassuring an abused woman that she is not alone and that the woman is not being singled out. A good sentence to use before asking the AAS questions is "Because domestic violence is so common in this country, we are asking all our patients questions about abuse" or "Because domestic violence is connected with so many health problems, we are asking all our patients questions about abuse." The AAS has excellent psychometric properties (Soeken, Parker, McFarlane, & Lominak, 1998). Nurse researcher Koziol-McLain and colleagues (2001) found a three-question adaptation of the AAS to have good sensitivity (i.e., identified the majority of battered women) and specificity (i.e., did not misidentify nonabused women) in emergency departments.

Because of perceived stigma and embarrassment, women are unlikely to volunteer information about abuse when they seek health care for themselves or their children; they are more likely to disclose information about abuse when a concerned health care provider poses questions in a nonjudgmental way. Lack of systematic screening in health care settings should be viewed as missed opportunities to begin to break the isolation that many abused women experience and to also perhaps save lives. In a recent nursing study of femicide, 47% of the women killed or the victim of attempted homicide by a current or former intimate partner had been seen in some health care setting the year before (Sharps, Koziol-McLain, Campbell, et al., 2001). Although battered women rarely report abuse to primary health care providers without being asked, both abused and not abused women say they think it would help battered women get help if women were routinely screened for IPV (Gielen et al., 2000; Glass, Dearwater, & Campbell, 2001). Even when the woman is not abused, asking the question as a routine part of nursing assessment educates her about the incidence and nature of the problem and can be an important nursing intervention at the primary-prevention level. Routine assessment for battering must be conducted in a nonjudgmental manner, in private, and with assurances of confidentiality. Battered women frequently feel shame over being abused and are appropriately frightened of the abuser's response if he discovers the violence has been discussed. In addition, battered women often have had previous experience with the health care system that has engendered mistrust. Therefore, the nurse must be aware of her own values in relation to violence against women in intimate relationships and be careful of her nonverbal cues and spatial separation between her and the woman.

Although it is often difficult to interact with clients privately in a busy trauma unit, any physical trauma to a female client, regardless of the plausibility of the explanation or solicitousness of the spouse, indicates private nursing assessment for possible abuse. Research has documented the failure of health care workers not only to identify battered women but also to rule out battering as the cause of trauma to a female patient, especially if she is pregnant (Sharps et al., 2001; Parker & McFarlane, 1991; McFarlane, Campbell, Sharps, & Watson, 2002). Because abuse is one of the primary causes of trauma to women in the United States, in emergency care, protocols must be established to keep any accompanying person in the waiting room until abuse is ruled out.

In studies of women coming to hospital emergency rooms and other health care settings, a majority of abused women are never clearly identified as such in the medical record (Glass, Dearwater, & Campbell, 2001). Nursing research found that a majority of abused women were not asked specifically if they had been abused when they sought health care. Studies found that health care to abused women is generally impersonal and insensitive to their needs, with minimal to no support given by health care providers. One of Drake's (1982) subjects said, "I just wish somebody would of come right out and asked me. I always hope they'll do that" (p. 45). Nurses must find a secluded place and do just that—ask. In prenatal-care settings, the pelvic exam can be a time to ask all family members to leave. The opportunity for privacy needs to be built into every female health history and exam according to the particular logistics of the setting so that a sudden excuse does not have to be invented.

The community-health nurse also finds privacy at a premium. The battered woman is usually reluctant to discuss the problem in front of her children, and the abusive spouse frequently finds a reason to be present when any helping professional is in the home. Suggesting a short walk with the wife, using the reason that the weather is fine or the nurse is restless, may be an effective way to create privacy. Going to the baby's room or the kitchen or to the bathroom with the woman to check an episiotomy or something else "private" can also create a secluded moment. A battered woman may sometimes resist the idea of home visitation; she has usually been warned to keep strangers out of the house. Meeting her at other locations, such as a restaurant, a social-service agency (e.g., Women, Infants, and Children), or a child-care center, may be a useful strategy to create privacy. Box 11-3 gives a shortened version of the Family Violence Prevention Fund Clinical Guidelines on Routine Screening, available in its entirety at http://www.FVPF.org.

When privacy has been obtained and a nonauthoritarian atmosphere created, sensitivity and directness are mandatory. However, although direct questions allow the client to disclose information about the abuse to the nurse, the nurse cannot expect the abused woman to always respond as directly. Battered women frequently use denial as a means of coping with the violence and may minimize its occurrence at first. In this situation, it is important to document the indicators of abuse, as well as the assessment process so that subsequent nurses and health care providers can add information.

If a woman discusses the abuse with a concerned professional, it should be remembered that the woman has chosen that professional for her disclosure. Therefore, it is unethical to only make an immediate referral to some other member of the health care team (e.g., a social worker) without assessing the situation further and discussing the woman's options with her. This is true even in a hectic emergency situation. A systematic nursing assessment of the abusive situation can be an intervention, increasing the battered woman's awareness of the seri-

---

BOX	11-3	**FAMILY VIOLENCE PREVENTION FUND CLINICAL GUIDELINES ON ROUTINE SCREENING (1999): ALL WOMEN AGED 14 AND OLDER***

PRIMARY CARE

- Every first visit for new chief complaint
- Every new patient encounter
- Every new intimate relationship
- All periodic exams (regular physical)

EMERGENCY DEPARTMENT AND URGENT CARE

- All females (at least age 15 through age 65), all visits

OB/GYN

- Every prenatal and postpartum visit
- Every new intimate relationship
- Every routine gynecological visit
- Every family planning visit
- Every STD-clinic visit
- Every visit to an abortion clinic

MENTAL HEALTH

- Every initial assessment (may take several visits for initial assessment, and women should be asked several times during the assessment in several different ways)
- Every new intimate relationship
- Annually if ongoing or periodic treatment
- Inpatient—as part of admission & discharge

---

*Short version–see http://www.fvpf.org for full guidelines.

ousness of the violence and of changes in abusive behavior over time. A non-threatening confrontation with information about a pattern of increasing severity and frequency helps the woman define the situation, often influences her decision-making, and can facilitate help-seeking behavior.

The abused woman who admits to being hit may minimize the seriousness of the problem. This often takes the form of blaming herself for the incidents, blaming her husband's alcohol use, asserting that the violence is permanently over, attributing its occurrence to a period of family stress, or using other forms of rationalization or intellectualization. It is useful to view minimization as partial denial, an appropriate reaction to a devastating situation, a traumatic-stress response, a necessary part of the grieving process, or any combination of these. Sensitive exploration of the history of abuse allows the nurse to gather data while helping the woman define the characteristics of the abusive situation and assists her in making decisions. As Goldberg and Carey (1982) suggested, "Assessment of the battered woman can be viewed as intervention and made an integral part of the therapeutic plan" (p. 66). This is especially important when the battered woman may not be seen again.

Findings in the history and physical examination that should alert the professional nurse to the possibility of wife abuse are presented in Boxes 11-4 and 11-5. No single at-risk finding in the tables necessarily indicates abuse, but several such findings warrant at least an at-risk nursing diagnosis. As with all assessments, the nurse must be systematic in collecting data, and all assessment data must be validated with the client. When violence or abuse is acknowledged by the client or strongly suggested by the nurse's assessment data, several areas of assessment specific to battered women must be carefully explored.

History

When violence has been indicated, the most effective means of obtaining the story of abuse is to use a communication model that allows the woman to talk about the problem from her perspective (Kinlein, 1977), "not interrupted" and "given time for full scope, emphasis, and even repetition" (p. 58). This can be initiated with a request to "tell me about the hitting" or another open-ended statement. If the woman asks where to begin, telling her "anywhere you would like" works well. If the information about abuse has come up in the middle of a systematic history, the nurse can indicate an interest in pursuing the topic further with the woman. The woman is given the choice of talking about it then or returning to the issue at the end of the more formal history.

The nurse's role during the narration is to listen empathetically and to record what is said as much as possible. This approach emphasizes the importance the nurse is imparting to the woman's words and provides a useful record for future reference. Specific documentation of the client's description of her situation is extremely important. It is particularly important to state in quotation marks who did it and when and where the woman says she was hit. (See Chapter 13 for specifics about documentation.) The nurse or the medical record may be needed in court to document the abuse, and both the abused woman and the nurse must be able to evaluate the history for patterns. The purpose of the record and its confidentiality and how she can obtain the record must be explained to the woman. Her greatest fear may be that the record will somehow be available to her spouse. Once she knows the record is available only with her con-

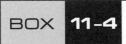

INDICATORS OF POTENTIAL OR ACTUAL WIFE ABUSE, FROM HISTORY

PRIMARY CONCERN/REASON FOR VISIT

- Unwarranted delay between time of injury and seeking treatment
- Inappropriate spouse reactions (e.g., lack of concern, overconcern, threatening demeanor, and reluctance to leave wife)
- Vague information about cause of injury or problem; discrepancy between physical findings and verbal description of cause
- Minimization of serious injury
- Emergency-room treatment for vague stress-related symptoms and minor injuries
- Suicide attempt; history of previous attempts

FAMILY HEALTH HISTORY/ FAMILY OF ORIGIN

- Traditional values about women's role
- Witnessing of spousal abuse or experienced child abuse (physical, sexual, or emotional)

CHILDREN

- Child abuse
- Physical punishment routine and severe
- Hostility of children directed against father
- Children seen by father as additional burden
- Unquestioning obedience expected from father
- Stepchild or stepchildren (her biological offspring, not his)

PARTNER

- Alcohol or drug abuse
- Machismo values
- Violence outside of home, including violence against women in previous relationships
- Low self-esteem, lack of power in workplace or other arenas outside of home
- Force or coercion in sexual activities
- Unemployment or underemployment
- Extreme jealousy (frequently unfounded) of female friendships, work, and children, as well as other men
- Stressors, such as death in family, moving, change of jobs, and trouble at work
- Abuse in childhood or witnessing of father abusing mother

HOUSEHOLD

- Poverty
- Aggression or violence for solving problems
- Isolation from neighbors, relatives; few friends; lack of support systems

PAST HEALTH HISTORY

- Fractures and trauma injuries
- Depression, anxiety symptoms, substance abuse
- Injuries while pregnant
- Spontaneous abortions
- Psychophysiological complaints
- Previous suicide attempts

(continued)

BOX 11-4	INDICATORS OF POTENTIAL OR ACTUAL WIFE ABUSE, FROM HISTORY *(Continued)*

NUTRITION

- Evidence of overeating or anorexia or bulimia as reactions to stress
- Sudden changes in weight

PERSONAL/SOCIAL

- Low self-esteem, poor evaluation of self in relation to others and ideal self, trouble listing strengths, frequent negative comments about self, doubt of abilities
- Feelings of being trapped, powerlessness, futility in making plans
- Chronic fatigue, apathy
- Responsibility felt for spouse's behavior
- Traditional values about home, a wife's prescribed role, the husband's prerogatives, strong commitment to marriage no matter what
- External locus-of-control orientation, loss of control over situation, fate or other forces determine events
- Major decisions made by spouse, far less power than he has in relationship, control of activities by spouse, money control by spouse
- Few support systems, few supportive friends, little outside home activity, discouragement of outside relationships by spouse or curtailment by self to deal with violent situation
- Physical aggression in courtship

SLEEP

- Difficulty sleeping
- Insomnia
- Sleep time in excess of 10 to 12 hours per day

ELIMINATION

- Chronic constipation
- Diarrhea
- Elimination disturbances related to stress
- Urinary-tract infections

ILLNESS

- Frequent stress-related illnesses
- Frequent colds and flu
- Treatment for mental illness
- Use of tranquilizers, mood elevators, or antidepressants

OPERATIONS/HOSPITALIZATIONS

- Hospitalizations for trauma injuries
- Suicide attempts
- Hospitalization for depression
- Refusals of hospitalization when suggested by physician

PERSONAL SAFETY

- Handgun(s) in home
- History of frequent accidents
- Lack of safety precautions

(continued)

BOX	11-4	INDICATORS OF POTENTIAL OR ACTUAL WIFE ABUSE, FROM HISTORY (*Continued*)

HEALTH CARE UTILIZATION

- No regular provider
- Mistrust of health care system

REVIEW OF SYSTEMS

- Headaches, undiagnosed gastrointestinal symptoms, palpitations, other possible psychophysiological complaints
- Sexual difficulties, husband is "rough" in sexual activities, lack of sexual desire, pain with intercourse, pelvic pain
- Joint pain or other areas of tenderness, especially at the extremities
- Chronic pain
- Pelvic inflammatory disease
- Neurological symptoms

sent, the record is a powerful resource in any future legal actions and a source of empowerment for the woman. The woman is more likely to need such records for custody actions than for criminal prosecution. After the narration, certain aspects of the situation should be explored in more depth, especially those that involve other health care problems (such as old, untreated injuries) or safety needs, for the woman to make a complete assessment. If follow-up is assured, these areas may be assessed in subsequent sessions, but they should not be forgotten.

Although the woman's feelings about the abuse need to be expressed, she may need to intellectualize or disassociate herself from her feelings to describe the situation. If she is not able to respond to sensitive questioning, it can be assumed that this process is necessary, at least temporarily. However, an abused woman may not describe her feelings because she assumes that her emotions are somehow unacceptable. She may fear the intensity of her feelings or find her fantasies of retaliation unacceptable. Whatever the feelings, the abused woman needs reassurance that it is normal for her to have strong and frequent socially undesirable emotions. It is often helpful for the nurse to repeat the whole gamut of feelings that other abused women described, from feeling angry, trapped, despairing, and hopeless to feeling great love for the abuser and confidence that violence will not recur. The nurse should also stress that conflicting emotions may be felt simultaneously and that the woman may frequently vacillate between them. Although the woman may not "own" her emotions at the time of assessment, should she later become aware of these reactions, it may be helpful for her to recognize their normalcy and acceptability.

Minimizing the abuse is done partly to avoid labeling the violence as abuse or battering. Most women who are physically or sexually assaulted (or both), even many times within the prior year, do not label themselves as abused or battered. In a nursing-research study, Campbell, Rose, Kub, & Nedd (1998) found that such women may label their situation as emotional abuse because they consider abused or battered women to be pathetic victims rather than the strong women they actually are. However, it seems that recognition of the situation as abuse is a turning point for these women. They reported that this recognition

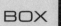

INDICATORS OF WIFE ABUSE FROM PHYSICAL EXAMINATION

GENERAL APPEARANCE

- Increased anxiety in presence of spouse
- Watching of spouse for approval of answers to questions
- Signs of fatigue
- Inappropriate or anxious nonverbal behavior
- Nonverbal communication suggesting shame about body
- Flinching when touched
- Poor grooming, inappropriate attire
- Overweight or underweight
- Hypertension

VITAL STATISTICS

- Overweight or underweight
- Hypertension

SKIN

- Bruises, welts, edema, or scars, especially on breasts, upper arms, abdomen, chest, face, and genitalia
- Burns

HEAD

- Subdural hematoma
- Clumps of hair missing

EYES

- Swelling
- Subconjunctival hemorrhage

GENITAL/URINARY

- Edema, bruises, tenderness, external bleeding

RECTAL

- Bruising, bleeding, edema, irritation

MUSCULOSKELETAL

- Fractures, especially of facial bones; spiral fractures of radius or ulna, ribs
- Shoulder dislocation
- Limited motion of an extremity
- Old fractures in various stages of healing

ABDOMEN

- Abdominal injuries in pregnant women
- Intra-abdominal injury

NEUROLOGICAL

- Hyperactive reflex responses
- Ear or eye problems secondary to injury
- Areas of numbness from old injuries
- Tremors

MENTAL-STATUS EXAMINATION

- Anxiety, fear
- Depression
- Suicidal ideation
- Low self-esteem
- Memory loss
- Difficulty concentrating

was accompanied by blaming themselves less for the violence, being more sure that their partner was the one who needed to change, and becoming less invested in the relationship, as compared to their state prior to recognition. In that research, many women said it was helpful for the nurse to point out that experts would label their situation as abuse or battering. Therefore, it may be therapeutic to point this out to women without forcing the label on them and to continue using terminology that the woman prefers.

Assessment of Danger

Violence that escalates over time or increases in severity must be described carefully. The Danger Assessment (Campbell, 1986, 1995) is a nurse-developed instrument useful in assisting the nurse and the battered woman to determine together the risk of homicide that exists in her particular situation. (See Appendix

C.) This 19-item instrument asks the woman to respond with yes-no answers to questions identifying the risk factors associated with the incidence of homicide in violent relationships; it takes approximately 10 minutes to complete. The instrument has been used in several research studies and has acceptable reliability and construct validity, but it has not been sufficiently tested to yield a cutoff score or concrete prediction (Campbell, 1992, 1995). In a recently completed 12-city study of femicide, each of the items significantly differentiated abused women who were killed from abused women in the same cities who were not. The instrument can be copied and used either clinically or in research, but users are asked to correspond thereafter with the author so that it can be developed further.

Initially, the nurse asks the woman to record all episodes of violence during the past year on a calendar and then, from looking at the calendar, to assess whether the abuse has become more frequent or more violent over time (items 1 and 2). Women can easily recall the approximate timing of abusive incidents (exact dates are not important) by anchoring them to holidays and other important events. This recording often helps the woman look at the pattern of abuse realistically if she has minimized its occurrence, and it is thus another instance of assessment as intervention.

After recording episodes on the calendar, the nurse informs the client that several risk factors for homicide in violent intimate relationships have been identified and invites her to see how many factors apply to her situation. Escalation of violence is identified as a serious risk factor for homicide in battering relationships, as is access to or the presence of a gun in the home. Threats of using a weapon or homicide often begin as abuse escalates and often precede lethal violence. Extreme substance abuse by the batterer (alcohol and certain drugs), forced sex, threats of lethal violence, stalking, extreme control of the woman's daily activities, extreme jealousy, and prior arrest for domestic violence are additional risk factors assessed by the tool. Research has indicated that abused women who killed their abusers were more likely than those who did not kill their husbands to have been threatened by their partners with lethal violence and to have threatened suicide themselves (Browne, Williams, & Dutton, 1998). Child-related factors, including battering during pregnancy, a stepchild (the woman's biological child but not his) in the home, and threats toward the children are additional factors the woman should consider while using the information generated by this tool for future decision-making. Threats or attempts of suicide are particularly important risk factors for femicide-suicide, a form of lethal domestic violence that makes up approximately 30% of intimate partner homicides of women. The separation of the woman from the abuser is the ultimate challenge to his desire for control, so the time immediately after she leaves is especially dangerous.

When the woman completes the Danger Assessment, she is encouraged to assess the degree of danger. If the woman and nurse validate the abuser's potential for committing lethal violence, the nurse is obliged to inform the woman that changing her own behavior within the relationship has been found to be basically ineffective in avoiding further incidents of abuse. However, she may be able to do things to increase her safety, like disarm or discard a weapon, ask police to impound any guns, or ask neighbors to call the police if they hear sounds of physical assault. Information about other alternatives also can be discussed, with particular attention on a plan for providing physical safety for the woman and her children. (See Box 11-6.) Because the woman may be most at risk for homicide when she

BOX **11-6**   **SPECIFIC CRITICAL SAFETY PLANS**

LEAVING

- If she plans to leave—she cannot tell him she is leaving face-to-face.
- She has to leave when he is not there, if at all possible. She could leave a note or call him later.

GUNS

- Have her remove or disarm guns.
- If he has been convicted for a domestic violence (DV) offense or has an Order of Protection out against him, he is not allowed to own a gun. Get the judge to have it removed!
- If no other action is possible, give her a child gun-safety pamphlet to take home.

BATTERER INTERVENTION

- Batterer intervention can work—it is worth a try—but often it takes a court order to get him there.
- If she has left, she can try to get him to go to batterer intervention.
- Make sure he completes batterer intervention before she returns.

ECONOMIC RESOURCES

- Have her put money aside—even just a little—every week.
- Help her get job training.

REACHING OUT—A REFERRAL IS NOT ENOUGH!

- Offer to call the police for her.
- Give her time and privacy with a phone.
- Dial the number and give her the phone.

National Domestic Violence Hotline at 800-799-SAFE.

leaves or lets the abuser know that she is leaving permanently, if the woman talks to the nurse about leaving, developing a plan for physical safety is necessary. If the abuse involves the children and the woman is unable to take action to provide for their physical safety, the nurse may need to call child protective services, the police, or both. There is usually sufficient evidence of old if not current physical injury to the child in such situations to warrant such actions. Immediate removal of the children and the woman to a shelter is another possibility.

After homicide risk has been assessed and if immediate danger is not present, the pattern of abuse can be examined to identify the events that trigger the abusive incidents. It is important during this part of the assessment to avoid blaming the woman. The focus of this assessment is on the stressors that occur within the relationship; seeing these helps the woman understand the mechanisms. It may also be useful to determine the amount of violence that occurred in the batterer's family of origin to help the woman connect his childhood learning with his present abusive behavior and thereby understand how deeply his behavior may be rooted in previous experience.

Social Support

Patterns of psychological abuse and controlling behavior, including jealousy and enforced isolation, should be explored with the woman. The pattern of abuse should be seen as part of the total relationship; doing so helps women to identify possible sources of feelings of entrapment, low self-esteem, and depression. Systematic assessment of personal networks and support systems are important to evaluate, especially when an abused woman describes isolation from family, friends, or both. (See Box 11-7.)

Findings related to personal networks of battered women indicate that a majority of battered women are not socially isolated, have the quantity of members in their personal networks similar to other women, and see them as frequently (McKenna, 1985). However, although the size of the network of an abused woman may be similar to that of another woman, the amount of support available to her is much less, and loss of network members is much greater. Box 11-7 lists several questions to explore with a battered woman to help her assess the support she may or may not have available to her through her personal network.

A health care provider needs to assess the reason for the loss of network members. Some batterers purposely isolate women from their social contacts, and, like the degree of violence, the enforced isolation begins subtly and increases over time. However, this is only one of the possible patterns. At least as often, the woman isolates herself from network members in a strategic effort to protect herself from any nonsupportive response from the network member. For example, the concerned family member who encourages the abused woman to leave her situation when she has not yet decided to deal with the violence by leaving is experienced as stressful rather than supportive. Minimizing contact with nonsupportive family members may be useful to the abused woman in maintaining her mental health. Assessment of social support can assist the woman in maintaining adequate supportive relationships while avoiding nonsupportive responses that increase her level of stress.

The woman's dependency on the marriage is also important to assess, both in light of the amount of loss she expects and in terms of her ability to leave. In a classic early study, Kalmuss and Straus (1982) identified two distinct areas of dependency on marriage (or an intimate relationship): objective dependence, or conditions that tie the woman to marriage in terms of economic survival (e.g., young children or few financial resources), and subjective dependence, the degree of her emotional investment. Using data on 2,143 couples, objective dependence was strongly related to abuse. Strong indications of both objective and subjective dependence on the marriage and heavy commitment to it would predict intense grieving reaction in the woman and less ability to contemplate leaving the relationship without interventions.

BOX 11-7   ASSESSMENT OF PERSONAL SUPPORT SYSTEMS

Ask the woman to make a list of the names of people in her life who are important to her. For each person, ask the woman:

- Does (s)he know about the abuse in your relationship with your partner?
- If *yes*, can this person be called on to help you in any way as you deal with this situation? If no, could this person be called on to help if (s)he knew about the abuse?
- If *yes*, indicate the type of support this person could be called on to provide (e.g., childcare, transportation, financial assistance, emotional support, and safe shelter).
- Are there any other people in your life who could be called on to help you deal with this situation?

The woman's perceptions about her children are also an important part of the history. Children of abused women are also frequently abused, probably more often and more seriously by the male partner but also by the woman (Edleson, 1999; Stark & Flitcraft, 1996). Indications of child abuse must be reported as they would in any other situation. The woman is frequently and justifiably concerned about the effect of the violence on the children, and the facts about intergenerational transmission of violence need to be shared. Conversely, she may describe her children as the reason that she stays in the relationship, and this needs to be carefully considered with her (Campbell, Rose, Kub, & Nedd, 1998). She may be able to outline, with the help of the nurse, the pros and cons of the relationship in terms of the children, which can be helpful in her assessment of the ramifications of the abuse.

Sexual Abuse

The possibility of sexual abuse needs to be explored with the woman. Research has indicated that sexual abuse occurs in at least 40% to 45% of battered women, but the woman will seldom initiate discussion about it (Campbell, 1989b; Campbell & Soeken, 1999a).

An introduction about the frequency of the problem can be useful in approaching the topic. The question "Does your partner (husband) ever force you into sex that you do not wish to participate in?" avoids language that the woman may not identify with and yet will explore experiences that would be labeled sexual abuse or marital rape. It is not important that the woman labels being forced into sex or sexual activities as abuse (unless she wants to bring criminal charges of marital rape against her partner), but she needs to disclose either emotional or physical distress from the sexual relationship. In two separate studies, it was found that women who were sexually and physically abused had significantly lower self-esteem than those who were physically abused only (Campbell, 1989b; Campbell & Soeken, 1999a).

Physical Symptoms and Conditions from Abuse

Many physical conditions may have direct links to physical abuse or be indirect sequelae related to the stress of physical and emotional trauma and fear. The most obvious health care problem for abused women is injury, with approximately 52% of abused women saying they were injured seriously enough from an abusive incident to need medical attention (Bachman & Saltzman, 1995). Such injuries have particular patterns that can be recognized. (See Chapter 13.)

In many well designed studies of women in a variety of health care settings, abused women have been found to have significantly more chronic health problems than nonabused women have, including significantly more neurological, gastrointestinal, and gynecological symptoms and chronic pain (Campbell, 2002; Campbell, Snow-Jones, et al., 2002; Coker, Smith, Bethea, King, & McKeown, 2000; Leserman, Drossman, & Hu, 1998; Letourneau, Holmes, & Chasedunn-Roark, 1999; McCauley et al., 1995; Plichta, 1996; Schei, 1991). Abused women have also been shown to visit health care professionals more often than women not battered and to incur more health care costs (Wisner et al., 1999).

In terms of mental health, abused women have significantly more depression, suicidality, and PTSD (posttraumatic stress disorder) symptoms, as well as problems with substance abuse (Golding, 1999). The forced sex that so frequently accompanies physical abuse contributes to a host of reproductive health problems, including chronic pelvic pain, unintended pregnancy, sexually transmitted diseases (STDs) including HIV, and urinary-tract infections (Campbell & Alford, 1989; Campbell & Soeken, 1999a; Letourneau et al., 1999; Maman et al., 2000). Like forced sex in abusive relationships, abuse during pregnancy is also a significant health problem addressed early on by nursing (e.g., Helton, 1986). Abuse during pregnancy has serious consequences for both the pregnant mother (e.g., depression and substance abuse) and infant (e.g., low birth weight and risk of child abuse; Gazmararian et al., 2000, and Murphy et al., 2001). See Chapter 4 for more information on abuse during pregnancy.

Although abused women have been found to be more frequently and severely distressed by physical symptoms of stress (Campbell, 1989a), the physical symptoms may be the result of damage from old injury as well as related to stress. For instance, a woman "slammed" against kitchen cabinets approximately once a month can suffer back or neurological damage from both impact and whiplash. This type of serious injury can be caused by the "pushing and shoving" that so often occurs in intimate relationships but sounds like a relatively mild instance of abusive tactics. Much is known about the neurological damage incurred by boxers, but an abused woman is more likely to be referred for counseling than for a neurological workup if she complains about frequent headaches (Diaz-Olavarietta, Campbell, Garcia de la Cadena, Paz, & Villa, 1999). These types of physical symptoms from injuries have been listed in Box 11-5.

Fortunately, as nurses become increasingly aware of the problem, they are taking active roles in identifying and providing services for battered women in the practice setting or in shelters for battered women and their children (Hollenkamp & Attala, 1986; Sheridan, 1998). Nursing care of survivors of intimate partner violence will improve as the theoretical explanations of the causes of, and women's responses to, intimate partner violence become increasingly informative. Theoretical work and empirical research will underpin the development of effective evidence-based nursing interventions.

Thus, the history part of the nursing assessment with an abused woman includes all the routine areas of questioning but also incorporates some areas specific to battering. (See Box 11-4 for indications of potential or actual wife abuse.) In the first narration, the woman may include at least some of the areas spontaneously, but if she does not the nurse must decide which additional areas to explore in light of time restrictions, possibilities of continued contact, and priorities suggested by the woman's verbal and nonverbal cues. The areas postponed in terms of history should be noted for further follow-up or passed on as topics to be covered in subsequent assessment by the professional to whom the woman is referred.

Physical Examination

The physical examination of the woman suspected of being abused should be conducted as any other physical assessment of an adult female. In addition to the standard protocol used for all clients, careful attention must be directed to any signs of injury, past and present, with exact measurement of even the most insignificant-looking bruise. A body map (see Abuse Assessment Screen, Appendix A) and photographs are valuable for recording the site of injuries. Because most injuries to the battered woman are to the face, chest, breasts, and abdomen, special attention should be paid to these areas (Stark et al., 1979). A thorough neurological examination may be indicated, as may be x-ray films for old and current fractures (Campbell & Sheridan, 1989; Diaz-Olivietta et al., 1999).

When conducting the physical examination, the nurse should remember that many conditions may be related to old injuries from abuse, and the nurse should ask specifically about the background of such conditions. For instance, hearing loss in one ear may be related to an untreated rupture of the tympanic membrane from a blow to the ear. The incidence of sexual abuse would indicate careful examination of the genitalia and a pelvic examination for physical signs of such. Marital rape has been associated with such physical problems as vaginal and anal tearing, hemorrhoids, and pain with intercourse and with the pelvic examination, and infections that may have resulted in pelvic inflammatory disease (Campbell & Alford, 1989). These types of findings on physical examination are listed in Box 11-5.

Extreme gentleness is important in light of the body-image damage that has been done. The general appearance of the woman should include observations about her behavior as well as physical appearance. Nonverbal behavior that indicates shame about her body is fairly common in battered women and understandable with respect to body-image insult. Other affective behaviors can give clues as to how the woman deals with feelings.

Mental Status Examination

During mental-status examination, signs of depression, high anxiety, low self-esteem, and PTSD (see Box 11-8) should be carefully noted (Woods, 1999). Especially when clients seem to overreact to apparently minor physical or emotional complaints, the nurse should remember that abused women tend to respond with greater than average anxiety to threats to their current well-being (Trimpey, 1989). This is understandable given the reality of threat and physical danger.

Several studies have described significantly higher levels of depressive symptoms in abused women when compared with samples of women in which the incidence of abuse is unknown (Campbell et al., 1996; Golding, 1999). When Campbell (1989a) compared abused women with other women having serious problems in an intimate relationship with a man, she found approximately equal mean levels of depression, suggesting that depression was related to grief and stress about the relationship ending rather than to being hit. However, the abused women were more likely to be seriously depressed. Depression is a common response to situational stress, especially when resources are inadequate or when multiple losses lead to prolonged grieving (Carpenito, 1992). Although not all persons who commit suicide are clinically depressed, thorough assessment of suicide potential is important. Because battered women are more likely to attempt suicide than are nonbattered women, suicidal intent must be considered as a real possibility (Stark & Flitcraft, 1996).

Nurses may assess self-esteem by asking the woman to list her strengths and weaknesses, by asking her to evaluate herself in comparison to her friends, or by inquiring about how near she believes she is to the person she would like to be. Another clue is if the woman blames herself for the abuse. Although a minority (20%) of women blamed themselves for their problems in the relationship in Campbell's (1989a) sample of battered women, those who did were more likely to be severely depressed and have low self-esteem. In light of the prevalence of low self-esteem in battered women, a more objective measure like the Culture-Free

BOX	11-8	POSTTRAUMATIC STRESS DISORDER (DSM-IV)

1. Existence of a recognizable stressor
2. Reexperiencing of the trauma as evidenced by at least one of the following:
   - Intrusive recollections of the event
   - Recurring dreams, nightmares
   - Sudden acting or feeling as if the trauma were recurring, stimulated by an emotional or environmental event
3. Psychological numbing as evidenced by:
   - Diminished interest in activities
   - Feelings of estrangement
   - Constricted affect
4. At least two of the following symptoms that were not present before the trauma:
   - Exaggerated startle reflex, anxiety
   - Sleep disturbance
   - Survival guilt
   - Impaired concentration or memory
   - Avoidance of activities that are reminders of the trauma
   - Intensification of symptoms by exposure to events that symbolize or resemble the traumatic event
   - Irritability, hypersensitivity

Self-Esteem Inventories (CFSEI) for Adults (Battle, 1981) may be used. When the setting does not allow for use of standardized tests to measure the response of the client, the woman's response to the structured interview questions should be carefully noted. When the setting does allow for use of a standardized instrument, it is recommended that the tool be an integral part of the nurse's interview rather than self-administered before the interview. This suggestion is based on research that indicated self-disclosure of highly sensitive information may be increased when the client interacts with a nurse who engenders a sense of trust and who responds in an accepting, nonjudgmental manner (McFarlane et al., 1991).

NURSING DIAGNOSIS

The nurse can best begin the diagnostic aspect of assessment by sharing with the abused woman her strengths as the nurse sees them. This is extremely important in terms of potential low self-esteem and the generally prevailing attitude of battered women that they will be condemned for their behavior—if not in terms of inciting the beatings in some way, then at least for not ending the relationship. Abused women are frequently extremely creative in finding ways to deal with a violent spouse and in bringing up their children with a minimum of damage. They need recognition of and support for those efforts. At the beginning of diagnosis, it is also helpful to explain how normal her reactions (such as depression) and behavior are in light of being beaten. The nurse must remember how much blame and fault-finding the woman usually receives from the batterer and to enthusiastically praise the woman. Clinical experience has shown that it is useful to record these strengths and show the woman that they are part of the record and therefore considered as important as any problems she may have. Gondolf

(1998) developed a more extensive strengths-oriented assessment of battered women that can be useful.

The next part of the diagnostic process is to ask the woman to list any concerns she has and what priority she places on them. To the nurse's surprise, the woman may focus on a problem that seems peripheral to abuse. This may be part of a testing process for the woman or may be what seems central to her at that moment. These concerns must be respected in deciding the course of nursing interventions. When the woman has listed the areas that she believes need attention, the nurse can add others, asking if the woman agrees that they also need inclusion. Then the nurse may need to explain the holistic nature of nursing; some women may think that the nurse is primarily interested in physical injury.

Another important aspect of the nurse's contribution to the diagnostic process is to help the woman determine patterns of stress-related symptoms. Battered women frequently report problems such as headaches, gastrointestinal symptoms, and heart palpitations. In one study, abused women were significantly more likely to have more frequent and more severe symptoms of stress than nonabused women (Campbell, 1989a). The woman may not see such complaints as related to the almost constant stress experienced and may need help in making the connection. The emphasis should be on the normalcy of these symptoms in her situation, although the possibility of further medical diagnosis and intervention should also be discussed. Symptoms may be related to old injuries or a decreased immune response that can also be the result of stress.

Nursing diagnosis of battered women may cover a range of concerns. A list of applicable nursing diagnoses (Box 11-9) and a sample nursing process (Box 11-12) are included in this chapter. Although other nursing diagnoses may be appropriate to specific abused women, the diagnoses listed will assist with many women attempting to deal with violence in intimate relationships.

PLANNING

The planning stage requires working with the battered woman to develop goals and interventions that seem appropriate together. Short-term goals should be fairly simple and concrete. Achievement of these first goals has immeasurable value in showing the woman that some of her problems can be solved, that she is capable of achieving solutions even in her restricted situation, and that working for long-term goals is also feasible. The battered woman may seem passive in the goal-setting phase because of her feelings of being trapped, her mistrust of the helping professionals, the protective mechanism of not looking toward the future, or any combination thereof. The nurse must recognize such behavior as normal and help the woman to formulate her own goals. This may be considered as partially an intervention; it is helping the woman develop problem-solving techniques.

Long-term goals may be more difficult for the abused woman to develop. The nurse must be careful not to prematurely impose a goal of leaving the abuser. A majority of abused women do eventually leave the violent relationship or manage to make the violence end (Campbell et al., 1994; Okun, 1986). Leaving the abuser or otherwise dealing with the violence is best considered a process. The woman may leave and return several times before leaving permanently. In one study, the average number of times women left and returned before making a final break was 5.2 times (Okun, 1986). Leaving and returning is

BOX 11-9   **NURSING DIAGNOSES TO CONSIDER WITH ABUSED WOMEN***

Ineffective coping related to response to identifiable situational stressors: The woman is unable to manage long-term situational stressors (relocation, inadequate finances, lack of support system, poor self-esteem).

Impaired adjustment related to response to multiple losses and inadequate support: During the period immediately following acute battering, woman experiences extended disbelief, shock, or anger and is unable to orient her thinking to the future.

Grieving related to actual or perceived loss related to wife abuse: The woman anticipates or is aware of losses (status, relationship, person) related to the abuse; when the grief is unresolved or prolonged, consider dysfunctional grieving as subsequent diagnosis.

Posttrauma response related to wife abuse: The type of violence experienced stimulates a sustained emotional response that interferes with interpersonal relationships and precipitates self-destructive behavior (suicide attempts, substance abuse); often seen in women who have a history of victimization (sexual assault, child abuse).

Decisional conflict related to wife abuse and conflict with personal values or beliefs: The woman finds herself unable to decide about a course of action because of the losses involved, or the decisions she perceives as necessary conflict with her values or the values of her support system.

Anxiety related to ongoing threat of wife abuse: Wife abuse threatens a woman's self-concept and interferes with her sense of security, roles, and values; fear may be a more useful diagnosis when the violence or threats of violence pose a direct threat to the woman's physical safety.

*Not inclusive of all diagnoses that might be used with abused women.

best understood as a healthy testing of the partner's promises to reform, of her children's ability to cope without their father, and of her economic and personal resources. The first few times she leaves, the woman may fully intend to return; she is making a point that the abuse needs to end, not the relationship. Later, she may entertain the notion of leaving for good, and she is more likely to use a shelter than go to family or friends. The battered woman may take months or years to reach the point of leaving permanently, and she may never reach it. She may, however, inquire whether the nurse believes this should be a goal, because she is often used to this advice. The nurse may need to explore her or his thinking on the subject. If the woman is not yet ready to contemplate the future, long-term goals may be set later in the course of the relationship.

Planning is mutual, with final decisions left to the woman. The nurse can offer support and suggested alternatives. It is difficult for nurses to imagine the battering situation, especially if unemployment, several young children, and a dearth of support systems accompany the problem. Clinical experience has shown that abused women have often thought of anything that traditional nursing has to suggest. The women, with encouragement to think as widely and fancifully as they can, usually discover the germs of effective solutions that can be refined, explored, and expanded with the nurse. Such a process can often be enjoyable for both the woman and the nurse. Nothing is more useful for raising self-esteem for the woman than determining her own solutions and being praised effusively for them.

NURSING INTERVENTION

Professional nursing interventions for the problem of wife abuse are based on the three levels of prevention. Identifying and caring for the individual battered woman is insufficient; nurses must seek the societal causes and work to eliminate their influence.

Primary Prevention

Primary prevention involves interventions at the societal level, identification of women at risk to become abused, and implementation of nursing care, both with those women at risk and with their potential abusers. Because wife abuse originates from social structures that disempower women and encourage controlling attitudes and behavior in men, prevention must start at this point (King, 1998).

Interventions at the Societal Level

Political activism is a mandatory role for nurses in changing the social structure so that all women have the means for economic independence and educational and political empowerment. Each individual nurse cannot be expected to take on every political cause that has impact on these issues. However, each nurse can be involved in one such issue and then at least vote and write to elected officials about the rest. Support for legislation and implementation that eliminates gender inequality in all of its aspects is an obvious starting point. Issues of equal compensation for work of comparable worth is an area of immense implication for the profession of nursing, as well as for the economic dependence of all women. The lack of affordable, responsible child care for working mothers also remains a significant block to economic independence for women. Private industry and government need constant prodding to make day care a reality for every woman who needs it. The lack of viable job training for women without advanced education or technical skills is an ongoing problem. Abused women are more likely to need welfare subsidy and have a more difficult time obtaining job training and viable work than nonabused women do. Nurses can join with other women in advocating change in these areas and can thereby realize the enormous strength of women working together, which is necessary in challenging deeply embedded values and structures.

This country has gone a long way toward eliminating sexism, yet vestiges continue to operate in subtle and insidious ways. Although there has been much improvement over the past decade, surveys of the American public continue to show that men across all the major ethnic groups are less concerned about domestic violence and less willing to do anything about it than are women (Klein, Campbell, Soler, & Ghez, 1997; Masaki, Campbell, & Torres, 1997). The child-rearing patterns of our culture are now emphasizing more male involvement, but full participation of fathers in all aspects of parenting has yet to be achieved. Boys can be encouraged toward this type of behavior in parenting classes in high school, and prenatal classes are also important in this regard. Fathers involved in labor and delivery may be more likely to be involved in child-rearing later. Nurses can also participate in public education to promote male participation in child-rearing; the proliferation of cable-television health programs presents excellent opportunities.

The male dominance and violence portrayed on television and in children's books must be protested frequently and vehemently. Pornography, especially that depicting violence against women, must be curtailed. Laboratory and field studies (Russell, 1993) have suggested that viewing erotic films depicting women as victims of violence increases men's aggression and acceptance of interpersonal violence against women. Erotica and pornography can be differentiated by the mutuality and reciprocity in sexual acts portrayed in the former and the humiliation and domination of women, if not actual violence, in the latter (Sandelowski, 1980). With these differentiations in mind, individuals can argue effectively against pornography without tangling with the issues of freedom of speech and open attitudes toward sex. Feminists advocate women banding together against pornography, demonstrating against movies depicting violent sex, confronting men who buy pornographic materials, and educating the public as to the dangers of such media (Russell, 1991).

The adult male in today's society often feels threatened. The feminist movement has challenged his traditional prerogatives, and economic malaise is eroding his chances to attain power and prestige in the work environment. He receives mixed messages in the media and from women as to whether strength and macho characteristics, or gentleness and advocating sexual equality, are preferable. Activities for health promotion for men should include supporting men's groups for discussion of the evolving male role and for helping men to get in touch with their feelings and learn to express them without aggression. The Family Violence Prevention Fund has started a new campaign for helping men reach out to young men and boys through parenting, sports, and other activities to teach them to become nonviolent. Nursing advocacy is also needed to create better school systems, less discrimination, job training, and job opportunities for young men in our society. Facing a future without viable opportunities to be productive or support a family, young men, especially those of minority ethnic groups and from poor backgrounds, often believe their only way of finding status is through a tough reputation that often includes controlling their female partners. Nursing assessment of individual men, including adolescents, should include a discussion of these issues and how the man deals with them. This is as important as assessing for physical problems.

Women also need help in overcoming psychological dependence on men. This need has been addressed well in women's support groups as an outgrowth of the women's movement. However, these groups remain predominantly organized and used by middle-class women. Poorer women generally do not perceive themselves as having the leisure time, the child care, or the transportation to take advantage of such groups and are not sure of their welcome. They are often overwhelmed by the problems of everyday living. However, discussions of women's roles and gaining support from each other can be part of groups that are organized around more "practical" aims, which can be held in poor neighborhoods with child care provided.

Waiting rooms of hospital and public-health clinics can be used to engage men and women in meaningful conversations on all types of issues. Professionals often complain that people do not take advantage of educational programs and discussion groups offered, and yet they allow the people they are trying to reach to sit for hours in a variety of waiting rooms or stand in endless lines to initiate contact with social and health services. The target groups are there; a more creative way than showing videotapes is needed to fill this time. Women who are clients of the mental health system need such discussions regardless of their symptoms. All women's roles are changing, and all women are dealing with this at some level. The women may not ask for "feminist therapy;" but mental health nurses should lead the struggle to ensure that therapy for women does not further cripple them with reinforcement of traditional psychiatric myths about female dependency. Problems in self-esteem and susceptibility to depression are natural outgrowths of growing up female in a sexist society.

School nurses and community-health nurses are in a good position to deal with these issues with adolescent girls. The high prevalence of dating violence should be discussed with these young women. (See Chapter 10.) Jealousy can be discussed and redefined as an issue of ownership rather than love. Adolescent mothers can be approached singly or in groups by maternal-child health nurses for discussion of issues related to dating, sexuality, and women's roles. These young women are at high risk of becoming caught in poverty and crippling of potentials. Dependence on a man can seem attractive as a way to escape, and such young women need help in growth before they can make wise decisions about intimate relationships with men.

Interventions with Women at Risk

No consistent factors have been identified as placing an individual woman at risk to be abused (Hotaling & Sugarman, 1990). However, women who are intimately involved with men displaying macho characteristics are at risk, especially those who are unemployed, lack power at work, are in high-stress situations, abuse alcohol, or were exposed to a violent home as a child. (Other characteristics indicating risk are in Boxes 11-4 and 11-5.) Recent evidence has suggested that abuse is more frequent in couples who are cohabiting, separated, or divorced than in those who are married (Dearwater et al., 1998; Hotaling & Sugarman, 1990). Thus, there is a need to assess all women for abuse, not just those who are married.

A woman at risk who has not been beaten may respond affirmatively to questions such as "Has your spouse ever threatened to hit you?" or "Have you ever been afraid that he would hit you?" It is useful to suggest a women's group for these women and to inform them that increased family stress may begin a cycle of battering; they need to know how to obtain crisis intervention in such a situation. It is also helpful to encourage women to plan a scenario of what they would do if they were beaten. This rehearsal usually lends support if beating occurs and does not frighten the woman unnecessarily as might be imagined; she may very well have thought of the possibility previously but, without support, has not thought it through completely.

Women at risk frequently subscribe to the myth that they can somehow save a man with problems—alcohol or drug abuse, a violent temper, or a rotten childhood—and that enough love and patience from her will cure him. Women need to understand that they cannot be held responsible for a spouse's behavior and that such problems require professional intervention, not just a partner's support. Convincing the man to accept help is, of course, a difficult issue. The man who exhibits a macho male identity finds it almost impossible to admit a need for help. The individual woman is the best judge of conditions under which the man may be willing to seek help, and the nurse can help her to create these conditions. An authoritarian message that help is necessary from a male physician can sometimes be useful in persuading the man. If the female partner thinks this would be helpful, the nurse can arrange it.

Other attitudes frequently displayed by the woman at risk for abuse are that all men are unreasonably jealous, at least occasionally resort to violence, and need to be dominant. Gentleness in male behavior may be woefully absent in her experience and community. A middle-class nurse from a different culture may be considered a useless source of information on male behavior in her world. Another nurse or health-team member from a similar background may be more persuasive. Even more useful is a group of women who are her peers, some of whom may have encountered or successfully demanded different standards of behavior. Such experiences can be difficult to arrange, but the results are worthwhile.

Assertiveness and leadership training is also helpful for both women who are at risk for battering and abused women. Assertiveness and leadership classes have been more prevalent for middle-class women than for those who are poor. Creativity is needed in making such classes available for the traditionally underserved. The classes could be held during lunch hours in workplaces like factories, office buildings, hospitals, and shopping centers where women are frequently employed; at neighborhood centers; or at Head Start classrooms when the children are occupied. Special care must be taken to be sure that poor women feel invited, that small groups of friends are encouraged to come, and that the relevance to their situation is emphasized.

Primary prevention can also take the form of fighting poverty at the societal level or helping the individual man or woman at risk to find a job (Raphael, 2000). It may also include promoting nonviolence in our culture and in individual families. Preventing wife abuse is certainly an almost overwhelming task, but fortunately others are involved. Nurses must band together with women and concerned men everywhere. Many groups of professionals can also be included—social workers, psychologists, concerned physicians, feminist lawyers, and some police. Coalitions of nurses and individuals from these groups can be formed. Nurses are welcome on boards of agencies and groups involved with wife abuse and can help set policy in this type of position. The opportunities for nurses to significantly make an impact on the quest to prevent the battering of women, both in terms of health promotion and identification and intervention for those at risk, are extensive and varied. Nurses can make a difference.

Secondary Prevention

Secondary prevention of wife abuse involves diligent efforts at early case-finding and interventions with women in the beginning stages of wife abuse. Women may be most receptive to intervention after an acute incident of violence that results in injury, but it is even more ideal to find her before an injury has occurred.

The emergency-department (ED) nurse is important in case finding. An estimated 14 to 18% of all women seen in emergency departments have been physically or sexually assaulted by an intimate partner in the prior year (Abbott et al., 1995). With that fact in mind, wife abuse should be ruled out before other causes of injury are investigated. Therefore, any male partner coming to an ED with an injured woman should be kept in the waiting room as a matter of policy until abuse is ruled out (Campbell & Sheridan, 1989). Questions about abuse should be direct, such as "Who hit you?" or "Who did that to you?" This approach minimizes the chances of the woman making up a story and conveys that the nurse is knowledgeable about abuse.

It is appropriate that the professional nurse takes responsibility for determining battering because the nurse is more likely to be female and therefore less threatening and because abuse, with all its psychological and social ramifications, is more logically within the wider scope of nursing than medicine (Warshaw, 1989). There may be a social work department that can help the woman also, but nurses should not make the referral until and unless the woman chooses to talk to a social worker. The woman may come to the ED with fairly minor injuries or other complaints in an attempt to seek help for the primary problem. It is tempting to treat such clients quickly with a lecture about the misuse of emergency rooms. A high index of suspicion for abuse in nurses will prevent these women from going away unserved.

Because the most frequent area of injury is the face, it is easy for both the woman and the emergency staff to focus on this type of obvious trauma and not conduct a complete physical examination. A superficial but bloody face wound may hurt more than the more serious head injury or internal injuries (Campbell & Sheridan, 1989). Given the high incidence of sexual abuse, a pelvic examination may be conducted if the woman so indicates.

If the injuries are serious enough to warrant hospitalization, this should be considered as beneficial in terms of protecting the woman temporarily and allowing her to really think, removed from the batterer and the stresses of home. The ED nurse can alert the inpatient staff of the possibility of abuse if it has not been confirmed, so that the woman's nurses can discuss the issue with her. Another alternative is to keep the woman in the emergency department for a few hours until the nurse has time to sit and talk with her. Often some privacy with a phone is a luxury that few women have at home; batterers are extremely surveillant and may monitor phone calls electronically. She could use the time to reach out for help to the National Domestic Violence hotline (800-799-SAFE) or local shelter or advocacy services.

An abused woman may also present herself to mental health facilities with a variety of psychiatric symptoms, including suicide attempts, in an effort to reach out for assistance. In clinical experience, battered women have often recounted how the psychiatric staff tended to "dope me up" as a primary intervention, which generally lessened their pain but also interfered with their resolve to take effective action. As soon as their symptoms subsided, they were usually released without any interventions to solve the underlying problems. This general course of events did not seem to alter whether they told of the abuse. Battering must be assumed to be a possible cause of or related to depression, anxiety, substance abuse, and marital problems, and it should receive specific inquiry and intervention. Researchers have begun to document the prevalence of abused women in both inpatient and outpatient mental health facilities (Dienemann, Campbell, Landenburger, & Curry, 2000).

Prenatal clinics, private obstetrical offices, childbirth-education classes, and inpatient postpartum floors are all places where nurses can be alert for wife battering (see Chapter 4), given the widespread incidence of battering during pregnancy.

In community-health nursing, nurses are in clients' homes and deal with families on a regular basis. In such settings, wife abuse may easily be revealed if the professional nurse is alert to the possibility and gently asks the right questions. Many battered women would be anxious to tell if asked empathetically in a safe and private situation. In birth-control clinics, community-health nurses may have contact with women in early stages of battering. A nursing study in a Planned Parenthood clinic demonstrated that 8.2% of 793 women responded that they were abused on the abuse-assessment screening questions shown in Appendix B. The actual prevalence was undoubtedly higher because nurses who interview women about abuse would discover more. This type of clinic is also an excellent setting in which to identify young women who are in relationships that are beginning to be characterized by violence and by excessive control by the man. Descriptions of the spouse making all the decisions about birth control or "forcing" the woman in any manner are indications that abuse may be present. Follow-up appointments for the woman are therefore important even if not mandatory in terms of the chosen birth-control method.

Coworkers typically know about abuse before it comes to the attention of professionals. A vigorous campaign of distributing information about wife abuse in the workplace, coupled with suggestions to approach the occupational-health nurse if abuse is known, can be useful for early identification. The woman may also be absent recurrently and show evidence of facial bruises, perhaps covered with heavy makeup. She may be defensive about questions regarding her absenteeism and indicate powerlessness in the relationship by saying she is not able to spend her salary according to her own desires, to work overtime, or to rearrange her schedule because of his objections. The workplace is an excellent setting to provide nursing care to a battered woman because of her separation from the spouse. (See http://www.fvpf.org for further information.)

Primary-care and managed-care settings and physician's offices are other health arenas where abuse, especially in middle-class homes, can be detected (King & Ryan, 1989; Jones et al., 1999). Battered women may often seek medical attention because of stress-related symptoms, chronic pain, or both. Nursing-assessment questions about abuse or careful review of physician's findings can identify the battered woman. Regardless of the setting in which abuse is identified, documentation is crucial. (See Chapter 13 for detailed instructions on documentation.) The record should clearly state who (by name) the woman says has injured her. This can be put in quotes after the phrase, "patient states" so there is no question of the nurse making a judgment about the perpetrator. In this way, abuse can be established for future court action, even if the woman states she has no intention of leaving or taking legal steps at the time of the nursing assessment. The court action for which the records are most often needed is a child-custody suit because the abuser often tries to obtain custody of the children if she leaves him. The woman may also decide later that she wants to press charges or may need the records in a court action against her for assault or homicide. The records should also contain a complete description of any visible signs of injury, old as well as new. These injuries should be recorded on a body map with the description, date of injury, and photograph, if possible. The nurse can discuss the record with the woman and how she can obtain it if she ever needs it. This gives her an important option and is therefore an empowerment strategy.

A Theoretical Framework for Intervention

To understand the abused woman, it is helpful to study her behavior in the context of the practice nursing theory developed by Landenburger (1989) that also has elements of similarity with a grieving framework (Campbell, 1989a; Flynn & Whitcomb, 1981). Her reaction can thus be seen as normal process in a situation of multiple and severe losses. In many societies, a successful marriage is often seen as the single most important achievement for women. This picture has changed somewhat in our country, but any battered woman is still dealing with the significant loss of the idealized version of marriage. The woman is typically thought to be responsible for the success of the marriage, and to acknowledge that it is in shambles entails considerable loss of self-esteem. Support for this interpretation was found in an early study (Campbell, 1989a) in which abused women and other women with serious problems in their primary relationships had similar scores on self-esteem and depression, though significantly lower than the instrument norms. For the abused woman, body-image loss because of the physical injuries and sexual abuse is also a part of the picture (Campbell, 1989b).

The abused woman has lost a great deal of trust in her mate and in the world as a safe place, and she has also lost her illusions that the man is basically good for her and an appropriate object of her love and affection. When she contemplates leaving the man, she must face the potential losses of status in marriage, financial security or some semblance thereof, a father for her children, her home, and various support systems. The tendency of many abused wives to stay married to their husbands, return to them after leaving, drop assault charges against them, and idealize them even after leaving has baffled and exasperated the scholars in the field and those working with battered women. This behavior can be perhaps best understood as a normal process of commitment to a relationship and then reaction to the multiple losses. Such reframing from a picture of victimization and pathology to one of normalcy and recognizing strengths has also been labeled a survivor framework (Gondolf, 1990; Hoff, 1988). The advantages of using such a framework are that it views the response patterns as essentially healthy and as a process to be worked through and supported by nursing care. Being perceived as survivors rather than victims is also an approach that most battered women prefer. Nursing researcher Jacqueline Dienemann (Dienemann, Campbell, Landenburger, & Curry, 2002) developed the Domestic Violence Survivor Assessment (DVSA) instrument to help the nurse and the woman identify her stage in the process.

Binding

Landenburger's (1989) practice theory of the process of entrapment in and recovery from an abusive relationship was derived from a grounded theory study of abused women and has support from several independent research projects (Landenburger, 1998). Her research indicates that a woman passes progressively through a process of binding, enduring, disengaging, and recovering. As with grieving, the process takes considerable time, and the behaviors vary in their appearance, sequence, intensity, and length of time required. Binding encompasses the initial development of the relationship and the beginnings of abuse within the relationship. As in any intimate relationship, the woman is trying to create a loving, long-term partnership. She has made a commitment to try to make this relationship work, and she works very hard at that, despite warning signals that begin to develop. She chooses to interpret the signs of ownership or jealousy that are almost always present as symbols of the love and attention she needs rather than as troublesome.

Similarly, all the authors who have traced the grief response have identified an initial period of shock and denial that follows significant loss. When the abuse first begins, the woman experiences a tremendous sense of loss of the idealized relationship she has worked to achieve. Other research has found that the battered woman may deny or minimize the importance of the initial battering in a variety of ways (Campbell et al., 1998; Merritt-Gray & Wuest, 1995). At first, the abuse is typically only a small part of the relationship (Landenburger, 1989). The woman may explain the occasional push or shove as a temporary aberration in an essentially loving relationship, or she may blame the stress that the man is currently undergoing or her own behavior. She may admit the violence but blame it on alcohol or a temporary loss of control in her spouse. He will typically blame factors that minimize his responsibility; this supports her denial. However, once a man has used violence with his wife, a psychological barrier seems to have been broken, and a pattern of abuse is started. The initial shock and denial of the woman, a perfectly normal response, may be perceived by the man as a form of acquiescence, a sign that the man's goals have been achieved, or both. Through no fault of hers, this may serve to reinforce his abusive behavior.

As the violence recurs, the impact and meaning become apparent. She begins to question what is happening as her attempts to make things right are obviously futile (Landenburger, 1989). For the woman, this is a transitional period into the next phase. The woman may experience many strong feelings. However, the intermittent pattern of some abuser's beatings may allow the woman to return to denial during quiescent periods. The feeling that first surfaces is sometimes anger, and the woman may try to fight back, either verbally or physically. This is a strategy that many abused women try at various points during the relationship; therefore her acts of aggressiveness should be interpreted in that light (Campbell, Rose, Kub, & Nedd, 1998). If the woman finds that fighting back only worsens the violence directed against her, she will stop and have to suppress her anger. In a traditional psychological interpretation, it can be predicted that the anger may be dealt with by turning it inward, by displacement onto others, by projection, or by developing somatic symptoms.

Enduring

In Landenburger's (1989) second phase, enduring, the woman sees herself as putting up with the abuse. Feeling responsible is an important aspect of this phase. The related concept of guilt is another strong feeling associated with loss and grief, and it has been noted in much of the literature that battered women frequently blame themselves for the abuse, at least at first. Their guilt is reinforced by the psychological abuse and blame dealt out by the spouse. However, in a sample of 97 battered women, only 20% blamed themselves for the abuse (Campbell, 1989a). As Landenburger found, many women who do not blame themselves for the abuse feel responsible in another way; they feel responsible for helping their partner or for staying in an abusive relationship. Bargaining is identified in a grieving framework, and the women in Landenburger's sample described a similar theme called "placating." The battered woman frequently makes a pact, either overtly or covertly, with her husband that she will correct whatever behavior he sees as a problem in return for an absence of violence. She also bargains with him about returning to him or staying with him only if he changes his behavior or seeks treatment for the violence or substance abuse (Campbell et al., 1998). This can be a very effective strategy for entering abusive men into batterer intervention. Gondolf (1988) found that the strongest predictor of women in shelters returning to their partner was that he was in counseling. However, as Gondolf (1988) pointed out, "Unfortunately batterers often use counseling as a form of manipulation . . ., dropping out as soon as the threat of separation is over" (p. 286).

The helplessness, despair, and loss of control, so often identified by abused women and clinically seen as depression, is a normal part of grieving. The period of enduring is extremely painful, as the woman struggles with her feelings of responsibility to the relationship and trying to determine why she is being abused. Women in both Landenburger's (1989) and Ulrich's (1998) samples described a loss or shrinking of self as the abuse continued and escalated. The battered woman doubts her ability to cope without the man and may feel totally worthless. She cannot be expected to make the difficult decisions and plans necessary for leaving when she is in this stage. Instead, she tries to hide the abuse and finds it difficult to disclose to anyone. This should also be interpreted as a normal desire to avoid the stigma associated with abuse and to protect her partner. Even to herself, she usually does not label what is happening to her as abuse or battering (Campbell, 1991; Campbell et al., 1998).

Disengaging

Acceptance of the loss, along with realistic plans for change either within the relationship or outside of it, comes slowly for most women. The degree of loss may prolong the time needed to opt for change. Some women may never work through the grieving process or are so traumatized that they are immobilized. However, most women next enter a stage of disengaging (Landenburger, 1989; Merritt-Gray & Wuest, 1995). They begin to identify with other women in similar situations through media accounts of abuse, friends or family members, or community or shelter support groups. (Those sources are therefore important adjuncts to other types of intervention, and the media should be encouraged to continue informed news coverage of abuse and abuse-related entertainment programs.) The abused woman for the first time may label what is happening as abuse and label herself as an abused or battered woman. Women in Campbell and colleagues' (1998) longitudinal study stated that this labeling process was accompanied by a significant change in how they thought about the relationship and what they did. They recounted shifts in blame from themselves to him, feeling like he was the one who had to change, not her, and deciding that the relationship would have to end.

In a nursing study of 51 women who had left abusers, Ulrich (1991) found that the two most frequent categories of reasons for leaving were safety and personal growth. The safety category included fearing for their own, others', or their children's physical safety or their children's emotional safety. The personal-growth category included sudden changes in awareness, having reached a personal limit, or being concerned for their own potential.

Women in the disengaging phase begin to actively seek help to end the relationship (Landenburger, 1989, 1998). Gondolf (1990) noted that women in his large sample of women in shelters more actively sought help as the abuse increased in severity and frequency. Bowker (1983) also noted that women's help-seeking switched from family and friends to more formal systems as time elapsed, and the more formal systems were found to be more helpful.

During disengagement, anger often reemerges and may become rage, and the woman may fantasize about killing her partner (Campbell et al., 1998; Landenburger, 1989). Her partner senses that she is close to a breaking point, and he often escalates his threats and violence to keep her in the relationship. These situations are extremely volatile, and serious injury or homicide of either partner may occur. This is the most dangerous part of the process but also the stage where the woman's self starts to reemerge.

Recovering

Progress is seldom direct and without vacillation between stages. The recovering phase includes the initial adjustment to leaving the relationship and may encompass a temporary return to him. It takes considerable work, effort, pain, and assistance from others for a woman to survive on her own (Landenburger, 1989, 1998; Wuest & Merritt-Gray, 1999). Part of the recovering phase is a struggle for survival, in terms of the necessities of life, dealing with her children's losses, and justifying her leaving to her partner, children, and critical others. Idealization of the spouse may be seen during this period, which is also characteristic of grieving. This mechanism is often difficult for professionals working with the abused woman to understand, and it may lead her to return to the spouse, especially if she is having problems with survival and depression. When viewed as a normal part of a process to be worked through, it is more acceptable. The response is also compounded by the fact that the man is not dead even if the woman has left him and that he constantly reappears in her life when she is psychologically vulnerable.

Part of this aspect of the recovery process is a search for meaning in the experience and her behavior, which includes determining why she stayed so long. Successfully working through the multiple losses and searching for meaning may well depend on the support given to the abused woman through the process (Wuest & Merritt-Gray, 2001). Nursing can be instrumental in providing that support.

Secondary-Prevention Nursing Interventions

Interventions at the secondary prevention level are based on an assessment of the point at which the abused woman is in her entrapment and recovery process. The early denial and minimization must neither be disparaged nor encouraged. The battered woman needs to know the facts about wife abuse—primarily, that it generally tends to escalate. During early abuse, she frequently wants to know if it is possible for the violent spouse to change. This is possible, but the woman should be aware that he must want to change and be willing to undergo intervention of some type. She needs to direct her efforts toward that end, rather than try to change her behavior to please him more, thinking she will thus avoid abuse.

A useful approach is to concentrate on assisting the woman to be as healthy as possible despite the batterings (Campbell & Soeken, 1999b). This usually seems logical to both the abused woman and the nurse, and it avoids such pitfalls as encouraging the woman to be more submissive. Areas of concern, such as low self-esteem and lack of assertiveness, can be approached in a variety of ways. Individual counseling aimed at raising self-esteem and teaching assertiveness skills can be useful, as can group and class situations. Once the abused woman feels better about herself, she may be able to set firm limits at home; but without these strengths, suggestions of such may be premature. Efforts to improve the health of the victim of early abuse can also focus on stress-related symptoms she may be experiencing. Relaxation training, exercise programs, role-playing, coping-skills development, and teaching the woman to be more in touch with her physiological self may all be helpful to her. Battered women may be kept socially isolated by the spouse or may find their support systems detrimental rather than helpful. The nurse can discuss the importance of positive support systems and problem-solve with her to try to find and develop new supportive networks or maintain existing ones. Alleviating some of the external stressors in the relationship, such as lack of child care or difficulties in finding financial resources, may be addressed through referral to social work or other community resources. The woman may need help in finding a job, which could be instrumental in improving her self-esteem and decreasing her economic dependence on the spouse. Many batterers find their spouses' employment threatening, but alleviation of some of the financial burdens may seem attractive enough to overcome their objections.

A woman in the early stages of battering frequently seeks some way of maintaining the relationship. Marriage or couple counseling may be dangerous to the woman. If she discloses the abuse in the sessions, she may be beaten for it; if she does not disclose, the therapist will not address the violence. However, if violence has only recently begun in the relationship, if the woman has been informed of and carefully considered the possible danger, and only if she has been assessed for the level of abuse in private and she and her partner are desiring of this intervention, it may be a potential recourse. The nurse can be instrumental in making sure the counseling is provided by someone knowledgeable about abuse, a clinician who is not interested in only keeping the couple together to the detriment of the wife. Rather than traditional marital therapy, models have been developed that are specifically designed for low-level-violence couples and have been evaluated as successful (Holtzworth-Munroe & O'Leary, et al., 2001). The man is encouraged to take responsibility for the violence (confrontation is used if necessary) and to learn new ways of dealing with anger and of thinking about and relating to his female partner. The couple is encouraged to expand their definitions of sex-role behavior and taught better methods of communication. Stopping the violence completely becomes the primary goal, and if this cannot be done by rebuilding the relationship the couple is helped with dissolution. Nurses can conduct this type of marital counseling themselves with proper background and training, or they can learn where such counseling is provided and work with the woman separately.

Besides interventions for individual abused women, the nurse should be concerned with institutional measures at the secondary prevention level. It is not enough that the nurse includes questions about battering in her own practice; protocols should be officially established so that all health professionals assess for abuse. The battered-woman's movement, several concerned physicians, the Nursing Network on Violence Against Women International, and the Family Violence Prevention Fund have been encouraging hospitals to have both protocols and training to systematically assess and intervene with these women. A classic early nursing research effort by Tilden and Shepherd (1987) found a significant increase in emergency nurses' documentation of battering (from only 9.2% of abused women documented as such to 22%) after staff training and implementation of a protocol. A later evaluation also showed significant improvement in attitudes of the medical and nursing staff as well as increased patient satisfaction in EDs that had utilized a "train the trainer" and system-change intervention to improve identification of IPV (Campbell et al., 2001).

In response to the work of the advocacy groups, in 1992 the Joint Commission on the Accreditation of Healthcare Organizations (JCAHO, 1997) adopted guidelines for written policies and procedures on family violence and sexual assault throughout the life cycle. (See Box 11-10.) Each revision since that time has strengthened the guidelines, which now include spouse and partner abuse as well as elder and child abuse. Member health care organizations are required to maintain appropriate family-violence referral lists, perform thorough assessment and documentation in every unit (including admission, discharge, and outpatient units) in the organization, and provide family-violence-intervention education to key personnel. Nurses also need to support training about abuse for the police, legal professionals, social workers, physicians, and clergy, as well as for nurses. Workshops for professionals and interested key people and public education on abuse are needed and can be conducted by nurses.

Tertiary Prevention

Tertiary prevention is aimed at helping the severely abused wife to first be safe and then to recover. The severely battered woman has been victimized by physical and psychological abuse for a significant amount of time and usually has experienced considerable physical and psychological damage. However, she has

---

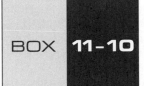

BOX 11-10 JOINT COMMISSION ON ACCREDITATION OF HEALTHCARE ORGANIZATIONS (JCAHO) GUIDELINES FOR WRITTEN POLICIES AND PROCEDURES (1997): CRITERIA NEEDED TO IDENTIFY POSSIBLE ABUSE VICTIMS

TYPES OF ABUSE TO BE ADDRESSED

- Physical assault
- Rape or sexual molestation
- Domestic abuse of elders, spouses, partners, and children

PROCEDURES FOR PATIENT EVALUATION

- Patient consent
- Examination and treatment
- Collection, retention, and safeguarding of specimens, photographs, and other evidence
- Notification/release of information to proper authorities
- Referral list of private and community-based family-violence agencies available through the hospital
- Medical record documentation that includes examinations, treatment, referrals to other care providers and community-based agencies, and required notification of authorities
- Training of staff in the identification and procedures needed to work with abuse survivors

PE (PHYSICAL EXAM SECTION) 1.8

- The hospital has objective criteria for identifying and assessing possible victims of abuse and neglect, and they are used throughout the organization. Staff is to be trained in the use of these criteria.
- The criteria focus on observable evidence and not on allegation alone. They address at least one of the following situations: physical assault, rape or other sexual molestation, domestic abuse, or abuse or neglect of elders and children.

From The Joint Commission Accreditation Manual for Hospitals, Update 3, 1997.

usually also developed strong resolve as a result of her ordeal and has many insights into her own nature and that of her husband. Tertiary prevention interventions are often performed in wife-abuse shelters or in mental health settings. The woman is usually experiencing many of the strong emotions associated with grieving and often can be helped at this point to achieve necessary acceptance of the losses and final resolution.

Harassment in Abusive Relationships

One of the difficulties in recovering from an abusive relationship is the harassment to which the abuser all too often subjects the woman, especially while she is trying to leave the relationship. The women in Campbell's (Campbell et al., 1994; Campbell et al., 1998) longitudinal study described the harassment and stalking as lasting anywhere from a month to several years, with an average of one year after they left the abuser. This behavior may make it more difficult for her to leave permanently (Wuest & Merritt-Gray, 1999). Studies have begun to address stalking (e.g., McFarlane et al., 2002), but only limited research focuses directly on harassment of battered women even though this behavior has been described extensively in much of the literature on abuse. None of the research instruments designed to measure various aspects of abuse contain items addressing harassment. Sheridan (2001) created the Harassment in Abusive Relationships: A Self-Report Scale (HARASS) instrument. Based on extensive interviews with battered women survivors and clinical experts on family violence, a list of harassing male behaviors that are applicable to many battering situations has been identified. (See Box 11-11.) The instrument can be used clinically as an assessment tool and as a stimulant for discussion in battered-women's support groups. Research has shown beginning psychometric support for its salience in homicide and attempted homicide situations (McFarlane et al., 2002), and future studies are planned.

The 10-Minute Intervention

Also called the "brochure-driven" intervention, the 10-minute intervention was developed by nurse researchers Judith McFarlane and Barbara Parker (1994) and has been tested with a quasi-experimental design with pregnant women (Parker et al., 1999). Women who completed the intervention were found to use significantly more safety behaviors and have less physical and psychological violence used against them six months and one year after the intervention. However, the intervention is not specific to pregnancy and can be used for safety planning in any setting.

The intervention uses a brochure that is a guide that the nurse can use to conduct the intervention with the woman. It can be duplicated and personalized for each woman and is available to be viewed on Microsoft Publisher at the Nursing Network on Violence Against Women, International (NNVAWI) website (http://www.nnvawi.org). It can easily be made specific to the locality where it is used before printing. It is also available through the March of Dimes.

The intervention first sets the abuse in context and then does a brief lethality assessment based on the Danger Assessment. The safety-planning portion is a choice-based system with several safety strategies offered for whether the woman is planning to stay with the abuser, work with the criminal-justice system, leave him, use shelter and advocacy-type services, or any combination thereof. The basic safety-planning options are presented in Box 11-6.

BOX 11-11	HARASSMENT IN ABUSIVE RELATIONSHIPS: A SELF-REPORT SCALE (HARASS)

My Partner or My Former Partner:

- Frightens people close to me.
- Pretends to be someone else in order to get to me.
- Comes to my home when I don't want him there.
- Threatens to kill me if I leave or stay away from him.
- Threatens to harm the kids if I leave or stay away from him.
- Takes things that belong to me so I have to see him to get them back.
- Tries to get me fired from my job.
- Ignores court orders to stay away from me.
- Keeps showing up wherever I am.
- Bothers me at work when I don't want to talk to him.
- Uses the kids as pawns to get me physically close to him.
- Shows up without warning.
- Messes with my property (for example, sells my stuff, breaks my furniture, damages my car, or steals my things).
- Scares me with a weapon.
- Breaks into my home.
- Threatens to kill himself if I leave or stay away from him.
- Makes me feel like he can again force me into sex.
- Threatens to snatch or have the kids taken away from me.
- Sits in his car outside my home.
- Leaves me threatening messages (for example puts scary notes on the car, sends me threatening letters, sends me threats through family and friends, or leaves threatening messages on the telephone answering machine).
- Threatens to harm our pet.
- Calls me on the phone and hangs up.
- Reports me to the authorities for taking drugs when I don't.

Mark how often each item occurs on the following scale:

0 = Never
1 = Rarely
2 = Occasionally
3 = Frequently
4 = Very frequently
NA = Not applicable

From Daniel J. Sheridan (2001). Reprinted with permission. Requests to use this instrument must be sent in writing to Daniel J. Sheridan, PhD, RN, Assistant Professor, Johns Hopkins University School of Nursing.

Nursing Roles in Shelters

Shelters for abused women have been established in most major cities in the United States and have been invaluable to battered women as a haven of physical safety for them and their children and as a setting for effective interventions of many types. Most shelters provide individual and group counseling; help with bureaucratic institutions, such as the police, the criminal-justice system, social-services organizations, child-care organizations, and organizations with programs for children; and aid the woman in making future plans, such as employment counseling and liaisons with housing authorities. Best of all, the women gain support and knowledge that they are not alone.

Unfortunately, many shelters are in difficult financial straits. Funding traditionally has been unstable, and most of the original government and private grants used for initial start-up have expired. Although financial support for battered-women's programs is provided by the Violence Against Women Act, these funds are only enough to fund basics such as food and shelter. Nurses are desperately needed at the policy-making level, on governing boards of shelters, on boards of social-service funding agencies, and at the state planning level to advocate the establishment of more shelters where they are needed and to ensure that existing shelters remain open and provide a full range of services.

Shelters are usually run with a combination of professional and volunteer staff, including social workers, occupational therapists, and child-care professionals as paid staff. In addition, many formerly abused women, feminists, nurses, lawyers, and others have been involved in the planning, operations, and volunteer services of shelters. Professional-education programs, including nursing programs, have found shelters to be an excellent clinical experience for students.

Health services are usually recognized as a necessary part of shelters, and they are obtained in a variety of ways. It is ideal to have a professional nurse as part of the paid staff of all shelters, and nurses involved in their planning can advocate this. When this is not feasible, community-health nurses can be contracted on a part-time basis, or arrangements can be made to refer women and children to nurse clinicians. However, in-house nursing care is preferable, considering the dangers involved whenever the woman leaves the shelter, the transportation difficulties, and the traditional mistrust of the health care system held by the poor and undeserved in general and battered women specifically. Nurses can fill the gap by volunteering at shelters and performing a variety of roles while there. Shelter staff may need some demonstration of the expanded autonomous roles of professional nursing. At first, they may envision the responsibilities of nurses as only that of monitoring blood pressure, teaching health classes, establishing first-aid procedures, and giving advice about the endemic children's diarrhea problems that come with change of diet and new environment. These roles may be important, but there is much more that nurses can do in wife-abuse shelters.

Nurses can successfully lead the support-group sessions conducted in most shelters. Several nursing experts have described models for groups of battered wives based on their experiences in a shelter (Campbell, 1986; Henderson, 1989). They suggest that the major goal be crisis intervention, allowing the women to initiate the topics and find their own solutions, finding meaning in the abusive experience, and offering and receiving peer support. The women come and go from the group because of their varying lengths of stay in the shelter, necessitating constant readjustment to differing stages of progress and different faces. Janosik and Phipps (1982) see this as an advantage because older group members can be role models for the newer members. The women may also be in a variety of phases of the entrapment and recovery process.

Nurses can also lead groups dealing with parenting issues or general health concerns that may include discussion of forced sex experiences. Clinical experience in shelters suggests that it is generally beneficial to allow the women to decide what areas to explore with the nurse, rather than using a set agenda. Topics may range from race relations among shelter staff and residents and among residents themselves to breast self-examination. Group sessions can be fun or serious depending on clients' needs. Flexibility and openness are important when the nurse is a group leader.

Women in shelters can also be seen individually for a variety of health needs. A shelter is a wonderful place to practice a range of nursing skills, from physical assessment to one-to-one counseling. Campbell and Humphreys (1987) and Hollencamp and Attala (1986) have described nursing care in shelters in detail.

The woman's length of stay in the shelter is variable, and the relationship with the nurse may be a single contact or may be of a fairly long-term nature. It is important to have a good community-resource network established with names and some knowledge of other nurses to whom women can be referred for follow-up. Once a battered woman has had beneficial contact with a nurse, she is usually enthusiastic about her long-term health care being handled by a nurse unless she has an acute problem needing medical diagnosis. Nursing often provides an excellent avenue through which she can meet her health care needs; battered women frequently express their pleasure with the woman-to-woman contact and the holistic possibilities of nursing care.

Tertiary-level individual interventions ideally start with building on the woman's strengths identified during the nursing assessment. It takes a great deal of courage to go to a shelter. One of the most poignant images from our clinical experience in shelters is the sight of the battered woman arriving, usually with several children in tow, at a completely strange place, with all of her hastily gathered belongings in a black plastic garbage bag. How many of us would be willing to leave our homes, with few if any financial or material resources and when we have been the victims of wrongdoing, and place our future in the hands of complete strangers? It is imperative to continually praise the abused woman for that act of courage alone.

Other strengths shown by the woman's appearance at the shelter include the mere fact of physical survival, the successful and often carefully planned escape, and the caring for the children shown by leaving. These need to be recognized as strengths and pointed out to the woman. Additional individual strengths found in assessment are important to stress to help combat the woman's feelings of being trapped and helpless. The strengths are a base for further developing problem-solving strategies. The woman may feel she has exhausted all her resources in just getting to the shelter and may need to be reminded that if she was able to do that she can do just about anything with a little help and a little time. The first few days at the shelter may need to be simply time to rest and recoup and gather her resources, in safety finally. The newly arrived shelter resident should not be expected to do much future planning until she has had a chance just to be relieved. However, her injuries need to be carefully documented for future legal proceedings. Because the nurse is often not present on her arrival, staff can be instructed how to measure and describe the physical problems. Photography of injuries is usually desirable. (See Chapter 13.) There also may be need for immediate medical intervention, and the nurse can be helpful in setting up protocols within the shelter and making contacts with the nearest emergency room.

Care for the physical injuries to battered women can require much ingenuity on the part of shelter staff and nurse consultants. Examples of women with injuries from clinical experience include a woman with a broken jaw that had been wired internally and set with a metal brace, a woman bleeding internally who had not been thoroughly examined in the emergency room, and a four-day postpartum mother who had been raped by her husband as soon as she got home from the hospital. The latter woman required hospitalization for hemorrhage, and she left her newborn baby and two siblings at the shelter. It is extremely helpful if the shelter has a nurse to call in such situations for consultation.

Other serious health problems can include medication for chronic diseases that has been left behind, dangerously high blood pressure necessitating transportation by ambulance, and severe asthma in a child. Chronic conditions are often exacerbated by the stress of the situation, and communicable diseases are common in communal-living situations as well as more common for those subjected to immune-system-depressing chronic stress. The nurse can devise a short health history form for the woman and her children that can be completed on arrival so that shelter staff members are alerted to health problems needing immediate attention. Women are also at high risk for AIDS because of unknown sexual infidelity of their partner, drug abuse, and the man's possible refusal to use a condom (Eby & Campbell, et al., 1995).

Individual nursing assessment can determine other physical health problems for which the woman seeks help for herself, her children, or both. It has been found helpful to announce a specific day and time that the nurse will be at the shelter to see any women who wish to seek care. Staff members can also make referrals for such problems as substance abuse or observable poor nutritional status. Communication with staff about health problems is important, and the regular shelter records of the women can be used to enter short nursing entries for assessment and interventions. With professional nursing care, the women have often found the shelter a good place to begin working on health problems that have been bothering them, which may or may not be directly connected with abuse.

The severely abused woman in a shelter is usually starting to experience strong grieving. Tears can be useful and healing, and the battered woman must not be hurried into decision-making activities until she has had a chance to mourn. Just as a grieving widow needs to talk about the deceased, the abused woman must be allowed to express herself fully about the man, including the good points and happy memories. Other residents and staff may not encourage this as much as they could; the shelter atmosphere sometimes is very much against all men, and this is natural.

The woman's anger also needs expression. The shelter, with its close living quarters, many responsibilities, and strong feeling tones, can sometimes be an explosive place. Children are noisy; people don't always attend to chores; and privacy is elusive. Anger that has built up over the duration of an abusive relationship can be released over a minor incident between residents, against staff, or against confused and restless children. The battered woman may feel resentful if she thinks staff and other residents are judging her for the way she has and is handling the abuse or for the way she mothers her children. The legal system and social-services system she has to deal with can also be frustrating. All these factors can underlie and trigger angry outbursts. These outbursts best handled as they occur, and the women involved are helped to see where the anger comes from and encouraged to express it verbally and assertively. This approach is helpful in both dealing with the situation at hand and in teaching the woman how to deal with anger constructively.

The guilt that the abused woman may feel is best dealt with by encouragement of expression first. As angry as it may make the nurse to hear the woman blame herself or worry about her spouse, this is a necessary part of grieving and recovery and cutting her off is not helpful. Again, assurance that this is normal is the beginning of intervention. Then the woman can be helped to review events, with an emphasis on the batterer's behavior, which helps her realize that usually what she said and did made no real difference in the final outcome. She also needs help in recognizing that no one can take responsibility for another's actions. She may need time to think through events again with this fact in mind.

The nurse's role in shelters can thus be seen as multifaceted. The nurse works as part of the shelter staff team, and the nature of her interventions is based on the needs of the staff and the residents. There is room for several nurses to work at once at one shelter, either in a rotating sequence or performing more specialized roles. Nursing roles may evolve over time, as staff and residents recognize what types of services are available. There is a definite need for nursing in all shelters, and nurses are urged to become involved.

Interventions in Mental Health Settings

The psychological consequences of living in an abusive relationship often lead women to seek help from mental health professionals. Although women with depression or anxiety disorders may clearly benefit from a variety of psychotherapeutic approaches, including psychotropic medications, specific attention to the underlying problem of abuse is often overlooked. Women's suicide attempts are another alarming manifestation of abuse that may come to the attention of psychiatric mental health nurses. Stark and Flitcraft (1996) found that battered women attempted suicide more frequently than nonbattered women did; in fact, 21% of the battered women had attempted suicide three or more times, compared to 8% of nonbattered women. Suicide risk was higher in African-American women than in Caucasian women.

The nurse may give tertiary-level interventions for abused women at both inpatient and outpatient mental health institutions. The middle-class battered woman may be more likely to seek help in these settings, or in a private psychiatrist's or psychologist's office, than in a shelter. The abused woman frequently presents with symptoms of depression, including suicidal intent, anxiety, or marital difficulties. Revealing the abuse and labeling it as such is the first task. The second is to assess the woman's danger, either from herself in terms of suicide or from the batterer, and to do crisis intervention if necessary on that basis. The third step is to assess for posttraumatic stress disorder.

Posttraumatic Stress Disorder (PTSD)

PTSD classification is useful in determining the seriousness of and treatment for the psychological effects of severe abuse. PTSD is a cluster of symptoms that arises from exposure to one or more severely traumatic events. The stressor is generally outside the range of usual human experiences. Any environmental stimulus perceived as dangerous, whether it produces physical injury or not, can be sufficiently traumatic to precipitate a posttraumatic stress disorder. The disorder has been noted in survivors of induced human trauma, such as war, assault, rape, incest, and wife abuse; and to natural catastrophes, such as fires, hurricanes, and earthquakes. Human-induced trauma is generally more difficult to recover from. The symptoms of PTSD, according to the DSM-IV, are listed in Box 11-8 (American Psychiatric Association, 1994).

The experience of a significant, recognizable stressor or trauma is followed by recurrent subjective reexperiencing of the trauma. It is important to realize that the reexperiencing can be of feelings associated with the trauma rather than actual flashbacks. For instance, one battered woman told of seeing a friend of her abusive husband in a shopping mall about six months after she left the husband and being overwhelmed with a terrible fear that she did not understand. There is also a general numbing of responsiveness, and cognitive or somatic symptoms of irritability, anxiety, aggressiveness, and depression may follow. As well as recurring dreams and nightmares, sleep disturbances such as insomnia often occur. Psychic numbing, or emotional anesthesia in relation to other people and to previously enjoyed activities, is also common. Alcohol and other substances may be used in an attempt to maintain control and soothe emotions.

Onset of PTSD varies among individuals and can be from a few hours or days to months or years after the stressor. Acute PTSD has an onset within six months of the traumatic event, and symptoms last for less than six months. Chronic PTSD, or the delayed stress response, is characterized by an onset of symptoms at least six months after the traumatic event, and symptoms last for at least six months. This type of PTSD is seen especially in Vietnam veterans, but it also has been reported in survivors of catastrophe and human-induced trauma. Symptoms are similar to those listed in Box 11-8, but they are more severe.

Victimization takes its toll, especially when it continues over an extended period of time, as with battered women. When individuals experience chronic victimization by someone close to them, the impact is intensified and complicated by the profound betrayal of trust. Many factors are important in the readjustment. The frequency, intensity, duration, and nature of the abuse affect the severity and duration of symptoms. PTSD stressors have been classified into two categories, bereavement and personal injury, with different types of symptomatology. Battered women experience both. Therefore, they can be expected to experience sadness over loss and discomfort over discovered personal vulnerability (bereavement), as well as fear of repetition of the event and feelings of responsibility (personal injury). Taking an active role during the trauma and immediately afterward has been linked to a better adjustment, but often abused women have been forced into a passive role. Lack of helpful support systems and socioeconomic problems have also been linked with slower and more difficult posttrauma readjustment. Finally, instead of the trauma being a single occurrence or time limited (tour of duty), abused women have continued exposure to the trauma over long periods of time. They have also often suffered multiple traumas such as childhood sexual assault as well as intimate partner violence, further worsening the PTSD. Thus, battered women may be suffering from serious PTSD, which obviously needs to be recognized (Woods, 1999).

PTSD is definitely responsive to treatment. The major focus in PTSD intervention is a combination of educating to normalize the reactions and provide information about PTSD and reprocessing the traumatic experiences. This explanation of the syndrome can assist women in their quest to make sense of their response to the abuse. Group treatment, such as in formalized treatment groups with mental health professionals as group leaders, is the treatment of choice. Sometimes antidepressants are prescribed to control intrusive thoughts and depression.

Other Mental Health-Related Interventions

Women with less serious symptoms can be treated in other types of groups. Consciousness-raising groups have been found to help women increase self-esteem, increase their sense of control, and significantly decrease depression. In such groups, women meet regularly to discuss and search for similarities among their personal experiences. Groups then use this knowledge of commonalities to develop an understanding of power relations between men and women and of the societal structures and processes that maintain these power relations. Such groups can be organized and led by nurses and held in mental health settings. Consisting of woman with various experiences, battered women can be referred to this type of group.

Individual therapy with abused women in mental health settings deals with many of the issues discussed in relation to individual interventions with women in shelters. Most domestic-violence experts recommend some sort of feminist therapy that explicitly addresses violence against women and the societal structures that support it.

Concomitant interventions for the abuser are necessary at the tertiary level. Both partners need to understand that the violence will escalate in severity and frequency if he does not receive interventions specifically for battering. If he refuses such intervention, and the confirmed abuser often will, the woman must be helped to understand that strategies designed to end the violence while remaining in the relationship are not likely to succeed. Abused women have no real control over their batterer's violent behavior. The nurse and abused woman should explore other options for her, and she should have a plan for escaping or otherwise staying safe if the situation becomes dangerous.

Interventions for Violent Men

It is ironic and aggravating that the abused woman must flee her home or be labeled as sick and receive treatment, while the batterer stays home and is seldom identified as needing interventions. Most abusers do not fit current definitions of mental illness, yet their behavior clearly must be changed.

Batterers may come to the attention of the mental health system through alcoholic-treatment programs, and specific questions about abuse should be included in the histories of such men. Their wives should also be asked about physical violence in the relationship, because the man frequently denies such occurrences or treats them lightly. It cannot be assumed that resolving alcohol problems will also solve the problems of violence in the relationship; specific interventions for abuse need to be implemented also.

There are now specific programs for abusive men in most localities, certainly a needed development. Many communities mandate batterer intervention through the law-enforcement system. Group treatment has been the avenue of choice, based on the Pence and Paymar (1993) model. Confrontation is used to get the abusers to admit their responsibility, and ways of dealing with anger besides hitting are taught. The men are also encouraged to get in touch with their other feelings and learn how to express them, and also to deal with changing sex roles, with parenting, and the difficulties of being a man today. To be effective, such groups must deal with attitudes as well as behavior. Research evaluation of batterer intervention has been mixed, and many of the research designs have been less than ideal. From the evidence accumulated to date, it appears that court-mandated participation is most successful; otherwise, most men drop out of treatment (Dutton, 1995). The majority of batterers significantly decrease the amount of both physical and psychological abuse that they use, even according to their partners (Gondolf & Jones, 2002; Dobash, Dobash, Cavanaugh & Lewis, 2000). Yet a certain percentage (about 20%) do not become less violent; in fact, those men assault their wives again almost immediately (Gondolf & Jones, 2002).

Male therapists or male and female cotherapists are generally used in leading such groups, to provide a role model and to better be able to challenge these men. Different types of groups may be needed for different types of batterers, depending on how traumatized they were as children and how much substance abuse is involved (Saunders, 1996; Holtzworth-Munroe et al., 2000).

The Nurse as Advocate

Where such programs for abusive men do not yet exist, the nurse can be instrumental in the community in advocating for their establishment. Once begun, nurses need to encourage them as a useful intervention for battering and to advocate their use to the police, lawyers, judges, and probation officers, as a mandatory alternative to jail or legal proceedings, if necessary. Establishment of these programs should work in conjunction with the formation of shelters for abused wives in all communities.

Advocacy also includes working at the local and state level to make it easier for abused women to find housing if they want to leave the abuser. Liaisons can be formed with shelters, other programs for battered women, and urban-housing and job-training programs. Vacant houses can be rehabilitated to provide a home for two abused women and their children. The women can receive support from each other, build on a friendship started in a shelter or group, and pool their resources to make a home. Advocacy and collaborations with public-housing authorities can also help the housing situation for battered women. When they understand the desperate need, the relationship between battering and welfare, and the funding restrictions that limit women's stay in shelters, they are often helpful in cutting red tape for battered women.

Advocacy can also take the form of working with the police and the legal profession. In addition, the nurse should discuss battering, and what battered women and their children need, with all her professional and social contacts. Shelters always need donations of time, money, supplies, clothing, and food. When talking about abuse, nurses frequently are told of personal battering by acquaintances and fellow professionals. As battering becomes more of a public issue, women feel more comfortable in talking about their own abuse. Advocacy for battered women and demonstration of knowledge on the subject of abuse become a novel means of case-finding and an opportunity for intervention.

EVALUATION

Evaluation of nursing care for abused women is based on achievement of goals set by the woman or group. When women formulate the goals, the nurse can avoid the trap of being dissatisfied with interventions that do not necessarily result in the woman leaving the relationship, even when in the nurse's view this would be the preferable outcome. The goals set for nursing care may be limited, depending on the amount of intervention possible. Achievement of the goals, however modest, can still be a powerful statement of possibilities to the battered wife. Praise for her progress, however small, can be an important reinforcer for the woman to seek further help and to have confidence in her own ability to address the underlying problems.

When working with battered women, the nurse needs to become accustomed to measuring gains in small steps and to deal with the women in a variety of stages of resolution. The nurse can begin to recognize that for every abused woman who is still in denial of the seriousness of abuse, another woman is close to rebuilding a healthy life for herself. It is easy for professionals to become discouraged when working with battered women; nurses express similar feelings when working with clients who have chronic health problems. These feelings can be dealt with by sharing with others who work with abuse and by taking pride in what has been achieved. Shelter staff also often need help with such feelings. Nurses can help by pointing out that women who return to the abusive relationship may still have gained a great deal of support and insight by staying in the shelter, feel less alone in dealing with the problem, know where they can go if they are in danger, and be farther along in their grieving process than when they first arrived.

During evaluation, the nurse may also need to deal with her own feelings of anger against the batterer, especially if the woman has not experienced them during the period of nursing intervention. This is a frequent dilemma of professionals dealing with abused women. If the nurse works in a shelter or with other professionals cognizant of wife abuse, it is appropriate for the nurse to delay her feelings of anger and discuss them later with her colleagues. Even if she does not have a good professional support system, it is important that the nurse not let her own anger show when she is with a woman not feeling anger. However, the feelings must be dealt with constructively, or the nurse will find anger against specific batterers becoming generalized to many men, and this will interfere with effective nursing practice. Even in shelters, the nurse and staff must be careful to deal with their understandably strong feelings in private, or the women will suspect that staff "talks about us" behind their backs. Working with abuse victims engenders many strong feelings, and the nurses and other professionals involved need to form their own support systems carefully so that they will not become incapacitated by the feelings or become "burned out." Evaluation includes the nurse's careful reevaluation of her own feelings and how they affect her nursing care.

Evaluation of nursing care with the battered woman includes making plans for the future. It is important for the woman who stays in the relationship to have a variety of choices of helpful services that she can rely on if she decides to seek further assistance. The nurse must make sure that the individuals to whom she refers the woman are knowledgeable about abuse and immediately can put the woman at ease.

SAMPLE NURSING PROCESS

A sample nursing process has been included to show how each of the four steps might be applied to a hypothetical case of wife abuse. (See Box 11-12.) The process is not intended to be applicable to all cases of battered women; instead, it is provided as an illustration of some of the aspects of wife abuse that might be

(text continues on page 356)

BOX **11–12**   **SAMPLE NURSING PROCESS** *(Continued)*

ASSESSMENT

BRIEF BACKGROUND

Anne is a 27-year-old African-American woman, married to John who is 28. They have two girls, ages 2 months and 3 years. In addition, Anne's 5-year-old son from a previous relationship lives in the home. She miscarried her 3rd pregnancy in the 6th month and within 2 months was pregnant again with the youngest child. Anne works as a sales clerk; John has been unemployed for 2 years. Anne was seen in the emergency department of the local hospital 1 week before this visit. She had multiple bruises, two fractured ribs, and disclosed to the emergency department that she had been beaten by her husband and was concerned about "his temper" but did not want to have the police called because she was afraid that would make John even more angry. Referral was made to the local Public Health Department, nursing division, for family visitation because of a high risk situation, with indications of domestic violence and potential child abuse, and also for follow-up care of her injuries and mental health concerns. Referral was also made to Anne's primary care provider, a Family Nurse Practitioner (FNP), for follow-up of her injuries and problems related to intimate partner violence, including potential mental health and gynecological problems.

The community-health nurse's (or FNP's) initial assessment of Anne includes but is not limited to the significant history and physical examination.

SIGNIFICANT HISTORY

There is a history of abuse over the last six years. Anne says that her husband is extremely jealous about her work relationships with other men and imagines that she is having affairs. Abuse has escalated over time in frequency and severity. Her husband beats her with fists and "shoves her around" at least once a month at current time. He has never used a weapon. Anne believes that being hit "now and then" often happens between men and women. She has not attempted to retaliate recently because the few times she has in the past, she was beaten more severely. However, she says she sometimes thinks about using violence in retaliation, including using the gun that he keeps in the bedside stand. She responds to a question about forced sex with great hesitancy and embarrassment that John "sometimes" forces her to perform sexual acts she is not comfortable with (particularly anal sex and sex with objects) by using threats such as, "you know what I can do to you if you don't make me happy," or, "You know how mad it makes me when you don't do what I want you to." She says she is afraid to ask him to use a condom because he says he wants to have a son and that he would think that she is unfaithful to him and might beat her up. At the same time, she knows about HIV and is concerned that John might have had sex with someone else when she was pregnant and right after the baby was born. She agreed to have sex with him again within 72 hours of the baby's birth because he insisted. She says it hurt her "a lot" and made her sad, and she did not go to her 6 week checkup with her midwife because she was embarrassed about how she might look "down there."

Anne reports severe headaches at least once a week. She also reports extreme soreness in her rib area and generalized fatigue because of "not sleeping well." She states that she wanted to get pregnant with their last child because John really wanted a son, and she thought the pregnancy would end the abuse. Anne appears to be somewhat confused and very disappointed that abuse has not ended, but says she loves John and wants the children to have a father and a happy home. She says she wants to get pregnant again because John wants her to, but does not know how she will work and care for all of the children. She says that she thinks the miscarriage may have been because of the beatings and the stress at home but says she did not feel "anything" when the miscarriage occurred and feels no sadness now because "they said it was another girl anyway." Anne also is worried that John is angry that the baby was another girl, and that he seems increasingly angry at all of the children, including her child, his stepson.

(continued)

BOX	11-12	SAMPLE NURSING PROCESS *(Continued)*

EXAMINATION

- General appearance: Energetic, neatly dressed young woman, average height and weight. Speaks quickly with many gestures; smiles when discussing pregnancy and the violence.
- Skin: 5cm oval-shaped contusion on left arm just above elbow, tender to touch.
- Musculoskeletal: Fracture of 9th and 10th right ribs was diagnosed by x-ray examination at ED visit 1 week prior. Rib area tender to the touch, and reported as very painful. Taping placed on ribs in ED has been removed because John wanted her to take them off—he said it was "ugly."
- Neurological: Alert, oriented to time, place, and person. Uses humor describing situation.
- Doesn't have many concrete plans for children. Unable to list personal strengths.
- Mental health: Sad affect.

NURSING DIAGNOSES, OUTCOMES, AND INTERVENTIONS

Nursing diagnoses (Carpenito, 1992) that could be used in this situation are described as follows.

DYSFUNCTIONAL GRIEVING

Dysfunctional grieving is related to loss of ideal relationship, loss of an unborn child, and wife abuse, as evidenced by prolonged denial and inability to discuss feelings.

SHORT-TERM CLIENT GOAL

Client will acknowledge the loss of the baby within two visits and express sorrow related to loss.

NURSING INTERVENTIONS

- Encourage client to express sadness about miscarriage. Encourage her to contact her sister whom she has identified as supportive and who called after the miscarriage.
- Form helping relationship with client.

LONG-TERM CLIENT GOAL

Client will acknowledge losses related to wife abuse and miscarriage and identify related losses.

NURSING INTERVENTIONS

- Discuss with client losses described by others in wife-abuse situations and in miscarriage situations.
- Encourage client to explore expectations of marriage and possible losses related to violence from spouse.

PAIN RELATED TO FRACTURE

Client's pain is related to fractured ribs as evidenced by client's report of extreme soreness and difficulty sleeping.

SHORT-TERM CLIENT GOAL

Client will report decreased pain in ribs and less difficulty sleeping within one week.

NURSING INTERVENTIONS

- Plan with client to have brief periods of rest throughout day.
- Tape ribs for support; provide extra tape and show client how to do it herself.
- Have client apply heat to area when resting to promote healing (showers/baths, heating pad/hot-water bottle).

ANXIETY RELATED TO POTENTIAL FOR VIOLENCE

Anxiety related to ongoing threat of physical violence (wife abuse) and potential for client use of violence as evidenced by headache, excessive rate of speech, thoughts of using violence, and insomnia.

(continued)

BOX **11-12** **SAMPLE NURSING PROCESS** *(Continued)*

SHORT-TERM CLIENT GOAL

Client will experience a decrease in anxiety-related symptoms within four weeks, specifically:
• Decreased incidence of headaches
• Reporting seven hours of sleep per night
• Reporting feeling less tension
• Decreased rate of speech
• Decreased thoughts of using violence

NURSING INTERVENTIONS

• Help client identify anxiety-producing situations and identify symptoms related to anxiety.
• Discuss current coping strategies with client and help her identify those that are effective.
• Teach client relaxation exercises to use daily before sleep and during rest periods.
• Help client plan a regular exercise regimen.
• Discuss sleep patterns with client and encourage sleep-enhancing mechanisms that she has used in the past.
• Discuss problems with using violence against John: potential for escalation, children witnessing.
• Assess for PTSD.

LONG-TERM CLIENT GOAL

Client will identify triggers to anxiety and institute stress-management strategies.

SELF-ESTEEM DISTURBANCE

Self-esteem disturbance is related to wife abuse as evidenced by inability to identify strengths.

SHORT-TERM CLIENT GOAL

Client will begin to increase self-awareness/self-exploration by the end of three weeks, as evidenced by:
• Comparing her own situation with situation of other women experiencing wife abuse.
• Identifying personal strengths used in dealing with her difficult situation.

NURSING INTERVENTIONS

• Encourage increased social interaction such as joining a woman's group.
• Discuss incidence of wife abuse and relationship to woman's role in society.
• Identify strengths observed and discuss these with client.
• Praise efforts at problem-solving.
• Explore feelings and behaviors with her.
• Help client identify what she can control and what she cannot.
• Be a role model in self-exploration.

LONG-TERM CLIENT GOAL

Client will increase self-esteem by the end of six months as evidenced by:
• Client being able to list at least 10 significant personal strengths.
• Client being able to identify long-term goals and confidently express realistic plans to achieve them.

NURSING INTERVENTIONS

• Continue to explore client's attitudes, feelings, and values with her.
• Help her to identify long-term goals and plans.

(continued)

BOX	11–12	**SAMPLE NURSING PROCESS** *(Continued)*

HIGH RISK FOR CONTINUED VIOLENCE AND INJURY

There is high risk for injury and continued abuse, including possible death related to wife abuse.

LONG-TERM CLIENT GOAL

Client will realistically assess danger and plan for safety by the end of four weeks, specifically:
- State realistically the pattern of abuse in the relationship.
- Identify husband's patterns of abusive behavior.
- Identify effects of violence on children.
- Establish plan for safety in case of future abuse.

NURSING INTERVENTIONS

- Share facts about wife abuse.
- Help client identify incidence and patterns of abuse using a calendar and body map.
- Discuss behavior of children in wife-abuse homes in general and assist her to compare that with behavior of her children. Offer referral to programs for children witnessing violence.
- Discuss risk of child abuse in abusive homes and offer referral to child abuse prevention services.
- Discuss characteristics of abusive men and relate that to husband's behavior.
- Discuss batterer intervention programs and how to persuade or mandate (through courts) John to join one.
- Identify community and personal resources for physical safety (e.g., a wife-abuse shelter, community support groups, national domestic violence hotline, or home of a supportive friend or relative).
- Discuss legal alternatives with her (protective orders, crime of wife abuse, divorce).
- Discuss safety strategies she can take if things become dangerous.
- Discuss neighbors who can be enlisted to call the police.
- Discuss safety strategies for children.

POTENTIAL FOR STDs AND HIV RELATED TO FORCED SEX

SHORT-TERM CLIENT GOAL

Client will obtain gynecological exam within 2 weeks.

NURSING INTERVENTION

- Coordinate care with gynecological care provider with communication of forced sex and lack of condom use as conditions so that client does not have to admit to this situation.

LONG-TERM CLIENT GOAL

Client will report successful nonviolent negotiation with John to use condoms and not force sex.

NURSING INTERVENTION

- Reiterate dangers of STD's and HIV.
- Role-play discussing safe and gentle sex with John, including appealing to his interest in satisfying sexual relationships, health care providers' insistence on condom use to prevent STD's and HIV no matter what.
- Brainstorm with Anne ways to approach John about these issues, including possibility of getting his brother (a close friend to both) to talk to him.

EVALUATION

Evaluation of nursing interventions is based on achievement of goals as perceived by client and nurse and takes place at intervals identified.

included in nursing care and as a suggestion of the wording of possible nursing diagnoses. Only a brief description of the case is presented. An in-depth assessment, including a complete history and physical assessment, would be indicated in most actual situations. Evaluations of nursing interventions are based on achievement of goals as perceived by client and as indicated by criteria met.

SUMMARY

Nursing care of abused women is based on thorough assessment, identification of strengths and areas needing nursing intervention, goal-setting and planning with the client, performing nursing interventions and working with other professionals in providing services, and evaluating outcomes. Primary prevention includes interventions with women at risk to be battered as well as assertive actions at the societal level directed toward attitudes that allow and encourage violence against women. Secondary prevention deals with active case-finding. A direct, knowledgeable, and empathic approach to women suspected of being abused is important. Nursing interventions at the secondary-prevention level are aimed at eliminating abuse before the patterns become entrenched. These interventions are performed in a variety of settings and follow the theoretical framework of accepting the woman at her current level of progress through the process of entrapment and recovery and sustaining the separation from an abusive relationship or otherwise ending the violence (Campbell et al., 1998; Landenburger, 1989; Merritt-Gray & Wuest, 1995; Wuest & Merritt-Gray, 1999). This has many characteristics of a grieving process, a reaction to multiple losses. Tertiary-level interventions may find the nurse providing care in shelters or in community-health settings or inpatient mental health settings. Nursing care at secondary and tertiary levels also includes advocacy for better services for battered women, their children, and batterers. The 10-minute intervention developed by nurses McFarlane and Parker (1994) has been shown to increase safety behaviors (McFarlane et al., 1998; Parker et al., 1999) and decrease future violence with pregnant women. But further empirical validation of this intervention and others is needed to document their impact and build practice theory to develop evidence-based practice.

References

Abbott, J. T., Johnson, R., Koziol-McLain, J., & Lowenstein, S. R. (1995). Domestic violence against women: Incidence and prevalence in an emergency department population. *Journal of the American Medical Association, 273*(22), 1763–1767.

American Association of Colleges of Nursing. (1999). *Violence as a public health problem.* Washington, DC: Author.

American Psychiatric Association. (1994). *Diagnostic and statistical manual of mental disorders* (4th ed.). Washington, DC: Author.

Bachman, R., & Saltzman, L. E. (1995). *Violence against women: Estimates from the redesigned survey,* Washington, D.C.: Bureau of Justice Statistics, National Institute of Justice.

Barcelona de Mendoza, V. (2002). Culturally appropriate care for pregnant Latina women who are victims of domestic violence. *Journal of Obstetric, Gynecologic and Neonatal Nursing, 30*(6), 579–588.

Battle, J. (1981). *Culture-free SEI self-esteem inventories for children and adults.* Seattle, WA: Special Publications.

Bohn, D. (1998). Clinical interventions with Native American battered women. In J. Campbell (Ed.), *Empowering survivors of abuse: Health care for battered women and their children* (pp. 241–258). Newbury Park, CA: Sage.

Bowker, L. H. (1983). *Beating wife-beating.* Lexington, MA: Lexington Books.

Browne, A., Williams, K. R., & Dutton, D. (1998). Homicide between intimate partners. In M. D. Smith & M.

Zahn (Eds.), *Homicide: A sourcebook of social research* (pp. 149–164). Thousand Oaks, CA: Sage.

Campbell, J. C. (1992). "If I can't have you, no one can": Power and control in homicide of female partners. In J. Radford & D. E. H. Russell (Eds.). *Femicide: The politics of woman killing* (pp. 99–113). New York: Twayne.

Campbell, J. C. (2002). Health consequences of intimate partner violence. *Lancet, 359*(9314), 1331–1336.

Campbell, D. W., & Gary, F. A. (1998). Providing effective interventions for African American battered women: Afrocentric perspectives. In J. Campbell (Ed.*), Empowering survivors of abuse: Health care for battered women and their children* (pp. 229–240). Newbury Park, CA: Sage.

Campbell, J. C. (1986). A support group for battered women. *Advances in Nursing Science, 8*(2), 13–20.

Campbell, J. C. (1989a). A test of two explanatory models of women's responses to battering. *Nursing Research, 38*(1), 18–24.

Campbell, J. C. (1989b). Women's responses to sexual abuse in intimate relationships. *Women's Health Care International, 10,* 335–346.

Campbell, J. C. (1995). Prediction of homicide in and by battered women. In J. Campbell (Ed.), *Assessing dangerousness: Child abuse, wife abuse, and sexual assault.* Newbury Park, CA: Sage.

Campbell, J. C., & Alford, P. (1989). The dark consequences of marital rape. *American Journal of Nursing, 89,* 946–949.

Campbell, J. C., & Campbell, D. W. (1996). Cultural competence in the care of abused women. *Journal of Nurse-Midwifery, 41*(6), 457–462.

Campbell, J. C., Coben, J. H., McLoughlin, E., Dearwater, S., Nah, G., Glass, N. E., Lee, D., & Durborow, N. (2001). An evaluation of a system-change training model to improve emergency department response to battered women. *Academic Emergency Medicine, 8*(2), 131–138.

Campbell, J. C., Rose, L., Kub, J., & Nedd, D. (1998). Voices of strength and resistance: A contextual and longitudinal analysis of women's responses to battering. *Journal of Interpersonal Violence, 13,* 743–762.

Campbell, J. C., & Sheridan, D. J. (1989). Emergency nursing interventions with battered women. *Journal of Emergency Nursing, 15*(1), 12–17.

Campbell, J. C., & Humphreys, J. (1987). Providing health care in shelters. *Response, 10*(11), 22–23.

Campbell, J. C., Kub, J., & Rose, L. (1996). Depression in battered women. *Journal of the American Medial Women's Association, 51* (3), 106–110.

Campbell, J. C., Miller, P., Cardwell, M. M., & Belknap, R. A. (1994). Relationship status of battered women over time. *Journal of Family Violence, 9,* 99–111.

Campbell, J. C., Snow-Jones, A., Dienemann, J. A., Kub, J., Schollenberger, J., O'Campo, P. J., & Gielen, A. C. (2002). Intimate personal violence and physical health consequences. *Archives of Internal Medicine, 162,* 1157–1163.

Campbell , J. C., & Soeken, K. (1999b). Forced sex and intimate partner violence: Effects on women's health. *Violence Against Women, 5*(9), 1017–1035.

Campbell, J. C., & Soeken, K. (1999a). Women's responses to battering: A test of the model. *Research in Nursing and Health, 22*(1), 49–58.

Carpenito, L. J. (1992). *Nursing diagnosis application to clinical practice.* Philadelphia: Lippincott.

Coker A. L., Smith, P. H., Bethea, L., King, M. R., & McKeown, R. E. (2000). Physical health consequences of physical and psychological intimate partner violence. *Archives of Family Medicine, 9,* 451–445.

Dearwater, S. R., Coben, J. H., Campbell, J. C., Nah, G., Glass, N. E., McLoughlin, E., & Bekemeier, B. (1998). Prevalence of intimate partner abuse in women treated at community hospital emergency departments. *Journal of American Medical Association, 280* (5), 433–438.

Diaz-Olavarrieta, C., Campbell, J. C., Garcia de la Cadena, C., Paz, F., & Villa, A. (1999). Domestic violence against patients with chronic neurologic disorders. *Archives of Neurology, 56*(June), 681–685.

Dienemann, J. A., Campbell, J. C., Landenburger, K., & Curry, M. A. (2002). The domestic violence survivor assessment: A tool for counseling women in intimate partner violence relationships. *Patient Education and Counseling, 46,* 221–228.

Dobash, R. E., & Dobash, R. P., Cavanaugh, K., & Lewis, R (2000). Changing violent men. Thousand Oaks, CA: Sage.

Drake, V. K. (1982). Battered women: A health care problem in disguise. *Image, 14,* 40–47.

Dutton, D. G. (1995). *The domestic assault of women.* Vancouver, BC: UBC Press.

Eby, K. K., Campbell, J. C., Sullivan, C. M., & Davidson, W. S. (1996). Health effects of experiences of sexual violence for women with abusive partners. *Women's Health Care International, 16*(6), 563–576.

Edleson, J. L. (1999). The overlap between child maltreatment and woman battering. *Violence Against Women, 5*(2), 134–154.

Fishwick, N. (1998). Issues in providing care for rural battered women. In J. Campbell (Ed.), *Empowering survivors of abuse: Health care for battered women and their children* (pp. 280–291). Newbury Park, CA: Sage.

Flynn, J. B., & Whitcomb, J. C. (1981). Unresolved grief in battered women. *Journal of Emergency Nursing, 7*(6), 250–254.

Family Violence Prevention Fund. (1999). *Preventing domestic violence: Clinical guidelines on routine screening.* San Francisco, CA: Family Violence Prevention Fund.

Gazmararian, J. A., Petersen, R., Spitz, A. M., Goodwin, M. M., Saltzman, L. E., & Marks, J. S. (2000). Violence and reproductive health: Current knowledge and future research directions. *Maternal Child Health Journal, 4* (2), 79–84.

Gielen, A. C., O'Campo, P. J., Campbell, J. C., Schollenberger, J., Woods, A. B., Jones, A. S., Dieneman, J., & Kub, J. (2000). Women's opinions about domestic violence screening and mandatory reporting. *American Journal of Preventive Medicine 19*(4), 279–285.

Glass, N. E., Campbell, J. C., & Dearwater, S. (2001). Intimate partner violence screening and intervention: Data from eleven Pennsylvania and California community hospital emergency departments. *Journal of Emergency Nursing, 27*(2), 141–149.

Goldberg, W., & Carey, A. (1982). Domestic violence victims in the emergency setting. *Topics in Emergency Medicine, 3,* 65–75.

Golding, J. M. (1999). Intimate partner violence as a risk factor for mental disorders: A meta-analysis. *Journal of Family Violence, 14*(2), 99–132.

Gondolf, E. W. (1988b). The effect of batterer counseling on shelter outcome. *Journal of Interpersonal Violence, 3*(3), 275–289.

Gondolf, E. W. (1990). *Battered women as survivors.* Holmes Beach, FL: Learning Publications.

Gondolf, E. W. (1998). *Assessing woman battering in mental health services.* Thousand Oaks, CA: Sage.

Gondolf, E. W., & Jones, A. S. (2002). The program effect of batterer programs in three cities. *Violence & Victims, 16*(6), 693–704.

Greenwood, G. L., Relf, M. V., Huang, B., Pollack, L., Canchola, J., & Catania, J. (2000). Battering victimization among a probability-based sample of men who have sex with men (MSM). *American Journal of Public Health.*

Hall, J. M. (1994). Lesbians recovering from alcohol problems: An ethnographic study of health care experiences. *Nursing Research, 43,* 238–244.

Helton, A. S. (1986). Battering during pregnancy. *American Journal of Nursing, 86*(8), 910–913.

Henderson, A. D. (1989). Use of social support in a transition house for abused women. *Health Care for Women International, 10,* 61–73.

Hoff, L. A. (1988). Collaborative feminist research and the myth of objectivity. In K. Yllö & M. Bograd (Eds.), *Feminist perspectives on wife abuse* (pp. 269–281). Beverly Hills, CA: Sage.

Hollencamp, M., & Attala, J. (1986). Meeting health needs in a crisis shelter: A challenge to nurses in the community. *Journal of Community Health Nursing, 39*(40), 201–209.

Holtzworth-Munroe, A., Markman, H., O'Leary, D., Neidig, P., Leber, D., Heyman, R., Hulbert, D., & Smutzler, N. (2001). The need for marital violence prevention efforts: A behavioral-cognitive secondary prevention program for engaged and newly married couples. *Applied & Preventive Psychology, 4,* 77–88.

Holtzworth-Munroe, A., Meehan, J. C., Herron, K., Rehman, U., & Stuart, G. L. (2000). Testing the Holtzworth-Munroe and Stuart (1994) batterer typology. *Journal of Consulting Clinical Psychology, 68*(6), 1000–1019.

Hotaling, G. T., & Sugarman, D. B. (1990). A risk marker analysis of assaulted wives. *Journal of Family Violence, 5*(1), 1–14.

Institute of Medicine. (2001). *Confronting chronic neglect: The education and training of health professionals on family violence.* Washington, DC: National Research Council.

Janosik, E. H., & Phipps, L. B. (1982). *Life cycle group work in nursing.* Monterey, CA: Wadsworth Health Sciences Division.

Joint Commission on the Accreditation of Healthcare Organizations. (1997). *Comprehensive accreditation manual for hospitals. Update 3.* Terrace, IL: Author.

Jones, A. S., Gielen, A. C., Campbell, J. C., Schollenberger, J., Dienemann, J. A., Kub, J., O'Campo, P., & Wynne, E. C. (1999). Annual and lifetime prevalence of partner abuse in a sample of female HMO enrollees. *Women's Heath Issues, 9*(6), 295–305.

Kalmuss, D. S., & Straus, M. A. (1982). Wife's marital dependency and wife abuse. *Journal of Marriage and the Family, 44*(2), 277–286.

King, M. C. (1998). The primary prevention of violence against women. In J. Campbell (Ed.), *Empowering survivors of abuse: Health care for battered women and their children* (pp. 177–189). Newbury Park, CA: Sage.

King, M. C., & Ryan, J. (1989). Abused women: Dispelling myths and encouraging intervention. *Nurse Practitioner, 14,* 47–58.

Kinlein, M. L. (1977). *Independent nursing practice with clients.* Philadelphia: Lippincott.

Klein, E., Campbell, J. C., Soler, E., & Ghez, M. (1997). *Ending domestic violence.* Newbury Park, CA: Sage.

Koziol-McLain, J., Coates, C. J., & Lowenstein, S. (2001). Predictive validity of a screen for partner violence against women. *American Journal of Preventive Medicine 21*(2), 93–100.

Landenburger, K. (1989). A process of entrapment in and recovery from an abusive relationship. *Issues in Mental Health Nursing, 10,* 209–227.

Landenburger, K. (1998). Explorations of women's identity: Clinical approaches with abused women. In J. Campbell (Ed.), *Empowering survivors of abuse: Health care for battered women and their children* (pp. 61–69). Newbury Park, CA: Sage.

Leserman, J., Li, Z., Drossman, D. A., & Hu, Y. J. B. (1998). Selected symptoms associated with sexual and physical abuse history among female patients with gastrointestinal disorders: The impact on subsequent health care visits. *Psychological Medicine, 28,* 417–425.

Letourneau, E. J., Holmes, M., & Chasedunn-Roark, J. (1999). Gynecologic health consequences to victims of interpersonal violence. *Women's Health Issues, 9*(2), 115–120.

Maman, S., Campbell, J. C., Sweat, M. D., & Gielen, A. (2000). The intersections of HIV and violence: Directions for future research and interventions. *Social Science Medicine, 50*(4), 459–478.

Masaki, B., Campbell, D. W., & Torres, S. (1997). Like water on rock. In E. Klein, J. C. Campbell, E. Soler, & M. Ghez (Eds.), *Ending domestic violence.* Newbury Park, CA: Sage.

McCauley, J., Kern, D. E., Kolodner, K., Dill, L., Schroeder, A. F., DeChant, H. K., Ryden, J., Bass, E. B., & Derogatis, L. R. (1995). The "battering syndrome": Prevalence and clinical characteristics of domestic violence in primary care internal medicine practices. *Annals of Internal Medicine, 123*(10), 737–746.

McFarlane, J., Campbell, J., Sharps, P., & Watson, K. (2002). Abuse during pregnancy and femicide: Urgent implications for women's health. *Obstetrics and Gynecology, 100*(1), 27–36.

McFarlane, J., Christoffel, K., Bateman, L., Miller, V., & Bullock, L. (1991). Assessing for abuse: Self-report versus nurse interview. *Public Health Nursing, 8,* 245–250.

McFarlane, J., & Parker, B. (1994). *Abuse during pregnancy: A protocol for prevention and intervention,* White Plains, NY: March of Dimes.

McFarlane, J., Parker, B., Soeken, S., Silva, C., & Reel, S. (1998). Safety behaviors of abused women after an intervention during pregnancy. *Journal of Obstetric Gynecology in Neonatal Nursing, 27*(1), 64–69.

McKenna, L. S. (1985). Social support systems of battered women: Influence on psychological adaptation. *Dissertations Abstracts International, 47*(5A), 1895.

Merritt-Gray, M., & Wuest, J. (1995). Counteracting abuse and breaking free: The process of leaving revealed through women's voices. *Health Care for Women International, 16,* 399–412.

Moss, V. A., Pitula, C. R., Campbell, J. C., & Halstead, L. (1997). The experience of terminating an abusive relationship from an Anglo and African American perspective: A qualitative descriptive study. *Issues in Mental Health Nursing, 18,* 433–454.

Murphy, C. C., Schei, B., Myhr, T. L., & Du Mont, J. (2001). Abuse: A risk factor for low birth weight? A systematic review and meta-analysis. *Canadian Medical Association Journal, 164* (11), 1567–1572.

Okun, L. E. (1986). *Woman abuse: Facts replacing myths.* Albany, NY: SUNY Press.

Orem, D. (1991). Nursing: *Concepts of practice* (4th ed.). St. Louis, MO: Mosby-Year Book.

Orlandi, M. A. (1992). Defining cultural competence: An organizing framework. In: *USDHHS: Cultural Competence for Evaluators (OSAP Cultural Competence Series).* Washington, DC: U.S. Public Health Service

Parker, B., & McFarlane, J. (1991). Identifying and helping battered pregnant women. *Maternal Child Nursing, 16,* 161–164.

Parker, B., McFarlane, J., Soeken, K., Silva, C., & Reel, S. (1999). Testing an intervention to prevent further abuse to pregnant women. *Research in Nursing & Health, 22,* 59–66.

Parse, R. R. (1987). *Nursing science, major paradigms, theories and critique.* Philadelphia: W. B. Saunders.

Pence, E., & Paymar, M. (1993). Education groups for men who batter. New York: Springer.

Plichta, S. B. (1996). Violence and abuse: Implications for women's health. In: M. M. Falik & K. S. Collins (Eds.), *Women's health: The Commonwealth survey* (pp. 237–272). Baltimore: Johns Hopkins University Press.

Raphael, J. (2000). *Saving Bernice: Battered women, welfare, and poverty.* Boston: Northeastern University Press.

Relf, M. V. (2001). Battering and HIV in men who have sex with men: A critique and synthesis of the literature. *Journal of the Association of Nurses in AIDS Care, 12*(3) 41–48.

Renzetti, C. (1992). *Violent portrayal: Partner abuse in lesbian relationships.* Thousand Oaks, CA: Sage.

Rodriguez, R. (1998). Clinical interventions with battered migrant farm worker women. In J. Campbell (Ed.), *Empowering survivors of abuse: Health care for battered women and their children* (pp. 271–279). Newbury Park, CA: Sage.

Russell, D. E. (1993). *Making violence sexy: Feminist views on pornography.* New York: Teachers College Press.

Sandelowski, M. (1980). *Women, health, and choice.* Englewood Ciffs, NJ: Prentice Hall.

Saunders, D. G. (1996). Feminist-cognitive-behavioral and process-psychodynamic treatments for men who batter: Interaction of abuser traits and treatment model. *Violence and Victims, 11*(4), 393–414.

Schei, B. (1991). *Trapped in a painful love.* Trondheim, Norway: TAPIR.

Sharps, P. W., Koziol-McLain, J., Campbell, J., McFarlane, J., Sachs, C., & Xu, X. (2001). Health care provider's missed opportunities for preventing femicide. *Preventive Medicine, 33,* 373–380.

Sheridan, D. J. (1998). Health care based programs for domestic violence survivors. In J. Campbell (Ed.), *Empowering survivors of abuse: Health care for battered women and their children* (pp. 23–31). Newbury Park, CA: Sage.

Sheridan, D. J. (2001). Treating survivors of intimate partner abuse. In J. S. Olshaker, N. C. Jackson, & W. S. Smock (Eds.), *Forensic emergency medicine.* Philadelphia: Lippincott Williams & Wilkins.

Short, L., & Rodriguez, R. (2002). Testing an intimate partner violence assessment icon form with battered migrant and seasonal farmworker women. *Women & Health, 35*(2/3), 181–192.

Soeken, K., Parker, B., McFarlane, J., & Lominak, M. (1998). The Abuse Assessment Screen: A clinical instrument to measure frequency, severity, and perpetrator of abuse against women. In: J. Campbell (Ed.), *Beyond diagnosis: Changing the health care response to battered women and their children* (pp. 195–203). Newbury Park, CA: Sage.

Stark, E., & Flitcraft, A. (1996). *Women at risk: Domestic violence and women's health,* Thousand Oaks, CA: Sage.

Stark, E., Flitcraft, A., & Frazier, W. (1979). Medicine and patriarchal violence: The social construction of a "private" event. *International Journal of Health Services, 9*(3), 461–493.

Sue, D. W., & Sue, D. (1990). *Counseling the culturally different: Theory and practice.* New York: Wiley.

Tilden, V. P., & Shepherd, P. (1987). Increasing the rate of identification of battered women in an emergency department: Use of a nursing protocol. *Research in Nursing and Health, 10,* 209–215.

Tjaden, P., Thoennes, N., & Allison, C. J. (1999). Comparing violence over the life span in samples of same-sex and opposite-sex cohabitants. *Violence & Victims, 14*(4), 413–426.

Torres, S. (1987). Hispanic-American battered women: Why consider cultural differences? *Response, 10*(3), 20–21.

Torres, S. (1991). A comparison of wife abuse between two cultures: Perceptions, attitudes, nature, and extent. *Issues in Mental Health Nursing, 12*(1), 113–131.

Torres, S. (1998). Intervening with Hispanic battered women. In J. Campbell (Ed.), *Empowering survivors of abuse: Health care for battered women and their children* (pp. 259–270). Newbury Park, CA: Sage.

Torres, S., Campbell, J. C., Campbell, D. W., Ryan, J., King, C., Price, P., Stallings, R., Fuchs, S., & Laude, M. (2000). Abuse during and before pregnancy: Prevalence and cultural correlates. *Violence and Victims, 15*(3), 303–322.

Trimpey, M. L. (1989). Self-esteem and anxiety: Key issues in an abused women's support group. *Issues in Mental Health Nursing, 10*(3–4), 297–308.

Turell, S. C. (2000). A descriptive analysis of same-sex relationship violence for a diverse sample. *Journal of Family Violence, 15*(3), 281–293.

Ulrich, Y. C. (1991). Women's reasons for leaving abusive spouses. *Health Care for Women International, 12*(4), 465–473.

Warshaw, C. (1989). Limitations of the medical model in the care of battered women. *Gender & Society, 3*(4), 506–517.

Wisner, C. L., Gilmer, T. P., Saltzman, L. E., & Zink, T. M. (1999). Intimate partner violence against women: Do victims cost health plans more? *Journal of Family Practice, 48*(6), 439–443.

Woods, S. J. (1999). Adaptation as a mediator of intimate abuse and traumatic stress in battered women. *Nursing Science Quarterly*.

Woods, S. J., & Campbell, J. C. (1993). Posttraumatic stress in battered women: Does the diagnosis fit? *Issues in Mental Health Nursing, 14*(2), 173–186.

Wuest, J., & Merritt-Gray, M. (1999). Not going back: Sustaining the separation in the process of leaving abusive relationships. *Violence Against Women, 5*(2), 110–113.

Wuest, J., & Merritt-Gray, M. (2001). Beyond survival: Reclaiming self after leaving an abusive male partner. *Canadian Journal of Nursing Research, 32*(4), 79–94.

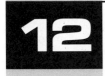

Nursing Care of Abused Women with Disabilities

• Dena Hassouneh-Phillips and Mary Ann Curry

A buse of women with disabilities is defined as a pattern of coercive and oppressive behavior that is harmful to their emotional, social, or physical well-being (Hassouneh-Phillips, 2000). This definition is broad enough to encompass the many forms of abuse women with physical disabilities experience, including psychological, physical, sexual, and financial abuse, as well as neglect and manipulation of assistive devices and medications (Hassouneh-Phillips & Curry, 2002; Nosek, 1996). The perpetrators may be intimate partners, family members, friends, caregivers, health care providers, transportation workers, and other service providers (Curry, Hassouneh-Phillips, & Johnston-Silverberg, 2001; Furey, 1994; Nosek, Howland, Rintala, Young, & Chanpong, 1997; Sobsey & Doe, 1991).

Whereas many of the forms of abuse women with disabilities experience are identical to those experienced by nondisabled women, the nature of their disabilities may place them at additional risk. Women with disabilities are more likely than nondisabled women to be abused by multiple perpetrators and to stay in abusive situations for longer periods of time (Nosek et al., 1997). Additionally, women with disabilities who depend on others for essential personal care may experience disability-specific forms of abuse, such as others threatening to deny essential personal care, intentionally placing belongings out of reach, or refusing to provide food and water (Powers et al., 2002). Unfortunately, because health care providers are often uninformed about the patterns and types of abuse women with disabilities experience, abuse assessment and intervention with this population in clinical settings is often lacking.

PREVALENCE

Only three published studies have examined the prevalence of abuse of people with disabilities who managed their attendant services through Independent Living Centers (Ulincy, White, Bradford, & Matthews, 1990). In the first study, 40% of participants reported an instance of theft, with the most frequently stolen items being money, jewelry, checks (attendant forged), prescription medications, television/stereos, and clothing. In addition, nine participants (10%) reported being both physically abused and robbed by an attendant. In the second study, a convenience sample of 439 disabled and 421 nondisabled women were surveyed about their abuse experiences. The incidence of abuse among women with and without disability was similar; 62% of both groups reported some type of lifetime abuse. Half of both groups had experienced physical or sexual abuse. Notable however, was the finding that women with disabilities were more likely to experience abuse by attendants and health providers and to experience abuse for longer periods of time than nondisabled women were (Young, Nosek, Howland, Chanpong, & Rintala, 1997). The third study examined abuse of women with cognitive or physical disabilities by personal assistance providers using a convenience sample of 200 women (Powers et al., 2002). Findings indicated that 67% of participants had experienced physical abuse, and 53% sexual abuse, at some point during their lifetimes.

Although these studies clearly indicate that abuse of women with disabilities is a serious problem, as do studies of nondisabled women, prevalence estimates across studies vary. Problems with sample size in the first study, the use of non-probability sampling in the second and third studies, differences in instrumentation, and the lack of a standard definition of abuse used across studies makes comparison of findings difficult at best. In addition to these methodological problems, there is a paucity of information available about the influence of demographic factors on women's risk for abuse. The limited information that is available, however, indicates that ethnicity and age do not affect women's risk. Unfortunately, the influence of disability type on women's risk for abuse remains completely unstudied, and no prevalence estimates in health care settings are available. Studies of men with disabilities who experience abuse are now in progress.

THEORETICAL FRAMEWORKS

Three theoretical frameworks have been applied or developed for use with abused women with disabilities: an ecological model, a theory of limitation, and a pathways-of-violence model. An overview of these theoretical frameworks is provided in Box 12-1.

Ecological Model

Curry, Hassouneh-Phillips, and Johnston-Silverberg (2001) used an ecological model to examine the environmental and cultural factors that contribute to the vulnerability of victims, the characteristics of victims that increases their vulnerability to abuse, and the characteristics of their offenders. Environmental and cultural factors identified by the model include pervasive discrimination, stigma, and marginalization of women with disabilities in institutions and in society at large. Characteristics that increase women's vulnerability to abuse include dependence on others for essential personal care, lack of education about appropriate sexual behaviors, a learned dissociation from any physical sensation as a result of perceiving their bodies marked as "public" by health providers, and a belief that experiencing any feelings, even if painful, is better than not feeling anything. Women with cognitive disabilities who use concrete thinking have limited experience or ability to use problem-solving skills and lack assertiveness; language and communication skills may also be limited. Finally, characteristics of offenders included in the model are the need for control, low self-esteem, exposure to abusive models, poor impulse control, anxiety, and antisocial behavior (Curry et al., 2001).

Theory of Limitation

Gilson, Cramer, and DePoy (in press) examined abuse experiences and service and resource needs of persons with disabilities. The investigators recruited

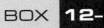

BOX 12-1   OVERVIEW OF THEORETICAL FRAMEWORKS AND MODELS OF ABUSE OF WOMEN WITH DISABILITIES

ECOLOGICAL MODEL
(Curry, Hassouneh-Phillips, & Johnston-Silverberg, 2001)

ENVIRONMENTAL AND CULTURAL FACTORS

- Discrimination
- Stigma
- Marginalization

CHARACTERISTICS THAT INCREASE WOMEN'S VULNERABILITY TO ABUSE

- Dependence on others for essential personal care
- Lack of education about appropriate sexual behaviors
- Dissociation from any physical sensation
- Belief that experiencing any feelings, even if painful, is better than not feeling anything
- Concrete thinking
- Limited experience or ability to use problem-solving skills
- Lack assertiveness, language skills, or communication skills

CHARACTERISTICS OF OFFENDERS

- Need for control
- Low self-esteem
- Exposure to abusive models
- Poor impulse control
- Anxiety and antisocial behavior

THEORY OF LIMITATION
(Gilson, Cramer, & DePoy, in press)

NATURE OF ABUSE

- Assault
- Neglect
- Restraint/control

WOMEN'S RESPONSES TO ABUSE

- Bad self
- Stuck
- Movement
- Unifying theme: the theoretical construct of limitation

PATHWAYS-OF-VIOLENCE MODEL
(Hassouneh-Phillips, 2002)

- Getting in
- Experiencing abuse
- Lack of intervention
- Staying in
- Breaking point
- Building support and ga ining strength
- Getting out

13 women and 1 man with physical, cognitive, or both physical and cognitive disabilities through the Centers for Independent Learning in their areas. Sampling included persons from both urban and rural settings, as well as three additional women who were not disabled. Using a feminist naturalistic design, the researchers conducted two focus groups using open-ended questions. Following thematic and taxonomic analyses, two overarching themes were identified: nature of abuse and responses to abuse.

Nature of abuse included assault, neglect, and restraint. Assault denotes direct emotional or physical abuse. Neglect refers to passive behavior on the part of perpetrators resulting in harm to women. Control/restraint describes the process through which the abuser deliberately limits women's physical, emotional, financial, or social options, resulting in harm.

Women's responses to abuse included bad self, stuck, and movement. Bad self describes the response of women with disabilities who accept the responsibility for their own abuse and attempt to change their behavior as a preventative mechanism. Stuck refers to women who become resigned to the abuse. Movement is defined as an active response to abuse in which women intend to engage in or actually engage in help-seeking behaviors.

The unifying theme for this grounded theory is the theoretical construct of limitation. Gilson and others (in press) reported that limitation was the single greatest factor that magnified seemingly ordinary situations into harmful ones, placing women with disabilities at risk for poverty and social isolation.

Pathways-of-Violence Model

The Women with Physical Disabilities' pathways-through-violence model emerged from preliminary findings of an ongoing qualitative study of abuse of women with physical disabilities (Hassouneh-Phillips, 2002). This model describes the process women go through as they enter, stay in, and eventually terminate abusive relationships. Constructs included in this model are getting in, experiencing abuse, lack of intervention, staying in, breaking point, building support and gaining strength, and getting out.

"Getting in" describes the women's processes of and risk factors for entering into abusive relationships. Women, particularly women with major mobility impairments, often have limited options for intimacy. When abusers offer the opportunity for intimate partner relationships, many women may be willing to ignore warning signs in order to experience intimacy. Women's risk factors for entering into an abusive relationship cited in the model include a history of childhood abuse, history of intimate partner abuse prior to the onset of disability, substance abuse, fear of being alone, poor parental relationships, comorbid mental-heath disorders, institutionalization, and dependency on others for essential personal care.

"Experiencing abuse" denotes the types of abuse a woman with disabilities experiences. Types are emotional, physical, sexual, financial, and disability-specific forms of abuse. Specific examples of various types of abuse are name-calling, theft of medication, forced sex, and abandonment or threat of abandonment to maintain power and control.

Once a woman with a disability experiences abuse, she often has nowhere to turn. In most areas, systems that address her specific needs are not in place. "Lack of intervention" describes the inadequacy of care systems to identify and intervene with women with physical disabilities. Common barriers to help-seeking identified by the model include lack of emergency back-up caregivers, lack of availability of caregivers in general, inaccessible shelters, inaccessible mental health services, and lack of awareness on the part of law-enforcement, health care, and social-service providers.

The problem of inadequate care produces factors that place a woman with disabilities at risk for remaining in abusive relationships for extended periods of time. "Staying in" describes these factors, which include low self-esteem, lack of social support, lack of resources, and receipt of essential personal care from an intimate partner.

The violence literature indicates that at some point most women eventually leave their abusers. "Breaking point" refers to the point in time when a woman begins to contemplate terminating her abusive relationship. This occurs when the harm associated with remaining in an abusive relationship outweighs any potential benefits. Sadly, many women may be willing to accept a certain level of abuse in exchange for intimacy, companionship, and personal care. When the abuse ceases to end or escalates to an unacceptable level, this trade-off becomes untenable.

Once a woman has reached the breaking point, she likely will begin the phase of "building support and gaining strength." She will start to build social networks, gain strength, actively seek safety, and deepen her resolve to leave. She could obtain alternative caregiver services, attend support groups or classes to bolster self-esteem and inner strength, and establish or strengthen ties with potential allies.

Finally, "getting out" means the process of leaving. This could be anything from refusing to utilize the services of a particular transportation worker to obtaining a divorce. Once out of her abusive relationship, a woman may then remain abuse-free, reenter the abusive relationship, or enter into a new relationship with a different abuser.

HEALTH EFFECTS OF ABUSE

In a Delphi study conducted by Berkeley Planning Associates, women with disabilities identified abuse as the most serious health issue they face (Berkeley Planning Associates, 1996). Unfortunately, very little information is available about the effects abuse has on the health of women with disabilities. What little information is available indicates that the effects are serious: abuse prevents women with disabilities from working, maintaining their health, and living independently (Powers et al., 2002).

Preliminary findings from Hassouneh-Phillips' (2002) qualitative study of abuse of women with physical disabilities are the only findings available that specifically address the health effects of abuse on this population. These findings indicate that the mental health effects include an increased risk for initiating or escalating alcohol or substance abuse, depression, suicidality, and posttraumatic stress disorder (PTSD). Regarding physical health, findings indicate that abuse may result in severe exacerbation of women's primary disabilities, malnutrition, disturbed sleep, skin breakdown, and urinary-tract infection. Finally, the social effects of abuse include fear and distrust of others, prostitution, homelessness, and severe isolation. These preliminary data indicate that abuse of women with physical disabilities severely impacts their ability to manage their primary disabilities, is associated with the onset of secondary comorbid psychological and physical conditions, and may place them at risk for severe social disadvantage.

BEHAVIORAL RESPONSES TO ABUSE

Due to both social devaluation and environmental access problems, women with disabilities often have fewer options for meeting potential partners than nondisabled women do. Often viewed as unattractive and incapable, women with disabilities wait longer in life to begin dating and to experience their first voluntary sexual contact. In addition, women with disabilities are less likely to marry than are nondisabled women (Fine & Asche, 1988). As a result, "a woman with a disability in a violent relationship may view it as her only opportunity to experience sexuality, marriage, childrearing, and other rites of womanhood. She may also have internalized her social devaluation to the point that she feels too inferior as a woman to merit a better relationship" (Gill, 1996b, p. 119). Thus, disabled women's behavioral responses to abuse are shaped by their social status and concomitant limited options for intimate and social connection.

In addition to having those limited options, women who rely on others for essential personal care also often have a difficult time finding caregivers. This shortage may result in women's willingness to accept anyone who is willing to take the job, including individuals with alcohol and drug problems, violent histories, and a criminal background. When abuse then occurs, women often seek replacement caregivers, only to find themselves in the same situation all over again. When an abusive intimate partner is also a caregiver, women with disabilities may be particularly at risk because of their desires for both intimacy and essential personal care.

In addition to the strong social factors associated with disability, women's individual histories also play a role. Women who were abused as children or who experienced domestic violence prior to the onset of disability may be particularly vulnerable to entering into abusive relationships. The increased likelihood of mental health disorders, low self-esteem, and alcohol and drug use among survivors of childhood and domestic violence, combined with the social devaluation of women with disabilities, places these women at increased risk for future victimization (Hassouneh-Phillips, 2002). Unfortunately, because no studies conducted to date have specifically examined the influence of culture, ethnicity, or disability type on the experiences of abuse of women with disabilities, the impact of these factors on behavioral responses to such abuse is unknown.

PRIMARY PREVENTION

Primary prevention of this abuse must address the social devaluation of this population and the need for adequate support services. Education of women with disabilities and their families, community advocates, and professionals and the creation of systems of care that support these women's ability to maintain independence are key to this endeavor.

One-on-one counseling in institutional and home settings, community-education classes, pre- and postsecondary education programs, distribution of educational literature, and the Internet are all educational opportunities for this female population and their families. Professional education should be included in nursing-, medical-, and dental-school curricula; in-service classes; and continuing-education offerings. Educational offerings should include information about patterns of victimization, abuse identification, and the health consequences of abuse for women with disabilities and their children. For the women and their families, information about ways to identify potential abusers while in the process of hiring caregivers and strategies to minimize caregiver strain and burnout may also be of value.

Currently, only a few established programs in the nation offer education about abuse of women with disabilities. The *It's My Right! Women in Charge* project is an educational outreach program sponsored by the Center for Self-Determination (CSD), which focuses on the problem of violence against women with developmental disabilities. Such women and professionals receive training and support via a formal curriculum designed to increase identification, prevention, and cessation of this abuse (CSD, 1999).

The *Stop the Violence, Break the Silence Training Guide and Resource Kit* offered by SAFEPLACE in Austin, Texas, consists of an abuse/violence prevention-and-education training guide and resource kit designed for use by persons with disabilities, family members, and professionals. The kit is based on the training materials of Disability Services ASAP, which operates a "national resource library of curriculum, videos, books, journals, anatomically correct models, etc. that promote abuse prevention/intervention strategies and education, and teaches the tenets of healthy relationships to people with disabilities" (SAFEPLACE, 2000, p. 3). Other programs include the Metropolitan Organization to Counter Sexual Assault (MOCSA) developmental-disabilities resource center in Kansas City, Missouri (MOCSA, 2001) and The Arc of Maryland's Gender Violence Prevention and Women with Developmental Disabilities project (Arc of Maryland, 2001). MOCSA provides a resource library, training and technical assistance, community education, and information and referral services to persons with disabilities experiencing abuse, and ARC offers a gender-violence-prevention curriculum for women and adolescent girls with developmental disabilities similar to other curricula previously cited.

Unfortunately, no established or standardized nursing-, medical-, and dental-school curricula addressing this type of abuse are available. Additionally, support systems that would enable women with disabilities who are dependent on potential or suspected abusers for essential personal care to terminate these relationships are severely lacking. To our knowledge, only two programs exist that provide women with disabilities the support services needed to get out of potentially abusive situations. The Domestic Violence Initiative for Women with Disabilities (DVI) is a domestic-violence program in Denver, Colorado, that serves the needs of this population (http://email.vs2000.org/ResourceDirectory/Provider/default.asp?ID=123.). The program offers peer support, domestic violence and disability education, information and referrals, small financial-aid grants, and court accompaniment. Abused Deaf Women's Advocacy Services (ADWAS) is a domestic-violence program that serves the needs of deaf and deaf/blind individuals (http://www.adwas.org/index.htm). Located in Seattle, Washington, ADWAS provides adult and child advocacy in the community, as well as community education and parenting information and support. ADWAS was recently funded by the Department of Justice to replicate its model program in other major cities across the country.

Recently, several federal agencies have begun considering ways to improve services for persons with disabilities who experience violence. In December 2001, the Violence Against Women Office conducted a focus group to gather data about unmet service needs, identify gaps in services, and discuss potential areas for future collaboration across agencies. Similarly, in May 2002, the Centers for Disease Control (CDC), National Institute of Health (NIH), National Institute for Disability and Rehabilitation Research, and several other organizations held a national meeting for the purpose of developing a national agenda to address the problem of abuse of people with disabilities. Although recent attention to the problem of abuse is heartening, work in this area is in its infancy.

SECONDARY PREVENTION

The routine screening and assessment of women with disabilities for past and current abuse has not been a priority for the disability community, domestic-violence advocates, or health care professionals. Advocates and professionals in the disability community have historically focused on obtaining access to basic health and social services and only recently have begun to address the urgent problems related to the abuse. Similarly, the domestic-violence community has primarily focused on outreach to and services for nondisabled women. This is due in part to the extremely limited financial resources and frequent staff turnover of most community-based domestic-violence programs. Thus, it is not surprising that advocates and professionals from the disability and domestic-violence communities rarely know about each other's programs and services, and both groups fail to detect women with disabilities who experience abuse. Finally, health care professionals have not paid attention to screening for abuse among women with disabilities, as they are more likely to focus on the health issues they assume are directly related to the disability. However, in many instances, these health issues are a result of violence, not the disability.

Methods of Screening

Women with disabilities generally have frequent contact with a wide variety of health professionals and disability- and social-service providers. Thus, there are many opportunities for screening and providing primary-prevention information about abuse. Nurses are uniquely positioned to provide leadership in this area because of their diversity of roles and workplaces. Examples of settings include hospitals, rehabilitation centers, skilled nursing facilities, outpatient clinics, disability-service agencies, and home health.

There are three primary methods of identifying abused disabled women: chart/record review (Box 12-2), clinical observation, and use of a screening tool. We encourage the simultaneous use of all three methods whenever possible. For example, a nurse in an outpatient clinic may note some "red flags" from a chart review, observe a troubling interaction between a woman with a disability and her partner, and then use a screening tool to ask specific questions. Because of the frequency of abuse against women with disabilities and its severe health consequences, all women with disabilities should be screened using one or more of the questions described in a following section. It is imperative to recognize that these women are exposed to many potential perpetrators, not just intimate partners. Therefore, it is also necessary to screen for abuse by paid and unpaid personal caregivers, family members, friends, health care providers, and transportation drivers.

| BOX | 12-2 | **IDENTIFICATION OF WOMEN WITH DISABILITIES WHO ARE EXPERIENCING VIOLENCE** |

CHART REVIEW

- Unexplained deterioration of health condition (e.g., uncontrolled diabetes, pressure sores, or seizure disorder)
- Delay in seeking treatment
- History of depression, drug use, or suicide attempts
- Unexplained weight loss or malnutrition
- Frequently missed or canceled appointments
- Unexplained bruises, fractures, & other injuries
- Frequent requests for medication refills due to loss or theft
- Unusual number of requests for equipment repair or replacement
- Skin breakdown
- Increased frequency of urinary-tract infections

CLINICAL OBSERVATION

- Partner or caregiver speaks for woman, contradicts, or minimizes what she says.
- Partner or caregiver attributes all of the woman's problems to her disability.
- Partner or caregiver is oversolicitous with care providers.
- Partner or caregiver is unwilling to let woman be alone.
- Partner or caregiver pushes woman beyond her physical limits (e.g., makes her stand long periods beyond her comfort level).
- Woman is obviously afraid of her partner or caregiver.
- Woman's appearance is unkempt.
- Woman is missing dentures, glasses, or hearing aids

Barriers to Screening

Nurses must recognize that women with disabilities have reported they believe it is important for health providers to screen for abuse, and in one study (Powers et al., 2002) more than half (62%) stated a preference for a nurse to conduct the abuse screening. Given the support for abuse screening, it is unfortunate that for many women distrust of clinicians may be a significant barrier to disclosure. Because women with disabilities generally have a great deal of exposure to health care providers, they are at increased risk for experiencing abuse perpetrated by clinicians and staff in health care settings. Powers and colleagues documented the following forms of maltreatment: ignored woman (58%); minimized complaint of pain (50%); didn't allow enough time to communicate (43%); insulted (40%); pushed beyond limits (40%); handled roughly (33%); and violated privacy (19%). Sadly, more obvious forms of abuse were also reported, including being touched inappropriately (12%) and forced sex (4%). Not surprisingly, women who are survivors of these forms of abuse perpetrated by health care providers may be hesitant to disclose abuse in health care settings.

For some women with disabilities, socialization that encourages them to accept maltreatment as normal and acceptable may be another barrier to disclosure. Moreover, because of isolation and repeated exposure to abuse, some women with disabilities may not recognize that they have been abused. For example, one woman reported that she didn't know it wasn't supposed to hurt when her hair was combed, as her childhood experiences had all been painful. These barriers underscore the importance of establishing rapport and developing trust with women with disabilities when screening for abuse in practice settings.

Communication Skills and Safety

All discussions with women must be conducted privately, not relying on a partner, caregiver, friend, or family member. If women require a professional interpreter, such as a sign-language interpreter, it must be done with the assurance of confidentiality. When talking with women who use wheelchairs, assume a position that allows level eye-contact, minimizing the need for them to look up. It is also important never to assume that because a woman has a physical disability she also has a cognitive disability.

When working with women with cognitive disabilities, allow them to speak for themselves and not rely on others for interpretation. Identify yourself, and speak clearly and directly to the woman using short sentences and simple language. Ask "who," "what," or "where" questions, and avoid confusing questions about time, sequences, or reasons for behavior. Be sensitive to guilt, self-blame, and fear of persons in authority. Most important, treat women with cognitive disabilities as adults and be fully present. Unfortunately, there is a misunderstanding that people with cognitive disabilities do not comprehend their experiences and are therefore unreliable reporters of mistreatment. Consequently, after being discounted over time, many women assume they won't be believed and stop trying to disclose their abuse. Therefore, it is essential that screening for abuse take place in an unhurried, trusting, confidential environment and that hurtful experiences, when disclosed, are validated as forms of abuse that the women did not cause or deserve.

Screening Instruments

Recent collaborations by nursing and disability researchers have resulted in two screening tools designed specifically for women with disabilities. Both tools were developed using qualitative interviews with women with disabilities. They each include the same two questions from the Abuse Assessment Screen (AAS) that ask about physical and sexual abuse as well as disability-specific abuse questions generated from the qualitative interviews.

The Abuse Assessment Screen-Disability (AAS-D) tool was developed and tested with 511 ethnically diverse women with physical disabilities who attended specialty clinics (McFarlane et al., 2001). Interviewers orally administered the four-item tool, which included the two AAS questions and two disability-related questions. The disability-related questions asked if anyone had prevented respondents from using assistive devices (e.g., cane or wheelchair) or had refused to provide an important personal need such as helping to take medication or get out of bed. Overall, 9.8% (n=50) reported abuse; 7.8% (n=40) reported physical or sexual abuse from the AAS, and an additional 2% (n=10) reported disability-related abuse. The primary perpetrator of physical or sexual abuse in general was an intimate partner, although health providers and family members were also identified. However, health professionals, intimate partners, and care providers were equally named as perpetrators of disability-related abuse.

The Abuse Assessment Screen for Women with Disabilities (Curry, Osh-wald, & Powers, in review) was developed from focus groups (Saxton et al., 2001) and data from surveys (Powers et al., 2002) conducted with women with physical or cognitive disabilities (see Appendix B). The eight questions include the two modified AAS questions, a question that asks if they feel unsafe with anyone, and five disability-specific questions. The AAS physical-abuse question was modified to read like so: "Within the last year, has anyone threatened or ac-tually hit, slapped, kicked, shoved, handled you roughly, or otherwise physically hurt you?" It was modified by including language about being threatened and handled roughly. The change reflects the descriptions from participants in the focus groups of how controlling and abusive the threat of being physically hurt was for them. Likewise, being handled roughly, which could result in a serious injury, was also frequently described as abusive. The AAS question about sex-ual abuse was modified accordingly: "Within the last year, has anyone touched you in a sexual way that you did not want or forced you to have sexual activi-ties?" The inclusion of being touched in an unwanted sexual way came from fo-cus group data that described how hurtful these touches were to women, with transportation drivers, personal-care providers, and health professionals being common perpetrators.

The five disability-specific questions cover manipulation of medication, fi-nancial exploitation, consistent emotional abuse, destruction of or withholding of assistive devices, and threat of or actual neglect with an important personal need. The latter two questions are very similar to the disability-related questions in the AAS-D that were just described.

The tool was field-tested with 47 ethnically diverse women with physical or cognitive disabilities who used some type of personal assistance. A majority of women described themselves as having a severe (47%) or moderate (43%) disabil-ity. All women were interviewed in-person using a protocol approved by an inter-nal review board.

Overall, 70% (n=33) reported experiencing one or more types of abuse within the past year. Five women (10.6%) reported physical or sexual abuse. This may have been higher than the 7.8% reported by McFarlane and colleagues (2001) because of the modifications made to the original AAS questions.

Fourteen women (30%) reported abuse related to assistive devices or neglect with personal needs, and one woman reported abuse related to manipulation of medication. This is considerably higher than the 2% disability-related abuse re-ported by McFarlane and others and may have been due to the inclusion of women with more severe disabilities.

Twelve women (25.5%) reported feeling unsafe with someone, 14 (29.7%) re-ported having valuables stolen, and 17 (36%) reported that someone close to them had yelled at them repeatedly or said things to put them down or hurt their feelings. Although financial and emotional abuse are also experienced by nondisabled women, we believe it is important to include these or similar ques-tions with women with disabilities. Women with disabilities are much more likely to be exposed to financial abuse, including theft of personal items and money, forged checks, credit-card and ATM-card abuse, and identity theft by caregivers, family members, and friends. Likewise, emotional abuse is not only common but also often described by women with disabilities as the most painful and disem-powering form of abuse.

ASSESSMENT

Once a woman with a disability has been identified as having experienced abuse, additional assessment is required. The type(s), frequency, and severity of abuse; impact on her disability and health; and the identity of the perpetrator(s) need to be assessed (see Box 12-2). Asking a woman to describe the abuse chronologically helps to identify patterns and possible escalation. It is important to validate and record her reports of threats of physical harm and threats of abandonment as abuse. For example, threats to refuse to let a woman out of her wheelchair all day or threats to leave a respirator-dependent woman alone at night are persuasive types of controlling and abusive behavior. Another powerful form of intimidation is to threaten to not provide or actually not provide essential personal care needed by a woman's children. If she is dependent on someone else to care for her children, the fear of losing her children makes it extremely difficult for a woman with a disability to seek help.

Risk Assessment

Assessment of the woman's potential for further harm is critical. The Risk Assessment checklist in Appendix B is based on the Danger Assessment (Campbell, 1995), focus-group and survey data, the clinical expertise of disability and domestic-violence advocates, and information from women with disabilities. The purpose of the checklist is to assess factors that might place disabled women at greater risk (Curry et al., in review). Some questions focus on the perpetrator, such as being someone who she depends on for care, who abuses alcohol, or who has access to a gun. Another set of questions focuses on the woman's situation, such as not having a back-up caregiver or having a health problem that could become serious if neglected. In a field-test of these questions with women with disabilities who had screened positive for abuse, 80% reported having a serious health problem that could become worse if neglected, and 60% reported they did not have an emergency back-up caregiver (Curry et al., in review).

If a woman reports past abuse, the nurse should determine if anyone was told and, if so, what the response was. Because women with disabilities often report not being believed when they disclose abuse, it is important to know what those experiences were and whether or not she was taken seriously. Nurses should inquire if her disability case manager had been told about the abuse and what if anything was done. A great deal of abuse—especially caregiver abuse—is handled within disability agencies by their own investigative units. Consequently, women with disabilities may never be referred to community-based domestic-violence programs or other external resources, including the criminal-justice system.

Mandatory Reporting

As mandatory reporters, nurses need to be aware of the particular requirements of their own state laws regarding reporting abuse against women with disabilities. In some states, mandated reporters are only obligated to report the abuse of people with developmental disabilities. Nurses need to know how developmental disabilities are defined in each state, as it may vary depending on age of onset of disability, IQ levels, and the current age of the victim. To complicate the matter further, there may be several investigative units within one state or jurisdiction depending on the type of disability. Consequently, crimes against persons with disabilities remain largely invisible and unappraised. Nurses can play an important role in raising awareness about the magnitude of the problem by diligently fulfilling their professional obligation to report these crimes.

We believe it is crucial to include the woman with disabilities in the reporting process. If she hasn't been told that you are a mandated reporter, explain what that means, making it clear that according to the law the abuse must be reported to the proper authorities. Then, invite her to join in reporting the incident so that she has an opportunity to take control of her situation. Ask her what she needs for you to do, such as talking to a particular case manager or notifying a nonabusing family member.

The assessment must be completely documented. A detailed description of the woman's experiences must be recorded as much as possible in her own words. A record of formal reporting needs to include the agency to which it was reported, the position of the person to whom it was reported, and the person's name.

PLANNING AND INTERVENTION

Planning and intervention strategies for women with disabilities who experienced violence is similar to the process used for nondisabled women, as it consists of determining available options and weighing the benefits and risks of each. However, women with disabilities may have fewer options and more challenges to consider, such as severity of the disability, level of dependence on caregivers, and scarce or nonexistent community resources. Critical factors in planning these interventions include:

- Empowering the woman to determine what she wants to do or have happen
- Determining her level of current risk or danger
- Imparting knowledge of available resources and services
- Planning for safety

As with nondisabled women, women with disabilities basically have three options:

- To stay with the abuser
- To leave the abuser
- To have the abuser removed from the place of residence

Stay With the Abuser

If the perpetrator is an intimate partner (IP), the woman may prefer the option of staying in the current relationship, particularly if the IP provides her with essential personal care. It is very likely the perpetrator has reinforced the belief that he is the only option for an intimate relationship, through put-downs about her lack of desirability, the demands of her disability, and her unworthiness.

Other aspects of the IP/caregiver relationship require consideration. If the IP is receiving funding from a state or private agency to provide caregiving, there may be overwhelming financial repercussions, as family income may depend in large part on this funding source. The IP may have legal authority over their joint finances and may be her legal guardian. If the woman and her abuser have children together, the possibility of losing custody to the abuser is very real.

The decision to stay with a perpetrator who provides personal care but who is not an IP is also made with difficulty. Powers and others (2002) identified the primary barriers to leaving an abusive relationship as not having a back-up caregiver, shortage of qualified caregivers, and fear of backlash if the abuse were to be reported. Going without essential care, being left all day in a wheelchair because the person from the agency didn't show up, having a cell phone taken away as punishment, and being admitted to a nursing home are real considerations in deciding whether to stay. Women may thus prefer to stay with an abusive caregiver.

Nurses must therefore be nonjudgmental. They should provide genuine reassurance to women that they are desirable, worthwhile individuals and they do not deserve the violence they are experiencing. Whereas this is true for all disabled women, it is particularly true for women with cognitive disabilities who may have experienced a lifetime of being told they are stupid and worthless. Finally, it is our experience that like most women who are experiencing violence, women with disabilities have remarkable strength and insight into what they need to do to survive.

Some form of risk assessment is needed to determine if there is danger of the situation becoming worse. We suggest using the Risk Assessment Questions found in the appendix. Information from the Risk Assessment can also be used to develop a safety plan for staying with the abuser or, if necessary, to encourage the woman to leave the abuser or have the abuser removed.

Safety planning for women who choose to stay can begin with determining what they believe they need to do to stay safe, such as finding a back-up care provider or finding a safe place to hide their medication. Another important step is developing a list of safe people they can talk to about the abuse and providing names and resources of community options, such as disability agencies, independent-living centers, and support groups. Obviously, knowledge of these resources is required and may require a fair amount of investigation to uncover. It is important to remind women that abuse is a crime, and they have the option of calling the police and filing criminal charges. A brochure with the screening and risk-assessment questions, empowerment messages, and suggestions for safety planning is available from the Oregon Health & Science University Center on Self-Determination (http://www.ohsu.edu/selfdetermination). A more extensive guide for personal safety planning for women who are living with their abuser is shown in Box 12-3. It was adapted from the materials produced by Personal Safety Awareness Center, a program of The Safe Place in Austin, Texas (http://www.austin-safeplace.org/services/psac/index.htm).

Leave the Abuser

Leaving the abuser is often an emotionally and logistically difficult choice for women with disabilities. Nurses are uniquely qualified professionals available to assist women with disabilities during this difficult time. Their knowledge of community resources and understanding of the physical and emotional needs of women with disabilities will be extremely useful. Finding a place to go, though a major consideration, is just one of many factors that need to be taken into account. Thus, whenever possible, nurses should encourage women with disabilities to develop a safety plan in preparation for leaving. The safety planning ideas in Box 12-4 were adapted from the materials produced by the Personal Safety Awareness Center, a program of Safe Place in Austin, Texas.

| BOX | 12-3 | **PERSONAL SAFETY PLANNING FOR EXPLOSIVE EVENTS** |

THINK AND PLAN AHEAD FOR PERSONAL SAFETY

- If cues suggest that the caregiver or IP is becoming angry and you feel afraid or unsafe, go to a place of safety or call someone you trust to come be with you.
- Plan for caregiver or IP to do intimate personal-care tasks when it feels safe.
- Try to have your form of mobility available (already be in your wheelchair, or have cane close by).
- Stay close to a phone. Keep cell phone safely tucked at side or close by (in wheelchair) with ringer turned off so abuser doesn't know you have it.
- If argument seems unavoidable, try to move into a room or area away from dangerous items such as knives or weapons. Try to stay near an exit if possible.
- Get out through an exit if possible. *Yell or make some loud noise if it is safe to do so.*
- Practice ahead of time how to get out of the home or get to a phone to call for help.
- Identify a friend or neighbor ahead of time you can call. Memorize that person's phone number or keep it in a safe place. Ask him or her to call 911 if that person hears a disturbance coming from your house.
- Contact the police when a crisis is not happening. Tell them about your situation. Ask them to send a patrol car by your house as often as possible. Many police will do this if they know you are a person with a disability.
- Figure out a code word or phrase you can use with your children, family, or neighbors to alert them to call 911 if you are in a violent situation.
- Plan ahead for where you will go if you have to leave home (even if you don't think that is possible).
- Use your own judgment and trust your feelings and instincts. If the situation is dangerous, consider giving the abuser what he or she wants, in order to calm him or her down. You have the right to protect yourself until you are out of danger.

When developing a safety plan for leaving, the nurse's primary role is that of advocate. The nurse and disabled woman may want to contact her disability case manager at the outset to learn what, if any, resources are available. In some instances, agencies have contracts with Visiting Nurse Associations or other agencies to provide emergency back-up caregivers. Unfortunately, this is often not the case, and there may be limited emergency funds available at the local level to assist women in leaving. Reporting the abuse to Adult Protective Services (APS) is another option, as in some cases this also is an avenue to resources. Nurses need to be aware, however, that many persons with disabilities have a fear of being reported to APS, may have negative past experiences with the agency, and may equate being reported with being put in a nursing home. Thus, unless the nurse is mandated in her jurisdiction to report the abuse to APS, the decision to contact the agency should be jointly made.

The nurse can also offer to call, or assist the woman in calling, local domestic-violence shelters and a crisis line to find out about available resources and space. If the shelter is not accessible or does not have immediate space, the people there should be asked if they can issue a hotel or motel voucher for an accessible room. The nurse may also need to assist in finding needed caregivers. If the woman has not made arrangements with friends or family members or if it is an emergency, temporary admission to a hospital, nursing home, or skilled-nursing facility may be the only choice.

BOX 12-4 SAFETY PLANNING WHEN PREPARING TO LEAVE

- Never let the abuser know of plans to leave; don't leave any clues like long-distance phone bills.
- Change your payee (if have one) on SSI/SSDI benefits to a trusted individual. Someone will need to contact Social Security Administration to change the payee name.
- Open a savings account in your name only. Have the benefits check directly deposited into that account.
- Plan for personal assistance. Ask several friends, family members, or faith-community members to help so one person is not overtaxed.
- Contact your case manager/caseworker to find out about back-up care.
- Obtain a post office box in your name, and hide the key or give it to a trusted friend or relative.
- Pack a bag with money, extra keys, medications, prescription numbers, spare adaptive aids or medical supplies, copies of birth certificates for you and your children, and a few spare clothes for you and your children. Leave those items with a trusted friend or relative.
- Figure out whom you could stay with (friends or family) or where you would need to go (accessible hotel or shelter).
- If you drive an adapted vehicle, make sure it is in good repair (make sure the abuser hasn't messed with it), and always keep it filled with at least a half tank of gas.
- Know your transportation options; apply for special transit services if available.
- Call your local domestic-violence shelter or the National Domestic Violence Hotline (24 hours a day, 7 days a week) at 800-799-7233 or TDD 800-787-3224 to discuss safety planning. Identify yourself as a woman with a disability so they can be the most helpful.
- Memorize your local domestic-violence or crisis hotline telephone number. Always carry enough money for a pay phone.
- Call the Adult Protective Services office in your area and report the abuse. Let them know your health and safety are at stake. They must take all self-reports. Ask what the investigation process will be like.
- When you leave, write a note to the abuser saying you went to a doctor's appointment or another place that will not make the abuser suspicious.
- If you use a credit card after leaving, make sure the bill will not be sent to the residence where the abuser lives or has access.
- If after you leave you need to telephone anyone who knows the abuser, be careful to block your call.

Other pragmatic issues that may need to be taken into account include accessible transportation, acquisition or transfer of durable medical supplies (such as oxygen or a commode), boarding of pets, accommodations in the new facility for a service animal, and access to interpreters. For all these reasons, nurses have to explore every imaginable possibility when assisting a woman when she chooses to leave the abuser. Nurses need to remind themselves and reassure the woman that leaving an abusive relationship may be one of the most difficult and bravest things the disabled woman has ever done. She needs reassurance that she knows the abuser best and is the authority on the steps that need to be taken.

It is crucial that the nurse advise the woman that the period immediately after leaving may be the most dangerous time for the safety of her and her children. She needs to have a plan of action if the abuser locates her, threatens her, or stalks her. She may want to obtain an Order of Protection, and the nurse should be prepared to facilitate the process if needed.

Remove the Abuser from the Residence

A majority of abused women with disabilities would prefer to remain in their own environments with whatever accommodations they require. If the abuser is an intimate partner and is unwilling to voluntarily leave, a temporary Order to Vacate or an Order of Protection may force the abuser to leave. Getting an order may be required if the abuser is not an intimate partner but has lived in the woman's home as her caregiver. We recommend that, with the woman's consent, nurses work closely with the woman's disability case manager, APS, or both when forcing an abuser out of the home. This is an extremely complex issue, which may require legal advice. For example, abusers have used laws regarding tenant's rights to remain in the residence against the victim's wishes.

Once the partner or caregiver leaves, safety issues need to reviewed. All locks should be changed, and the woman should obtain an Order of Protection if she has not already done so. If the abuser is an intimate partner, pressing charges may serve as a deterrent to future violence, and the abuser may be subject to court-mandated treatment programs. If the abuser is a paid caregiver hired through an agency or state provider, the abuse should be reported to the proper authorities. Unfortunately, however, even when reported, the lack of formal systems for maintaining records often results in these offenders frequently being rehired.

FOLLOW-UP AND EVALUATION

Nurses may have only limited contact with the woman, such as during an inpatient hospitalization, or have the opportunity to remain in contact over an extended period of time, such as in a specialty clinic. In the case of limited contact, the evaluation may consist of making sure the woman has a list of community resources and determining if the nurse, or another professional such as a community-health nurse, can call the woman to inquire about her well-being. If the woman does agree to subsequent follow-up, it is important to obtain safe phone numbers, good times to call, and a back-up plan if the abuser answers the phone.

For cases in which continued follow-up is possible, we recommend that the nurse and the woman jointly decide on realistic goals and the methods of evaluation. For example, a realistic goal for a woman with a cognitive disability may be to develop a plan for staying safe when she commutes from her group home to a sheltered workshop. The goal-setting may include listing safe places to go if harassed, such as a fast-food restaurant, and deciding who it is safe to tell if she is in trouble, such as a bus driver or police officer. As another example, a nurse may assist a woman with multiple sclerosis develop a detailed safety plan for leaving an abusive IP who also provides essential care. A mutually determined method of evaluation may be that the woman has called area shelters to inquire about physical accessibility and the nurse has inquired about services available through APS. An example of a nursing process is displayed in Box 12-5.

NURSING ADVOCACY AND FUTURE DIRECTIONS

The seriousness of the problem of abuse among women with disabilities confirms the need for universal screening for abuse with every client contact in reha-

(text continued on page 381)

BOX 12-5   SAMPLE NURSING PROCESS

ASSESSMENT

BRIEF BACKGROUND

Sandy is a 42-year-old European-American female who sustained a C5-6 spinal-cord injury at the age of 26. Sandy is a survivor of childhood sexual abuse and, prior to the onset of her disability, domestic violence. She has a past and current history of alcoholism and illicit drug use. Sandy presents to your office with complaint of a right-shoulder injury following an assault perpetrated by her boyfriend/caregiver.

Throughout Sandy's visit, the nurse is careful to avoid "taking-over" her care, making sure Sandy is in charge of all decisions that affect her life to the extent possible. The nurse begins the assessment by eliciting Sandy's story. While listening to Sandy, the nurse assures Sandy that she is believed, provides emotional support, and is careful to avoid blaming her in any way for the abuse. Elements of Sandy's history the nurse gathers include, but are not limited to, the significant history and physical exam.

SIGNIFICANT HISTORY

Sandy reveals that the injury occurred in her van yesterday at noon and the perpetrator's name is George Smith. George was trying to prevent Sandy from driving to the police station and in doing so threw her out of her wheelchair and proceeded to beat and choke her. Sandy's shoulder hit the floor of the van when she was thrown out of her wheelchair. She is not sure, but it is possible that she might have hit her head as well. Currently, Sandy's sole abuser is George, who is both her caregiver and intimate partner. Sandy relies on George for daily personal care such as toileting and bathing. She reports that George over the past year has abused her emotionally, physically, and in ways that are disability-specific. Examples of the abuse she has experienced include name-calling, hitting, confining her to bed, denying her access to her wheelchair, and stealing of prescription narcotics. When the nurse asks how the abuse affects Sandy's ability to manage her primary disability, Sandy reports that while partnered to George, she has become increasingly depressed, increased her use of alcohol, experimented with IV drug use (given and administered to her by George), and unintentionally lost 20 pounds. Sandy asks that the nurse not contact her disability caseworker because her abuser is paid by the state to provide her care and she is afraid that reporting the abuse would endanger this funding. Sandy reports that she has become increasingly isolated and has been evicted from two apartments due to her abuser's drug use and violent behavior over the past year. Sandy's lethality assessment reveals that her risk for lethal violence is low.

PHYSICAL EXAM

In addition to gathering Sandy's history, the nurse performs a physical exam. The nurse performs an examination of Sandy's shoulder, neck, elbow, wrist, back, chest, abdomen, and other proximal extremities looking for hidden injuries. Because Sandy is not sure whether or not she hit her head, the nurse also performs a thorough neurological examination. During the physical exam, the nurse considers the pattern of Sandy's injury and the extent to which the injury appears consistent with her story. The nurse further assesses the extent to which Sandy's injury may affect her ability to use her wheelchair, shift her position in her wheelchair, and perform wheelchair transfers. Finally, the nurse asks Sandy for her consent to take photographs of her visible injuries. Sandy agrees and signs a written consent. With the help of a scale, the nurse then proceeds to photograph Sandy's injuries. The nurse is careful to take close-up, mid-range, and full-body shots. After completion of the physical exam, the nurse ascertains that Sandy has a right-shoulder strain with no other observable injuries and no new neurological deficits. Sandy's ability to use her right

(*continued*)

BOX **12-5**   **SAMPLE NURSING PROCESS (*Continued*)**

arm is reduced, thereby making use of her wheelchair, shifting position in her chair, and wheel-chair transfers painful and difficult.

NURSING DIAGNOSES, OUTCOMES, AND INTERVENTIONS

Nursing diagnoses that could be used in this situation include the diagnoses described as follows.

ADULT VIOLENCE

Adult violence is related to unequal power relationships and dependency on abuser for essential personal care.

SHORT-TERM CLIENT GOAL

Maintain safety.

LONG-TERM CLENT GOAL

Remain free of abuse.

NURSING INTERVENTIONS (RELATED TO BOTH SHORT-TERM AND LONG-TERM GOALS)

- Provide Sandy with information about the cycle of abuse and its health consequences.
- Work with Sandy to create an individualized safety plan. (See Boxes 12-3 and 12-4.)
- Provide resource information that includes information about domestic violence and disability community resources, and the accessibility of these resources for women who use wheelchairs.
- Encourage Sandy to call 911 if she fears for her safety.
- Encourage Sandy to change her locks if she wishes to separate from George.
- Arrange for back-up caregiver services to minimize dependence on abusive care providers in the future.
- Refer Sandy to a domestic-violence support group to work through emotional issues related to abusive experiences.
- Work with Sandy to increase the size of her social network.

IMPAIRED MOBILITY AND SELF-CARE ABILITY

Her impaired mobility and ability to engage in self-care activities are related to her existing spinal-cord injury and her recent shoulder injury.

SHORT-TERM CLIENT GOAL

Promote shoulder healing and self-care activities.

NURSING INTERVENTIONS

- Discuss shoulder-mobility limitations to avoid aggravation of the injury.
- Provide shoulder support.
- Outline potential changes in Sandy's personal-care routines based on her new temporary shoulder limitation.
- Discuss strategies for maximizing Sandy's self-care abilities.

LONG-TERM CLIENT GOAL

Return shoulder to previous level of function.

NURSING INTERVENTIONS

- Arrange for primary-care follow-up for ongoing evaluation and management of Sandy's shoulder injury.

(continued)

BOX 12-5 SAMPLE NURSING PROCESS (*Continued*)

- Arrange referral to occupational or physical therapy if deemed necessary following the initial stages of healing.
- Reinforce the importance of using her safety plan to reduce the likelihood of future injury.

UNMET PERSONAL-CARE NEEDS

Unmet personal-care needs are related to abuse and neglect perpetrated by current caregiver.

SHORT-TERM CLIENT GOAL

Obtain immediate personal-care assistance services from a safe and competent provider.

NURSING INTERVENTIONS

- Assess the level, type, and frequency of personal assistance needed.
- Explore options for immediate back-up caregiving services available in the community.

LONG-TERM CLIENT GOAL

Obtain personal-care assistance from safe and competent providers over the long term.

NURSING INTERVENTIONS

- Discuss long-term caregiving resources and options available in the health system and community.
- Refer Sandy to a caregiver-management community course to promote effective hiring and communication skills for use with future caregivers.

SUBSTANCE ABUSE

Substance abuse is evidenced by escalating and unsafe use of alcohol and illicit drugs.

SHORT-TERM CLIENT GOAL

Consider treatment options.

NURSING INTERVENTIONS

- Discuss the impact of alcohol and drug use on Sandy's health.
- Encourage Sandy to seek treatment.
- Discuss treatment options available to Sandy for alcohol and drugs.
- Refer Sandy to an appropriate alcohol and drug treatment center.
- Provide Sandy with information about Alcoholics Anonymous or 12-step programs in her community.
- Provide Sandy with information about community substance-abuse programs specifically designed for people with disabilities.

LONG-TERM CLIENT GOAL

Abstain from alcohol and drugs.

NURSING INTERVENTIONS

- Help Sandy make a commitment to long-term abstinence.
- Maintain a solid support system.
- Begin psychotherapy to deal with the traumatic effects of childhood sexual abuse and promote use of healthy coping skills.
- Counsel Sandy to avoid spending time with individuals who drink or use drugs excessively.

EVALUATION

Evaluation of nursing interventions is based on achievement of goals as perceived by Sandy and as indicated by the criteria met.

bilitation, health care, and other professional settings. Service providers seeking to intervene with abused women must be aware of the resources available in their communities to facilitate appropriate referrals in their local areas. The development of resources and improvement of services for women with disabilities who have been abused are essential precursors to effective abuse intervention (Nosek, Howland, & Young, 1997; Swedlund & Nosek, 2000). Collaboration with domestic-violence shelters to provide personal-assistance providers and replace medications and assistive devices left behind when abused women are forced to leave their homes is also necessary. Additionally, collaboration with law enforcement and other professionals should occur to facilitate removal of abusers from women's homes and provide essential personal care services in emergency situations.

In addition to improved services, research is needed to support evidence-based practice. Qualitative studies are needed to investigate the cultural contexts of abuse of women with disabilities both within the dominant culture and within various ethnic cultures. In addition, research that focuses specifically on the abuse experiences of women with different types of physical, cognitive, and psychiatric disabilities has to be conducted. More information about abuse within specific settings is also needed. Future quantitative research efforts should include identification of risk factors for abuse, examination of the direct and indirect effects of abuse on women's health, and additional studies to test the validity of the AAS-D and the Abuse Screening Tool Specific for Women with Disabilities. Abuse interventions using RN, Nurse Practitioner, and interdisciplinary models of care must be developed and tested. To ensure that future research findings are accurate and empowering to the women, it is essential that women with disabilities are involved at all levels of this important work.

Future directions in the care of abused women with disabilities must use a collaborative model, with the women at the center. Researchers have the obligation to elevate the issue to the same level of public awareness as violence against women in general and to conduct collaborative research that includes violence and disability researchers and women with disabilities. Service providers must work to increase the implementation of model programs and improve the quality and accessibility of health care and other services abused women with disabilities need. Educators must ensure that content on abuse of women with disabilities, and the social context of disability, is included in nursing-, medical-, and dental-school curricula, and they must provide community education about this issue. It is incumbent on nurses to be involved in all these endeavors to ensure that women with disabilities have access to the quality care they deserve and the knowledge and resources needed to end abuse in their lives.

References

Arc of Maryland. (2001). *Gender violence prevention and women with developmental disabilities* [Online]. Available: http://www.thearccmd.org/Programs/GenderViolence/gender_violence.htm.

Berkeley Planning Associates. (1996). *Priorities for Future Research: Results of BPA's Delphi Survey of Disabled Women*. Oakland, California: Berkeley Planning Associates.

Campbell, J. C. (1995). *Assessing dangerousness: Violence by sexual offenders, batterers, and child abusers*. Thousand Oaks, CA: Sage.

Center for Self-Determination, (1999). *Women with developmental disabilities violence project* [Online]. Available: http://www.ohsu.edu/selfdetermination/violence.shtml.

Curry, M., Hassouneh-Phillips, D. & Johnston-Silverberg, A. (2001). Abuse of women with disabilities: An ecological model and review. *Violence Against Women*, 7(1), 60–79.

Curry, M., Oshwald, M., & Powers, L. (in review). The development of an abuse screening tool specific for women with disabilities. *Journal of Aggression Maltreatment and Trauma.*

Fine, M., & Asch, A. (1988). Introduction: Beyond pedestals. In M. Fine & A. Asch (Eds.), *Women with disabilities: Essays in psychology, culture, and politics* (pp. 1–37). Philadelphia: Temple University Press.

Furey, E. M. (1994). Sexual abuse of adults with mental retardation: Who and where. *Mental Retardation, 32,* 173–180.

Gill, C. (1996). Becoming visible: Personal health experiences of women with disabilities. In D. Krostoski, M. Nosek & M. Turk (Eds.), *Women with physical disabilities: Achieving and maintaining health and well-being* (pp. 5–16). Baltimore: Paul H. Brookes.

Gilson, S., Cramer, E., & DePoy, E. (in press). (Re)Defining abuse of women with disabilities: A paradox of limitation and expansion. *Affilia: Journal of Women and Social Work.*

Hassouneh-Phillips, D. (2000). *Pilot study: Women with physical disabilities: A narrative study of abuse experiences.* Unpublished manuscript, Oregon Health Sciences University, Portland.

Hassouneh-Phillips, D. (2002). [Women with physical disabilities' experiences of abuse]. Unpublished raw data.

Hassouneh-Phillips, D. & Curry, M. (2002). Abuse of women with disabilities: State of the science. *Rehabilitation Counseling Bulletin, 45*(2), 96–104.

McFarlane, J., Hughes, R., Nosek, M., Groff, J., Swedland, N., & Mullens, P. (2001). Abuse Assessment Screen-Disability (AAS-D): Measuring frequency, type, and perpetrator of abuse toward women with physical disabilities. *Journal of Women's Health & Gender-Based Medicine, 10,* 861–866.

Metropolitan Organization to Counter Sexual Assualt, (2001). *The MOCSA Developmental Disabilities Resource Center–A sexual abuse prevention and information program for persons with disabilities* [Online]. Available: http://www.mocsa.org/services.htm.

Nosek, M. A. (1996). Sexual abuse of women with physical disabilities. In D. M. Krotoski, M. A. Nosek,, C. A. Howland, D. H. Rintala, E. M. Young & G. F. Chanpong (Eds.), *National study of women with physical disabilities: Final report.* Houston, TX: Center for Research on Women with Disabilities.

Nosek, M., Howland, C., & Young, M. (1997). Abuse of women with disabilities: Policy implications. *Journal of Disability Policy Studies, 8,* 157–176.

Powers, L., Curry, M., Oschwald, M., Maley, S., Saxton, M., & Eckels, K. (2002). Barriers and strategies in addressing abuse: A survey of disabled women's experiences. *Journal of Rehabilitation, 68*(1), 4–13.

SAFEPLACE (2000). Stop the violence break the silence: A training guide and resource kit. Available online: http://www.austin-safeplace.org/programs/disability/stopTV.htm.

Saxton, M., Curry, M., Powers, L., Maley, S., Eckels, K., & Gross, J. (2001). "Bring my scooter so I can leave you": A study of disabled women handling abuse by personal assistance providers. *Violence Against Women,7*(4), 393–417.

Sobsey, D., & Doe, T. (1991). Patterns of sexual abuse and assault. *Disability and Sexuality, 9,* 243–259.

Swedlund, N., & Nosek, M. (2000). An exploratory study on the work of Independent Living Centers to address abuse of women with disabilities. *Journal of Rehabilitation, 66*(4), 57–64.

Ulincy, G. R., White, G. W., Bradford, B., & Matthews, R. M. (1990). Consumer exploitation by attendants: How often does it happen and can anything be done about it? *Rehabilitation Counseling Bulletin, 33,* 240–246.

Young, M. E., Nosek, M. A., Howland, C. A., Chanpong, G., Rintala, D. H. (1997). Prevalence of abuse of women with physical disabilities. *Archives of Physical Medicine and Rehabilitation Special Issue, 78,* S34–S38.

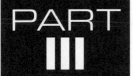

PART III

Nursing Education, Policy, and Future

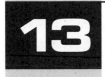

Legal and Forensic Nursing Responses to Family Violence

- Daniel J. Sheridan

Family violence, in all its forms, is now a crime in all states. For example, regardless of whether it is child abuse, dating violence, intimate partner violence, elder abuse, or the abuse of vulnerable people with cognitive, mental health, or physical disabilities, it is a crime to push, slap, punch, kick, or injure anyone. Many forms of familial or institutional neglect are also potentially criminal in nature.

Forensics pertains to the law and the courts; however, it is not limited to the criminal courts. Nurses who work with survivors of family violence throughout the life cycle may be asked to testify in a variety of courts, including criminal, family, guardianship, juvenile, and probate courts. This chapter introduces basic abuse-related legal definitions and applies the principles of forensics to nursing practice with abused and neglected patients.

DEFINITIONS OF ABUSE AND NEGLECT

Child Abuse

Although Caffey first described child abuse in 1946, Kempe, Silverman, Steele, Droegmueller, & Silver (1962) are credited with coining the phrase "Battered Child Syndrome." In the 40 years since Kempe and colleagues' salient work recognized abuse of children as a major public-health problem, in every state laws have been enacted that not only make abuse of children illegal but also mandate health professionals, social-service workers, and teachers, to name a few, to report suspected abuse to various county or state child protective agencies.

Despite efforts to drastically reduce child abuse, it is still endemic. There are more than 3 million referrals to child protective agencies annually with more than one third of these cases substantiated (Administration of Children, Youth and Families, 2000). The American Medical Association estimates there may be as many 2 million cases of child abuse annually in the United States that result in the deaths of more than 1,000 children (Administration of Children, Youth and Families, 1998; Berkowitz, Bross, Chadwick, & Whitworth, 1992a). It is generally believed child abuse and neglect is grossly underreported.

Legal definitions of child abuse are unique to every state and can be quite complex. However, there are enough similarities between states to discuss more generic, clinically useful definitions. For example, child abuse could be defined as physical injury of a child (under the age of 18) by a parent, household member, or other person who has permanent or temporary custody or responsibility for supervision of the child (Suggs, Lichenstein, McCarthy, & Jackson, 2001).

The American Medical Association (Berkowitz et al., 1992a) defines child abuse as "inflicted injury to a child and can range from minor bruises and lacerations to severe neurologic trauma and death" (p. 8). The Criminal Code of Oregon (2002) defines child abuse, in part, as "any assault . . . of a child and any physical injury to a child which has been caused by other than accidental means, including injury which appears to be at variance with the explanation given of the injury" (p. 561). The Criminal Code of Oregon (2002) further defines as child abuse such acts as any mental injury causing observable and substantial mental impairment, rape, sodomy, incest, unlawful sexual penetration or sexual abuse, sexual exploitation, negligent treatment and maltreatment, substantial threats of harm, and buying or selling a person. The Criminal Code of Oregon (2002) allows, as do laws in all states, reasonable discipline of a child, including corporal (physical) punishment, as long as the discipline does not inflict physical injury.

Child Neglect

Although child abuse is much easier to identify because of visible trauma to the body, the Administration of Children, Youth and Families of the U.S. Department of Health and Human Services (1999) estimates child neglect is much more common. Underdiagnosis and underreporting of possible neglect is common because providers often attribute the neglectful behaviors to parental lack of resources or ignorance. It is much more difficult to measure neglect, especially what appears to be minor neglect. Usually only severe or life-threatening forms of neglect get reported to child protective services because overworked and short-staffed protective-service response systems only act immediately on the most severe of neglect cases.

Neglect, which can be physical, social, or emotional, often is defined in deprivational terms and involves actual or potential harm. Providers are often accused of failing to provide a needed item or service, or an act was omitted that resulted in actual or potential harm and that a parent or parent-figure would reasonably have provided.

Neglect is reportable to child protective services anytime there is a failure on the part of the parent or person acting as parent to provide basic emotional support, food, clothing, shelter, or medical care. Actual harm does not need to have occurred for neglect to be reported (Suggs et al., 2001). Missing one pediatric appointment is usually not grounds for calling the protective-service hotline. However, a pattern of missed appointments without reasonable explanations can be an indication of a child at risk of harm.

Seldom is it clear which cases of possible neglect should be reported to protective services and which should not (Suggs et al., 2001). Most hospitals have created Suspected Child Abuse and Neglect (SCAN) teams that meet on a regular basis to discuss reported cases of abuse and neglect and to review, as a group, possible neglect cases. In-house SCAN team membership will vary among institutions; however, it is common to have at the table a pediatrician, registered nurse, social worker, therapists, hospital attorney, chaplain, and security officer. Representatives from local law enforcement, criminal prosecutors, and protective-service administrators may also participate in the SCAN meetings.

Some examples of reportable medical neglect include but are not limited to failing to provide reasonable dental care, immunizations, ordered prescription or over-the-counter medication, needed eyeglasses, hearing aids, and assistive devices, such as a wheelchair. Although the perpetrators of child abuse and child sexual assault are mostly male, the perpetrators of child maltreatment are often women (Suggs et al., 2001). Maternal contributions to child neglect include mother's age, mental illness, alcohol and drug use/abuse, and a severe lack of resources.

As with child abuse, the nurse does not need to prove neglect has occurred prior to making a report to child protective services. Despite the less-than-clear guidelines that determine what is neglect, it would be prudent for the nurse to report all cases of suspected neglect to child protective services.

Leaving a vulnerable child unattended or in an area where the child is at risk of harm is also neglect. This may include intentionally leaving a five-year-old home alone all day or having one's children living in a home where illegal drugs are manufactured or sold (Criminal Code of Oregon, 2002).

Child and Adult Sexual Assault

Known or suspected child sexual assault is reportable as child abuse and usually receives a high-priority response from child protective services, especially if there are injuries or physical evidence consistent with sexual abuse. Sexual assault is not limited to penetration of body cavities. It also includes any form of sexual contact or behavior by an adult or sibling toward a child. Each legal jurisdiction has specific laws that define all the different types of child sexual abuse, from acts that are criminal misdemeanors to different levels of felonies. In general, child sexual assault is perpetrated by an adult, young adult, or another child against a child who is not developmentally prepared and cannot give informed consent (Berkowitz, Bross, Chadwick, & Whitworth, 1992b).

There is a proliferation of trained sexual-assault nurse examiners (SANEs) providing highly specialized medical forensic examinations of adults and children suspected of being sexually assaulted. Many conditions mimic physical child abuse, child neglect, and especially child sexual assault. Bays (2001) has written one of the most comprehensive chapters about conditions mistaken for child physical abuse that should be a must-read for any nurse who is part of the team assessing and documenting possible child abuse, child neglect, and child sexual assault.

Girardin, Faugno, Seneski, Slaughter, and Whelan (1997) compiled an extensive collection of images of sexual-assault-related trauma to adult patients. The International Association of Forensic Nurses recently developed an examination/certification examination for Adult Sexual Assault Examiners and is developing a similar exam for nurses who conduct sexual-assault examinations of children who may have been assaulted.

Intimate Partner Violence

Intimate partner violence is often defined as the physical, emotional, sexual, or financial abuse of an intimate or former intimate partner (Sheridan, 2001). Whereas emotional and financial abuse of an intimate partner is significant, it is usually not part of a forensic response. It is not illegal to call your partner mean names. It is not against the law to control all the assets within a family. However, it is illegal to verbally threaten someone with bodily harm. It is a forensic matter when during a divorce proceeding one fraudulently hides one's assets to keep one's soon-to-be ex-partner from getting an equitable portion of the joint assets.

When intimate partner abuse or domestic-violence legislation was being written in the late 1970s and 1980s, most states adopted a series of civil protective orders designed to provide various legal safeguards to abused partners. These legal remedies are frequently called Domestic Restraining Orders or Orders of Protection. In many states, violating one of these civil protective orders can put the violator at risk of being arrested and charged with a crime. The protective orders can grant a variety of remedies to the abused person. In addition, for example, protective orders can give the victim temporary custody of the children; require the reported perpetrator to leave the home (temporarily); require the reported perpetrator to stay hundreds of feet away from the victim's home, workplace, or school; prohibit the reported perpetrator from harassing or interfering with the personal liberty of the victim; or any combination thereof. Over the past 25 years, the concept of protective orders has been expanded to provide additional legal protection to children and the elderly.

Elder Abuse

Definitions of what constitutes elder abuse and at what age one is considered elderly vary from state to state and from study to study (Geroff & Olshaker, 2001). In general, most laws consider elder-abuse survivors to be aged 65 and older. The terms elder "abuse" and elder "mistreatment" are often used interchangeably; however, abuse generally refers to physical violence whereas mistreatment includes neglect (Geroff & Olshaker, 2001).

In 1992, the American Medical Association, in its elder-abuse treatment guidelines, identified a variety of abuses and neglects inflicted on the elderly (Arvanis, et al.). See Table 13-1. In general, elder abuse is divided into three categories:

- Elder physical and emotional abuse
- Neglect
- Financial exploitation

The plight of abused elders was first brought to the medical community's attention in the mid-1970s when two British medical journals published practice-based articles on "granny battering" (Baker, 1975; Burston, 1975). Elder abuse affects a disproportionate number of women for two reasons. First, women live

Table 13-1 • American Medical Association Definitions of Elder Abuse

TERM	DEFINITION
Physical abuse	Acts of violence that may result in pain, injury, impairment, or disease
Physical neglect	Failure of the caregiver to provide the goods or services that are necessary for optimal functioning; or, avoidance of the older adult
Psychological abuse	Conduct that causes mental anguish in an older person
Psychological neglect	Failure to provide a dependent elderly individual with social stimulation
Financial or material abuse	Misuse of the elderly person's income or resources for the financial or personal gain of a caretaker or advisor
Financial or material neglect	Failure to use available funds and resources necessary to sustain or restore the health and well-being of the older adult
Violation of personal rights	Ignoring the older person's rights and capabilities to make decisions for himself or herself

Adapted from Aravanis, S. C. et al. (1992). *Diagnostic and treatment guidelines on elder abuse.* Chicago: American Medical Association.

longer than men; thus, there are more women available to be abused. Second, a significant proportion of elder abuse is intimate partner violence grown older. Women battered by intimate partners in their 20s, 30s, 40s, and 50s become elder-abuse survivors in their 60s and older.

Elder abuse patients present with a variety of physical-abuse and neglect symptoms, with many of the physical symptoms similar to naturally occurring changes related to aging. Fractures that look traumatic in nature could be from underlying disease. What may appear, at a glance, to be severe (traumatic) bruising, may in fact be a form of ecchymoses called senile purpura. (See Figure 13-1.)

Anytime one suspects family violence in any of its forms, however, especially for possible elder-abuse patients, it is prudent to ask the provider to obtain baseline lab values. Relatively common tests such as a complete blood count (CBC) with platelets, basic chemistry profile (CHEM-7, albumin, protein, BUN, and creatinine), coagulation panel, liver profile, and urinalysis may provide evidence of malnutrition and dehydration. Grossly abnormal hematological findings may detract from a finding of abuse and support an underlying medical condition. As with the evaluation of suspected child abuse, the suspected elder-abuse patient should receive a thorough radiographic evaluation to look for a pattern of multiple fractures in various stages of healing (Geroff & Olshaker, 2001). Pertinent findings on history and physical examination are shown in Box 13-1.

Abuse of Vulnerable People With Disabilities

In recent years, states have begun to pass legislation making abuse and neglect against people with physical, cognitive, and mental health disabilities re-

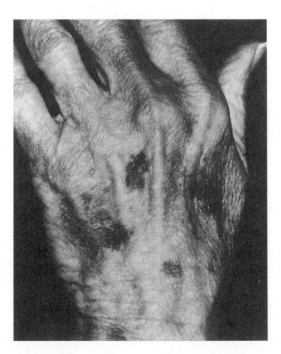

FIGURE 13–1 • Senile purpura.

BOX 13-1	PERTINENT FINDINGS ON HISTORY AND PHYSICAL EXAMINATION

PHYSICAL ABUSE AND NEGLECT

Patterned Injuries: Slap marks, fingertip-pressure bruises, rope or ligature marks on wrists/ankles, bite marks, immersion line

Bruises: Especially on areas of the body not over bony prominences, multiple stages of healing

Wounds: Laceration, abrasion, puncture, especially if untreated or in various stages of healing; decubiti

Head injury: Traumatic alopecia, scalp swelling

Burns: Cigarette marks, scald burns with an immersion line, absent satellite splash burns

Fractures: Spiral/oblique orientation without a given twisting mechanism, multiple fractures of different ages, mechanism not consistent with history

Subdural Hematoma: From violent shaking with cerebral atrophy, as well as from direct blow

Nutrition: Dehydration, cachexia, weight loss, electrolyte abnormalities, fecal impaction

Drug Levels: Subtherapeutic or toxic, or presence of a drug not prescribed

Disease Patterns: Untreated chronic disorders, excessive exacerbations of chronic disease

Poor Hygiene: Filth, soiled with excrement, infestation, dental caries

Personal Effects: Inadequate clothing, shoes, glasses, hearing aid, dentures

Living Conditions: Fire hazard; infestation; inadequate heating, air conditioning, or plumbing

PSYCHOLOGICAL ABUSE AND NEGLECT

Communication: Ambivalence, withdrawal, poor eye contact, cowering, noncommunicative

Mood/Affect: Agitation, depression, passivity, anxiety, hopelessness

Behavior: Fear, apprehensiveness, shame, paranoia, infantile behavior

Motor: Involuntary movement, rocking, sucking, trembling

Psychosomatic: Poor appetite, disturbed sleep patterns, posttraumatic stress disorder (may result from physical abuse as well)

Interactions: Caregiver insists on remaining with patient at all times, elder fearful of caregiver

SEXUAL ABUSE

Wounds: Located over breast or genitalia

Infection: New sexually transmitted disease without reported sexual activity

Bleeding: Unexplained vaginal or anal bleeding

Pain/Tenderness: Noticed during pelvic or rectal exam

ABANDONMENT

Institutional Desertion: Leaving an elder at a hospital without means of return

Public Desertion: Leaving an elder at a public location to be picked up by police or emergency medical service; homelessness

SELF-NEGLECT

Many of the above

---

portable to protective-service agencies. Many elder-abuse reporting acts were expanded to include vulnerable people, or specific statutes were developed to address the abuse and neglect of vulnerable people.

As a former abuse investigator for people with cognitive and mental health disabilities, I can say that the plight of these abused and neglected patients is hidden behind the closed doors of family homes, private homes, group homes, and institutions. In assessing for family violence throughout the life cycle, verbal histories from the victims are a key part of most investigations. Very young children and the confused or comatose elderly are not able to verbalize what happened. Most patients with cognitive and mental health disabilities either are not verbal, or their verbalizations are not necessarily credible from a legal perspective.

Evaluation of possible abuse and neglect is often based on a thorough review of care records, interviews with direct-care givers, and, when available, a forensic review of the injuries to help determine if the injuries are consistent (or not consistent) with the history of occurrence provided by the caretaker(s). A growing number of forensically trained advanced-practice nurses, including me, provide abuse-and-neglect forensic-consultation services to investigators of elder and vulnerable-person abuse.

MANDATORY REPORTING OF ABUSE

Children

All states have some form of mandatory reporting of suspected child abuse or neglect by a variety of people such as health professionals, police officers, social workers, and educators. Most of the reporting statutes protect the mandated reporter from being successfully sued if the report to child protective services was made in good faith and without malice. Failing to report child abuse can result in fines, notification of one's professional licensing board, of both.

Much controversy exists about reporting child abuse and neglect, especially when significant medical evidence supports the need to report. Unfortunately, it is not unusual for providers to delay a call until they have more proof that abuse or neglect have taken place. Most reporting statutes clearly state that one must call the child protective-services hotline if one has reasonable cause to suspect abuse may have occurred. Any discussion about whether one should call signifies reasonable cause to report.

Child protective-service hotlines vary by location. Many states have established a county-by-county notification system, whereas others have a statewide, central hotline that prioritizes all calls prior to forwarding approved cases to the appropriate county investigative system. Children who are considered most at risk are evaluated and investigated first. An at-risk, abused child hospitalized in a controlled environment may be deemed less at risk than that child's siblings still inside the reportedly abusive home. It is fairly common for nurses to become confused and frustrated with the prioritizing of child protective services.

Hotline numbers should be prominently posted somewhere in the treatment area and in the child abuse/neglect policy and procedure. Although the notification of the child protective-services hotline can be delegated to a designated person, hotline personnel usually prefer to talk with the professional who has the most firsthand information as to why the call needed to be made.

Anytime the nurse calls the hotline, he or she should document the following in the progress note:

- The reason(s) for the call
- The time of the call
- The full name of the person who took the call
- The response of the child-protective-service worker to the call (i.e., accepted or not accepted)

When suspected abused and neglected children are in the treatment area, some states allow certain professionals to take emergency, temporary protective custody. In some states, only the child protective-service worker can take temporary custody; in others, a police officer can also take custody of the child. In addition, some states allow physicians to take emergency, temporary custody of children, especially if it is thought the child will be removed from the health facility by possibly abusive or neglectful parents before the police or child protective services arrive.

When the decision has been made to call child protective services, it is recommended the parents be notified of the decision if it is believed that notifying them does not place the child, mandated reporter, or other staff and patients at risk. If the health facility has in-house security officers, it would be prudent to have them nearby during the notification process.

All but eight states have mandatory reporting statutes that require health professionals to report suspected abused and neglected elders to adult protective services (Geroff & Olshaker, 2001). As with mandatory reporting of child abuse, the reporter does not have to have proof that elder mistreatment has occurred before one's mandate to report is triggered. All that is needed to report elder mistreatment is reasonable cause to suspect abuse or neglect (physical, emotional, or financial) might have occurred. Most elder-abuse mandatory-reporting statutes provide immunity from being sued as long as the report was made in good faith without malice. Like child abuse, in most states, failing to report suspected or known elder abuse can result in a fine, sometimes brief jail time, and notification of one's professional licensing board.

Intimate Partner Violence

Most states have some type of law requiring health providers to report domestic violence to some state agency. For example, a recent Oklahoma law requires notification of domestic violence to the state health department (for data purposes), and Illinois has been requiring police notification of all suspected crime victims and perpetrators for more than 40 years. In most states, a police-notification requirement for domestic abuse is limited to patients with injuries from a weapon, such as a gun, knife, or other deadly object (Hyman, Schillinger, & Lo, 1995).

In the mid-1990s, California passed legislation making it mandatory for health providers to not only report domestic violence to the police but also to provide the police a detailed report of what the patient (victim) said about the suspected crime. Four other states (Kentucky, New Hampshire, New Mexico, and Rhode Island) have mandatory-reporting statutes specifically tailored to intimate partner violence (Hyman et al., 1995).

Battered-women's advocates have voiced concern that mandatory reporting of domestic violence places abused women (the largest percentage of abused intimates) at further risk of harm because of possible retaliation by the abuser (Hyman et al., 1995). In a case-controlled study of more than 200 abused women, almost 50% preferred it be the women's decision to call the police, and about 66% of the abused women voiced concerns that mandatory reporting to police by health professionals would (and is) preventing women from disclosing the true nature of their injuries (Gielan et al., 2000).

Studies are being developed to explore if there is a link between mandatory reporting of intimate partner violence and increased risk of harm to abused patients (Hyman et al., 1995). The nurse needs to know if he or she is practicing in a state that has mandatory reporting of all forms of intimate partner physical violence. The controversy of mandatory reporting should not prevent the nurse from conducting routine screening for abuse using reliable and valid assessment tools. Not screening and documenting intimate partner violence in the health record may place the nurse and the healthcare institution at risk of civil suit for failing to provide a minimal standard of care.

The Abuse Assessment Screen (AAS), created and modified by nurse clinicians and researchers, is one of the most widely used intimate partner-violence screening tools. (See Appendix A.) It was first developed by Helton (1987) as a nine-question screen, then modified by the Nursing Research Consortium on Violence and Abuse as a five-question screen (Sheridan, 2001). In a classic study, McFarlane, Parker, Soeken, & Bullock (1992) effectively used a three-question version of AAS to identify women being beaten while pregnant, and McFarlane, Greenberg, Weltge, and Watson (1995) effectively shortened the AAS to a two-question reliable and valid screen. Other reliable and valid clinical screens for intimate partner abuse include the Partner Violence Screen (Feldhaus et al., 1997) and Hurt, Insulted, Threatened, & Screamed, or HITS (Sherin, Sinacore, Li, Zitter, & Shakil, 1998).

Because intimate partner abuse can escalate to domestic homicide or homicide/suicide, lethality screening is needed for all patients who screen positive for intimate partner violence. Two reliable and valid screens for increased risk of domestic homicide patients are the Danger Assessment (Campbell, 1995) and the Harassment in Abusive Relationships: A Self-Report Scale, or HARASS (Sheridan, 1998, 2001).

Use of Hearsay Evidence

Hearsay, in general, is defined as something one has heard but does not know for sure is true. Hearsay evidence refers to what a witness has heard someone else say rather than on what he or she actually heard or saw him- or herself. It is secondhand or greater information.

In general, hearsay statements, whether they are made to a friend at school or to the nurse are usually not allowed in court, even if the statements were meticulously documented verbatim by the professional. Myers (2001) used a classic example of a child sexual-abuse case to illustrate hearsay problems. A four-year-old girl tells the health professional, "Daddy put his pee-pee in me down there (pointing to her genitalia). Then he took it out and shook it up and down until white stuff came out" (p. 545). Unless the prosecuting attorney carefully established the legal grounds by which to use this documented statement as an exception to hearsay, there is an excellent chance the judge would not allow the health professional to testify about this compelling, but none-the-less hearsay, statement made by the child. Statements are hearsay if the following requirements are met (Myers, 2001):

- The child used words to describe something that happened.
- The child spoke those words before the case went to trial, and someone who heard those words repeated them.
- The child's words were introduced in court to prove what the child said actually happened.

Excited Utterance as an Exception to Hearsay

One of the most common exceptions to hearsay is excited utterances, statements made immediately after a startling event. Myers (2001) outlined seven factors that increase the likelihood of an excited utterance being allowed as testimony in court:

Nature of the event. Judges realize there are some situations that are more alarming than others are. The more likely a judge will find the events emotionally shocking, the more likely the statement made by the patient will be usable in court.

Amount of time between the crisis event and the patient's statement. If there has been very little time between when the reported event occurred and the time the statement was made, judges are more likely to consider the statement as a hearsay exception. This time period can be from several minutes to hours, if accompanied by symptoms consistent with being excited or agitated.

Symptoms of being emotionally upset. Statements made by victims who have documented behavioral symptoms such as, crying, sobbing, shaking, and cowering have more of an impact on judges allowing them as excited utterances.

Speech patterns. Documenting if the victims speech was pressured or hurried suggests a heightened emotional state and contributes to the likelihood the statement will be usable as an excited utterance.

Spontaneity of the statement. Unsolicited statements are more likely to be viewed as part of the criteria for an excited utterance versus documented answers to series of routine screening questions on abuse and neglect.

Number and type of questions used to collect a more thorough history. Even if the victim made an initial spontaneous statement, the number and nature of the follow-up questions could adversely affect the usefulness of the statements as excited utterances. For example, if the victim was asked a series of leading or suggestive questions by the interviewer after hearing the first spontaneous statement, all of the statements would be disallowed.

First safe opportunity. If a victim has been under the control of or held captive by the reported perpetrator, statements made to the first person the victim sees when safe may qualify as an excited utterance, especially if accompanied, for example, by heightened emotional affects and pressured speech.

Statements Made to Health Professionals for Diagnosis and Treatment

Many states have exceptions to hearsay for statements made to a health professional (physician, nurse practitioner, physician assistant, registered nurse, therapist, or technician) when the statements are related to possible injury from the reported criminal act(s). The courts are more likely to hold reliable statements made to health professionals because the patient has an interest in being truthful to receive the best and most appropriate medical care. However, statements made during the course of psychotherapy are not as likely to be allowed as exceptions to hearsay (Myers, 2001).

Myers (2001) discussed points of interest to the health professional regarding the likelihood statements made for diagnostic and treatment purposes can be used in court:

- Before any specific questions are asked about the reported crime, the provider needs to preface questioning with the need for accuracy on the part of the patient in order to provide the most accurate care.
- The health information documented in the record must be pertinent to the reported crime. If the patient is being seen for pain in the left big toe but reports her ex-boyfriend struck her face five times with a closed fist, it would be difficult to connect the two in a logical way to allow the assault-related statement to be used an exception to hearsay.
- If the victim identifies the perpetrator, there needs to be a logical reason to write the reported assailant's name in the chart. Naming the battered women's ex-husband as the reported perpetrator could easily be argued as necessary for safety-planning for the victim and her children.

Fresh Complaint of Sexual Assault

In some states, if a victim states he or she was just raped or sexually assaulted, that statement may be considered a fresh complaint of rape or sexual assault. The fresh statement may be an exception to hearsay, especially if there is corroborating evidence (Myers, 2001).

The Residual Child and Elder Hearsay Exceptions

Many states have a residual hearsay exception that is written in broad-enough language to allow attorneys to argue in court that hearsay that does not fit in a specific allowed category could be used in a particular case. An increasing number of states are beginning to pass legislation to allow hearsay evidence from children and the elderly if the professionals who interviewed them can articulate why the statements made to them by the reported victims were credible and reliable.

Documenting the following type information may be very helpful in allowing child or elderly hearsay into court (Myers, 2001):

- Consistency of statements
- The affect of the patient
- Medical evidence of abuse
- Spontaneity of the patient's statements
- The patient's belief that telling the truth could result in corporal punishment or punitive sanctions

FORENSIC TERMINOLOGY

The misuse of basic forensic definitions in nursing documentation can be used by attorneys to question the accuracy and reliability of the nurse's overall assessment and written documentation. Table 13-2 lists common definitions

Table 13-2 • **Common Definitions of Forensic Terms**

	ENCYCLOPEDIA AND DICTIONARY OF MEDICINE, NURSING, AND ALLIED HEALTH	TABER'S CYCLOPEDIC MEDICAL DICTIONARY
Abrasion	A wound caused by rubbing or scraping the skin or mucous membrane	The scraping away of skin or mucous membrane as a result of injury or by mechanical means
Avulsion	The tearing away of a structure or a part	Tearing away forcibly of a part or a structure
Bruise	Superficial discoloration due to hemorrhage into tissues from ruptured blood vessels beneath the skin surface without the skin being broken	A traumatic injury (usually to the skin but some times to internal organs) in which blood vessels are broken but tissue surfaces remain intact, causing discoloration, swelling, inflammation, and pain
Burn	Injury to tissues caused by contact with dry heat (fire), moist heat (steam or liquid), chemicals, electricity, lightning, or radiation	Tissue injury resulting from excessive exposure to thermal, chemical, electrical, or radioactive agents
Contusion	An injury to tissues without breakage of skin where blood accumulates in surrounding tissues, producing pain, swelling, and tenderness; a bruise	A bruise
Cut	*See Incision*	Separating or dividing of tissues by use of a sharp surgical instrument such as a scalpel
Ecchymosis	A hemorrhagic spot, larger than a petechia, in the skin or mucous membrane, forming a nonelevated, rounded, or irregular blue or purplish patch	A bruise—that is, superficial bleeding under the skin or mucous membrane
Hematoma	A localized collection of extravasated blood, usually clotted, in an organ, space, or tissue	A swelling comprised of a mass of extravasated blood, usually clotted, and confined to an organ, tissue, or space, caused by a break in a blood vessel
Hemorrhage	The escape of blood from a ruptured vessel; can be external, internal, or into the skin or other tissues	To burst forth blood loss
Incision	A cut or wound made by a sharp instrument	A cut made with a knife, electro-surgical unit, or laser, especially for surgical purposes
Indurated	Hardened; abnormally hard	Hardened
Laceration	The act of tearing; a wound produced by the tearing of body tissue, as distinguished from a cut or incision	A wound or irregular tear of the flesh
Lesion	Any pathological or traumatic discontinuity of tissue or loss of function of a part; broad term including wounds, sores, ulcers, and tumors	A circumscribed area of pathologically altered tissue; an injury or wound
Petechia	Minute, pinpoint, nonraised, perfectly round, purplish red spots caused by intra-dermal or submucous hemorrhage, which later turn blue or yellow	Small, purplish, hemorrhagic spots on the skin that appear in patients with platelet deficiencies or febrile illness
Puncture	The act of piercing or penetrating with a pointed object or instrument	A hole or wound made by a sharp, pointed instrument
Purpura	A hemorrhagic disease characterized by extravasation of blood into the tissues, under the skin and through the mucous membranes, and producing spontaneous ecchymoses and petechiae on the skin	Any rash in which blood cells leak into the skin or mucous membranes, usually at multiple sites. Purpuric rashes are often associated with disorders of coagulation or thrombosis. Pinpoint purpuric lesions are called petechiae; larger hemorrhages into the skin are called ecchymoses
Wound	A bodily injury caused by physical means, with disruption of the normal continuity of structures	A break in the continuity of body structures caused by violence, trauma, or surgery to tissues

Table 13-3 • **Forensic Health Definitions**

FORENSIC TERM	DEFINITION
Nonindurated	Opposite of indurated; soft
Patterned injury	Imprint or pattern to tissue, usually skin, that suggests an object was used or by what mechanism the injury occurred
Pattern of injury	Injuries in various stages of healing; for example, broken bones, lacerations, or contusions

from *Taber's Cyclopedic Medical Dictionary* (Venes & Thomas, 2001) and the *Encyclopedia and Dictionary of Medicine, Nursing, and Allied Health* (Miller & Keane, 1978). Table 13-3 features common forensic health definitions that do not appear in these dictionaries. Samples of injuries and suggested descriptions are included in the Figures 13-2 through 13-11.

DOCUMENTATION

Documentation of family violence should be both written and photographic.

Written Documentation

Written documentation of histories of abuse should be as verbatim as possible. Because of time constraints in clinical settings, it is often impractical to chart extensive histories of abuse verbatim. Therefore, it is recommended the nurse chart verbatim the exact statements as to who caused the injury and any direct threats of harm the victim reports being made by the reported perpetrator (Sheridan, 2001).

The nurse needs to avoid biased or pejorative terms in her or his notes such as "patient refused," "patient uncooperative," or "patient noncompliant." For example, instead of charting "patient refused to talk with police about the assault," the nurse should chart in a more objective manner "patient did not want to talk

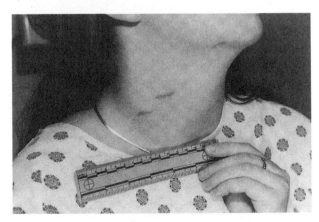

FIGURE 13-2 • Patterned, fingernail-like scratch abrasions to the right lateral neck and chin from strangulation mechanism of injury.

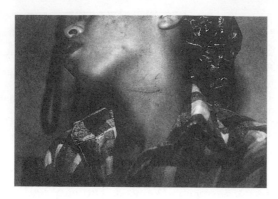

FIGURE 13-3 • Patterned, fingernail-like scratch abrasions to the left lateral neck from strangulation mechanism of injury.

with the police." If one charts "patient claims she was assaulted by her brother," the word "claims" suggests the nurse did not believe the patient. When charting abuse histories in the nursing record, it is best to preface the statements with "Patient said" or "Patient states."

Many providers chart minimally on family-violence cases in hopes they will not be called to testify. As one who has survived testifying in multiple court cases on a variety of abuse cases, I can say that it is better to have written one's original notes in detail. In fact, detailed documentation of abuse histories in the medical record has been highly recommended by the American Medical Association for more than 10 years (Flitcraft, Hadley, Hendricks-Matthews, McLeer, & Warshaw, 1992).

In addition to writing thorough and objective histories of abuse, the nurse should also use body maps and forensic photography to document abuse injuries and injuries from possible neglect. A multitude of body/injury maps are available to the nurse. However, if a body map is used, it should be one that has been officially approved by the institution's forms committee. A medical-records clerk may remove forms from the chart that are not officially approved by a given institution.

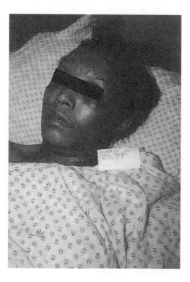

FIGURE 13-4 • Patterned, punch-like abrasion from a ring with stone to the mid-forehead; sutured partial avulsion injury to the nose; punch-like contusion to the left eye involving the sclera; and strangulation-related abrasions to the neck.

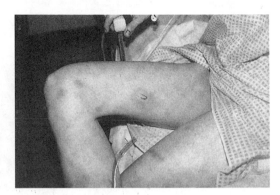

FIGURE 13-5 • Patterned, punch-like contusion to right medial thigh with a patterned imprint abrasion from ring with stone; patterned, fingertip-like contusions to right medial knee and left anterior medial thigh from a reported marital rape.

Forensic Photography

Photographs of abused patients support the cliché that pictures speak a thousand words. Whenever a suspected survivor of any form of family violence has visible injury, it is imperative the injury be photographically documented in the medical record (Sheridan, 2001). For adult abuse survivors, a signed consent-to-photograph form is recommended (see Figure 13-12). However, injuries to abused and neglected children, elderly, and the disabled can be photographed without consent in most states as part of the ongoing investigation. Consent is waived because the person who would have to grant consent is often the suspected perpetrator of abuse and neglect or may have failed to protect the patient from abuse and neglect. The most common types of cameras used in health care settings include Polaroid, 35 mm, and digital.

Polaroid Systems

Polaroid manufactures a variety of camera systems. If a Polaroid system for forensic photographic documentation of injury and neglect is available for use in one's work setting, it is recommended to buy a Spectra Law Enforcement Kit, a Macro5 Kit, or both. The Spectra system has a built-in lens that automatically is in focus from infinity to as close as two feet. The Spectra system comes with two

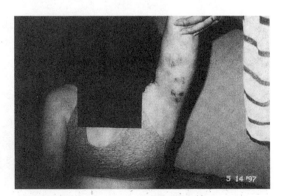

FIGURE 13-6 • Multiple, patterned, fingertip-like contusions to the left upper arm.

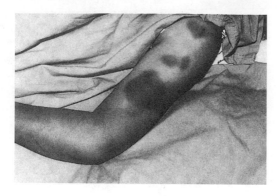

FIGURE 13-7 • Multiple patterned, punch-like contusions to the left upper arm.

lens adapters that allow one to take additional photographs from approximately 10 inches and 4 inches from the wound, respectively. The Macro5 has five built-in lenses that are preset to take images from a distance of 52 inches (0.2×), 26 inches (0.4×), 10 inches (1×), 5 inches (2×), and 3 inches (3×). Focusing the Macro5 is easily accomplished by observing converging white lights.

The advantages of Polaroid photography include its ease of use. Point the camera, and push the shutter button, and within a few minutes an in-focus color image will develop. Additional images can be immediately taken to ensure the injury has been adequately documented. Loading film into Polaroid cameras is fast and easy.

Disadvantages of using a Polaroid system include the cost of film. Whereas the Spectra camera system is approximately $250 and the Macro5 approximately $700, the cost of each Polaroid photograph averages a little more than $1. However, even if 20 Polaroid images of an abused patient are taken, the cost of the film is the least expensive part of the overall medical/nursing evaluation. Furthermore, if at least one of the Polaroid prints is useful in substantiating abuse or convicting a perpetrator of a criminal offense, the money would be well spent. Other disadvantages of Polaroid photography include the absence of negatives to make additional prints or to enlarge existing prints for court-demonstration purposes. These disadvantages have been lessened with the development and proliferation of high-quality, inexpensive color photocopiers and digital scanners.

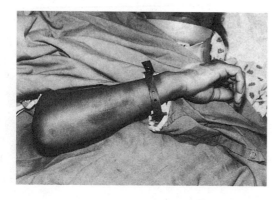

FIGURE 13-8 • Patterned, defensive, posture-like contusions to ulnar surface of the right arm.

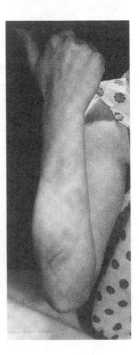

FIGURE 13-9 • Patterned, defensive posture-like contusions to the right lower arm.

35-mm Color Photography

The forensic gold standard for photographically documenting abused and neglected patients is a 35-mm camera (Besant-Matthews & Smock, 2001). Disposable cameras and inexpensive 35-mm cameras that have a fixed focal length of only four feet should never be used for forensic photography. The quality of the photographs and the inability to obtain, in-focus, close-up images of injuries or the sequelae of medical neglect makes cheap cameras forensically useless.

Scores of good 35-mm cameras are on the market from a variety of major manufacturers. There is a wide variance in price; however, a decent 35-mm camera with zoom capabilities, an adequate flash, and focal length of at least two feet before using macro-lens adapters can be purchased for around $300. Many cameras with variable lenses will allow one to zoom in and out. The 100–105-mm

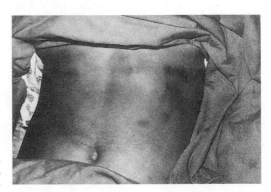

FIGURE 13-10 • Patterned, hidden, punch-like contusions to the upper abdomen, lower anterior chest.

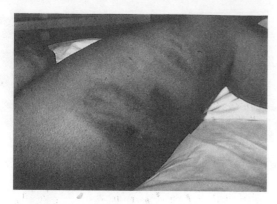

FIGURE 13-11 • Patterned, foot kick/stomp-like contusion to the right, superior lateral thigh, pushing blood outward from the point of impact, and patterned, foot kick/stomp-like contusion to the right inferior lateral thigh.

lens is among the most popular and is ideal for general patient, injury, and autopsy photography (Besant-Matthews & Smock, 2001). Most 35-mm cameras on the market today have "automatic" features that make their use much more user friendly than cameras of days gone by.

Advantages of 35-mm photography are many and include the ability to make duplicate copies from negatives and to enlarge the images for court-demonstration purposes. The quality of 35-mm images is usually superior to Polaroid images, especially if quality, high-resolution film is used. It is recommended that one use 35-mm print film.

The disadvantages of 35 mm include time delays between taking the photograph and getting the film developed and empty or damaged negatives. With the proliferation of one-hour photo-development stores, the time delay in developing film is less of a disadvantage than it was previously. If the film is not correctly threaded into the camera spool or is not totally rewound before opening the camera back, the images will be either never recorded or overexposed prior to development.

When using 35-mm print film, use 12-exposure film with a recommended film speed of ISO 200 to 400. There should never be more than one victim or case on a role of film. Most injuries to a particular victim can be adequately recorded on one roll of 12-exposure film. If the abused patient has multiple injuries, use multiple roles. A forensic nurse who photographs the scene(s) of suspected abuse or neglect would be better off using rolls of 24-exposure print film. Never waste remaining shots on a roll of film on silly or extraneous poses; simply rewind the roll of film whenever finished taking pictures of injuries from all viewpoints.

In recent years, the market has been flooded with all types, shapes, and sizes of digital cameras at prices that make them affordable to most people. Digital cameras do not use film; rather, they capture and store data bits on disks or memory files within the camera. The data bits can then be transferred to a computer for processing and storage. Digital photographic images are rapidly becoming part of forensic investigations in many jurisdictions.

The advantages of digital are many. One instantly knows if the injury being photographed is captured or not. The stored images can be reproduced and printed as often as needed and as large as needed. The digital images can be electronically transmitted almost instantly via the Internet for expert forensic consultation. If taken correctly, digital images approach the quality in detail of 35-mm prints.

University of Louisville Hospital

PHOTOGRAPH/INTERVIEW CONSENT

Medical Record No.
Name
Unit/Bed

Date	Unit	Name of Patient

I, _____, authorize the party named

below to photograph, videotape and/or interview _____

while a patient at University of Louisville Hospital. I release University of Louisville Hospital from any and all

liability which may arise from the use of these photographs, tapes or interviews. I waive all rights I may have

for any claims for payment in connection with any exhibition, televising or publication of said photographs.

X	TYPE OF CONSENT	YES	NO
	1. Interview		
	2. Photograph		
	3. Video Taping		
Please indicate location where photographs/tapes will be stored (cannot be stored in Medical Records)			

X	PURPOSE OF CONSENT	YES	NO
	1. Public Relations Purposes (newspapers, radio, television)		
	2. Legal Purposes		
	3. Educational Purposes		
	4. Personal Reasons		

Name of Person Conducting Photo/Taping/Interview Session	Title of Person		
Name of Organization Being Represented			
Address of Organization	City	State	Zip Code	Telephone No.
Signature of Patient/Legal Guardian	Date	Relationship to Patient	
Witness	Title		Date

ULH/600-113(10/96)

FIGURE 13-12 • Consent-to-photograph form. From Olshaker, J. S., Jackson, M. C., & Smock, W. S. (2001). *Forensic emergency medicine*. Philadelphia: Lippincott Williams & Wilkins.

Disadvantages of digital photography are also many. A good digital camera costs more than $500 and is usually more complex to use than other modes of photography. Training all staff who may have to use the digital camera can be a challenge. Furthermore, a system needs to be developed within clinical settings to transfer the data from the camera to a computer. The data then need to be stored (burned) on a CD-ROM that will serve as the "negative." Someone has to print the images onto special paper via a quality color printer using special computer software. In addition, digital cameras can be easily stolen from the clinical sites. This is true of all cameras, but because digital cameras are usually small and in high demand, they are especially susceptible to theft.

Another major disadvantage to using digital cameras as part of a forensic medical documentation is the ease in which the images can be altered or manipulated. Despite the possibility of image alteration, more and more courts are allowing digital images, especially if the images are immediately stored on an unalterable disk.

Rule of Thirds

No matter what type of camera is used for forensic documentation, the images of the abused/neglected patient should be taken using a concept called rule of thirds. The very first photographic image should be an overall image of the patient, preferably from head to toe. Each injury should have a minimum of three images recorded. The first should be from several feet away so the injury is clearly in context as to who the victim is and where on the body the injury is located. The second image should cut the distance by a third and be more focused on the injury. The last image with regular lenses should again be cut by another third. This image should be at distance of about two feet from the actual injury. If one is using a camera system that allows for the use of macro lenses, closer images of the injury should be taken, especially if the close-up views document the presence (or absence) of trace evidence or a patterned injury.

Avoid Being an "Expert" in Photography

No matter what camera system is used, the nurse should never describe him- or herself as an expert photographer, even if the nurse is quite knowledgeable about cameras and photography. When on the witness stand, and especially during a hostile cross-examination, it is best to keep the questions focused on the actual injuries and one's nursing assessment and not on the technologies and idiosyncrasies of photographic techniques. A minor error in the nurse's testimony on photographic theory can allow the attorney to question the standard of nursing care. In general, if a nurse takes a picture, he or she has only to testify that the injuries depicted in the photographic are a true and accurate likeness of what he or she saw and treated on the date and time of health services.

All photographic images need to labeled with, at least, the following information:

- Patient's name
- Patient's medical identification number
- Patient's date of birth
- The date and time of the photograph
- The name of the photographer
- The body location of the injury
- The forensic case number (if known)

Consent Issues

Most states allow photographs of suspected abused and neglected children without consent of the parents, as part of the ongoing investigation. For the seriously injured, unconscious, or cognitively impaired patient, implied consent is a legal construct that allows providers to take photographs immediately. This is especially important if waiting for the patient to improve to the point to give informed consent would result in the inability to photographically document the injury or trace evidence (Besant-Matthews & Smock, 2001). Efforts to subsequently obtain signed consent either from the later cognitively improved patient or from a family member should be made and documented in the health record.

In all cases in which signed consent to photograph has been obtained, the completed form must be part of the official health record according to the institution's policy and procedure. Failure to have the consent in the health record may prevent the medical images from becoming part of a court proceeding.

SUMMARY

The nurse, no matter where he or she practices, is in a unique position to be one of the very first people outside the abusive home or institution to learn about the severe physical, sexual, and psychological trauma being inflicted to vulnerable patients. Most nurses have had little to no training in the forensic identification and documentation of abuse survivors. Forensic nursing is the fastest growing specialty in nursing, and this chapter is only an introduction to basic forensic-nursing skills. Readers interested in ongoing educational and career opportunities in forensic nursing should explore the website for the International Association of Forensic Nursing (http://www.iafn.org).

References

Administration of Children, Youth, and Families. (1999). *Child maltreatment 1997. Reports from the states to the National Child Abuse and Neglect Data System.* Washington, D.C.: U.S. Department of Health and Human Services.

Administration of Children, Youth, and Families. (2000). *Child maltreatment in 1998. Reports from the states to the National Child Abuse and Neglect Data System.* Washington, D.C.: U.S. Department of Health and Human Services.

American Medical Association. (1992). *Strategies for the treatment and prevention of sexual assault.* Chicago: Author.

Aravanis, C., Adelman, R. D., Breckman, R., Fulmer, T. T., Holder, E., Lachs, M., O'Brien, J. G., & Sanders, A. B. (1992). *Diagnostic and treatment guidelines on elder abuse and neglect.* Chicago: American Medical Association.

Baker, A. A. (1975). Granny battering. *Modern Geriatrics, 5,* 20–24.

Bays, J. (2001). Conditions mistaken for child physical abuse. In R. M. Reece & S. Ludwig (Eds.), *Child abuse: Medical diagnosis and management* (pp. 177–206). Philadelphia, PA: Lippincott Williams & Wilkins.

Berkowitz, C. D., Bross, D. C., Chadwick, D. L., & Whitworth, J. M. (1992a). *Diagnostic and treatment guidelines on child physical abuse and neglect.* Chicago: American Medical Association.

Berkowitz, C. D., Bross, D. C., Chadwick, D. L., & Whitworth, J. M. (1992b). *Diagnostic and treatment guidelines on child physical abuse and neglect.* Chicago: American Medical Association.

Besant-Matthews, P. E., & Smock, W. S. (2001). Forensic photography in the emergency department. In J. S. , M. C. Jackson, & W. S. Smock (Eds.), *Forensic emergency medicine* (pp. 257–282). Philadelphia, PA: Lippincott Williams & Wilkins.

Burston, G. R. (1975). Granny-battering. *British Medical Journal, 3,* 592.

Caffey, J. (1946). Multiple fractures in long bones in infants suffering from chronic subdural hematoma. *American Journal of Roentgenology, 56*(2), 163–173.

Campbell, J. C. (1995). Prediction of homicide of and by battered women. In J. C. Campbell (Ed.), *Assessing dangerousness: Violence by sexual offenders, batterers, and child abusers* (pp. 96–113). Thousand Oak, CA: Sage Publications.

Campbell, J. C., Soeken, K. L., McFarlane, J., & Parker, B. (1998). Risk factors for femicide among pregnant and nonpregnant battered women. In J. C. Campbell (Ed.), *Empowering survivors of abuse: Health care for battered women and their children.* Thousand Oaks, CA: Sage.

Criminal Code of Oregon. (2002). Salem, OR: Legislative Counsel Committee.

Feldhaus, K. M., Kozoil-McLain, J., Amsbury, H. L., Norton, I. M., Lowenstein, S. R., & Abbott, J. T. (1997). Accuracy of 3 brief screening questions for detecting partner violence in the emergency department. *Journal of the American Medical Association, 277*(17), 1357–1361.

Flitcraft, A. H., Hadley, S. M., Hendricks-Matthews, M. K., McLeer, S. V., & Warshaw, C. (1992). *Diagnostic and treatment guidelines on domestic violence.* Chicago: American Medical Association.

Geroff, A. J., & Olshaker, J. S. (2001). Elder abuse. In J. S. Olshaker, M. C. Jackson & W. S. Smock (Eds.), *Forensic emergency medicine* (pp. 173–202). Philadelphia, PA: Lippincott Williams & Wilkins.

Gielan, A., C., O'Campo, P. J., Campbell, J. C., Schollenberger, J., Woods, A. B., Jones, A. S., Dienemann, J. A., Kub, J., & Wynne, C. (2001). Women's opinions about reporting domestic violence screening and mandatory reporting. *American Journal of Preventive Medicine, 19*(4), 279–285.

Girardin, B. W., Faugno, D. K., Seneski, P. C., Slaughter, L., & Whelan, M. (1997). *Color atlas of sexual assault.* St. Louis, MO: Mosby.

Helton, A. (1987). *Protocol of care for the battered woman.* White Plains, NY: March of Dimes Birth Defects Foundation.

Hyman, A., Schillinger, D., & Lo, B. (1995). Laws mandating reporting of domestic violence: Do they promote patient well-being? *Journal of the American Medical Association, 273*(22), 1781–1787.

Kempe C. H., Silverman, F. N., Steele, B. F., Droegmueller, W. & Silver, H. K. (1962). The battered-child syndrome. *Journal of the American Medical Association, 181*(1), 17–24.

McFarlane, J., Greenberg, L., Weltge, A., & Watson, M. (1995). Identification of abuse in emergency departments: Effectiveness of a two-question screening tool. *Journal of Emergency Nursing, 21*(5), 391–394.

McFarlane, J., Parker, B., Soeken, K., & Bullock, L. (1992). Assessing for abuse during pregnancy: Severity and frequency of injuries and associated entry into prenatal care. *Journal of the American Medical Association, 267*(23), 3176–3178.

Miller, B. F., & Keane, C. B. (1978). *Encyclopedia and Dictionary of Medicine, Nursing, and Allied Health.* Philadelphia, PA: Saunders.

Myers, J. E. B. (2001). Medicolegal aspects of child abuse. In R. M. Reece & S. Ludwig (Eds.), *Child abuse: Medical diagnosis and management* (pp. 545–562). Philadelphia, PA: Lippincott Williams & Wilkins.

Sheridan, D. J. (1998). *Measuring harassment of abused women: A nursing concern.* Unpublished doctoral dissertation, Oregon Health Sciences University, Portland.

Sheridan, D. J. (2001). Treating survivors of intimate partner abuse. In J. S. Olshaker, M. C. Jackson & W. S. Smock (Eds.), *Forensic emergency medicine* (pp. 203–228). Philadelphia, PA: Lippincott Williams & Wilkins.

Sherin, K. M., Sinacore, J. M., Li, X.-Q., Zitter, R. E., & Shakil, A. (1998). HITS: A short domestic violence screening tool for use in a family practice setting. *Family Medicine, 30*(7), 508–512.

Suggs, A., Lichenstein, R., McCarthy, C., & Jackson, M. C. (2001). Child abuse/assault–General. In J. S. Olshaker, M. C. Jackson & W. S. Smock (Eds.), *Forensic emergency medicine* (pp. 151–171). Philadelphia, PA: Lippincott Williams & Wilkins.

Venes, D. & Thomas, C. L. (Eds.). (2001). *Taber's Cyclopedic Medical Dictionary* (19th ed.). Philadelphia, PA: FA Davis.

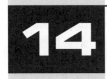

Future Directions

• Angela Henderson, Rachel Rodriguez, Terry Fulmer, and Janice Humphreys

Family violence is a major health concern. This is true not only in North America but also around the world (Heise, 1994; Heise, Raikes, Watts, & Zwi, 1994); indeed, it has been labeled "the intolerable status quo" (Bunch, 1997, p. 40) and identified as a violation of human rights of enormous proportions (Renzetti, Edleson, & Kennedy Bergen, 2001). Family violence has also been identified as an important area for the involvement of health care professionals, including nurses, but health care professionals have not always been effective in this work (Butler, 1995; Pahl, 1995). Family violence, in all its forms, affects everyone on all levels. It restricts and injures people. It severely curtails the functioning of families and limits their capacity as the main support of the individual and their effectiveness as contributors to the community. Communities are forced to commit scarce financial, legal, and social-service resources to deal with its various manifestations (Handivsky & Greaves, 1996; Johnson & Sacco, 1995; Zorza, 1995). Lastly, we fall short as moral and ethical individuals and as a culture when we fail to effectively address the needs of some of society's most disadvantaged members, those affected by family violence.

Taking action, of course, is not easy. If it were, the problem of family violence would have been resolved years ago. Preceding chapters have explored the theoretical background of aggression, violence, and abuse, and explored family violence in relation to individuals and families at all stages of life. The legal and forensic nursing responses to family violence have been discussed. This chapter focuses on nursing's future directions in the field of family violence. Implications for nursing practice and education, research ethics, and health policy are explored in this context. A number of ideas and assumptions should be kept in mind throughout this chapter. They provide a framework with which to understand the complexity of these issues and a context in which to understand the nursing-care needs of survivors of family violence.

First, nurses should function in multidisciplinary teams in which the contributions of all members are understood and valued. Interdisciplinary collaboration is becoming the norm. It is a particularly vital notion, however, with regard to the people who have experienced family violence. A multidisciplinary approach, when working with those experiencing abuse, helps to ensure a coordinated response and makes it less likely that people fall through the cracks. It also increases the possibility of devising complex, multifaceted interventions geared to a specific individual. This is particularly important because individuals in complicated situations are likely to be in involved in several different systems.

Second, nurses must understand the larger picture. They work within but one part of the health care system; that system operates as part of a larger whole. Health care institutions, health care providers, administrators, and policymakers confront ever more stringent restrictions on health care spending, thereby limiting the resources needed to address family violence. At the same time, community resources, such as shelters, women's centers, child-care agencies, and convalescent homes, also face cutbacks and, in some cases, closure at a time when their clients' situations are becoming more acute and more complex (Agnew, 1998). This raises several questions. To what extent do individuals act under their own control and to what extent are their actions mediated by their circumstances? How do health care providers set priorities when allocating increasingly scarce resources? Whatever policy decisions, actions, and services are decided on, the scarcity of funds is the context in which they will be implemented. In providing health care services, it is important to remember that globalization and highly mobile societies influence us all. We are all part of an international community in which the members of different cultures and nations are interacting with and affecting each other, moving freely from place to place. This is a strength in many ways, but it also increases the complexity of health care delivery for providers, decision makers, and policy designers. In such a climate, the many skills that nurses possess—listening, communicating, teaching and supporting—will be increasingly valuable.

Third, in recognizing the complexity of an individual's circumstances, nurses must understand that many factors influence an individual's ability to act independently or in his or her best interest. Poverty, health status (mental and physical), race, class, creed, language ability, substance abuse, sexual orientation, and urban or rural residence all have profound implications for an individual's ability to access the services and resources he or she needs (Radomsky, 1995; Russell, Hightower, & Gutman, 1996). For example, no one is simply an abused woman; she is an abused poor woman, African-American woman, or Punjabi-speaking mother of five living with her husband's parents. All of these circumstances contribute to her unique situation and should be taken into account when designing interventions to meet her needs.

Lastly, because nurses and other health care providers working in the field of family violence may not have always been effective, nursing must address the reasons for that lack of effectiveness. It is clear from nurses' accounts that there are many reasons, some of which are structural, environmental, and personal (Henderson, 2001a; 2001b). Because many of them are personal, nurses working with survivors of family violence, or indeed those who work in any sensitive area, must willingly explore their own beliefs, values, and influences in relation to the topic to ensure their personal biases do not negatively influence their approaches. As you read this chapter, reflect on the issue under discussion and be aware of your reactions to it. Introspection is an essential part of effective nursing, particularly so when caring for family-violence survivors who frequently are embarrassed or ashamed by what they consider a stigmatizing condition and who are acutely sensitive to a caregiver's demeanor.

These then are some of the complex factors that complicate working with people experiencing family violence. Paradoxically, they are also factors that suggest some of the most effective solutions to the problems of individual patients or clients. Accounting for these issues when planning your nursing approach means, for example, that you understand the importance of knowing about local resources that are open to new clients. It means automatically considering which other professionals are needed in the situation and what their contributions should be. It means understanding the impact of language barriers or religious beliefs on an individual's willingness to take specific actions on their own behalf. Lastly, it means recognizing one's own particular "buttons" and understanding their influences on your approach to a situation. Consideration of all these areas will enable nurses to take a nonjudgmental and supportive approach to planning excellent nursing care.

NURSING THEORY AND FAMILY VIOLENCE

The development of nursing theory of domestic violence is evolving, although considerable work remains to be done. Much of the research to date has studied women's experiences and explanations about their violent relationships and their experiences and behaviors related to leaving their abusers. Examples of some recent contributions to nursing-theory development follow.

A case study by Belknap (2000) presents an interpretive reading of one woman's story using Gilligan's theory of moral reasoning. Throughout the article, Belknap described "Eva's story" (p. 1), the account of a Mexican-American woman who survived years of severe abuse at the hands of her mother's boyfriend. By conducting four interpretive readings, Belknap described the different levels of moral transitioning that Eva went through as she described her abuse and the decisions she made as she moved through, and eventually out of, the relationship. This study, along with other work by Belknap, offers nurses a theoretical grounding in moral decision-making that provides insight into battered women's decision-making.

Clark, Pendry, and Kim (1997) discussed an emerging theory of freedom-seeking behavior in their study of homeless women in a domestic-violence shelter. In-depth interviews with four black women and three white women reported patterns in their violent relationships and their "awakening" (p. 6) when they decided to leave their abusers. Four patterns of violence emerged from the data. The first, appearing in the early stages of the relationship, was described as "Camelot and broken promises" (p. 4). In the second phase, there was increased isolation and shame associated with the physical signs of abuse. This phase also included harassment and humiliation. The third phase was marked by themes of power, placation, and terror. Finally, the awakening, a realization that the woman must end the relationship, was accompanied by "murderous thoughts, and escape" (p. 6). These four phases, and the emerging theory of freedom-seeking offered by Clark and others, can assist nurses in assessment and intervention by understanding which phase a battered woman is in and which strategies may be the most helpful.

The work of Wuest and Merrit-Gray (1999) is beneficial in understanding how a woman sustains separation from her abuser and reclaims her sense of self. In this grounded-theory study, the authors described one of the stages in the process of reclaiming the self, the stage they call "not going back" (p. 5). Within this stage are two subprocesses identified by these researchers as "claiming and maintaining territory and relentless justifying" (p. 6). Claiming and maintaining territory involves finding a safe and stable place to live. Relentless justifying describes how women gain and maintain their credibility as survivors of abuse and, therefore, justify themselves as deserving of assistance and support. According to the authors, "previous research has begun to clarify how women prepare to leave abusive relationships and the crises involved in leaving" (p. 12). The process of not going back is one part of the explanatory theory developed by

Wuest and Merritt-Gray for the purpose of furthering nurses' understanding of the long-term process of leaving a violent relationship.

Kearney (2001) discussed the results of a grounded-theory approach to analyzing 13 qualitative research studies (of which 7 were nursing research); her goal was to synthesize the results into a theory of "women's experiences in violent relationships that would be grounded in diverse qualitative reports and relevant across geographic and sociocultural contexts" (p. 270). This analysis produced a model she described as "enduring love" (p. 279). Enduring love can further the nurse's role as an advocate for battered women through an increased understanding of the abusive relationship's dynamics. Kearney added that the theory of enduring love is not presented as new or original, as it was crafted from the work of others. Rather, she invited challenge and refutation. By discussing the limitations of this analysis, the author opened the door for continued discourse and further research regarding theory development in this area.

Although some of the previous examples included women of color, theory development lacks nursing research that includes women of color and other marginalized women, such as lesbians, immigrants, and sex workers. Further research is also needed regarding women who choose to stay in violent relationships. For example, understanding the sociocultural underpinnings of how intimate relationships are formed in a particular group can contribute to nursing's understanding of how women will view their options when a relationship becomes violent.

Developing and testing nursing theory in the area of domestic violence is critical to designing and evaluating appropriate nursing interventions for the care of battered women.

NURSING RESEARCH AND FAMILY VIOLENCE

Nurses have conducted some of the most important research in the area of family violence. Nursing has a holistic focus, one that enhances the complexities of individual and family functioning. These characteristics among others make the profession particularly well-suited to conduct meaningful research in the area of family violence. Over the years, nurses have made significant contributions in all of the areas of family violence discussed in this book.

Major advances in nursing research in the field of family violence over the past decade were summarized in two recent reviews (Campbell & Parker, 1999; Humphreys, Parker, & Campbell, 2001). As these authors pointed out, both qualitative and quantitative approaches have been used extensively to document various aspects of the issues. Over the past decade, qualitative methods have illustrated the perspective of adult survivors of family violence, of children who either witness or are the direct recipients of abuse, of members of culturally diverse groups, of those in same-sex relationships, and of those providing services to survivors (Arroyo & Eth, 1995; Henderson, 2001b; Johnson & Ferraro; 2000; Renzetti et al., 2001).

Research into violence during pregnancy and battered women's psychological responses to abuse have received considerable attention. Research into violence during pregnancy accounts for 20% of all the reviewed nursing research. The largely qualitative research into women's psychological responses to violence is particularly rich and remarkably similar across multiple studies. International studies on intimate partner violence are beginning to appear in the literature, and research that addresses the unique experience of ethnically diverse women is occurring with greater frequency (Humphreys, Parker, & Campbell, 2001, p. 277).

Nurse researchers have been particularly instrumental in showing the efficacy of universal screening for abuse during pregnancy, during visits to emergency departments, and at other points where women encounter health care professionals (Grunfeld, Hotch, & MacKay, 1996; Shepard, Elliott, Falk, & Regal; 1999). It is clear that universal screening is an important tool that should be used in every health care encounter, in all settings, and with people in any type of family constellation. Nursing recognizes that violence can occur in any relationship, that many people presenting for reasons unrelated to abuse will nevertheless be experiencing it, and that there is a "lack of personal or demographic characteristics that can identify women more likely to be abused" (Campbell & Parker, 1999, p. 555). Nursing research has been successful in illustrating that screening improves identification of and intervention with abused women and in showing that education of health care professionals improves screening rates. Research has also shown that women want to be asked the question and that nurses can be enormously effective in working with abused women and their children (Campbell, 1998; Davies, Lyon, & Monti-Catania, 1998).

Much of the earlier work was conducted with small samples using descriptive approaches, and these studies have helped to build a rich, client-centered base of knowledge about client perspectives. Studies using quantitative methods are increasing as larger population-based studies, longitudinal studies, and predictive studies are undertaken. Recognizing the important contribution that qualitative and quantitative research both make in the area of family violence has been a particular strength of nursing research over the years.

Ethics

The topics that are receiving research attention are becoming increasing sophisticated, subtle, complex, and, therefore, more demanding in terms of planning and execution. This evolution requires recognizing the importance of ethics in nursing on violence (Campbell & Dienemann, 2001). Several characteristics of violence research raise ethical concerns and dilemmas, including safety issues, both in relation to those experiencing the violence and those conducting the research, the vulnerability of the research population, the sensitive value-laden nature of the topic, particular subtleties with regard to informed consent, confidentiality, and dissemination of findings. As Campbell and Dienemann pointed out, there is often no obvious "right" answer to ethical questions, and "resolution depends on reflexive contemplation of the context, ethical principles and viewpoints of participants, as well as the experience and best judgment of the researcher" (pp. 57–58). As research in family violence increases in sophistication, so will the level of complexity increase in relation to the ethical issues involved. Those contemplating research in this area must think through these issues before embarking on their studies.

Safety

Clearly, safety is a major concern when working in the area of family violence. It is important, for example, to recognize that violent individuals tend to have poor impulse control and feel justified in their violence. A violent tendency and lack of impulse control is a dangerous combination and may place at risk both those who are recipients of such violence, based simply on their participation, and those who conduct the research. For this reason, researchers must pay particular attention to designing safety protocols in anticipation of problems. When conducting research in family violence, the level of physical danger should not preclude a study but it should emphasize the importance of careful planning. Every phase of the process needs to be considered from the perspective of safety. How will research participants be recruited? How will research assistants be trained? How will people get to the interviews? How will they get home again? How will one know if it's safe to talk when conducting a telephone interview? How will one store, analyze, and disseminate the findings in such a way as to ensure confidentiality? How will one help research assistants and research participants recognize the need for safety? All these points must be considered when developing a protocol for safety.

Vulnerability

Those who experience family violence are vulnerable. Not only are women and children individually vulnerable but the population of which they are a part may also have particular vulnerabilities that make research with them particularly challenging. Several examples help illustrate this point. Members of diverse populations may be reluctant to talk with researchers because they are loath to expose the group to negative judgment from a dominant culture. Women in rural areas may be worried that, if they talk to researchers, the whole community will be aware of the meeting. The experiences of those who do not speak English may be missed by researchers because appropriate translators are unavailable. This list illustrates the complexity of women's experiences and emphasizes the need to recognize that individuals live in complicated circumstances.

Given the statistics on abuse and violence, research participants are not the only ones who should be considered when planning studies. There may be vulnerable individuals among the research assistants and the support staff and among the principle investigators. Protocols for safety should include plans for regular check-ins with all members of the research team and also should include a mechanism whereby individuals can initiate a debriefing if they become upset during a particular interview. It is easy to forget how distressing it might be, for example, to be alone and typing an interview with an abused women if one is unfamiliar with such content.

Violence Research and Values

All research is value laden in that it comes from a particular interest area and is initiated by a researcher working from a particular perspective, within a particular framework, and with a set of particular, potential outcomes in mind. All research should have as its goal the improvement of the human condition, whether by knowing more about it, showing the efficacy of some intervention, or illustrating relationships between factors. Many researchers in the field of violence research work within paradigms that are openly emancipatory. One of the most recognized tenets of such paradigms is that research must have the potential to improve the conditions of the research participants and the groups they represent; indeed, the group is often included in the design and conduct of the research (Campbell & Dienemann, 2001). In this paradigm, the obvious overlap between research as an academic enterprise and research as a political act is much more explicit. On one hand, this is a strength because it should help ensure relevant, practice-grounded research. On the other hand, it theoretically raises concern that personal biases and convictions might be allowed to contaminate the scientific rigor of studies. This makes the process of researcher reflexivity extremely important in studies coming from an emancipatory framework and also underlines the importance of critically assessing the procedures used and the claims made for research findings.

Informed Consent, Confidentiality, and Dissemination of Findings

Because of the sensitive nature of the information being gathered in family-violence research, issues of informed consent must be given careful consideration. It may not always be clear to participants, or indeed to the researcher, what is being consented to. For instance, material under discussion tends to be more personal, is covered in greater detail, and is often being discussed with someone with whom a participant has developed a closer relationship than is common in most research. Researchers must be sensitive to the need for ongoing informed consent because, though such in-depth interviews may be empowering, the potential to reveal more than was intended and the potential for subtle coercion are always issues. Some recollections may be triggered during an interview that a participant has long since forgotten, is distressed by, and did not anticipate talking about. Verifying that a participant is still comfortable with the topic under discussion is a good strategy. A participant may not regret disclosures until after an interview is over, so it important to inform participants that they can withdraw consent after the interview or that they can withhold a particular piece of information. It is also a good strategy to ask research participants to paraphrase the consent form as they are signing it so that the researcher can be sure they understand its implications. Lastly, it is a good idea, as part of the consent process, to discuss how the information will be disseminated with participants. This strategy can help researchers to understand the particularly sensitive parts of a story. This understanding can be crucial in the dissemination phase, particularly in relation to qualitative articles, when the inclusion of a good, "juicy" verbatim story can be a strong temptation.

Future Directions

A number of areas appear to be particularly relevant for future nursing research in family violence. Several of these derive from the previous discussion of ethics. For example, there is increasing interest in participatory-action research in which the impetus for the research comes from and is grounded in the community. Indeed, this approach is often considered by community activists to be a necessary and defining characteristic of emancipatory approaches. Although there is inherent value in involving the community, defining the strengths and limitations of such collaborations and explicitly outlining guidelines under which such studies can work need consideration. Attention to the conditions in which participatory approaches are best used will result in relevant and timely studies.

In many areas of research, multidisciplinary collaboration is becoming the norm. Increasingly funding institutions insist, as a condition of funding, that researchers show that truly collaborative partnerships exist. In family-violence research, such partnerships can yield particularly rich results because survivors are, over time, so often in contact with different components of the system. A woman and her children, for example, may be in contact—at the same time—with the health care, social-welfare, and criminal-justice systems as well as with community grass-roots organizations. It is clearly in everyone's best interest that the various systems understand and respect the contributions of each other. Collaborative research can help explicate and clarify these contributions because a researcher can often bring together so many disparate groups.

In recognizing the importance of multidisciplinary collaboration, research must also focus on the intersection of social, criminal, and health policy. Recognizing the influence of such factors as poverty and homelessness on health, coupled with an understanding of factors like violence on a family's likelihood to be poor or homeless, will help in recognizing the huge impact of violence in families' lives. Nursing, with its focus on the factors influencing individual and family functioning and on those factors' influence on health, is in a good position to initiate, coordinate, and conduct research from such a holistic standpoint.

Nurses, for the same reasons, are well-positioned to undertake research into the impact of violence on the lives of individuals and families who face special challenges. Such challenges might include, for example, being a visible minority or a recent immigrant, being unable to speak English, being disabled, and being in some other marginalized group, such as lesbians or those who live in a rural community. Nurses are used to working with individuals with complex health concerns and so are well-positioned to understand the importance of research integrating the impact of violence with other intersecting concerns.

Nurse researchers must continue valuing the qualitative and quantitative approaches to research and using them both in the generation and testing of interventions designed to address family violence. Ongoing longitudinal studies are needed in which interventions are identified, tested, evaluated, and refined in all areas of family-violence research. Interventions are needed in primary, secondary, and tertiary prevention and must be rigorously tested and systematically integrated to form a foundation for evidence-based practice. Program-evaluation research also needs to be conducted to evaluate the efficacy of programs aimed at survivors of family violence.

NURSING PRACTICE AND FAMILY VIOLENCE

Family violence can only be addressed when there is vigilant screening and assessment to impact the progression and outcomes. To date, little has been required in undergraduate education, and only recently, in certain states, has mandatory education on the topic of child abuse and neglect been required for professionals. Every curriculum at all levels should have required content on family violence with appropriate education related to theory, research, and practice responsibilities, including available screening and assessment instruments. Some literature suggests that single-item screening is effective with women, but its effectiveness across all age groups is yet to be tested (Wasson et al., 2000).

Whether an individual uses single-item screening or a more extensive screen, however, screening and assessment must take place in all care settings and across all age groups. The importance of creating systems that require screening and assessment as a part of standard practice must be underscored. The content for screening and assessment protocols may vary according to age groups. For example, child-rearing patterns will be particularly important to understand when child abuse is suspected. Conflict resolution and conflict tactics, however, should be addressed in all age groups. The Conflict Tactic Scale (CTS) created by Straus (1978) should be a required screen whenever there is a suspicion that violence may evolve from volatile situations.

Standardized protocols are extremely useful to practitioners who are uncertain as to what information they should gather. Although such protocols are sometimes limiting, they create an approach that engages practitioners who are not yet comfortable with routine screening for family violence. It is highly unlikely, in the absence of protocols that are required for family-violence screening, that the engaging will take place at all.

Each encounter with the health care system provides an opportunity for family-violence screening and assessment. Hospitals, community-based organizations, and home visits each afford an opportunity not only to observe for high-risk situations but also to specifically ask whether a client would like to discuss any violence or mistreatment. This is not simply an emergency-department issue once symptoms have presented. Proactive screening in all settings will provide an important opportunity for clinicians and patients to discuss this taboo issue.

Further, family-violence screening should not be limited to traditional family constellations. Domestic violence in lesbian, gay, transgender, and bisexual communities needs specific, research-based practice protocols. Adolescents living together should be approached with the same screening and assessment rigor as used with other age groups. College campuses have seen an increase in violent behavior between partners, and efforts should be made to work more closely with these institutions and all occupational-health service officers to get procedures in place to stem the tide of family violence.

Mandatory reporting laws for abused children and older adults are currently in effect in most states, and, while they provide some impetus for intervention, no systematic research studies explain the impact of mandatory reporting on outcomes related to family violence. This is an important issue that should be addressed in the very near future.

Intervention

Intervention strategies should be carefully crafted to recognize the autonomy of individuals. Respect for self-determination may prevent patients from withdrawing once a patient seems concerned that family-violence histories are being taken. A high degree of discomfort and shame is related to being victimized, particularly if a loved one is the perpetrator. Careful attention should be paid to older adults with cognitive impairment because it has been proven that they are at higher risk for mistreatment and will be unlikely to give a comprehensive health history.

Protocols for safety planning must be in place to insure that appropriate actions can be taken once family violence is detected. Knowledge of safe havens and shelters, along with any costs, is important information in the planning process. In some instances, a protective-service admission may be required in a hospital setting until a safe haven can be found. When victims of family violence refuse intervention, it is important to provide them with a list of appropriate telephone numbers and shelters in the event that they decide to accept intervention later. The importance of documentation cannot be overstated, and such documentation should be carefully scripted within the context of existing protocols. If no such protocol is available, administrators should be asked for guidance to insure a consistent approach that is acceptable to practitioners and legal counsel alike.

Diversity

The issues of diversity and vulnerability with regard to marginalized individuals are often given lip service without careful analyses and planning. To date, little information explains how people behave in different cultures and what is acceptable to other cultures. In the United States, however, assault and battery is against the law, and this should be a guiding principle. Sensitivity to diversity can still be present, even when national norms of the United States are respected. Elderly immigrants, for example, are at multiple risk given language barriers, atypical social norms, potential financial constraints, and living arrangements that might include living with violent family members. Maintaining contact, providing multilingual documents that list contact information for safe havens and care planning, and assuring all people that they have a place to contact when they need support are important aspects of comprehensive nursing care for those who may be victims of family violence.

Professional nurses must stay abreast of the latest developments and professional practice guidelines as discussed in national forums such as the American Nurses Association and the American Medical Association. Advance-practice nurses and nurse scientists with expertise in family violence need to participate in policy discussions to inform interdisciplinary groups on "best practice" in nursing for family violence.

NURSING: EDUCATION AND FAMILY VIOLENCE

Family violence in all its forms affects up to 25% of all people in some way over their lifetime. There are multiple negative physical and mental health effects of such exposure, and a systematic response is needed from health professionals (Institute of Medicine, 2002). Nurses are a formidable workforce within the health care system and, because of their close emotional and physical connections with patients, are a critical cornerstone of any health response to the issue. Research has consistently shown that, while individual nurses are often enormously helpful to individual patients who have experienced violence, their response as a group is patchy, inconsistent, and often unhelpful (Campbell & Parker, 1999). Research has also shown that the more education on violence professionals receive, the more likely they are to suspect its effects in their patients and to respond appropriately (Humphreys et al., 2001; Tanner, 1993).

Increasingly, specific content on family violence is being integrated into nursing curricula. Not all forms of violence, however, are included to the same extent. Since the 1970s, child maltreatment has been included in almost all programs. Although progressively more content on intimate partner violence is reported, such programs are still in the minority, and elder abuse continues to be the least addressed in nursing programs (Institute of Medicine, 2002; Woodtli & Breslin, 1996). This content must be included in nursing curricula. Nursing intervention in family violence falls clearly within the profession's mandate, and the failure to address the issue systematically is unacceptable. Because the field of family violence is enormous and the amount of information practitioners must assimilate is so large, it is impossible to prepare nurses for every task that they may encounter in their practices. It is equally clear that nurses are more likely to suspect violence as an issue, to screen, to identify, and to intervene if they have received specific education on the topic. This paradox must be considered carefully by nurse educators, and it may hold true for any sensitive value-laden topic that nurses struggle with in their practices (Whitley, Jacobson, & Gawrys, 1996).

Why has nursing failed to address this destructive health issue? There may be many reasons. Nursing and nurses exist as part of a wider society and are influenced by values and beliefs. As part of the broader health care field, nursing is dominated by a generally conservative, white, middle-class, male value system. In addition, the health care system is physician dominated. Though the number of women becoming physicians is increasing, medicine is still a male profession. In contrast, regardless of the specific male/female ratio, nursing is a female profession.

In the second half of the 20th century, the development of nursing knowledge became more focused on medically defined topics. As such, it is often taken for granted that nurses take direction in large part from physicians. As nurses became more technically proficient (a development initiated to a large extent by the demands of wars), many of the traditional nursing-education focuses began to take a back seat to technological demands. Some of these changes have also been driven by the demands of the workplace. In times of cutbacks and restructuring, employers want new employees to "hit the ground running," and that means a great deal of time in nursing programs must be spent on physical and technical skill development.

Recently, however, nursing seems to be reclaiming its holistic orientation and is increasingly focused on the psychosocial needs of the patient, often in the context of health promotion, harm reduction, or population health. This would seem to be the ideal time to include family-violence content in nursing curricula. It is also critical that such content consider several factors in this book, such as a multidisciplinary focus, an understanding of the broader picture, and a focus on diversity and complexity in people's circumstances.

Because it is so important that nurses function in multidisciplinary teams, when working with family violence it is critical that they learn how to contribute effectively. It means understanding and valuing each profession's input and valuing and promoting nursing's unique contributions. Nurses understand well how family violence can affect an individual's day-to-day life. Understanding the normal development of individuals and families provides an excellent basis for working with families experiencing violence. Nursing education also emphasizes a nonjudgmental approach to working with people, a strategy vitally important to the success of any work with survivors. As such, nursing has a unique perspective that will strengthen the work of any multidisciplinary team, providing that nurses are prepared to work assertively and collaboratively.

Nurses have a role in coordinating the various professionals and organizations working with their patients. When people enter the health care system for the first time, it is easy for them to become inundated with advice and confused by the input of many people. Nurses can advocate for patients, interpret different professional perspectives for them, and, understanding of the demands of everyday life, help them prioritize and plan. In the context of family violence, advocacy, long recognized as a nursing skill, makes an enormous difference. For example, nurses are well-placed to advocate on behalf of children who witness the abuse of their mothers, both by helping mothers with parenting concerns, which can be overwhelming when so many competing demands beset them, or by interpreting child behavior for teachers (Humphreys, 1998).

Nurses are also familiar with the complexities of language barriers and being unfamiliar with one's rights. Nursing educators must become more conscious of integrating policy analysis and political influences on health into nursing curricula. Nurses are in a perfect position to influence policymakers so that patients, who might be overlooked in planning because of unique characteristics and circumstances, are less likely to fall through the cracks. But such political awareness has not been traditionally included in nursing curricula. Incorporating such content into a program that emphasizes an integrated approach to analyzing issues on the micro, meso and macro levels and provides students with the skills to do so would be a great step forward.

Effectively intervening in family violence requires skills that are well within the purview of nursing yet are more complex than those required in most interactions. This is because these skills require nurses to be aware of their own beliefs and values as they affect the interaction. Nurses are socialized into their families first, their communities and societies second, and their profession last. As they mature they are exposed to the values of their surroundings as everyone else is, and they internalize those values just as unconsciously. So, for example, if a nurse grows up in a family in which the prevailing beliefs are traditional, conservative, white, middle-class, and male in orientation, then that viewpoint will be integrated into a worldview. To challenge that view will require an active, purposeful approach and is not easily accomplished in the absence of support. Yet nursing is a profession in which practitioners are able to relate to their patients' worldviews, and that requires them to accept others and to consider and be open to other viewpoints. The development of such a viewpoint can be facilitated in a nursing program that encourages a commitment to lifelong learning and an understanding of the importance of knowing one's self when it comes to effectively caring for those experiencing family violence—or indeed any sensitive and difficult topic.

The effectiveness of nurses in caring for those experiencing family violence is related to two other areas: acknowledging and understanding the impact of family violence in the personal lives of nurses and acknowledging and understanding the impact of intervening in emotionally challenging patient situations in work circumstances that are usually not particularly supportive. These two areas overlap in that there is a need to provide student nurses with the necessary skills to explore their own personal values and beliefs by using a mechanism that provides individual support and supervision. Such a mechanism can decrease the negative, emotional impact of practice in such a personally demanding profession, particularly when practice relates to sensitive and potentially personal topics.

Nursing continues to be a primarily female profession. There is no reason to believe that the prevalence of abuse among nurses would be lower than in any other group of women, and, as it turns out, the prevalence may be well above the average (Henderson, 2001b; Janssen, Basso, & Constanzo, 1998; Moore, 1998). It follows, then, that if there are ongoing effects of violence that need to be considered when working with survivors, we should be assessing student nurses (Bohn & Holz, 1996). Assessment and intervention with this group is important for two reasons: first, because everyone should be assessed for such experiences, and second, because the presence of such a history seriously affect a nurse's ability to work effectively with survivors.

In the same way nurses must be helped and supported in the personal exploration of their own beliefs and values, how they acquired them and whether they continue to espouse them, they must understand the implications of those beliefs and values on their practice. There is perhaps no other profession with the exception of psychotherapy where such an understanding is crucial to how its practitioners subsequently approach their work. Nurses clearly understand the need for such exploration (Henderson, 2001a). Such work, however, is demanding and requires specific skills on the part of those working with the students. Nursing programs must make a real commitment to such an approach, but the potential, positive impact of this investment goes far beyond those working directly with survivors of family violence.

With regard to future directions in nursing education in family violence, educational policymakers must provide the necessary leadership; professional organizations at the federal, state, or provincial levels must send clear messages to their constituents regarding appropriate levels of preparation for their members and such directives must be mandated and enforced. Nursing curricula must be evaluated "to determine their impact on the practices of health care professionals and their effects on family-violence victims. Evaluation must employ rigorous methods to ensure accurate, reliable, and useful results" (Institute of Medicine, 2002, p. 158). Leadership is also an issue in health care settings. Health care administrators must provide ongoing educational forums to keep practitioners abreast of new developments in the field of family violence and to alert them to agency requirements regarding assessment, identification, and intervention.

NURSING: PUBLIC POLICY DEVELOPMENT AND FAMILY VIOLENCE

The impact of public policy on nursing's ability to provide culturally relevant and accessible care to a diverse population of battered women is becoming increasingly important. This section focuses on the different aspects of public policy and their impact on the provision of nursing care. Although the following examples are based on policies that were developed in the United States, this discussion aims to motivate nurses worldwide to understand the intersection of multiple social-policy issues and their impact on the provision of nursing care to battered women.

The multifaceted nature of nursing's work in public policy is rooted in the reality that domestic violence is socially situated. In other words, a violent relationship is only one layer in the life of a battered woman and her family. Legislation related to issues such as health care, welfare, housing, and immigration can collectively impact a woman's decision to stay with or leave her abuser.

Health Care

Current policy issues related to domestic violence include the following: mandatory reporting by nurses and physicians, universal screening, and confidentiality and privacy of a battered woman's medical records. Mandatory reporting by health care professionals is currently in place in six states across the country. This legislation has created controversy because of the potential negative consequences for battered women. Domestic-violence advocates have stated that mandatory reporting may deter women from seeking health care services, whereas others have argued that legislation can take the burden of reporting off a woman. Recent research with battered women has shown that women have mixed responses to the question of mandatory reporting. Sachs, Koziol-McLain, Glass, Webster and Campbell (2002) conducted a large (n=845) population-based study of women's risk for intimate partner violence. Abused women in the study were significantly less likely to support mandatory reporting of domestic violence by health care professionals as compared to nonabused women (59% versus 73%, $p < 0.01$). Reasons that endorsed support included: abused women would find it easier to get help (81%) and would like health care personnel to call the police (68%). Reasons that endorsed opposition included: women would be less likely to disclose abuse (77%), would resent someone else having control (61%), and reporting would increase the risk of perpetrator retaliation (44%). The researchers concluded that most women support mandatory reporting by health care personnel. However, abused women were significantly less supportive than those not abused.

In another study of battered women in shelters (Smith, 2000), 74% of the sample (n=241) supported mandatory reporting by health care professionals, although few believed that the laws would benefit them directly. Most felt that the law would benefit other women. One particularly troubling finding was that 20% of women in the sample reported that they would be less likely to seek health care if mandatory-reporting laws were in effect.

Universal screening by health care providers has wide support, although questions remain. Who should screen? How often? In what settings? A bill is currently in Congress, HR 4032: Domestic Violence Screening and Treatment Act (2002), that would "provide coverage under the maternal and child health block-grant program, the Medicaid program, and the Federal employees health-benefits program" (p. 1). It would provide for routine verbal screening for domestic violence by a provider, danger assessment for women who screen positive for domestic violence, and treatment such as safety planning, health education, and counseling.

Confidentiality of patient medical records is guided by the Health Insurance Portability and Accountability Act (1996) (HIPPA) and the rules implemented in April of 2001. Under these rules, an individual's medical information is protected from inappropriate or inadvertent misuse by health care providers, insurance companies, and employers. Nurses should be aware that, although these laws are a significant step in protecting the privacy of battered women, some domestic-violence advocates are suggesting even stricter provisions for protection (Family Violence Protection Fund, 2001).

Welfare

The elimination of the Aid to Families with Dependent Children (AFDC), or "welfare," in 1996 brought about significant changes in the lives of poor women and their children. The Personal Responsibility and Work Opportunity Reconciliation Act of 1996 (PRWORA) included a provision entitled Temporary Aid to Needy Families (TANF), which replaced the AFDC program. With it came employment requirements and a five-year limit on a person's ability to receive these benefits. Requirements for mandatory training and employment (which could place a woman at increased risk of danger from a perpetrator) and the five-year limit had a significant impact on a woman's decision to stay with her abuser or to leave.

As a result, the Family Violence Option (FVO) was created to provide a safety net for battered women. The FVO is "a state option included in the TANF statute that allows states to screen for victims of domestic violence, provide services, and grant waivers of program requirements where the requirements would endanger or penalize victims" (NOW Legal Defense and Education Fund [NOWLDEF], 2001). A review, current as of April 2002, is available through the NOWLDEF for nurses to determine if their state has adopted the FVO.

Proposed legislation promoting marriage is another public-policy issue associated with welfare reform that could have a significant effect on battered women. The Personal Responsibility, Work, and Family Promotions Act (HR 4700, 107th Congress, May 2002) is one of several bills before Congress to promote marriage, fatherhood, the reduction of nonmarital births, and divorce reduction. This legislation is directly tied to the re-authorization of TANF. Individual states have also been allowed to create their own programs around marriage promotion tied to TANF benefits. Nurses should fully assess the impact of this type of legislation on the safety of battered women.

Housing

Aside from the more commonly known problems battered women face in finding safe accommodation for both the short and long term, "one strike and you're out" policies present in federal housing programs have created additional hardships (National Organization of Women Legal Defense and Education Fund, 2001, July 10). This zero-tolerance policy places battered women at risk for eviction because of their partners' violent behavior. Several national forums have been held recently to address the housing problems that battered women face.

A recent article by Menard (2001) summarized the different aspects of housing problems for battered women and outlined three specific policy recommendations. The recommendations are: "review and modify, as necessary, existing housing policy and programs to increase their responsiveness to women with abusive partners or ex-partners; promote policies and programs that increase all women's access to safe, affordable, and stable housing, as well as housing assistance and support services when necessary; publicize more widely information on available subsidized and nonsubsidized housing and housing-assistance programs, as well as services and protections available to domestic-violence victims" (p. 4). Nurses should follow the progress of these policy recommendations, as they will have important consequences for safety planning with battered women.

Immigration Issues

Battered immigrant women face unique challenges to their safety. Because their ability to remain in the United States is often tied to their relationship with their partners, abusers often use this as a weapon to keep women from reporting violence or seeking services. Until the passage of the Violence Against Women Act of 1994, battered immigrant women, especially undocumented women, were at the mercy of their abusive partners. Specific provisions under the act, known as the Battered Immigrant Women's Provisions, have assisted providers of domestic-violence services to offer legal protection for these women. In 1999, the Battered Immigrant Women Protection Act of 1999 was passed by Congress to provide even more protection for this vulnerable group of women (National Organization of Women Legal Defense and Education Fund, 2001, July 10). Although it is beyond the purview of nursing practice to understand every aspect of these provisions, nurses serving immigrant populations understand that battered immigrant women, regardless of their immigration status, have a legal right to protection under the law and access to shelter.

The previous examples are intended to help nurses understand the interconnectedness of different areas of public policy as they relate to the care of battered women. Universal screening of women is only the first step in providing care. When a woman screens positive for domestic violence, it is important for a nurse to understand the implications of other policies in developing a plan of care. Although nurses should be aware that these policies exist, there is a need to work in multidisciplinary teams to offer women the best and safest possible alternatives.

SUMMARY

Great strides have been made to end family violence, but there is a long way to go. Nonetheless, it is important to remember the successes and victories that have been achieved. Because of the efforts of dedicated practitioners, researchers, legislators, and activists, both in North America and around the world, the commitment to end family violence is now solidly on the global agenda. It is hoped that the commitment to this work will continue and that there is a general recognition that people can only reach their full potential as contributing members of society when their rights are respected and they feel safe and cared about. Until that goal is achieved, nurses will continue to be in the forefront of this work, as they have been from the beginning.

References

Agnew, V. (1998). In search of a safe place: *Abused women and culturally sensitive services.* Toronto, Canada: University of Toronto Press.

Arroyo, W., & Eth, S. (1995). Assessment following violence-witnessing trauma. In E. Peled, P. G. Jaffe, & J. L. Edleson (Eds.), *Ending the cycle of violence: Community responses to children of battered women* (pp.27–42). Thousand Oaks, California: Sage.

Belknap, R. (2000). Eva's story: One woman's life viewed through the interpretive lens of Gilligans' theory. *Violence Against Women, 6*(6), 586–605.

Bohn, D. K., & Holz, K. A. (1996). Sequelae of abuse: Health effects of childhood sexual abuse, domestic battering. *Journal of Nurse-Midwifery, 41*(6), 442–456.

Bunch, C. (1997). The intolerable status quo: Violence against women and girls. In *The progress of nations, 1997* (pp. 40–45). New York: UNICEF.

Butler, M. J. (1995). Domestic violence: A nursing imperative. *Journal of Holistic Nursing, 13*(1), 54–69.

Campbell, J.C. (Ed.). (1998). *Empowering survivors of abuse: Health Care for battered women and their children.* Thousand Oaks, CA: Sage.

Campbell, J. C. & Dienemann, G. D. (2001). Ethical issues in violence against women. In C. M. Renzetti, J. L. Edleson, & R. Kennedy Bergen (Eds.), *Sourcebook on violence against women* (pp. 57–72). Thousand Oaks, CA: Sage.

Campbell, J. C., & Parker, B. (1999). Clinical nursing research on battered women and their children. In A. S. Hinshaw, S. L. Feetham, and J. L. F. Shaver (Eds.), *Handbook of clinical nursing research* (pp. 535–559). Thousand Oaks, CA: Sage.

Clark, P., Pendry, N., & Kim, S. (1997). Patterns of violence in homeless women. *Western Journal of Nursing Research, 19*(4), 490–500.

Davies, J., Lyon, E., & Monti-Catania, D. (1998). *Safety planning with battered women: Complex lives/difficult choices.* Thousand Oaks, CA: Sage.

Family Violence Prevention Fund. (2001). *Accessing HIPAA: How federal medical privacy regulations can be improved* [Online]. Available: http://www.endabuse.org.

Grunfeld, A., Hotch, D., & MacKay, K. (1996). Identification, assessment, care, referral, and follow-up of women experiencing domestic violence who come to the emergency department for treatment. In M. Russell, J. Hightower, & G. Gutman (Eds.), *Stopping the violence: Changing families, changing future* (pp. 76–83). Vancouver, Canada: Benwell Atkins.

Handivsky, O., & Greaves, L. (1996). The economic costs of violence against women. In M. Russell, J. Hightower, & G. Gutman (Eds.), *Stopping the violence: Changing families, changing futures* (pp. 139–146). Vancouver, Canada: Benwell Atkins.

Heise, L.L. (1994). Gender-based abuse: The global epidemic. In A. J. Dan (Ed.), *Reframing women's health: Multidisciplinary research and practice* (pp. 233–252). Thousand Oaks, CA: Sage.

Heise, L. L., Raikes, A., Watts, C. H., & Zwi, B. (1994). Violence against women: A neglected health issue in less developed countries. *Social Science and Medicine, 39*(9), 1165–1179.

Henderson, A. D. (2001a). Emotional labor and nursing: An under-appreciated aspect of caring work. *Nursing Inquiry, 8*(2), 130–138.

Henderson, A.D. (2001b). Factors influencing nurses' responses to abused women: What they say and do, and why they say they do it. *Journal of Interpersonal Violence, 16*(12), 1284–1306.

Humphreys, J. (1998). Helping battered women take care of their children. In J. C. Campbell, (Ed.), *Empowering survivors of abuse: Health care for battered women and their children* (pp. 121–137). Thousand Oaks, CA: Sage.

Humphreys, J., Parker, B., & Campbell, J. C. (2001). Intimate partner violence against women. In D. Taylor and N. Fugate Woods (Eds.), *Annual review of nursing research* (pp. 275–306). New York: Springer.

Institute of Medicine. (2002). *Confronting chronic neglect: The education and training of health professionals on domestic violence.* Washington, DC: National Academy Press.

Janssen, P. A., Basso, M. C., & Constanzo, R. M. (1998). The prevalence of domestic violence among obstetric nurses. *Women's Health Issues, 8*(5), 317–323.

Johnson, H., & Sacco, V. F. (1995). Researching violence against women: Statistics Canada's national survey. *Canadian Journal of Criminology, 37*(3), 281–304.

Johnson, M. P., & Ferraro, K. J. (2000). Research on domestic violence in the 1990s: Making distinctions. *Journal of Marriage and the Family, 62,* 948–963.

Kearney, M. (2001). Enduring Love: A grounded formal theory of women's experience of domestic violence. *Research in Nursing and Health, 24,* 270–282.

Landenburger, K. M., (1993). Exploration of women's identity: Clinical approaches with abused women. *Clinical Issues in Perinatal and Women's Health Nursing, 4*(3), 378–384.

Menard, A. (2001). Domestic violence and housing: Key policy and program challenges. *Violence Against Women, 7*(6), 707–720.

Moore, M. L. (1998). Attitudes and practices of registered nurses who have experienced abuse/domestic violence. *Journal of Obstetrical and Neonatal Nursing, 27*(2), 175–182.

National Organization of Women Legal Defense and Education Fund. (2001, July 10). *Zero tolerance policy affects domestic violence victims, civil rights groups charge in Oregon* [Online]. Available: http://www.nowldef.org.

Pahl, J. (1995). Health professionals and violence against women. In P. Kingston & B. Penhale (Eds.), *Family violence and the helping professions* (pp. 127–148), London: Macmillan.

Personal Responsibility, Work, and Family Promotion Act, HR4700, 107th Congress. (2002).

Radomsky, N. A. (1995). *Lost voices: Women, chronic pain, and abuse.* Binghamton, NY: Harrington Park Press.

Renzetti, C. M., Edleson, J. L. & Kennedy Bergen, R. (Eds.), *Sourcebook on violence against women.* Thousand Oaks, CA: Sage.

Russell, M., Hightower, J., & Gutman, G. (Eds.). *Stopping the violence: Changing families, changing futures.* Vancouver, Canada: Benwell Atkins.

Sachs, C. J., Koziol-McLain, J., Glass, N., Webster, D., & Campbell, J. (2002). A population-based survey assessing support for mandatory domestic violence reporting by health care personnel. *Women and Health, 35,* 121–133.

Shepard, M. F., Elliott, B. A., Falk, D. R., & Regal, R. R. (1999). Public health nurses' responses to domestic violence: A report from the enhanced Domestic Abuse Intervention Project. *Public Health Nursing, 19*(5), 359–366.

Smith, A. (2000). It's my decision, isn't it? A research note on battered women's perceptions of mandatory intervention laws. *Violence Against Women, 6*(12), 1384–1402.

Straus, M. A. (1978). The Conflict Tactic Scale. In J. Touliatos, B. Perlmutter, & M. Straus (Eds.), *Handbook of family measurement techniques.* Newbury Park, CA: Sage.

Tanner, C. (1993). Nursing education and violence against women. *Journal of Nursing Education, 32*(8), 339–340.

Wasson, J. H., Jette, A. M., Anderson, J., Johnson, D. J., Nelson, E. C., & Kilo, C. M. (2000). Routine, single-item screening to identify abusive relationships in women. *Journal of Family Practice, 49*(11), 1017–1022.

Whitley, G. G., Jacobson, G. A., & Gawrys, M. T. (1996). The impact of violence in the health care setting upon nursing education. *Journal of Nursing Education, 35*(5), 211–218.

Woodtli, M. A., & Breslin, E. (1996). Violence related content in the nursing curriculum: A national study. *Journal of Nursing Education, 35*(8), 367–374.

Wuest, J., & Merritt-Gray, M. (1999). Not going back: Sustaining the separation process in leaving abusive relationships. *Violence Against Women, 5*(2), 110–133.

Zorza, J. (1995). How abused women can use the law to help protect their children. In E. Peled, P. G. Jaffe & J. L. Edleson (Eds.), *Ending the cycle of violence: Community responses to children of battered women* (pp. 147–169). Thousand Oaks, CA: Sage.

Abuse Assessment Screen

1. WITHIN THE LAST YEAR, have you been hit, slapped, kicked, or otherwise physically hurt by someone?   YES   NO

    If YES, by whom? _____

    Total number of times _____

2. SINCE YOU'VE BEEN PREGNANT, have you been hit, slapped, kicked, or otherwise physically hurt by someone?   YES   NO

    If YES, by whom? _____

    Total number of times _____

MARK THE AREA OF INJURY ON THE BODY MAP.
SCORE EACH INCIDENT ACCORDING TO THE FOLLOWING SCALE:

1 = Threats of abuse including use of a weapon

2 = Slapping, pushing: no injuries and/or lasting pain

3 = Punching, kicking, bruises, cuts and/or continuing pain

4 = Beating up, severe contusions, burns, broken bones

5 = Head injury, internal injury, permanent injury

6 = Use of weapon; wound from weapon

SCORE
_____
_____
_____
_____
_____
_____

If any of the descriptions for the higher number apply, use the higher number.

3. WITHIN THE LAST YEAR, has anyone forced you to have sexual activities?   YES   NO

    If YES, who? _____

    Total number of times _____

Developed by the Nursing Research Consortium on Violence and Abuse.
Readers are encouraged to reproduce and use this assessment tool.

1. DURANTE EL ÚLTIMO AÑO, fué golpeada, bofeteada, pateada, o lastimada fisicamente de alguna otra manera por alguien?   SI   NO

   Si la respuesta es "SI" por quien(es)_____

   Cuantas

2. DESDE QUE SALIO EMBARAZADA, ha sido golpeada, bofeteada, pateada, o lastimada fisicamente de alguna otra manera por alguien?   SI   NO

   Si la respuesta es "SI" por quien(es)_____

   Cuantas veces? _____

EN EL DIAGRAMA, ANATÓMICO MARQUE LAS PARTES DE SU CUERPO QUE HAN SIDO LASTIMADAS. VALORE CADA INCIDENTE USANDO LAS SIGUIENTE ESCALA: GRADO

1 = Amenazas de maltrato que incluyen el use de un arma   _____

2 = Bofeteadas, empujones sin lesiones fisicas o dolor permanente   _____

3 = Moquestes, patadas, moretones, heridas, y/o dolor permanente   _____

4 = Molida a palos, contusiones several, quemaduras, fracturas de huesos   _____

5 = Heridas en la cabeza, lesiones internal, lesiones permanents   _____

6 = Uso de armas; herida por arma   _____

Si cualquiera de las situaciones valora un numero alto en la escala.

3. DURANTE EL ÚLTIMO AÑO, fuè forzada a tener relaciones sexuales?   SI   NO

   Si la respuesta es "SI" por quien(es)_____

   Cuantas veces? _____

APPENDIX B
Abuse Assessment Screen for Women With Disabilities

Screening Questions

In the last year, has anyone you know:

- Made you feel unsafe?
- Yelled at you over and over again or hurt your feelings?
- Refused or neglected to help with an important personal need such as using the bathroom, eating, or drinking?
- Damaged or kept you from using a phone, wheelchair, cane, walker, or other assistive device?
- Refused to give you your medication, kept you from taking it, or given you too much or too little?
- Stolen money, valuables, equipment, or medication; forged checks; or used your credit/debit card or information about you without your permission?
- Threatened or actually hit, slapped, kicked, pushed, shoved, restrained, or otherwise physically hurt you or handled you roughly?
- Touched you in a sexual way you did not want or forced you to have sexual activities?

Risk Assessment

Women with disabilities who have been abused need to know that some things may make their situation more dangerous.

You may be at greater risk if the person who is hurting you:

- Is someone you depend on for care
- Is drunk often or uses drugs
- Threatens to hurt or actually hurts your pets or children
- Hurts you more often or severely
- Keeps you from getting services or health care
- Controls most of your daily activities
- Threatens to kill themselves or others
- Can get a gun

Or if you:

- Don't have a back-up caregiver
- Have difficulty getting out of the house
- Are unable to call for help
- Have a health problem that can become serious if neglected, such as diabetes, skin sores, or epilepsy

APPENDIX C
Danger Assessment

Several risk factors have been associated with homicides (murders) of both bat-terers and battered women, in research conducted after the murders have taken place. We cannot predict what will happen in your case, but we would like you to be aware of the danger of homicide in situations of severe battering and for you to see how many of the risk factors apply to your situation.

Using the calendar, please mark the approximate dates during the past year when you were beaten by your husband or partner. Write on that date how bad the incident was according to the following scale:

1. Slapping, pushing; no injuries and/or lasting pain
2. Punching, kicking; bruises, cuts, and/or continuing pain
3. "Beating up"; severe contusions, burns, broken bones
4. Threat to use weapon; head injury, internal injury, permanent injury
5. Use of weapon; wounds from weapon

(If *any* of the descriptions for the higher number apply, use the higher number.)

Mark "Yes" or "No" for each of the following. ("He" refers to your husband, partner, ex-husband, ex-partner, or whoever is currently physically hurting you.)

_____ 1. Has the physical violence increased in severity or frequency over the past year?

_____ 2. Has he ever used a weapon against you or threatened you with a weapon?

_____ 3. Does he ever try to choke you?

_____ 4. Does he own a gun?

_____ 5. Has he ever forced you to have sex when you did not wish to do so?

_____ 6. Does he use drugs? By drugs, I mean "uppers" or amphetamines, speed, angel dust, cocaine, "crack," street drugs, or mixtures.

_____ 7. Does he threaten to kill you and/or do you believe he is capable of killing you?

_____ 8. Is he drunk every day or almost every day? (In terms of quantity of alcohol.)

_____ 9. Does he control most or all of your daily activities? For instance: does he tell you who you can be friends with, when you can see your family, how much money you can use, or when you can take the car? (If he tries, but you do not let him, check here: _____)

_____ 10. Have you ever been beaten by him while you were pregnant? (If you have never been pregnant by him, check here: _____)

_____ 11. Is he violently and constantly jealous of you? (For instance, does he say "If I can't have you, no one can.")

_____ 12. Have you ever threatened or tried to commit suicide?

_____ 13. Has he ever threatened or tried to commit suicide?

_____ 14. Does he threaten to harm your children?

427

_____ 15. Do you have a child that is not his?

_____ 16. Is he unemployed?

_____ 17. Have you left him during the past year? (If have _never_ lived with him, check here___)

_____ 18. Do you currently have another (different) intimate partner?

_____ 19. Does he follow or spy on you, leave threatening notes, destroy your property, or call you when you don't want him to?

_____ **Total "Yes" Answers**

Thank you. Please talk to your nurse, advocate or counselor about what the Danger Assessment means in terms of your situation.

Copyright 1985, 1988, 2001 by Jacquelyn C. Campbell.

Index

Note: Page numbers followed by "b" indicate boxed material; those followed by "f" indicate figures; those followed by "t" indicate tabular material.